Injured Brains of Medical Minds

Injured Brains of Medical Minds

Views from Within

Compiled and edited by

NARINDER KAPUR

Wessex Neurological Centre, Southampton General Hospital
Department of Psychology, University of Southampton

Oxford   New York   Tokyo
OXFORD UNIVERSITY PRESS

1997

This book has been printed digitally and produced in a standard specification in order to ensure its continuing availability

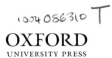

OXFORD
UNIVERSITY PRESS

Great Clarendon Street, Oxford OX2 6DP

Oxford University Press is a department of the University of Oxford.
It furthers the University's objective of excellence in research, scholarship,
and education by publishing worldwide in

Oxford New York

Auckland Bangkok Buenos Aires Cape Town Chennai
Dar es Salaam Delhi Hong Kong Istanbul Karachi Kolkata
Kuala Lumpur Madrid Melbourne Mexico City Mumbai Nairobi
São Paulo Shanghai Taipei Tokyo Toronto

Oxford is a registered trade mark of Oxford University Press
in the UK and in certain other countries

Published in the United States
by Oxford University Press Inc., New York

Original material and selection © N. Kapur 1997

The moral rights of the author have been asserted

Database right Oxford University Press (maker)

Reprinted 2003

ISBN 0-19-852144-8

Printed in Great Britain by

Antony Rowe Ltd., Eastbourne

To the authors of these papers,
for their courage and foresight.
To my wife Ritu, and my children
Sarina, Soniya, and Shashi, for their love and support.

Preface

You would certainly make very clever doctors of men who from their earliest years, besides acquiring scientific knowledge, had come in contact with very many cases, and who had themselves suffered from every malady, and were not constitutionally very healthy.

(Plato)

While a vast amount has been written by researchers and clinicians about brain damage and its consequences for patients, surprisingly little has been written from the perspective of the individual brain damaged patient. Awareness of psychological deficit after brain injury[1] is an increasingly important topic in the study of brain–behaviour relationships (e.g. Marcel and Bisiach 1988; Prigatano and Schacter 1991). Doctors and other clinicians who become patients provide a unique perspective of the healer who now needs to be healed. With the recent interest in accounts of brain injury or illness that emphasize the experience of the sufferer (Gardner 1977; Sacks 1985, 1995), the perspective of the healer-turned-patient is all the more worthy to report. In the area of psychiatry, an attempt has already been made to harness the views of health workers who have suffered a mental illness (Rippere and Williams 1985). In specific fields of handicap such as stuttering, there are accounts by sufferers who also have clinical or medical qualifications (Speech Foundation of America, 1972). The aim of this book is to try and rectify the gap in the neurological literature by bringing together in one volume a series of personal papers, around fifty in all, that report the experiences of doctors/clinicians/scientists who have been afflicted with a brain illness or brain injury. To my knowledge, this has never been done before. The major purpose of this book is therefore archival—providing a record of accounts of brain injury written by a particular category of sufferer, many of these accounts having been published in scattered sources, across different time periods. A second aim of the book is to provide commentaries on the articles. These commentaries are intended to: (1) highlight signs or symptoms that may be of particular note to a neuroscientist, clinician, or informed reader; (2) consider some of the observations reported in the articles in the light of current theory and data in the clinical neurosciences; and (3) comment on the implications of the observations for the management of neurological patients. The *specific commentaries* following each paper offer comments that relate to individual articles. For a few chapters in the book, there are more general issues that arise and that form a common thread throughout articles within a chapter. In such cases, the articles lend themselves to more detailed discussion, and I have therefore added a further, *general commentary* at the end of that particular section. Finally, it is also important to see if broader lessons can be learned across the eight topics of the book, and to set these self-report articles in the context of other self-reports. I have tried to do this in the *Overview* chapter at the end of the book.

---

[1] The term 'brain injury' is used in this book in a generic sense, and includes brain damage from whatever aetiology.

Much of the data in this book is by its very nature unique, since the cognitive and psychosocial observations emanate from single cases, and there are the obvious limitations of generalization that are associated with single-case studies and with introspective accounts. My own commentaries on the papers in this book are, of course, largely determined by the length and content of the articles written by the individual sufferers themselves. The shorter articles, in general, only warrant brief comments. Some of the papers have a distinct cognitive orientation, while others have a much more clinical perspective in mind. Where the cognitive symptoms described by the writers have helped to illuminate issues in cognitive science, I have tried to make appropriate observations. Other authors have given greater attention to the general problems of adjusting to the specific handicaps that they have had to overcome, adapting to their changed role in society, etc., and in these cases my comments have been more general ones.

In view of the wide range of articles that a book of this type will perforce encompass, I have divided the book into three parts: *Part I* includes articles that have a cognitive bias. *Part II* is organized along clinical-neurological lines. *Part III* comprises the *Overview* chapter. I am aware that some of the readers of this book may include non-specialists and also undergraduate students—to this end, I have provided a brief introduction and reading list for each of the topics covered in Parts I and II.

Each paper in its own right represents a fascinating insight into the effects of brain damage on the individual, covering areas that are often neglected in standard textbook accounts of the effects of brain disease and brain injury. With his/her own particular specialist knowledge and experience, each author of an article has been able to provide a unique cognitive and psychosocial perspective on the impact of brain pathology. Although most of the authors of the papers in this book were doctors, medical students, nurses, or clinical psychologists, I have also included a few articles by experimental psychologists and biological scientists, since they have provided a similar and revealing perspective to the neurological symptoms that they suffered.

The large majority of the articles reprinted in this book deal with self-reports by individuals on the transient or permanent brain dysfunction that they suffered. I have included a few exceptions to this, where the medical mind in question could not, for reasons of the disease process itself, recall or recount his/her symptoms. One is the story of an attack of transient global amnesia, as told by a physician who examined the patient, a surgical colleague, during the episode of the surgeon's memory loss (Klawans). The second is an account by the wife of a professor of medicine who developed Alzheimer's disease (Morgan). In addition, I have included the remarkable descriptions by Hughlings-Jackson of his two medically qualified patients who suffered from memory loss associated with temporal lobe epilepsy, one of whom published a specific article about his condition ('Quaerens')—this article is also reprinted in the book. In all of these cases, the perspective of the carer/ informed observer is given due prominence—this perspective is often missing from accounts of the effects of brain pathology. These particular articles provide some invaluable and unique observations of the behavioural changes associated with the condition in question, many of which were beyond the awareness of the sufferer.

Where particular papers permit me to do so, in my commentaries I have tried to indicate the clinical and theoretical implications of the articles. Just as important are examples in the papers that may be used as illustrations for teaching. What could be a more telling demonstration of unilateral visual neglect than Sir Peter Medawar's description (p. 284) of nurses helping themselves to chocolates that were located on the left side of his bed, in the area of his defective vision? What could be a more graphic example of the distinction between 'procedural' and 'episodic' memory than the experience of the surgeon during his attack of transient global amnesia (p. 23), when he could readily remember the surgical procedures for terminating a gallbladder operation, but had no recollection whatsoever of the episode a few minutes earlier when he removed the gallbladder? There are numerous such examples in this book, examples that I hope will provide a useful source of teaching material across the range of specialities within the clinical neurosciences.

Southampton   N.K.
March 1996

REFERENCES

Gardner, H. (1977). *The shattered mind. The person after brain damage.* Routledge & Kegan Paul, London.

Marcel, A. J. and Bisiach, E. (ed.) (1988). *Consciousness in contemporary science.* Oxford University Press.

Plato *The republic,* (trans. A. D. Lindsay, 1976), p. 93. Dent, London.

Prigatano, G. P. and Schacter, D. L. (ed.) (1991). *Awareness of deficit after brain injury.* Oxford University Press.

Rippere, V. and Williams, R. (ed.) (1985). *Wounded healers. Mental health workers' experiences of depression.* Wiley, Chichester.

Sacks, O. (1985). *The man who mistook his wife for a hat.* Duckworth, London.

Sacks, O. (1995). *An anthropologist on Mars.* Picador, London.

Speech Foundation of America (1972). *To the stutterer* (Publication No. 9). Speech Foundation of America, PO Box 11749, Memphis.

Acknowledgements

I am grateful to the Nuffield Foundation for providing funds for research towards the preparation of this book.

I am very fortunate to have had the benefit of colleagues' comments on part or all of draft versions of the book. I would therefore like to thank—Professor Frank Benson, Mr Jason Brice, Dr Chris Colbourn, Dr Bill Gibb, Dr Peter Halligan, Dr Lee Illis, Dr Mark Manford, Professor Alan Parkin, Professor John Richardson, Dr Pam Thompson and Dr Barbara Wilson. Dr Macdonald Critchely very kindly gave me the benefit of his vast experience and pointed out several articles that no on-line search facility on earth could have retrieved. Within my own department, I thank Lynn Hoggarth, Pat Abbott, and Susan Rossell for all their efforts over the past few years. I am grateful to Vanessa Whitting and her colleagues at Oxford University Press for making the transition from manuscript to book a smooth and enjoyable one. Dr Elizabeth Moore and Dr Chris Colbourn kindly helped with the design of the jacket cover.

A number of organizations have assisted with parts of the research required for this book, including the British Medical Association, the Royal Society of Medicine, the Wellcome Institute Library, London, and the Rockefeller Library of the National Hospital for Neurology and Neurosurgery. I am grateful to these and to other bodies, and to my own invaluable resources in Southampton, namely the Wessex Medical Library and the Teaching Media Unit.

This work would not have been possible without the foresight and courage shown by the authors of the articles in putting down on paper their experiences and thoughts, so that others might benefit from their suffering. I hope that readers of this book will share the sense of wonder and privilege that I found when reading these papers. I am indebted to the various copyright holders for granting me permission to reproduce articles and illustrations for the book. If I have made any errors or omissions in copyright approval, I apologize for these in advance. (As in the case of my previous book, my royalties from this book will be going to charity. I am grateful to the Arpana Hospital Trust, Karnal, India for agreeing to use my royalties for their health care work in northern India.)

After writing my first book eight years ago, I promised my family that I would not write another. I ask their forgiveness for breaking this promise! I thank them for their forbearance over the past three years that I have spent researching and writing this book.

Contents

PART II: Clinical conditions

4 *Parkinson's disease*   165

5 *Brain tumour*   217

6 *Stroke*   243

PART III: **Overview**

9 *Overview*   399

PART I

Cognitive disorders

Memory disorders 1

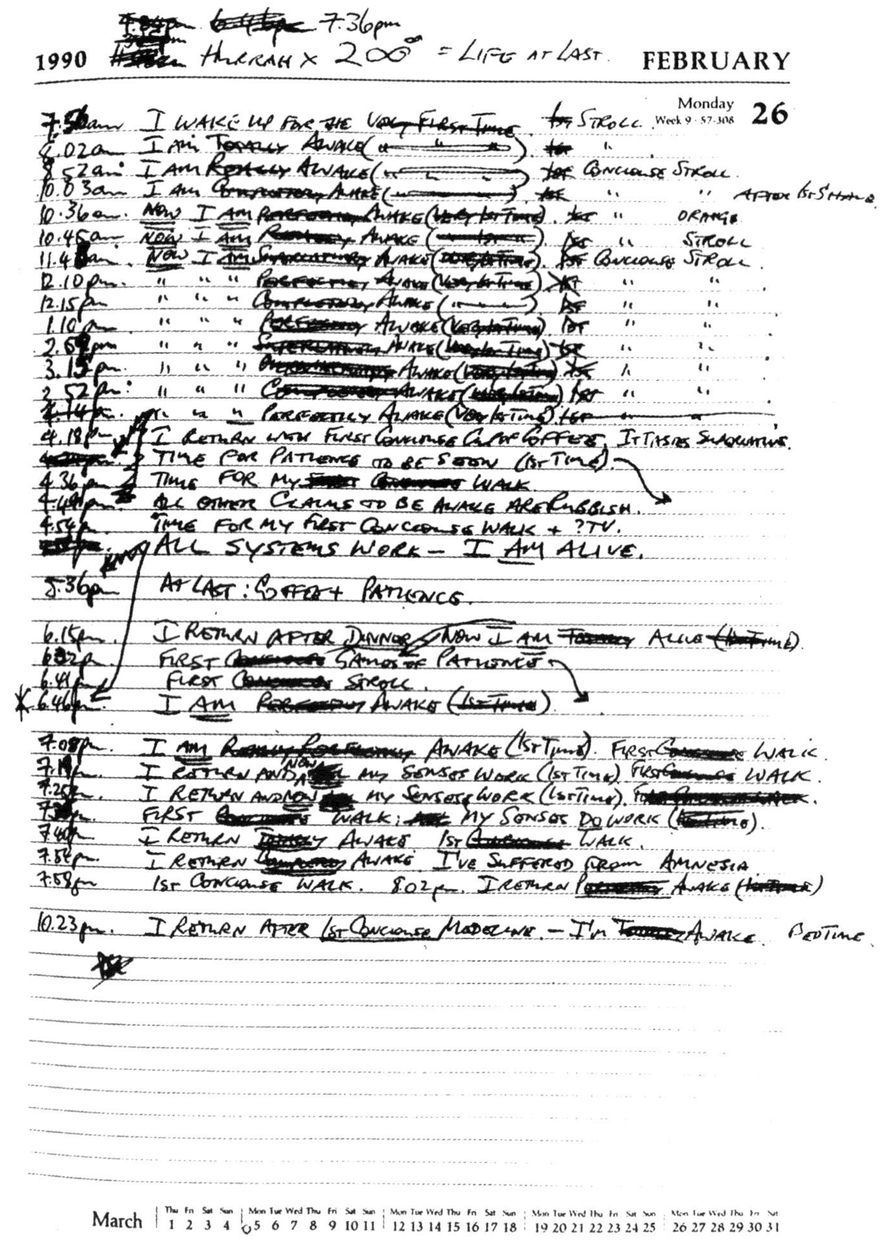

Figure 1. A sample page from the diary of a 51-year-old very severely amnesic patient. He was a professional musician who suffered bilateral temporal lobe damage following herpes simplex encephalitis. Note his persistent belief that he has just woken up and is experiencing events for the very first time, and that he is only just 'consciouse' [conscious] of what is going on around him. His case is described in more detail elsewhere (Wilson *et al.* 1995; Wilson and Wearing 1995).

INTRODUCTION

Memory difficulties are among the first signs of a disease process taking place in the brain, and they are also one of the major, residual sequelae of a brain illness or brain injury. One of the main reasons for this is that a large number of brain areas are involved in putting information into memory, in ensuring that it is stored adequately, and in retrieving it successfully. Thus, memory requires the use of one or more sensory modalities, systems relating to attention/concentration, language processes, and also mechanisms that cover functions such as arousal, motivation, use of strategies, etc. It is, therefore, no wonder that when damage to the brain does occur, for whatever reason, then memory functioning is likely to be disrupted.

There is still some disagreement amongst memory researchers as to the best ways in which to classify and label the different types of memory functions that exist. I will outline one of the most recent attempts at classifying memory (Schacter and Tulving 1994), as it is one that perhaps commands the broadest support at present. The classification itself is based on the results of research in normal and neurological subjects, where one type of memory appears to be governed by rules that do not apply to other types of memory, and where one type of memory may be disrupted after a brain lesion, while the other types of memory continue to function normally. It is worth bearing in mind that with advances in memory research, this classification may well change and become more refined over the coming years.

Schacter and Tulving (1994) distinguish between five memory systems:

1. *Episodic memory*—this relates to memory for discrete events that occurred at a particular time and in a particular place. It could refer to a message you were told half an hour earlier, or to a memorable event from your childhood.

Structures deep in the brain, such as the hippocampus, fornix, mammillary bodies, and thalamus, appear to be critical for this form of memory. The terms 'limbic system', 'diencephalic system', and 'limbic-diencephalic system' are variously used to refer to a network of structures that includes these particular areas as well as neighbouring structures (see Mishkin and Appenzeller 1987 and Aggleton 1991 for more detailed discussion of the anatomy of episodic memory disorders).

2. *Semantic memory*—this refers to our knowledge of facts, both about the world (e.g. who Winston Churchill was), and about ourselves (e.g. our name and address). This memory system is also implicated in our ability to use language, in particular word-finding ability, and in our ability to recognize everyday objects and to recognize familiar faces.

Semantic memory is more closely related to neocortical areas, especially the association areas of the cortex, than to deeper structures.

3. *Primary memory*—in cognitive psychology, this memory system is also known as 'working memory' and 'short-term memory', and it refers to the memory we use when we have to store or manipulate information in our mind over short intervals. This may happen when we are solving an arithmetic problem, keeping track of a conversation between several people, or trying to retrace a path that we just followed.

Neocortical areas are also considered to be critical for these memory functions, and it is thought that the frontal areas of the brain in particular may play an important role in this type of memory.

4. *Perceptual representation memory*—this essentially refers to the perceptual traces that are left in the brain after a particular experience. One way to think of this system is when you see a new model of car for the first time. It attracts your attention, and you probably spend some time looking at it. The next time you see it, even if only for a short time, your brain will respond in a different way to seeing it, usually taking less time or requiring less information than before to recognize it as familiar. This faster processing by your brain will occur, even if you cannot explicitly recall having seen the car before, that is the faster reaction time may occur below the level of conscious awareness. The primary sensory cortices, and adjacent areas of cortex, are thought to be the major sites for this type of memory system.

5. *Procedural memory*—this usually refers to our memory for how to do things, such as how to ride a bike or how to pronounce a difficult word when reading.

The areas of the brain that are involved in procedural memory may well depend on the particular content of the memory process in question—in the case of motor skills, it is thought that the cerebellum may play an important role, though it is likely that for this type and other types of procedural memory there is also a close interaction with primary motor and association areas of the cortex.

It follows from a classification such as the one outlined above that there will be a wide range of memory disorders that result from brain pathology. The memory system that is most frequently involved when neurological patients complain of everyday memory difficulties is the episodic memory system, and the self-report articles that follow are largely concerned with episodic memory symptoms. Memory disorders may be chronic—as in the case of the **Meltzer** article and the **Morgan** article, or transient—as in the case of the article written by **Klawans** and also the account by **Dr X**. Dr X's account consists of two articles, the first written by him shortly before his consultations with me, and the second article that comprises a transcript of my interviews with him and with his wife.

Episodic memory disorders include the classical amnesic syndrome, where there is severe loss of memory for recent events, but where other cognitive functions are broadly intact, and mild and moderate everyday memory difficulties, such as the residual sequelae of a significant head injury. These milder memory impairments are much more common than the classical amnesic syndrome, but they have been the subject of fewer research studies.

Semantic memory loss may take the form of word-finding difficulties in patients with dysphasia, or the inability of some patients to identify objects or familiar faces. In cases of dementia, both semantic and episodic memory loss may be present, and in the later stages of the illness there may be severe impairment of memory. In the article by **Morgan**, the patient with presumed Alzheimer's disease suffered a total loss of familiarity recognition for his wife.

In the case of both episodic and semantic memory disorders, it is important to distinguish between memory loss for events and facts that were retained before the occurrence of a brain injury/brain illness—*retrograde amnesia*; and memory loss for those facts and events that were experienced after the occurrence of the brain injury/brain illness—*anterograde amnesia*. Some patients, such as **Meltzer**, may have both forms of memory loss, while in other cases only one or other type of memory loss may occur.

In addition to the specific commentaries that follow each article, I have also included a general commentary at the end of this section.

REFERENCES

Aggleton, J. (1991). Anatomy of memory. In *Memory disorders. Research and clinical practice* (ed. T. Yanagihara and R. C. Peterson), pp. 23–61. Marcel Dekker, New York.

Mishkin, M. and Appenzeller, T. (1987). The anatomy of memory. *Scientific American*, **256**, 80–89.

Schacter, D. L. and Tulving, E. (1994). What are the memory systems of 1994? In *Memory systems 1994* (ed. D. L. Schacter and E. Tulving), pp. 1–38. MIT Press, Cambridge, MA.

Wilson, B. A. and Wearing, D. (1995). Prisoner of consciousness: a state of just awakening following herpes simplex encephalitis. In *Broken memories* (ed. R. Campbell and M. Conway), pp. 14–30. Blackwell, Oxford.

Wilson, B. A., Baddeley, A. D., and Kapur, N. (1995). Dense amnesia in a professional musician following herpes simplex viral encephalitis. *Journal of Clinical and Experimental Neuropsychology*, **17**, 668–81.

FURTHER READING

Baddeley, A., Wilson, B., and Watts, F. (ed.) (1995). *Handbook of memory disorders*. Wiley, Chichester.

Campbell, R. and Conway, M. A. (ed.) (1995). *Broken memories. Case studies of memory impairment*. Blackwell, Oxford.

Kapur, N. (1994). *Memory disorders in clinical practice*. Lawrence Erlbaum, Hove, UK.

Parkin, A. (1987). *Memory and amnesia*. Blackwell, Oxford.

Rose, S. (1992). *The making of memory*. Bantam, London.

Poor memory: a case report

Malcolm L. Meltzer

Malcolm Meltzer (who died in 1987) was a psychologist, attached to the Psychology Department of George Washington University, Washington, DC, USA. His research included topics in the area of community psychology. In 1974 he had a cardiac arrest, and because of anoxia, the cardiac arrest resulted in brain damage.

I. PAST MEMORY

The loss of past memory was not as extreme as it is in amnesia. When I came out of the coma I had been in for 6 weeks, I knew who I was, and I knew that I was a husband, a father, and a psychologist. I knew my family, but I had difficulty recognizing some of my friends. In the beginning I thought I had two children, but I have but one. I thought my daughter was 13, but she was 15 at that point. I also thought I was 33, but I was 44.

During the drive home from the hospital (after 11 weeks), I saw that I did not recognize the route home, even though it was a route quite familiar to me. At that point, I realized that some of the geography of the city was lost to me. But I did recognize my home and the neighborhood when we arrived there. My house was familiar to me, but I didn't remember where some things were kept and how some things were used. I had to relearn how to play the stereo, set the alarm clock, use the calculator, change a razor blade, etc. All of these things were relearned, but because of the short-term memory problem, it often took several trials to relearn and keep these things in mind.

The feeling engendered by this inability to do things done in the past was that of incompetency. When should bills be paid? What is used to fix a broken chair? When should the oil be changed in the car? Where is the best place to buy a new washing machine? What kind of machine would be best? How do you get from one place to another? When guests come, how do you prepare some drinks that might be requested? What must be done to ready the house for winter? Which are good places to go for a vacation? How do you get there? Where do you stay? What have you enjoyed and not enjoyed in previous vacations?

So, many things I had learned and that had made me feel like a competent person seemed to have been lost, and I wondered if I could be an adequate husband, father, or worker again. Combined with this, I felt to some extent that I had lost my identity. This was not total or extreme, but there were some questions in my mind about beliefs, values, and purposes in life. In addition, I felt that I had lost some of my cultural background when I had difficulty remembering some of the customs, traditions, and beliefs of the groups to which I belonged. This produces a feeling of being somewhat alone.

II. SHORT-TERM MEMORY

This information about short-term memory function was collected in a 2-week period in April 1975, 6 months after the cardiac arrest. I carried pencil and paper and wrote down each indication of memory difficulties. The information is organized into five categories: Cognition, recreation, living, interpersonal relationships, and personality.

A. Cognition

Organization of thinking was hampered. Problem solving often involves the organization and reorganization of data. The sequences or the relationships of the data must be coordinated, but I had trouble keeping the facts in mind, which made it difficult to organize them. Sometimes I had decided beforehand that a particular fact or idea was important and must be included in making a decision, but then the idea was lost, or if written down, the importance of it was lost. Sometimes this resulted in the usual organic confusion.

To problem solve effectively, it is important that all the variables be included and the way things have worked in the past be considered. But the history of the variables may be lost and then some of the variables to be considered may not be remembered and included. Deficits in past and present memory combine to make it difficult to think in an orderly way. Too much is missing.

Then when you are on the track of something, any distraction can cause a loss of train of thought, and that means you need to start over again. Of course many distractions come from the outside, but many distractions can be inner. The difficulty in remembering and thinking is constantly in your field of awareness, and it often intrudes as you are thinking. Once again the train of thought is broken and you go back to the beginning.

Difficulty in conceptual thinking has been considered a hallmark of some types of organicity. Sometimes it was hard to think conceptually, and it was easier to deal with things at a concrete level. But it appears that memory is a crucial part of conceptual thinking. How is it possible to organize, to see similarities and differences, or to extract the essence from a variety of objects or events when you cannot keep the objects or events in mind? Comparing things along a number of variables is difficult to do when you cannot retain the variables or retain the comparison after you have made it.

Therefore, thinking becomes a real effort and sometimes there is no reinforcement if you lose the product of your labor by not remembering the conclusion or decision you have made. It is difficult to exclude negative thoughts when you are faced consistently with evidence that your memory is poor. These thoughts act as a distraction and they interfere with the train of thought. The slightest distraction may mean that you have to remind yourself of what you are thinking. Soon you become reluctant to reason some-

thing out. What's the use? You decide that you can't do it, so stop thinking and accept the simplest solution.

B. Recreation

The memory (or cognitive) problem interferes with the ability to understand and enjoy a variety of activities.

Movies and TV watching become work. If it is a story, the trouble is remembering the beginning of the story or who the characters are. If it is a complicated plot, it is hard to follow or understand. Even if it is a simple plot, you may be puzzled about the people together in the second act if you forget that they smiled knowingly at each other in the first act. And you can't enjoy the story by talking about it with friends because you don't remember enough about it to talk about it.

In terms of sports on TV there is trouble remembering which team is which, which team is ahead, which players did the scoring, and how it all relates to their past performance. The thrill of the moment is still there, but part of the excitement is relating it to past performances and to the situation as a whole. Some of those things are missing, and missing also is the pleasure of sharing these experiences with friends.

Reading becomes difficult (partly because of a perceptual problem) because the meaning of some words has been lost and rereading is necessary to remember what already has been read even in the same paragraph. Rereading is also necessary because the ideas that are being expressed may not be understood since the sequence of thoughts can't be kept in mind. Especially difficult were complex and scientific materials, often because the words or terms were understood but they could not be related to other things. The terms or words lacked the richness of meaning they once had.

Playing games, once a pleasure, also became work. The game enjoyed most in the past was a form of duplicate bridge. Memory and cognition are crucial in bridge and it became difficult to remember things like the bidding sequence, the meaning of some bids, what has already been played, what is still out, and the strategy decided upon to play the hand.

Sight-seeing also becomes a chore. I had trouble remembering where I just was and what I had just seen. Seeing the sights had less meaning because I had trouble relating them to the history of the place or to other places. There was some joy in rediscovering places I had previously visited, but with new places, and some of the old ones, the unfamiliar stimuli were confusing and the awareness of the memory problems intruded on the pleasure of being on a vacation.

C. Living

This section relates to a number of activities that have to do with daily living and that were hampered by the memory deficit.

Directions, geography, locations, and the way to get around were difficulties that recurred. Even inside a building, getting lost was commonplace, and sometimes it took days for me to figure out and remember how to get out of a building. In taking walks, even in a familiar neighborhood, I could get lost. In taking a bus, I occasionally would get on the wrong bus or get off at the wrong stop. Remembering the right bus number was difficult. I started driving again about a year after being discharged from the hospital, and at first I needed to get instructions and directions from others on how to get to places not far from where I live.

One role in being the 'man of the house' is being able to take care of some things that have to do with the operation of the house or the family. It was difficult to play that role. Taking care of financial matters was especially difficult. I couldn't keep in mind information about interest rates, types of accounts, types of stock, or bonds, and I kept forgetting what my family already had in terms of these things. Since my arithmetic and spelling skills were hampered, I was reluctant to take over responsibility for things like paying bills, filling out the income tax, or dealing in any way with finances.

I never had been especially competent at repairing or building things, and the memory problem made it even more difficult. There was trouble remembering where things were kept and how things were used. Simple things like how to tie a tie or change a razor blade had to be relearned. Things that were slightly more complicated were relearned, but there was difficulty retaining new learning. I had trouble remembering where things were kept or where I put them to use them later. Losing or misplacing things was a regular occurrence.

Sometimes I didn't remember if I had already done something, like on two occasions I wasn't sure if we had had dinner yet. Dates, phone numbers, license plate numbers, and addresses were hard to keep in mind. Sometimes I wasn't sure what day of the week it was.

D. Interpersonal relations

Having conversations could become a trial. Often in talking with people I was acquainted with, I had trouble remembering their names or whether they were married or what our relationship had been in the past. I was worried about asking how someone's wife is and finding out that I had been at her funeral 2 years ago. So there was the worry of saying the wrong thing to people, and this made me cautious and reticent in my interactions with others.

But there were other reasons to be reticent. Often if I didn't have a chance to say immediately what came to mind, it would be forgotten and the conversation would move to another topic. Then there was little for me to talk about. I couldn't recall much about current events or things I read in the paper or saw on TV. Even juicy tidbits of gossip might be forgotten. So in order to have something to say, I'd tend to talk about myself and my 'condition'. My conversation became rather boring.

Interacting with others often made me anxious because I would worry about appearing too organic or might act improperly in some way. I was reluctant to make a suggestion for fear that it might be inappropriate. I was fearful of making a promise to do something because I was worried I might forget to do it. So being quiet and playing it safe became the watchwords.

E. Personality

The terms that best describe me during this period are passive, dependent, self-conscious, and withdrawn. But none of these was to an extreme degree. I was active in many ways and I stayed involved as much as I could stand it. But in comparison to the way I used to be, I became a narrow, passive, dependent person.

I was less confident that I could handle things so I resisted trying some things or getting involved in some things. I was more cautious than I had been, and I waited for other people to suggest things. There was more dependency on others and more expectation that others would take care of things. There was less willingness to take responsibility or to make decisions. Along with this was a tendency not to speak my mind, not to stand up for what I thought.

Also there was less involvement with friends and family. It was hard to follow up on things that had been planned, it was difficult to know what role I should play, and there was an unawareness of how to participate in things. In whatever I was doing, I was repeatedly reminded of how poor my memory was, and this led me to pay less attention to what was happening around me. Often I was locked in self-preoccupation, and too often this increased my degree of depression.

But on the positive side, I also became more sympathetic, more accepting of things, and more patient. This became more possible because at that point I wasn't supposed to be assertive or responsible or productive.

III. REHABILITATION

The first step in the rehabilitation program designed by my wife and me was to review my life to find out what I had done and what kind of person I had been. Of course, I had not lost a great deal of this information, but I had lost enough to make the review interesting and sometimes surprising. I looked at picture slides, college and high school year books, past appointment books, and folders in my file cabinet. I talked with my wife and daughter about things we had done together and I talked with friends about the 'old days'. Much of my talk with family and friends during the first few months of my being home from the hospital was related to the past. In general, I got good news. My wife, daughter, and I have had a good life, and I had been doing good and interesting work. This served as a strong base to start on and helped me from getting too depressed.

The second step was starting to get involved in things. About 6 weeks after leaving hospital, I began to come in to my office at the university. I talked with faculty members and students, and I sat in on some classes and meetings.

The third step was to try to see what I could do in terms of work. Early in the spring of 1975 I began to supervise the therapy and diagnostic work of a few graduate students. It was extremely difficult to do, and I learned what anxiety really is. But it was important to do because I learned that I still was a clinical psychologist and that I had not lost all of my skills and knowledge. At this point, I also started to seek professional help. I contacted the university reading center and arranged to see a remedial reading teacher. My reading was evaluated to be ranging from about the seventh- to ninth-grade level, and I had difficulty with speed and comprehension. The teacher arranged a graded program to help with this. I met with her twice a week for $3\frac{1}{2}$ months. It was extremely difficult to do because I was still easily confused, mixed up, and I had difficulty remembering what we were doing and how we were doing it. But my reading did improve, and more important, I felt that I had someone to work with and something was being done. This work was especially helpful because the teacher obviously involved herself in the work, and she tried to help me with my memory in addition to my reading. She looked into the literature about memory, and she designed some exercises to help with that too. At this early point in rehabilitation, the relationship with the teacher was most important, and I also was able to see some improvement in my reading ability. This work stopped at the beginning of the summer because the problem was no longer the reading itself, but memory and cognition.

During this period I returned to the weekly duplicate bridge game I had been playing in for a number of years. It was extremely difficult, and I could not play unless I took a tranquilizer. I lost regularly. But after about 6 months I started to win more often than I lost. I feel that the bridge playing was important in my rehabilitation. Like muscles are strengthened by exercise, the brain must be stimulated, and there is nothing more stimulating than duplicate bridge.

Along with the help in reading, I returned to the hospital as an outpatient to see the physical therapist who had helped me so much while I was hospitalized. I was barely able to walk because of muscle weakness, and her work with me led to great improvement. But my legs were still a little weak, and once again the exercises she arranged led to further improvement. As with the reading teacher, the relationship with the physical therapist and the feeling that something was being done were most important.

Also in the spring of 1975, I heard of a neurologist who was conducting research on short-term memory, and I volunteered to be a S in this study. He accepted me, and it was agreed that he would teach me some strategies to deal with my memory difficulties when the research data were collected. After 4 months, he told me that my short-term memory was normal and that I should just relearn the things I had forgotten. The psychologist who worked with the neurologist did explain to me that my short-term memory was not 'normal', but the problem was that the loss of so much past memory meant that I had lost the 'pegs' to attach new information to. My short-term memory was poor, but it was poor because my long term-

memory was poor. This obviously made sense, but I got no help in how to deal with it. Relearning was being done all along, but it was difficult for two reason: The loss of 'pegs' meant that comprehension of abstract material was especially difficult and retention of such material was also unlikely. I got no help in how to relearn.

The fall of 1975 was a depressing period. I had some unrealistic fantasies that things would be magically different after 1 year, but the improvement was not as great as I hoped for, and I was without any professional help. But three things happened near the end of 1975. I was able to arrange to work with a psychologist at the Howard Rusk Rehabilitation Center at NYU Medical Center. After some evaluation, she set up some exercises to help me with the perceptual problem that was interfering with my relearning. I had been aware of the perceptual difficulties, but I had not realized how this impaired my ability to relearn things. Exercises and strategies she developed or suggested led to improvement in perception, memory and cognition.

Second, at the beginning of 1976, at the suggestion of the psychologist at NYU Medical Center, I began to see a psychotherapist to help me with the emotional side of things and to make plans for the future. This helped me to try things and to understand more realistically my situation.

Third, at the beginning of 1976, I started to work as a volunteer 3 days a week at a community mental health center. The beginning was very difficult. I couldn't remember people's names or faces, and it took me 2 weeks to learn how to get out the building. But I was with mental health people, some whom I knew, and they understood the difficulties that I was having. Mainly, my work was supervising the clinical work of the junior staff members and students. I also saw a couple of patients.

In 1977 I decided I was ready for work and opened an office for the practice of psychology. That continued until 1980, when I returned to the faculty of the university with which I had been associated. At this point, I am able to do many of the things that were impossible to do early after the cardiac arrest, and while some of my abilities have not returned, enough has returned so that I can function in my present work setting.

IV. RECOMMENDATIONS FOR PATIENTS AND THERAPISTS

Following are some of the things that I have learned that seem important in rehabilitation work with patients with memory problems. Of course, many of these may be important in rehabilitation for a number of different kinds of problems. First, some suggestions for the patient:

1. It is important to stay involved in things. It is easy to withdraw because of the difficulty and embarrassment of being involved with people. The embarrassment will come when you do not recognize or remember the name of someone you have known well. More embarrassment comes when you ask someone how his wife is, and it turns out that she has been dead for 3 years. Anxiety comes when you are asked a question or to do something you have been able to answer or do before. Also, it is uncomfortable to be with a group of people and to have nothing to say. But you do need the stimulation, and you need to prevent yourself from withdrawing into a state of self-preoccupation. The stimulation helps bring back old memories. These old memories have not been erased, but the problem is how to retrieve them. Being involved helps.

2. Do try things even though you feel that you won't be able to do them. Of course, try things that are at a lower level than you were able to do before. Try again a few weeks later, and then try again. Realizing that you now are able to do something you couldn't do before is very encouraging.

3. Do try to find some things that you can do fairly well. It is important to feel competent at some things, even though those things may not be related to your previous work.

4. Write everything down. If you do want to remember something, make a note of it as soon as possible.

5. Keep notes on your progress. It is important to keep progress notes because you will not remember what it was like a few months before. By keeping the notes on what you have and have not been able to do at a particular point and then at a later point, you will be able to see the progress. The steps in improvement are very small and slow, and you will not be able to recognize the improvement unless you have notes over time.

6. Do not try to conceal the memory problem. If you do try to conceal it, you will be even more anxious, and you may do some ridiculous things in trying to cover it up.

7. In conversations, you may feel that you don't remember something, but the first thing that pops into your mind is often the correct thing. Take a chance. Say it.

8. Do not keep thinking you will be returning to the same level at which you were previously. Set some smaller goals for yourself, and think about some things you might want to do and be able to do in the future. If it turns out you're able to do more, that would be a happy surprise. But if you set larger goals, you are likely to become depressed.

9. Read some success stories of people who have overcome intellectual difficulties (Moss, 1972), and read some books on training memory (Lorayne & Lucas, 1974).

10. Say 'be patient' to yourself every time you find you cannot do something. You must wait, things will be better.

11. Accept the difficulty of things and learn to live with the anxiety you feel when you try to do things. Tranquilizers may be helpful. Things will be easier, but this will change slowly, very slowly.

Now, some suggestions for the rehabilitation therapist:

1. Talk slowly and try to avoid complicated sentences. The patient will have difficulty holding things in mind, and may have lost the meaning of some words. Do ask him to review what is important for him to remember.

2. Accept the fact that it may take several trials and repetitions before the patient keeps the information in mind.

3. Provide the patient with a place he can work alone, a place without distractions or interruptions.

4. Recognize that the patient may have visual memory difficulty in addition to auditory ones. This means that he will have difficulty recognizing materials and equipment already used several times. He may not recognize you. Things should be kept in the same place.

5. Establish sub-goals and keep records that can be shown to the patient so that he can see the progress being made.

6. No matter how high the patient's premorbid intelligence might have been, he may have difficulty understanding instructions that seem simple. Memory is a key part of cognition, and do check to see if the patient is understanding what is being asked of him. Ask the patient to review and repeat the instructions.

7. Understand his negativistic and hostile behavior as attempts to show himself and you that he is a competent person who can accomplish and control some things. If he makes you angry, he still can do something.

8. Do find some things that the patient can be competent at.

9. Do not minimize or deny the patient's difficulty with memory. ('Oh, I have a poor memory too. I never remember where I put things.') Give honest evaluations, and do not water down the difficulty.

10. Realize that the patient may feel alone and incompetent, and more important than the rehabilitation techniques used is the relationship with you—somebody who is interested and cares.

11. In terms of techniques for helping short-term memory, there are few established methods. Memory is not a single factor, but one that is related to learning, perception, and attention. Often, things are not remembered because they are not learned or perceived to begin with. The first principle is pay attention. The second principle to teach is, intend to remember, expect to remember. If the expectation is one of forgetting, forgetting is more likely. Third, select the parts or items that are most important to remember. For example, in reading a newspaper article, select the items or information that is most important to remember. Fourth, try to relate the items or information to something already known. Connect it. Don't just let it sit there. Think about it. Fifth, review what is to be remembered. Write it down or think about it as often as possible.

One word about practice in memorizing. Earlier in this century, school children were made to do a lot of memorizing in order to strengthen their ability to remember things. Apparently this did not work. Memorizing by itself was not useful. What was useful were techniques for learning and remembering, techniques such as attending, selecting, relating, and organizing things learned. Reading Hunter (1957) is useful.

One final note. Help for me has come from a number of sources. In the early stage of my rehabilitation, most important were the physical therapist and the reading teacher. Later, two psychologists helped me with the cognitive and emotional problems. Of little help were the two neurologists I saw. Both suggested that I just relearn what I had forgotten, but they didn't recognize or appreciate the learning problems that I had, and they were unable to suggest strategies for relearning. Of course, being a psychologist myself, I was more able than some others to help myself and to find the resources available for rehabilitation. Finally, most important of all have been my wife and daughter, not only with the emotional support but also with the retraining and rehabilitation over this period. Without them, I am not sure how much rehabilitation would have taken place.

REFERENCES

Hunter, L. M. L. (1957). *Memory: facts and fallacies*. Penguin Books, Baltimore.
Lorayne, H. and Lucas, J. (1974). *The memory book*. Ballantine, New York.
Moss, C. S. (1972). *Recovery with aphasia*. University of Illinois Press, Urbana.

(Meltzer 1983)

COMMENTARY

In terms of severity of brain insult, the illness sustained by Meltzer was a particularly severe episode, with a coma duration of six weeks. If this had been a head injury, it would have been classified as a 'very severe' injury. We do not have any neuroanatomical information, apart from the indication that there was specific damage to the right hemisphere. As in most cases of severe hypoxia, one would have expected bilateral cerebral pathology, with an emphasis on the hippocampus and the so-called watershed areas separating the distribution of the middle and posterior cerebral arteries. Although focal damage limited to the hippocampus has been noted in some cases of cerebral hypoxia (e.g. Zola-Morgan *et al.* 1986), it is important to note the significant degree of variability in cases of hypoxia, both in the severity of the memory loss and in the presence of coexisting cognitive deficits (Hopkins *et al.* 1995). A positron emission tomography study of patients with a post-anoxic syndrome following cardiac arrest yielded evidence of widespread abnormalities in the cortex, in subcortical structures, and also in white matter areas (DeVolder *et al.* 1990). In Meltzer's case, the long period of coma (six weeks), and the significant retrograde amnesia in the early recovery period, both point to the presence of pathology over and above discrete lesions to the hippocampus.

In his everyday adjustment, Meltzer appeared to have difficulties that were additional to his memory deficits, such as impaired reading, problem-solving symptoms, and some perceptual difficulties. His reading difficulties had at least three components—a perceptual component, a difficulty in comprehension of words/phrases, and a difficulty in retention of what he had read. Meltzer's reading difficulties point to the presence of some left-sided pathology in addition to the more focal right-sided lesions that are indicated in the article. A mild difficulty in scanning words/sentences might be expected to follow right-sided damage alone, but the extent of reading difficulties noted by Meltzer point to the presence of bilateral pathology. The difficulty in retention of what he had read, and therefore the difficulty in comprehension of complex sentences, would be readily explicable in terms of his anterograde memory loss that was secondary to limbic-diencephalic pathology alone. It is likely that this pathology, combined with bilateral cortical damage, resulted in the reading difficulties that he experienced.

In the case of Meltzer's problem-solving symptoms, there is a possibility that these may have been due in part to a dysexecutive syndrome that was secondary to frontal lobe damage—such damage is occasionally seen after hypoxia (Hopkins *et al.* 1995). However, there is no doubt that his memory deficits played a major part in his problem-solving symptoms—his retrograde and anterograde amnesia meant that he had difficulties in knowing the past connotations of items, in being able to hold a number of thoughts in memory at the same time, and in keeping track of thoughts after a period of distraction.

The major part of his problems arose directly from his memory difficulties. What is particularly notable in this case study is the loss of past memories and the impact that this had, not only in its own right, but also in its interaction with new learning. It is difficult to be certain of the duration of his retrograde amnesia, which appeared to have 'shrunk' or recovered over the first year after his hypoxic event, but in the early stages—around six weeks after the onset of the brain illness—he thought that he was eleven years younger than he really was. A second major theme is the effect of his memory loss on his social interaction and his emotional well-being—areas that have been somewhat neglected in research on memory disorders.

Meltzer's loss of past memories had, at least in the initial stages, major impacts on his sense of identity, and this resulted in some feelings of isolation. In the early recovery period, he found that he had forgotten what were his beliefs, values, customs, traditions, etc.—sets of personal knowledge items which all contribute to one's sense of identity and one's place in society. It seemed that, in technical jargon, both his 'personal semantic' memory and 'autobiographical events' memory were affected in the early stages.

The loss of past memories was particularly interesting in the wide range of skills that were temporarily lost—finding his way about familiar routes, knowing how to operate things such as the stereo, calculator, alarm clock, etc. He also noted that solving problems required both holding in short-term memory the variables in question and also being aware of past experience in the use of these variables—since he had both anterograde and retrograde memory loss, Meltzer suffered a double blow in some problem-solving settings. There was also loss of memory for familiar people, in particular, memory loss for information about such people, in addition to memory loss for their name. In the initial stages of recovery, there were major deficits in tackling particular situations and in initiating behaviours that would previously have been taken for granted and would have been performed automatically (e.g. When should bills be paid? When should oil be changed in a car? Which are good places to go for a vacation? Where is the best place to buy a new washing machine?). Certain memories were less likely to be lost than others, for example, familiarity in respect of his house and its immediate locality was relatively preserved, whereas memory for other routes in his locality was lost. Note that Meltzer's retrograde amnesia did have some adverse effect on his ability to retain new information: 'My short term memory was poor, but it was poor because my long term memory was poor' (p. 12). In his own words, he did not have the 'pegs' from his long-term memory on which he could hang new information that had to be learned. In the research literature, group studies of alcoholic Korsakoff patients have shown a rather weak relationship between severity of anterograde amnesia and severity of retrograde amnesia (Shimamura and Squire 1986). In contrast, those single-case studies with particularly severe anterograde amnesia (e.g. Damasio *et al.* 1985; Wilson *et al.* 1995) also have a marked degree of retrograde amnesia. My own clinical experience would appear to tie in with Meltzer's observations—where a patient with anterograde amnesia also has significant retrograde memory loss, it does tend to act as a handicap in attempts to learn new information, either incidentally or in rehabilitation settings.

Although as clinical neuropsychologists we tend to conclude that reasoning and problem-solving ability are unaffected in cases of pure amnesia (where tests such as IQ tests are performed well), the report by Meltzer brings home the point that many reasoning and problem-solving situations will require some degree of 'working memory' and that in this sense general cognitive functioning may often be affected to some degree by marked memory impairment.

In general, learning *how* to perform tasks is retained in amnesia, and what is lost is recollection of the original learning experience. In Meltzer's case, he did lose memory for certain skills—it may be that the particular skills that were lost were ones that had recently been acquired (e.g. the stereo and the alarm clock, that he had difficulty in operating, may have been recently used for the first time, and the 'engrams' relating to the storage of relevant perceptual-motor sequences may therefore not have been as firmly entrenched as some other skills). It is possible that his right temporo-parietal damage, perhaps in combination with cerebellar pathology, resulted in his loss of certain premorbid perceptual-motor skills. A patient that my colleagues and I reported a number of years ago, who suffered memory loss following a penetrating paranasal snooker cue injury that affected limbic-diencephalic structures (Dusoir *et al.* 1990), also complained that he initially had significant difficulty in using a calculator with which he had been proficient before his injury. Although associations of deficits is much less significant than dissociations between deficits, the coexistence of loss of such 'procedural skills' suggests that there may be an overlap of mechanisms underlying loss of autobiographical, episodic memory (e.g. recollecting work or family experiences), loss of factual memory (e.g. when should oil be changed in a car?) and loss of skill knowledge (e.g. knowing how to operate a mechanical/electronic device). Note that Meltzer was able to relearn his lost skills, presumably to the same level of proficiency as before, even though it took a number of relearning trials—in spite of his marked anterograde memory impairment, relearning was possible. This may have reflected both the presence of some minimal representations of the 'engrams' for the particular skill, and/or the fact that learning of such perceptual-motor skills is usually intact in amnesic patients. In my own studies of patients with retrograde amnesia (Kapur 1997), I have often found that patients may be able to relearn facts and skills that have been lost, but they will not be able to relearn the vividness of the original experiences that have been erased from their memory. An analogous observation, though dealing with anterograde amnesia, has also been reported in a moving account by a pathologist, who described a form of paraneoplastic limbic encephalitis that was associated with Hodgkin's disease in his 15-year-old daughter (Carr 1982). After recovery from a devastating period of amnesia, the child was able to relearn factual material that had been lost, but she was never able to recall the 18-month period of her life during which her memory was severely impaired.

Meltzer's paper is a useful reminder of the variability in the extent of functional recovery that may exist after brain damage, both between patients and also across functions within a particular patient. In his particular case, after emerging from coma he could recognize his family but not some of his friends, and when going home a few weeks later his home and neighbourhood were familiar to him but not the route home nor some of the geography of the city. His recovery period appeared to stretch over a number of years—it was five years before he could return to his original university position, and some improvements appeared to continue to occur well into the second year of recovery. This is a useful reminder that, although most neuropsychological recovery does take place in the first 6 to 12 months, in some cases it can continue for years afterwards.

Meltzer thought that most of his loss of premorbid memories reflected loss of retrieval—whether this is specific to the type of brain insult that he sustained is open to question. Some authors (e.g. Volpe *et al.* 1986) have argued that cerebral hypoxia results in selective loss of memory retrieval functions, while leaving recognition memory relatively spared. Meltzer remarked on the influence of his poor short-term memory on his thinking and on his problem-solving ability, and this is something that has also been rather neglected in published studies of memory loss. Even in this very 'cognitive' area of handicap, Meltzer noted side-effects on his emotional adjustment—at times he became passive, he had feelings of depression, and he lacked in confidence. In the case of conversational settings with a number of other people present, difficulties arose due to a combination of emotional/motivational factors (e.g. feeling of caution, a tendency to withdraw) and cognitive factors (e.g. keeping track of a conversation, not making a promise in case it might be forgotten). In the case of personality/temperament changes, there were some positive changes—thus, he now felt more sympathetic with others, he was more accepting, and he was more patient.

One of the most interesting facets of Meltzer's paper is his advice to patients and to therapists. There are several strands that emanate from this. He strongly advocates a positive approach, with participation in any cognitive or other activities that may be of benefit. He stressed its importance in two ways—first, he felt that something was being done to help him, and secondly he found it valuable to build up a relationship with his therapists. Some of the general lessons he feels he has learned in relation to rehabilitation are found in many accounts of therapy after brain injury, but they are worth repeating—the systematic documentation of progress, the setting of realistic goals, being positive in the sense of trying/making guesses when encountering a retrieval difficulty, being patient, and accepting that some degree of anxiety will inevitably be present during the process of rehabilitation.

There are also general guides for the therapist—talking slowly and repeating instructions, making sure that there is inclusion of some activities that the patient can perform without error, being prepared for some anger and hostility but not to over-react to this, etc. His recommendation with regard to 'error-free' learning finds a ready counterpart in current memory rehabilitation research, where 'error-free' training paradigms have in certain contexts yielded much better learning and delayed retention than 'error-full' training paradigms (Wilson *et al.* 1994). There are a few general points that do stand out—his praise for the role of therapists and psychologists (with rather negative comments on what neurologists could offer!), the support given by his family, and his advice that patients should read literature relating to their handicaps.

In terms of specific retraining procedures, it is interesting that Meltzer found playing bridge an important part of his rehabilitation. 'Like muscles are strengthened by exercise, the brain must be stimulated, and there is nothing more stimulating than duplicate bridge' (p. 12). At first glance, this advice does go against accepted practice in memory therapy (Wilson and Moffat 1992), that memory or other cognitive functions are not like muscles—more practice does not make for better memory. Meltzer does in fact appear to accept this towards the end of his article—he refers to earlier memory research which found that memorizing by itself was not useful, and that what *was* useful were techniques such as good concentration, relating bits of information to each other, and organizing things to be learned. The particular memory strategies that Meltzer recommends echo what is often espoused in memory therapy, but they are worth repeating—ensure good concentration and motivation, select what is important in the mass of material to be remembered, relate new information to old, and regularly review/rehearse what has been learned.

REFERENCES

Carr, I. (1982). The Ophelia syndrome: Memory loss in Hodgkin's Disease. *Lancet*, 1, April 10. 844–5.

Damasio, A. R., Eslinger, P. J., Damasio, H., Van Hoesen, G. W., and Cornell, S. (1985). Multimodal amnesic syndrome following bilateral temporal and basal forebrain damage. *Archives of Neurology*, **42**, 252–9.

DeVolder, A. G., Goffinet, A. M., Bol, A., Michel, C., De Barsy, T., and Laterre, C. (1990). Brain glucose metabolism in postanoxic syndrome. A positron emission tomographic study. *Archives of Neurology*, **47**, 197–204.

Dusoir, H., Kapur, N., Byrnes, D. P., McKinstry, S., and Hoare, R. D. (1990). The role of diencephalic pathology in human memory disorder: evidence from a penetrating paranasal brain injury. *Brain* 113, 1695–1506.

Hopkins, R. O., Gale, S. D., Johnson, S. C., Anderson, C. V., Bigler, E. D., Blatter, D. D., *et al.* (1995). Severe anoxia with and without concomitant brain atrophy and neuropsychological impairments. *Journal of the International Neuropsychological Society*, **1**, 501–9.

Kapur, N. (1997). Autobiographical amnesia and temporal lobe pathology. In *Classic case studies in the neuropsychology of memory* (ed. A. J. Parkin). Psychology Press, Hove, UK. In press.

Shimamura, A. P. and Squire, L. R. (1986). Korsakoff's syndrome: A study of the relation between anterograde and remote memory impairment. *Behavioural Neuroscience*, **100**, 165–70.

Volpe, B. T., Holtzman, J. D., and Hirst, W. (1986). Further characterization of patients with amnesia after cardiac arrest: Preserved recognition memory. *Neurology*. **36**, 408–11.

Wilson, B. and Moffat, N. (1992). *The clinical management of memory problems* (2nd edn). Chapman & Hall, London.

Wilson, B., Baddeley, A., and Evans, J. (1994). Errorless learning in the rehabilitation of memory impaired people. *Neuropsychological Rehabilitation*, **4**, 307–26.

Wilson, B. A., Baddeley, A. D., and Kapur, N. (1995). Dense amnesia in a professional musician following herpes simplex virus encephalitis. *Journal of Clinical and Experimental Neuropsychology*, 17, 668–81.

Zola-Morgan, S., Squire, L., and Amaral, D. (1986). Human amnesia and the medial temporal lobe region: Enduring memory impairment following a bilateral lesion limited to field CA1 of the hippocampus. *Journal of Neuroscience*, 6, 2950–67.

'Did I remove that gallbladder?'

Harold L. Klawans

Professor Harold Klawans wrote this article about his colleague, a general surgeon, who suffered an attack of transient global amnesia. Professor Klawans himself is a distinguished Professor of Neurology, and works at the Department of Neurology, Rush-Presbyterian-St Luke's Medical College, Chicago, USA.

Ken Keltner's* name is not a household word. It never has been and never will be. After all, the names of only a select number of surgeons ever fall into that category, and most of them are cardiovascular surgeons: DeBakey, Christian Barnard. Ken Keltner is a general surgeon: gallbladders, hemorrhoids, and hernias are his turf—with varicose veins for variety—not coronary artery bypasses or heart transplants or valve replacements. Nothing that glamorous.

By the time he came to see me as a patient in 1986, we'd known each other professionally for over twenty years. We were not friends but professional colleagues who respected each other and had shared patients off and on for two decades. Ken is well respected as a general surgeon. He doesn't teach or do any research. He doesn't even have a faculty appointment at any of Chicago's six medical schools. But he does general surgery better than most surgeons, including those with appointments at the various medical schools. In his own part of the world, the far western suburbs of Chicago, he's considered a doctor's doctor, one of those rare individuals other doctors trust to operate on them and members of their own families.

Ken arrived at my office at five minutes to eleven, accompanied by a nurse named Joan Gordon. Both were still garbed in their green surgical scrub suits. Ken looked tired. His face, which often appeared boyish for a man in his middle fifties, now clearly showed his age. He walked with his usual rapid, confident stride, but something was different. Normally when Ken Keltner walked into a room, everyone felt his presence, his strength

* All names have been changed for the purpose of this article.

of personality. But this time it was almost as if no one had entered my office.

I greeted him by name as one colleague to another, and he in turn greeted me by name. I was glad that he could do that much. I'd been prepared for the worst. When Joan called, she'd told me that Ken had had a stroke and was completely delirious.

Before I had a chance to say anything more, he asked two questions. He asked them in rapid succession without waiting for any reply in between. 'Where am I? What's happening to me?'

His voice was flat. It betrayed no emotion at all—no fear, no concern, no bewilderment. Nor did his eyes. Nor his face. The most I could sense was a mild degree of curiosity, not a driving interest—far from it. It was more like a totally detached curiosity as if he were pursuing some minor academic point about gallbladder surgery, something he probably ought to know but nothing that would affect his life or alter his behavior.

He repeated his two questions once again: 'Where am I? What's happened to me?'

Once again he didn't pause in between for a reply. And for the second time, it seemed that the process of asking was more important to him than any answers his questions might evoke.

'You are in my office, Ken,' I replied. 'I'm going to examine you.'

He nodded as if he understood what I said to him.

I paused.

He asked his two questions once again: 'Where am I? What's happening to me?'

My answer had not gotten through. He might have understood it briefly, but that understanding had not been incorporated into his consciousness.

'Where am I? What's happening to me?'

Once again I answered his questions and watched him nod in return. Before he got a chance to ask them again, I asked Joan to describe what she had observed.

The story she told me was a remarkable one. Even though she'd never received any training in neurological nursing and she didn't really understand what had happened, she was able to reconstruct what had happened in minute detail. She'd sensed right at the beginning that something was not right and had tried hard to notice and remember exactly what happened.

They'd been in the operating room for over an hour and a half. It was the same OR [Operating Room] they worked in together three mornings a week, week after week, year after year. In addition to Joan, who was the scrub nurse, three people were in the OR: Ken Keltner, the anesthetist, and the patient, Vera Bickford. Ken was removing her gall-bladder. The operation had gone smoothly and quickly. He was a quick surgeon; he made decisions rapidly, and his hands moved quickly.

Then he did something he rarely did. He looked up at the clock on the wall of the operating room. Joan looked, too. It was 9:43. They'd begun the operation at 8:05.

'One hour and thirty-eight minutes,' he said. She couldn't remember the last time he'd cared how long an operation had taken. 'I'll be done in another five or six minutes,' he continued.

That was obvious to her. They had done hundreds of gallbladders together. All that was left to do was to suture Mrs. Bickford's abdominal wall closed.

'Skin to skin in one hour and forty-three minutes', he said.

'Not bad', she replied.

'Not bad at all,' he echoed. 'Especially for a fifty-eight-year-old general surgeon who works without residents.'

She could not remember his ever having said anything like that. Working at a hospital without residents was his own choice. And she hadn't known that he was fifty-eight. She'd thought he was younger than that.

This was, he told her, the sixteen hundred and forty-second gallbladder he'd removed

during his career as a general surgeon. At one time he'd debated putting metal tags on each gallbladder as he removed them. Metal tags with consecutive numbers. They did that with the duck at that restaurant in Paris. 'What was the name of that restaurant?' he wondered out loud.

Joan had no idea. She'd never been to Paris. By now she was afraid something was wrong. Ken was normally all business during an operation, and this was not business. The operation had come to a standstill, work remained to be done.

'It's on the Left Bank,' he mused. 'Just beyond Notre Dame, with a great view of the back of Notre Dame.'

She knew what she had to do. She handed him the forceps with the needle and suture already loaded into it. He took it just as he always had and put in the first suture. And the second. And the third. It would take a total of about nine or ten more. Then Mrs. Bickford would have a nice thin scar.

'What was the name of that restaurant?' he asked again.

'Which one?'

'The one with the numbered ducks.'

'The one in . . .'

'Where was that restaurant?'

She handed him another suture, and he put it in.

'What restaurant?' he asked.

Joan had no interest at all in restaurants, in Paris or not. She wanted to know why Ken Keltner was thinking about restaurants instead of this operation. And the next one. Did he remember that he had another operation to do immediately after Mrs. Bickford? On somebody named Mitchell? She reminded him.

He looked at her blankly.

He couldn't have forgotten, thought Joan. He never forgot anything about his patients. Perhaps he hadn't understood. 'What's our next operation?' she asked as cheerfully as she could.

'A hernia,' he said. 'Or a vein stripping. Or something.' He couldn't remember.

She looked at the half-closed wound. He had put in five sutures. That left about six more to go. And he was just standing there as if he had no idea what he should do next. He looked up at her.

The nurse smiled at him.

'Did I take out that gallbladder?' he asked.

Joan was so startled she couldn't make any reply.

'Did I take out that gallbladder?' he repeated.

'Yes,' she said. 'Everything went well.'

'Good,' he said. Then after a pause, 'Did I take out that gallbladder?'

'The operation's almost over,' she said. She reached over and picked up the gallbladder that had been removed about twenty minutes earlier and showed it to him. 'Here's the gallbladder. You see that it's been removed.'

'Yes,' he nodded. Ken stood there motionless.

Joan still did not know what was wrong, but she knew that something was. And it was serious. A stroke she thought. He must be having a stroke. 'You are closing up,' she said, taking complete charge of the operating room. 'You have already put in about five sutures. Take the forceps and put in another one.'

'Yes,' he said. 'Closing up. I see.'

Ken began to put in the next stitch. Joan watched him critically. As far as she could tell, he did it as deftly and quickly as ever. The distance from the previous one was perfect, and so was the closure of the wound— excellent opposition of the two sides, no excess puckering. He was a meticulous surgeon. That, she told me, was why she liked working with him, why she'd been working with him for a dozen years. That was also why she'd let him take out her own gallbladder three years ago.

He was done tying the knot. He should have started the next stitch. Instead he asked the same question: 'Did I take out that gallbladder?'

'Yes,' she replied.

'Oh,' he nodded. 'What am I doing now?'

'You are closing up.'

'Oh,' he said with almost a touch of insight.

'Closing up,' she repeated.

'Closing up,' he said.

'Put in the next suture,' she instructed him.

Ken went back to work. Once again Joan scrutinized his every move. If he did anything wrong, she'd have to call for help, to get someone else into the OR to close up. She wanted to avoid that if she possibly could, but she couldn't endanger the patient in any way.

Ken stopped. He had put in one more perfect suture, and he once again began his litany. 'Did I take out that gallbladder?'

There was one difference this time. He did not wait for an answer before he asked his second question: 'What am I doing?'

Slowly, carefully, and firmly, Joan answered his questions and told him what to do. Once again he followed her instructions.

The process went on. Suture. Knot. Questions: 'Did I take out that gallbladder? What am I doing?' Instructions. Suture. Questions.

By the time they'd finished, he'd added a third question to his routine: 'Where am I?'

Finally, he had put in the last suture. Joan had talked him through the operation. Mrs. Bickford's abdomen was closed. The scar was straight. The two sides were aligned perfectly. Ken had closed Mrs. Bickford's surgical incision as well as he had closed up any gallbladder Joan had assisted him on in the last dozen years. Technically his hands had performed their job as well as ever. Joan looked at the clock. It had taken ten minutes, about five minutes longer than it should have. It had seemed far longer than that to her. She was thankful that he'd been able to finish the operation.

That was when she had called my office and told my secretary that she was bringing Ken in to see me. She was sure that he had had a stroke—a small stroke, but nonetheless a stroke.

Ken had stood there quietly throughout Joan's entire description of what had happened to him, not interrupting her even once. This was a man who normally was impatient with long, drawn-out explanations, always anxious to get to the bottom line, but he'd said nothing. He had to have heard every word she'd said. Had he understood it all? Had he understood any of it? Did he now understand what had happened to him and what was happening to him?

His expression had not changed a bit. He still had the same detached yet mildly curious look on his face. His repertoire also remained the same: 'Where am I? What's happening to me?'

Obviously, any attempt to derive further information about the present episode from him would be an exercise in futility. Facts obtained through language, the way most of us learn most of what we ever learn, were not being learned by Ken. Despite being told numerous times that he had successfully removed Mrs. Bickford's diseased gallbladder, he didn't know that he had removed it. And showing him the gallbladder hadn't helped either; the nonverbal stimulus had made no difference. So his problem was not merely a failure to understand language.

His problem was learning and memory. Ken could not learn new facts. He could not incorporate what he heard or saw or felt into his memory.

And his problem extended beyond brand new facts or experiences. He had been in my office at least a dozen times before, yet he didn't know where he was. Two days a week for the past twenty years or more, he had been operating in the same operating room in the same hospital; yet once this episode had taken hold, he didn't know where he was or what he was doing.

Memory is a complex and only partially understood activity of the brain. Neurologists often divide it into three separate components: immediate, recent, and remote. While these three functions are often defined as separate entities, they actually are not. They blend into each other, and any such divisions are arbitrary at best.

Immediate memory is the ability to recall something as soon as it has been learned or presented. This is formally tested by asking a patient to repeat a three-digit number.

Try it: 2–7–1.

Close your eyes, and repeat the number. Child's play, right?

Then four digits: 6–3–2–8. Then five. Then six. Then seven: 9–4–2–8–0–1–0. For that one, I always use my own phone number. That way I don't forget what number I've given the patient.

Next I show the patient three objects and ask him to name them—a key, a quarter, and a comb, or whatever else is in my pocket at the time. I then put the objects back in my pocket and ask the patient to name them again. So much for testing immediate memory.

'Where am I?' Ken asked for the fortieth time.

'Ken,' I said forcefully, 'you are in my office.'

He nodded.

'Now,' I asked, 'where are you?'

'Where am I?'

There was no need for numbers or keys. His immediate memory was not functioning at all.

Recent memory involves the ability to recall after a time delay. The delay can be one of minutes or hours or days. Any definition of when immediate recall ends and recent memory begins is arbitrary, but most authorities agree that any recall that occurs after a delay of several minutes is a function of the process of recent memory. Recent memory requires some sort of chemical change that can persist for hours or days. Immediate recall requires no such long-lasting alteration.

How is this tested? What were those three objects I named for you and then put back in my pocket five minutes ago? A key, a quarter, and a comb. Don't feel bad if you missed one or two. I hadn't asked you to remember them.

Next I ask the patient about recent events in his life. What did you have for lunch? For dinner last night? What did you do last night?

The segment of Ken's recent memory that covered the time for which he had no immediate recall could not be functioning. If a patient is unable to recall the names of three objects immediately, then there is no way he will be able to come up with those names after a delay of five or ten minutes.

But his defects in recent memory were more extensive than that. He didn't even recall starting the operation, and that had been before this episode had begun.

Did he know what he'd had for breakfast?

He didn't.

Or what he'd done the night before?

He had absolutely no idea. Recent memory was part of the problem.

But what about Ken's remote memory? *Remote memory*, which is what we usually consider memory, encompasses the ability to recall after weeks and months. The chemical process may involve the production of new proteins within the brain; in any case, remote memory does involve a rather persistent or permanent chemical change.

I was certain that this type of memory was at least partially functioning. Why? Because he recalled facts that he had learned in the past. He had recognized me. He had seen me, known who I was, and recalled my name. His simple 'Harold' had shown that he could recall faces and names and could connect the two. His nonverbal recall of faces worked, and so did his memory for names.

I also knew that he had retained other types of information. According to Joan, he had closed the incision as technically well as ever. His technical skills had been retained, although she had had to tell him what to do. He did not know where he was or what he had to do; he could not see the open wound and understand that he had to suture it shut. But the ability of his brain to direct his hands and fingers in the appropriate way had been preserved; each suture was perfectly placed.

He could remember faces and names and skills. The fact that at least parts of his remote memory were preserved did not surprise me, for certain aspects of remote memory are almost impossible to destroy. People always remember who they are. Ken did; he never asked, 'Who am I?' (The only exceptions are patients with severe psychiatric disorders and characters in soap operas. My definition of a soap opera is an art form that allows a patient to develop total amnesia and yet form new memories.) And people always recognize loved ones and people they have known for years. Ken remembered people he knew; he never asked Joan who she was.

But was his remote recall completely intact? That was the next question I had to ask.

There are always two steps in making a neurological diagnosis. The first step is to define precisely the nature and extent of the neurological dysfunction. The neurologist does this by taking a careful history and then performing a neurological examination. Once this is completed, the doctor knows what is working inside the brain and what isn't. By applying his knowledge of the anatomy and physiology of the brain, he can tell where the lesion is and whether there is more than one area of abnormality. This is the key step and requires no knowledge of diseases.

Once this question is answered, the doctor can address the second question: What caused the abnormal function? Thus, the process boils down to two questions:

1. In what way is the brain not working right?

2. What is causing that malfunction?

Taking the first step—defining the way or ways in which Ken's brain was malfunctioning—involved answering two questions:

1. What were the nature and extent of his memory loss? Was it limited to learning and immediate or very recent memory, or was his memory for events that occurred long ago also affected to any measurable degree?

2. What were the nature and extent of any other neurological symptoms he might have developed?

While the first question may seem difficult to answer, it is in fact quite simple. All it requires is some general knowledge and a bit of bravado. There are events and facts that no healthy adult with a normal brain should ever forget. They vary with the experience and educational level of the individual patient, and of course the examiner does not always know the answers, but that shouldn't prevent him from asking the questions. Few patients fabricate answers. Those who do are readily given away upon careful questioning.

What questions does everyone know? Where he was born, the date, the name of the hospital, his mother's first name. As the testing goes on, the questions get more difficult: the names of his brothers and sisters, the birth order and relative ages of his siblings, his mother's maiden name. The list can go on and on, and of course can result in a virtual biography: name of grammar school, name of high school, job history, social history, names of his children, dates of their births, and so on. He should have been able to answer them all.

This approach has its limits, however. Much of this material is 'overlearned', so a patient can recall these facts but still have serious gaps in his memory. Therefore, questioning the patient about less overlearned facts is often a better technique to detect less overt degrees of remote memory loss. For some reason, the classic neurological approach to this has been to ask the patient to perform tasks such as listing the names of the presidents backward starting with Reagan.

Try it—without looking at the list that follows.

Not so easy was it? I never expect a patient to list presidents before 1900. But even with that limitation, it still isn't so simple to do. The correct answer is:

Reagan
Carter
Ford (so easily forgotten)
Nixon
Johnson
Kennedy
Eisenhower
Truman
Roosevelt
Hoover
Coolidge
Harding
Wilson
Taft
Roosevelt

The problem is that lots of people never *cared* who the president was, and besides, many who did can't name them in reverse order. After all, how well did you do? And you thought you were one of those who cared.

I remember one particular patient I saw in consultation about ten years ago. The residents had asked me to see him just to make sure they had not missed anything. He was about eighty, and when admitted to the hospital with pneumonia he'd been confused. As his pneumonia had cleared, however, so had his confusion. But the house staff was very concerned about his memory loss. He couldn't list a single past president. In fact, he didn't even know who the current president was. Nor did he know the name of the current or past governors of Illinois. (Since Illinois has had a series of governors who are singularly forgettable, that may not have been a fair question.)

He *did* know the deceased mayor of Chicago, Hizzoner Mayor Daley. But everyone knew him, even patients with significant degrees of dementia. For a Chicagoan, knowing Daley's name was like knowing one's own name or place of birth. Such material is not just learned once and then stored in the brain; it is overlearned and rarely if ever, forgotten.

Why? Overlearned facts are probably stored in multiple areas of the brain. Single strokes cannot remove all of the traces. Since the chemical changes that underlie these facts have been so reinforced over the years, few, if any, diseases can undo them.

For this patient, Mayor Daley was the only political figure who crossed the line and became overlearned. The old man could not think of the name of one other politician. Not FDR. Not JFK. Only Richard J. Daley. Hizzoner would have been proud.

The old man wasn't sure he had ever heard the name of any other mayor of Chicago. Certainly the name Michael Bilandic, then the mayor of Chicago, was unfamiliar to him. But then Bilandic, the successor to Daley, was singularly forgettable.

Giving up on politics, I started with the biographical questions. The old man got them all right. He gave brief, sharp, rapid answers. The medical students and residents were surprised.

I stopped when I learned he had had only two years of schooling, in rural Georgia. What next? His lack of formal education was a barrier to formal intellectual testing. 'Are you a baseball fan?' I asked.

He was.

'Cubs or Sox?'

'Cubs.'

'What happened in 1938?'

'The homer in the dark to win the pennant.'

'Who hit it?'

'Gabby Hartnett,' he answered. 'Why, everybody knows that.'

Everybody doesn't. In fact, no one else in the room did, aside from the patient and me. 'Gabby died,' I informed him. I guessed that he wouldn't know. The ex-Cub Hall of Fame catcher had died only ten days earlier.

He looked at me with astonishment. 'When?' he asked.

'Last week.'

'I didn't know.'

Of course not. He'd been incommunicado inside an oxygen tent.

There was little more to test. To test his more recent memory, I asked him about the last season's Cub players, and he passed with flying colors. 'Did you ever know the names of the presidents?' I asked.

'Only one.'

'Grover Cleveland.'

He nodded.

One of the residents remained skeptical. He was obviously not a baseball fan and certainly not a Cub fan. He wanted to know how I could be certain the patient hadn't lied to me about the facts of his own history.

I couldn't prove it, but I knew. Even the most ardent baseball fan knows his mother's name better than Gabby Hartnett's, and no disease that I ever heard of erases the former from a patient's memory before the latter. Besides, he made an association that no patient with significant memory loss or dementia could make.

'What was that?' the resident said.

'Alexander,' I said.

The resident was lost.

'Grover Cleveland Alexander was a pitcher, one of the greatest ever. A Hall of Famer, like Gabby Hartnett. Alexander was named after a president, Grover Cleveland. And that was the one president the patient knew.'

Unfortunately, not everyone is a baseball fanatic. There are, however, events that

allow the questioner to tell whether or not a patient's memory is intact. Events that should be recalled in full detail by all normal adults.

Try answering these questions in as much detail as you can. Choose the right ones, depending upon your age: What were you doing when you heard that Kennedy (the president, not Bobby) had been shot? What do you recall about that weekend? What were you doing when you heard that Martin Luther King, Jr., was killed? What do you recall about that weekend? VJ day? VE day? Roosevelt's death (FDR, not Teddy)? Roosevelt's funeral? Pearl Harbor? Lindy's landing in Paris? Or, more recently, the first space walk? The *Challenger* disaster?

That was a lot easier than the reverse-order list of presidents, wasn't it? Such questions, therefore, are more likely to differentiate normal from abnormal.

To test the extent of Ken Keltner's memory loss, I started with Kennedy's assassination.

Ken knew precisely what he had been doing on that fateful day. He'd just finished surgery, a gallbladder followed by a double hernia repair. He left the postoperative area and went to the waiting room to talk with the relatives of his patients. The TV was on, and the relatives were huddled around it. They told him what had happened. They hardly asked him about the operations. He remembered seeing the building on TV. The Texas School Book Depository. He remembered Oswald and Ruby. And seeing Ruby kill Oswald. So much for 1963.

He also remembered less shocking events in clear detail—the Army–McCarthy hearings, the ticker tape carrying names of each American POW crossing the thirty-eighth parallel from North Korea to freedom. His remote memory was obviously intact.

I asked him to describe a gallbladder operation, from incision to closing. He did it without hesitation. It was like listening to someone read from a textbook of surgical techniques. 'When did you do your most recent gallbladder surgery?' I asked.

He wasn't sure.

'How about your most recent hernia?' I asked.

Same response.

'Appendix?'

'I did one on Christmas Eve,' he said.

That was the last operation he could remember. He remembered it, and everything that had happened before it, quite well. But after that—zero. He remembered nothing.

The rest of his exam was entirely normal. There was no weakness or paralysis, no sensory loss, no incoordination, no abnormalities of his balance or gait, no speech difficulties, no difficulty identifying objects, following instructions, or spelling words either forward or backward.

I was done. I told him not to worry, he was going to make a complete recovery. He shrugged. Did he have any questions, I asked.

Yes, he did. 'Where am I? What's happening to me?'

I told him, and he asked again. I knew further reassurance would not help. I stepped outside his room, counted to ten, and walked back in. I said hello.

He smiled and said hello. He recognized me and called me by name. 'When did I see you last?' I asked.

'About a month or two ago. At a meeting. Don't you remember? One of the guys wasted so much time. You were far too patient with him.'

I did remember—almost as well as he did. The meeting had been about two months ago, before Christmas. Before the appendectomy he had been able to recall.

The answers to all these questions enabled me to complete the first step of neurological diagnosis—determining the nature and extent of the brain malfunction. Ken Keltner had a circumscribed defect of memory. The rest of the functions of his brain were completely normal. Defining the nature and the extent of this defect had also given me the diagnosis, for only one disorder does this.

Dr. Kenneth Keltner, general surgeon, was in the midst of an attack of one of medicine's most startling syndromes, transient global amnesia, or TGA as it is called by those who love acronyms. A little over thirty years ago, two American neurologists from Boston, C. Miller Fisher and Raymond D. Adams, coined the term *transient global amnesia* to describe self-limited episodes in which the only major alteration in behavior is a marked disruption of memory. (The French use a different term to describe the same event: *ictus amnésique*, or amnesic attack. No one uses an acronym for this; it's one of the advantages of being French.)

Episodes like this occur in middle age or later life. They start abruptly, as did Ken's; one moment the patient is normal, the next moment he isn't. Often they start after emotional or physical stress. Sometimes they don't.

Others, not the sufferer, notice TGA. The patient's behavior may change. He may become restless, bewildered, or unusually quiet. His mind may start to wander. That was what Joan Gordon had noticed first. Dr. Keltner, usually all business during an operation, had started to wonder about the time, the length of the operation, the number of gallbladders he had removed in his career, the name of a French restaurant. Then the patient begins to ask questions. The questions always have to do with the present or the immediate past. And the patient repeats the questions over and over again, no matter how many times they are answered.

The questions are usually similar: Where am I? What's wrong? What's happening to me? At times they are tied to recent events: Did I take out that gallbladder?

Aside from learning and memory, the patient is normal, as was Ken. The sufferer cannot lay down new memories and often cannot recall events of the past few hours, days, or even weeks. But he can read, write, calculate, and even perform such skilled tasks as suturing an abdomen. Although Ken could not recall that he had to close Mrs. Bickford's abdomen, when told to do so, he put in the stitches with his usual skill.

Attacks of transient global amnesia are short and self-limited. They come on unexpectedly and depart on their own—hence the term *transient*. An episode usually lasts only a few hours, rarely hanging on for a day or two. All types of learning and recall are involved. The patient cannot remember what he sees, reads, hears, smells, tastes, or feels—

hence the term *global*. There is often some retrograde loss of memory, an inability to recall events that took place immediately before the attack began—hence the term *amnesia*. This usually goes back for hours and days, but sometimes can extend back far longer. The last operation Ken could recall had taken place six weeks earlier.

When the episode is over, the patient is able to function as well as he could previously, with a major exception: He has absolutely no memory for the event itself, and he may have a short additional period of retrograde amnesia for the days or hours preceding the onset. Aside from this permanent memory gap, everything is back to normal.

Once he recovers, the patient is often quite concerned, of course. He is aware that something has happened to him and left him with a blank spot in his life. The family members who witnessed what actually happened are far more frightened, often petrified. They all have the same worries, and they all ask the same questions: Was it a stroke? Is it a warning that the patient will have a stroke? Was it the beginning of epilepsy? Was it the beginning of Alzheimer's disease? Will it come back? If it does happen again, can it be permanent? Irreversible?

Mrs. Keltner arrived at my office just as I finished examining her husband. She asked me about him, and I told her what I had told him. She talked to him and then asked me the usual barrage of questions.

I tried to answer them all, but it wasn't easy. There's a lot we don't know about transient global amnesia, but we do know enough to reassure the families that none of their fears are justified. That's what I told Mrs. Keltner. Her husband had not had a stroke. This was not a warning sign. He wasn't destined to have a stroke. It wasn't the beginning of some sort of epilepsy or Alzheimer's disease. It would probably never happen again. Even if it did, it would go away again. Less than 10 percent of patients have a second episode, and it's rare to have more than two or three such attacks. No one's life has become a series of gaps due to recurrent experiences of TGA. It comes and goes, and when it goes, it's gone.

But she persisted. What had really happened to her husband?

That question was harder to answer. The fact is that we don't really know. We only have some theories. Once again I told Ken that he would recover, but it made no difference. I reassured his wife once again. I'm not sure she believed me at first—like most wives of physicians, she took whatever any physician said skeptically—but at least she did not repeat her questions. She let it go at that.

What causes an episode of TGA? For some reason, and the reason may not be the same in all patients, the areas of the brain that are critical for the registration of memory and for memory retrieval turn off only to turn on again. How could this happen? We aren't sure. The key to understanding TGA may be the fact that such episodes often are precipitated by specific events. These events include a wide variety of acute stresses, such as:

- Immersion in very cold water. An interesting example of this was at one time labeled 'amnesia by the seaside'. While it has usually involved saltwater, episodes have followed a swim in fresh water or even a pool.
- Sudden exposure to cold.
- Sudden immersion in a hot bath or shower.
- Physical exercise or exertion.
- Sexual intercourse.
- Sudden emotional stress. This includes a long list of activities, from receiving an obscene phone call to witnessing the death of a spouse.
- An acute painful experience such as a dental extraction.

Memory is a complex process that involves wide areas of the brain. Two of the most important areas are regions on the undersurface of the temporal lobes at the base of the brain. Destruction of one of these causes no permanent memory loss, but destruction of both causes total inability to ever lay down a new memory.

To know what can suddenly turn off memory, we would have to understand what turns it on, and we don't know that.

Memory, like most mental functions, turns off when we sleep and turns back on each morning as if the same activating system that alerts consciousness switches memory back into gear. But memory doesn't always switch on simultaneously or completely. We all have had times when our memory did not turn on. We wake up in the morning, and for a few moments we don't know where we are or what we're supposed to do. Then it clicks in; we remember. This also happens at other times, often when we're drowsy and suddenly need to function alertly. The mind is a blank; including the memory. Then all of a sudden everything switches back on. The switching on of memory every morning when we wake up is so automatic that we take it for granted, like a car shifting gears by itself.

Sometimes, however, the switch fails. Often this failure is caused by some acute, unusual stress. How? Why? I have no idea. It's as if our gears become worn with age and less reliable, so that a sudden shock can shift us from one gear to another temporarily, until our gears fall back into place.

The analogy, while crude, isn't totally inappropriate. Deep within the substance of the brain is a network of cells called the *reticular activating system*. One of the functions of this system is to maintain consciousness. It also supplies a necessary input that drives many of the brain's functions. One of these is consciousness itself, another is attention, and a third is learning and memory. The reticular system, when active or 'switched on', supplies drive to the rest of the brain.

So that's what happened to Ken. The drive for learning and memory got switched off. The parts of his brain that underlie memory were left intact, so his remote memory was normal.

Ken was admitted to the hospital, and over the next six hours his memory recovered completely except for a gap of some forty-eight hours. We did all the right tests (more to reassure the patient and his wife than for any other reason): CT scan, NMR scan, EEG. The results were all normal. The next day we discharged Ken. Within two days he was back at work in the OR.

I still see him about once or twice a year. And each time he asks me, with a twinkle in his eye, 'Did I remove that gallbladder?' I nod. And he says, 'Damn right. Skin to skin in less than two hours—without a brain. Not bad for a general surgeon.'

NOTE

There is no single entirely satisfactory review of transient global amnesia. The interested reader could start with the following:

Caplan, L. B. (1985). Transient Global Amnesia. In *Handbook of clinical neurology*, Vol. 45 (ed. P. J. Vinken, G. W. Bruyn, and H. L. Klawans), pp. 205–18. Elsevier, Amsterdam.

(Klawans 1988)

COMMENTARY

Klawans' account of his surgical colleague who was suffering an attack of transient global amnesia (TGA) provides a unique glimpse into the world of a TGA patient, and mirrors some of the detailed case histories that have been published (e.g. Hodges 1991). The account of TGA fits with most of the established features of TGA, and is unlike other conditions such as transient epileptic amnesia (Kapur 1993).

It is interesting that Klawans' patient actually looked and behaved differently from the moment he walked into Klawans' consulting room. Klawans described this as a 'totally detached curiosity' (p. 21). It is seldom that the clinician sees an amnesic patient whose demeanour and behaviour were previously familiar to him, and so these observations are particularly interesting in this regard.

The first observations of the TGA attack were made by the patient's theatre nurse, as the attack had happened towards the end of the surgical procedure. She had worked with him for 12 years. It was slightly atypical remarks (about the duration of the operation, his age, etc.) that first made her wonder if something was wrong, rather than a full-blown amnesic symptom. The inappropriate nature of these and subsequent remarks, and the fact that his mind seemed to be wandering alerted her that something was seriously wrong—these are to some extent non-memory symptoms, and have seldom been reported in other accounts of TGA.

The observation that the patient appeared to have a naming difficulty (p. 22) and a reduction in the fluency of his output (p. 23) highlights the verbal/left temporal lobe bias that is evident in some studies of TGA (Hodges and Oxbury 1990; Kapur *et al.* 1996). It is also noteworthy that he could carry out remaining aspects of the surgical procedure flawlessly. As has been noted in most TGA studies, the performance of an over-learned perceptual-motor skill is often spared in TGA (Caplan 1985). Klawans remarked—'Ken had closed Mrs. Bickford's surgical incision as well as he had closed up any gallbladder Joan had assisted him on in the last dozen years. Technically his hands had performed their job as well as ever' (p. 23). Note, however, that the surgeon suffering the TGA attack did take twice as long as usual to finish off the procedure, partly due to his incessant questioning and the reassurance that he had to be given, rather than any apparent deficiency in his surgical skill at the time. In addition to the preservation of well-established 'old' memories, there is now some preliminary evidence to suggest that patients during an attack of TGA may be able to learn new information, and to retain this information over intervals as long as one week (Kazui *et al.* 1995). In a study carried out in my laboratory (Kapur *et al.* 1996), the patient was not only able, during the TGA episode, to show improvements over a series of learning trials in her ability to identify pictures from their fragments, she also showed evidence of having retained some of this learning one week later, even though she had amnesia for having seen me before and for having done any of the tests a week earlier!

The fact that the surgeon was able to recognize Klawans as familiar, and able to greet him by name, highlights the focal nature of the amnesia that afflicts patients with TGA—it contrasts nicely with the observations of a patient with prosopagnosia, who could barely recognize faces of friends as familiar, but with verbal cues could readily recall details related to specific events that occurred in respect of these individuals (Temple 1992). These contrasting cases provide a form of double-dissociation between 'visual semantic memory' on the one hand, and 'verbal episodic memory' on the other hand.

Premorbid memories were also affected to some degree (p. 27–8), and this reinforces the observations of some degree of retrograde amnesia during the acute period of TGA (Evans *et al.* 1993). Note that the patient appeared to have loss of familiarity recognition of the operating theatre and of Klawans' office, suggesting a fairly significant retrograde amnesia.

Allowing for the nuances of terminology, Klawans' conclusion that immediate memory was not intact (p. 24) is interesting and may possibly need some qualification. Immediate memory, in the form of repetition of a relatively short sequence of items immediately after it has been heard/seen, would usually be intact in TGA patients. However, where there is even a short delay of a matter of seconds between presentation of stimuli and their recall, this form of 'short-term' memory tends to be affected in some severely amnesic patients such as those with TGA. The severity of the patient's amnesia is indicated by the observation (p. 28) that he did not re-member seeing Klawans before, even ten seconds after Klawans left the room and then returned.

Much of the patient's very well-established premorbid knowledge was intact, such as his knowledge of himself, his ability to recognize his family, friends and colleagues. Over-learned facts were not destroyed, and Klawans offers the hypothesis that 'overlearned facts are probably stored in multiple areas of the brain' (p. 26). Note that during the TGA episode the patient retained a 'flashbulb' memory for what he was doing around the time of Kennedy's assassination, and he could give a detailed verbal description of what was involved in a gallbladder operation. The latter probably comes under the rubric of 'over-learned facts', and the former may reflect the fact that events that are highly emotionally significant to an individual are usually retained, even if they are not 'over-learned' in the traditional sense.

The precise pathophysiological mechanisms underlying TGA remain an enigma, though some clues have emerged in recent years. It would seem likely that some form of vasospasm accompanies the onset of TGA, and that this results in a tempo-rary disruption in blood supply to, and therefore ischaemia of, temporal lobe struc-tures. This vasospasm would usually arise from branches of the posterior cerebral artery, although in some cases it may occur from the anterior choroidal artery. While medial temporal lobe structures have been implicated by most research studies (e.g. Kazui et al. 1995), it is worth noting that a few studies have also remarked on the involvement of thalamic (Goldenberg et al. 1991) and frontal lobe (Baron et al. 1994) structures in TGA. It is likely that in a typical TGA episode medial temporal lobe or other limbic-diencephalic structures will invariably be affected, with both the extent of limbic-diencephalic and lateral temporal lobe/frontal lobe involvement being dependent on the severity of the attack, and also perhaps on the individual cerebral vasculature in question, since this can vary from person to person. The pattern of pathophysiological disturbance will in turn determine features such as the severity of retrograde amnesia that is present, and the presence of deficits such as a mild naming difficulty.

There is a close relationship between the incidence of TGA and a previous history of migraine (e.g. Zorzon et al. 1995). Cerebral blood flow studies of patients under-going a migraine attack have pointed to an imbalance in activity between brain-stem nuclei that play a role in control of vascular supply to the brain (Weiller et al. 1995). It remains possible that a similar study of patients undergoing a TGA attack might reveal a focus in the brainstem as the primary trigger that sets off the chain of neurochemical/neurophysiological events that result in such a devastating episode of memory loss. Indeed, one study has reported a case where an episode of TGA occurred shortly before a stroke that involved the brainstem (Howard et al. 1992).

REFERENCES

Baron, J. C., Petit-Taboué, M. C., Le Doze, F., Desgranges, B., Ravenel, N., and Marchal, G. (1994). Right frontal cortex hypometabolism in transient global amnesia. A PET study. Brain, 117, 545–52.

Caplan, L. B. (1985). Transient global amnesia. In Handbook of clinical neurology, Vol. 45 (ed. P. J. Vinken, G. W. Bruyn, and H. L. Klawans), pp. 205–18. Elsevier, Amsterdam.

Evans, J., Wilson, B., Wraight, E. P., and Hodges, J. R. (1993). Neuropsychological and SPECT scan findings during and after transient global amnesia: evidence for the differential impairment of remote episodic memory. *Journal of Neurology, Neurosurgery and Psychiatry*, **56**, 1227–30.

Goldenberg, G., Podreka, I., Pfafflmeyer, N., Wessely, P., and Deecke, L. (1991). Thalamic ischaemia in transient global amnesia: a SPECT study. *Neurology*, **41**, 1748–52.

Hodges, J. R. (1991). *Transient amnesia*, Saunders, New York.

Hodges, J. R. and Oxbury, S. M. (1990). Persistent memory impairment following transient global amnesia. *Journal of Clinical and Experimental Neuropsychology*, **12**, 904–20.

Howard, R. S., Festenststein, R., Mellers, J., Kartsounis, L. D., and Ron, M. (1992). Transient amnesia heralding brain stem infarction. *Journal of Neurology, Neurosurgery and Psychiatry*, **55**, 977.

Kapur, N. (1993). Transient epileptic amnesia: An update and a reformulation. *Journal of Neurology, Neurosurgery and Psychiatry*, **56**, 1184–90.

Kapur, N., Abbott, P., Footitt, D., and Millar, J. (1996). Long-term perceptual priming in transient global amnesia. *Brain and Cognition*, **31**, 63–74.

Kazui, H., Tanabe, H., Ikeda, M., Nakagawa, Y., Shiraishi, J., and Hashikawa, K. (1995). Memory and cerebral blood flow in cases of transient global amnesia during and after the attack. *Behavioural Neurology*, **8**, 93–101.

Temple, C. M. (1992). Developmental memory impairment: Faces and patterns. In *Mental lives* (ed. R. Campbell), pp. 199–215. Blackwell, Oxford.

Weiller, C., May, A., Limmroth, V., Juptner, M., Kaube, H., Schayck, R., *et al.* (1995). Brain stem activation in spontaneous human migraine attacks. *Nature Medicine*, **1**, 658–60.

Zorzon, M., Antonutti, L., Mase, G., Biasutti, E., Vitrani, B., and Cazzato, G. (1995). Transient global amnesia and transient ischemic attack. Natural history, vascular risk factors, and associated conditions. *Stroke*, **26**, 1536–42.

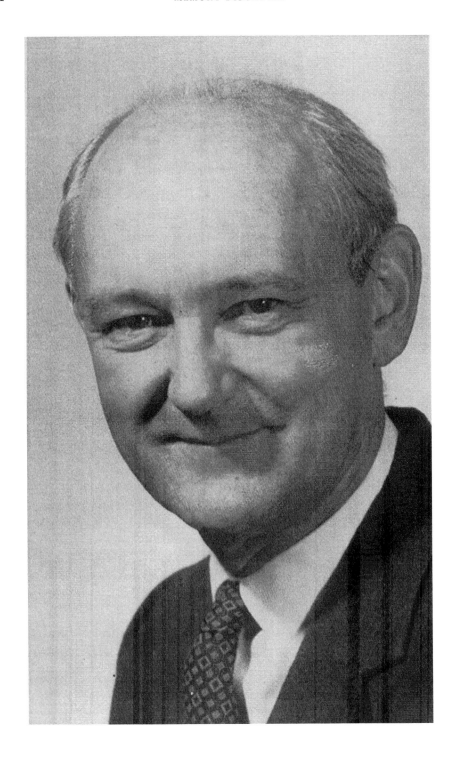

Figure 2. Professor Hugh Morgan.

Looking after a patient with Alzheimer's disease

Mrs M. J. Morgan

Mrs M. J. Morgan wrote this article about her husband, Professor Hugh Morgan (born 16 June 1916, died 25 July 1995). From 1952 to 1968, Hugh Morgan was Professor of Medicine at the University of Khartoum, Sudan. From 1968 to 1981, he was Honorary Professor of Medicine at the University of Birmingham.

My personal experience of looking after my husband with Alzheimer's disease may, I hope, help others to understand what the carer goes through and the sort of help that is needed.

When diagnosis was made I was intensely shocked, but as Hugh was present I had to hide my tears until he was asleep that night. I then spent what seemed like all that night in tears. It felt as I imagine it must if your partner suddenly dies. If the general practitioner could involve the community psychiatric nurse early on it would be a tremendous help and support for the carer to have the disease explained and to understand that it is a terminal illness for which, at the present time, there is no cure. The duration and speed of deterioration, however, can vary enormously. It helps greatly to be warned what may happen next. The carer is then prepared, and this makes coping with the distress easier.

Carers need reassurance that it is a disease and not a disgrace. They need to be encouraged to talk about it and not try to hide it and hope it will go away. A sense of humour helps. I was very fortunate in that Hugh has a wonderful temperament, totally courteous, polite, and considerate at all times, and did not become aggressive. Walking in Solihull one day, a car parked beside us and a gentleman got out, when to his obvious amazement he found himself being shaken warmly by the hand with the comment 'How nice to see you again.' It was obvious to me that he had never seen Hugh before. Another hazard was queuing at the till in a shop. I thought that Hugh was just behind me but had not bargained for his natural reaction of always letting ladies go first. I looked round to find him several ladies back, busy trying to carry some other lady's basket—I had a distinct feeling she thought he was trying to steal something.

It helps to talk about these episodes with friends and not bottle it up. Being able to laugh with someone is very therapeutic, even though sadly it is not funny. Peoples' lack of understanding because the patient looks normal produces a lot of stress. The look of normality is there only because of hard work in constantly supervising washing and dressing.

PRACTICAL TIPS

There are many practical tips such as changing locks on bathroom and lavatory doors so that they can be opened from the outside; leaving landing and lavatory lights on at night; having a night light in the bedroom; and locking doors to rooms not required. The patient may have a compulsive desire to hide things; maybe he thinks he is putting them in a safe place. Hugh carefully collected dead leaves and put them in drawers—all drawers. He also mixed things up. Early on he would spend hours 'sorting' slides. I presumed that he thought he was preparing a lecture, but the result was that thousands of slides both clinical and social are mixed up all over the house in odd places. This was when I realised that locked doors would help. He never objected when he found a locked door, he just went to another.

If a marriage partner has the disease normal marriage has ended—including the physical relationship. If the healthy partner does not understand what is happening he or she may well get the feeling, 'What's the matter with me?' You are in fact a widow or widower but can't have a funeral and be allowed to grieve. The carer has to make all the decisions with no discussion or understanding any more. I think I have changed a great deal in the past seven years because of this. My life until then had been listening while first my father and then Hugh did the talking. The carer needs warning that patients feel alarmed when they first find they do not know where they are and hence follow the carer everywhere. This made me get irritable at times until Hugh confessed to a friend that he was frightened when out as he did not know which country he was in. It was only when he saw a police officer or a letterbox that he knew he was in England.

It was a terrible shock for me when my husband no longer recognised me. It happened one night in the bedroom. He was rooted to the spot and wouldn't get into bed. Then he said, 'I can't get in because I don't know who is going to get in the other side.' This was like being hit on the head as it brought home forcibly that he no longer knew who I was. The carer should be warned that this will happen.

The carer may not have heard of the attendance allowance; I hadn't until the community psychiatric nurse told me to apply. I would make a plea that when assessing a patient the interviewer gives the carer a chance to talk without the patient being present. I was not given the chance, and this caused me great distress. I thought that Hugh would understand what I was saying and could be hurt by it at the time, even though he probably forgot three minutes later. The patient needs to be told about enduring power of attorney as soon as the disease is diagnosed if not before because he or she has to understand and sign the document. It saves a lot of problems later. The Alzheimer's Disease Society or Citizens Advice Bureau will explain.

RELIEF AND GUILT

I was at first horrified at the idea of Hugh going to a day centre. My community psychiatric nurse, however, talked it through with me, and I realised it was to give me some relief. In the event it was splendid as Hugh thought he was there as the doctor, and the staff did not disillusion him. He thought he was in the ward and sometimes would comment, when I collected him, that sister had been rather bossy that day.

It would help if the general practitioner could give the carer the address and telephone number of the local office of the Alzheimer's Disease Society—the sooner the better. They give a lot of helpful advice. The carer needs early warning that eventually the patient could be permanently in hospital. I was told at the beginning that when the doctors thought that Hugh should be cared for in hospital I was not to argue. I therefore had some years to accept the idea, which was not easy. When the time came, to my great surprise, my first feeling was of relief but this was followed swiftly by enormous guilt. I have now, after more than two years, lost the guilt as I realise he is far better cared for in hospital than I could do at home 24 hours a day. Many people have a horror of their loved ones being in a psychiatric hospital because they still think of the old Victorian lunatic asylum. Many people have come to me and said, 'Wouldn't he be better in a private nursing home dear?' I explain that he could not have better care than he is getting and that most nursing homes are not equipped or the staff not trained to look after someone with dementia.

Carers need help to accept the fact that when their partner no longer recognises them it is not wrong to allow the patient to be in hospital. In fact if they refuse they could end up there as well. Help is also needed so that the carer does not think they must visit every day. Visiting is distressing, but the patient does not know who the carer is anyway. I was advised always to have a friend with me when I visit, which I did once a fortnight at first. Now, on advice, I go once a month: it is like visiting a mobile corpse— Hugh is not there, only his body. The main reason for visiting is to support the staff, who understand why I do not visit often. I suspect that some of the younger staff find it hard to understand that to me my husband, who does not know me, has been dead for some years. For months now no communication has been possible when I visit.

Research is essential, and if the general practitioner thinks that the carer would be helped it is a good idea to talk about a postmortem. I saw an article in the Alzheimer's Disease Society's magazine, and it is now all arranged. For me it has helped to feel that maybe some good might come from years of sadness.

(Morgan 1989)

COMMENTARY

Memory difficulties are the hallmark of patients suffering from Alzheimer's disease—in the early stages of the illness, memory symptoms may be similar to those described by Meltzer and may comprise moderate or marked difficulties in retaining new information and in retrieving well-established knowledge. However, as the disease progresses, memory impairments represent part of a more global deterioration in cognitive and everyday functions. At this time, the needs and the perspective of the carer are just as important, and the observations made by Morgan are particularly valuable in this respect.

Morgan, speaking of her husband's diagnosis, points to the importance of counselling at the time of diagnosis. A diagnosis of Alzheimer's disease is in effect a diagnosis of a terminal illness, one that does not have any active medical treatment, and for many patients and their carers it hits them as hard as would a diagnosis of cancer. An appropriate level of counselling, without burdening the patient/carer with too much information, is therefore important, since uncertainty breeds fear, both in the carer and in the patient, and fear breeds distress. Morgan gives a number of useful tips that help when looking after someone who is 'confused', such as locks on bedroom/bathroom doors, etc. Reminding the patient which country he/she is in, something that one would usually never think about, may be important in a condition such as Alzheimer's disease. A further dramatic symptom that is largely unique to Alzheimer's disease, although usually only in the later stages of the illness, is the loss of recognition of the carer.

Morgan makes the important point that, when being interviewed by care staff, it is both helpful and less distressing if the patient is not present—the carer can talk more openly about her concerns and her needs. Relief for the carer is important for most crippling neurological conditions, but with the psychological symptoms associated with Alzheimer's disease, such relief is all the more necessary.

The dilemma of deciding where the patient should go in the terminal years of his illness, and how to cope with visits to see the patient, are well covered by Morgan. The importance of staff who are trained to look after someone with dementia and to offer counselling to family members also comes across in this article.

Busman's holiday

Dr X

Dr X was, at the time of the onset of his illness, a consultant psychiatrist. During his career, he did in fact have a special interest in neuropsychiatric conditions.

I lay in the neurosurgical ward recovering from insertion of my ventriculo-peritoneal shunt and listening to the incessant talk of my neighbour. He had decided that as we shared a battle-front we were the best of friends. Much disclosure on his side called for me to reveal my way of life—as a doctor—to which he retorted 'Oh, so it's a busman's holiday'!

I developed hydrocephalus at the age of 53 as a consequence of aqueduct stenosis, having by then been a consultant psychiatrist for some years. The precipitant for ultimate aqueduct failure remains a mystery.[1] The clinical picture in the final phase conformed to that for 'normal pressure hydrocephalus', with memory impairment, ataxia and the start of urinary incontinence. However, the clinical picture was far from clear until the final phase. Certainly it was not clear to me or to the colleagues who recognised me as being unwell. In this cautionary tale my medical training did not help me understand my illness and those around me did not perceive its nature either.

In retrospect I can date the first event in the illness as four months before the ultimate surgery last April. The dinner party had started late and the coffee had yet to come when I sank asleep on the accommodating shoulder of the senior lady on my right. It was all laughed off as the result of a long day. Thereafter I struggled on, still thinking that the effect of age on memory was more severe than others had ever revealed. And then I concluded that I was suffering from stress-induced depressive illness, there being some work-related pressures. How conveniently one finds evidence to support the theory upon which one has settled. My good GP was a fellow traveller with the conclusion,

[1] This was later found to be a mid-brain tumour.

and when I fell asleep at the wheel causing a mercifully slight incident, he supported my notion of treatment with a selective serotonin re-uptake inhibitor (SSRI) and some time off. Even the start of ataxia, with particular difficulty in moving forward out of chairs, I ascribed to an unusual SSRI side-effect. An observant colleague similarly noted occasional report of ataxia as a side effect.

I remain indebted to the team in the psychiatric unit where I became a patient for first seeing the organic nature of my disorder and to the NHS neuro-surgical team who followed through with scan and then with surgery. My clinical colleagues with generous self-critical hindsight recalled after the event that my gait had changed, becoming a little high stepping, that my complaint of hiccoughs had been a pointer away from depression and that my handwriting had charted motor decline. Once the organicity of the case was recognised, I myself should have been wondering where the tumour was. And yet, as my psychiatrist commented, it was almost as though the hydrocephalus had 'leucotomised' me, sparing me from such appropriate worry.

Anyone in doubt as to the meaning of the term 'busy' might visit a neurosurgical recovery ward at night. My respect for the nurses there endures. There arose for me the question, of course, as to whether I was a doctor or a patient. This was thrown into sharp focus by the disturbance of a fellow patient determined to walk home one night with tubes and all, the whole situation coming close to one in which the duty psychiatrist might be called. The ward team's whispered discussion was amplified by the ancient building and thus I heard that sedation was being considered with an utterly homeopathic dose of major tranquilliser, there being the prospect of a long disturbed night for us all. I decided that I had no advisory function in this unit and that such situations occur in many surgical wards on many nights. My decision to remain passive in my status as a patient was followed by the crisis blowing over somehow.

The shunt insertion was immediately effective. In the following days I could remember my PIN number once again and the phone numbers of old friends. My family recognised me as 'sharp' once again. Psychometric testing produced a flattering result sufficient to support my return to work. I returned on a part-time basis, four months after surgery. However, problems persisted. I was given to short sleeps lasting a few minutes in idle moments. There was no ictal basis for these. Yet they would lead to embarrassment in company, for example in lunch-time meetings. Furthermore I had suffered on two occasions from global amnesia lasting 24 hours. The occurrence of a third bout with ataxia after return to work pointed to shunt malfunction and the need for surgical revision.

Shunt revision involved two visits to theatre, some six months after the initial surgery. This was in the hands of a different neurosurgeon. I am now in a convalescent phase once again some three months after the revision. Impairments have receded: ataxia

went immediately, exceptional sleep capacity is lessening and short-term memory is now close to normal. However, it is only now that zest and spontaneity are returning and only now that I experience a full emotional range. Immediate as the effects of successful surgery have been, true recovery has been gradual.

I have some observations about the neurosurgical experience. While recovering in my neurosurgical bed and as news came through the headphones of messy injuries in the Gorazde enclave, I reflected that I was fortunate to have the hole in my head made with such skill! Shunts are wonderful for ensuring survival. It came as a surprise that the peritoneal end led to extra girth and a need for trouser enlargement. There's the overall point: that recovery from any form of surgery to the cranium is a gradual matter, more gradual than one might at first think. This point is not universally accepted. The neurosurgical team first involved saw freedom for me to resume work some six or eight weeks after initial surgery.

There is a further point concerning the family's role in such a disorder: I have had to overcome natural independence, learning to rely upon my family not only for valued support but for realistic feedback about my performance.

(Dr X 1995)

CLINICAL INTERVIEWS

First amnesic episode: interview with Dr X

NK   The first episode that happened in June 1994—what's your last memory of things that happened before that episode?

Dr X   Being at home and setting off for a scan at the hospital.

NK   That was at Winchester I think, wasn't it?

Dr X   Yes.

NK   So your last memory is being at home and just getting ready to set off, which would have been just an hour or so before the scan itself?

Dr X   Yes.

NK   OK, and your next memory after the episode is what? What's your first memory after the episode?

Dr X   The next morning.

NK   The next morning. OK. The scan was in the afternoon do you think?

Dr X   I can't remember.

NK   So anyway most of the day is gone, plus an hour before the episode, essentially?

Dr X   Yes.

Mrs X's account of the first amnesic episode

NK   Let's just concentrate on the episode then—the first episode?

Mrs X It was approximately a month after neurosurgery, it started one evening when we went to our daughter's school, for a concert. My husband had been actually quite active physically in the morning, he'd used our garden strimmer. He had a rest in the afternoon and was looking forward to the evening. He actually prepared the evening meal. The first half of the concert went fine. After the interval when we sat down he fell asleep. I nudged him and when he woke up he woke unusually, his responses weren't as normal . . .

NK   In what sense were they not normal?

Mrs X It was as though he was in a daze.

NK   How long had he been asleep for?

Mrs X I would say about five minutes.

NK   Were there any specific behaviours during that evening of the concert which were abnormal? You say that when he woke up from that sleep he wasn't quite right, but were there any involuntary movements, or him saying the wrong things, or doing any inappropriate things, or short term memory loss, or . . .

Mrs X No, not on that occasion . . .

NK   How did you know that there was something wrong then?

Mrs X The fact that he wasn't tuned in to what was happening on the stage. Normally he enjoys concerts. He would have made observations on our daughter's performance, about other performers, as he did in the first half of that concert. From the moment of sleep on it was as though he was not part of that occasion. He was very depressed after this occasion that he couldn't remember our daughter's performance, and, of course, she found it very hard to come to terms with.

We sat through the rest of the concert, but when I tried to speak to him he did not respond as usual. We actually went downstairs and saw several people afterwards and among those people was Dr Z who works here. I was interested to see that socially he had a conversation, so he seemed to be all right then. On the way home, he complained of feeling sick and having a headache. By the time we got home I was quite worried about him. I thought he was tired. The next day when we woke his responses were very strange. That day, anyway, he was due to have a scan of his tummy to look at the peritoneal end of his shunt.

NK   That was in Winchester, yes?

Mrs X This was in Winchester. He stayed in bed all morning because it was as though he was very sleepy. At one time when I went in to tell him something I could tell his eyes were not right, they stared at me in a rather frightening manner and this happened several times after that before the next bouts of neurosurgery. Again, I had to explain to him that we were going into Winchester for a scan.

NK   But he didn't realize that?

Mrs X He knew beforehand, but nothing I said seemed to register.

NK   Yes, OK.

Mrs X I got him to the scan . . .

NK   Now during this time was he confused in the sense of saying the same thing over and over again?

Mrs X Absolutely. Yes.

NK   So when did that start?

Mrs X All that day.

NK   All that day?

Mrs X Yes.

NK   From the beginning of the day?

Mrs X From the beginning of the day.

NK   So from when he woke up you mean?

Mrs X From when he woke and as I say he was not well the night before. He'd had this strange sleep at the concert.

NK   So he would ask the same question again and again. What sorts of questions would he ask, what sorts of things would he say to indicate that his memory was poor?

Mrs X 'Why am I here?' 'What are we doing here?' I'd explain why. This was at home and also at the hospital and by this stage, socially it was becoming embarrassing for other patients sitting in the waiting area.

NK   He was able to recognize you OK?

Mrs X Yes.

NK   Yes, and did he have any word-finding difficulties in the sense of difficulty in finding the right words to describe what it was he wanted to say or anything like that or was he OK?

Mrs X He was OK, so much so that when we went in to have the scan he had actually met the radiologist on a previous occasion. The strange thing was that he remembered that occasion.

NK   When was that?

Mrs X It must have been five years earlier I should think, at a dinner party. He remembered that incident and reminded the radiologist of that time.

NK   During that time did he have any difficulty in remembering things that had happened during the previous few days or few weeks? Was there any amnesia or was it just purely the short-term repeating of things?

Mrs X It was just the short-term. I think the fact that he remembered the occasion that he met the radiologist is interesting.

NK   Was there a specific thing that you did, that he said, or that you asked him, that indicated to you that his memory for the previous few weeks was pretty OK? Did he remember the concert, going to the concert the day before?

Mrs X No, not at all that day.

NK   So then, did it stretch back to one day or did it go back several days, his memory loss?

Mrs X Quite a while.

NK   How long do you think, a few weeks do you think?

Mrs X Yes, I would say so. I didn't talk to him too much as it was clear . . . and it was such hard work just trying to get him to concentrate on getting him to the scan.

NK   But there was no other indication? You must have talked about the concert the previous day, because he doesn't remember going to the concert, but there was no other indication that he had memory loss for earlier events? Was there any other indication that he had memory loss for the previous few days, few weeks, or few months?

Mrs X No clear indication.

NK   While he was having the scan he was still a bit confused was he?

Mrs X Absolutely. It was only the next day when he woke up that he seemed absolutely his old self.

NK   OK, and the next day he had memory loss for the previous day and the day of the concert.

Mrs X And the evening of the concert from the time he fell asleep during that concert.

Second amnesic episode: interview with Dr X

NK   The next episode then, when was that please?

Dr X   The next episode was also during the summer months. It was on a day when our children were out sailing with friends and we went to Lymington to meet them. And we were very gently entertained to supper by these friends who were very tactful and I was unable to remember any of the outing at all. I couldn't remember the journey to Lymington, being in Lymington, meeting the friends. I had a dim recollection of meeting a man and he looked a bit like Hattersley, the Labour politician. I was able to comment on that to my wife who confirmed that it was a correct impression.

NK   OK. What's your last memory before that episode?

Dr X   I can't . . .

NK   You can't remember? You don't remember setting off to Lymington. Do you remember anything of that morning or the previous day?

Dr X   I remember the previous day, I remember seeing my daughter off on this journey. She went off for the day's sailing . . .

NK   That would have been in the evening she went off?

Dr X   Early in the day we went away, we went across Winchester to the house of friends to leave my daughter there and I recall that.

NK   OK, but there is nothing else of that day and nothing of the next day, so basically one and a half days have gone there?

Dr X   Yes.

NK   OK, right. Do you remember the following day pretty OK, or nothing much?

Dr X   Once recovery had occurred then all was well.

NK   But there was nothing specific?

Dr X   No.

Mrs X's account of the second amnesic episode (two consecutive episodes)

NK   OK, right, fine, let's go on to the next occasion then please?

Mrs X That was on a Friday and he woke up and I could tell he was having a similar performance—he didn't know what was happening that day, he was repeating himself. When I tried to explain what we were doing it was as though it wasn't registering in his memory.

NK   And did he seem to lose the previous day or few days as well or was it just short term?

Mrs X   It was just short term.

NK   Was there any specific thing that you did ask him about the previous few days that told you that his previous day's memory was OK or did you not? Was there no opportunity?

Mrs X   I was so worried about the state that he was in I didn't want to tax him.

NK   OK, but it wasn't that, in conversation, something cropped up that indicated that he had, or had not, a memory for the previous day?

Mrs X   Conversation was difficult.

NK   Difficult just because he was repeating himself?

Mrs X   Yes, and all he wanted to do was sleep.

NK   Did he have any difficulties in finding the right words to describe what he wanted to say or when he did talk he was he OK?

Mrs X   He did have difficulty in finding words and tended to repeat what I had said.

NK   On this occasion, or on the previous occasion, did he have a normal night's sleep? I know that on the evening of the concert he wasn't quite right, but as far as you can see that night plus the night of the second episode, preceding the second episode was his sleep normal?

Mrs X   Normal deep sleep.

NK   OK, there's no evidence of him thrashing about?

Mrs X   No, absolutely not.

NK   OK, carry on, so . . .

Mrs X   So, that was on the Friday and on the Saturday again he woke quite normally as though nothing had happened, he had just missed a day.

NK   So is it fair to say then that on the first day the episode of confusion, in the sense of repeating himself, etc., lasted from first thing in the morning until last thing at night?

Mrs X   Until late at night, he gradually seemed to come to in the evening.

NK   OK, so you're talking of about 12 hours?

Mrs X   Yes.

NK   And the next occasion was also about 12 hours?

Mrs X   Also 12 hours. He woke up seemingly OK on the Saturday. We went to collect Pippa from some friends who suggested that we went out in the evening. As we were driving away I realized that he was slipping into this state that I was now becoming familiar with.

NK   This was the evening of the attack?

Mrs X   The evening, the Saturday evening.

NK   The following day?

Mrs X   Yes, the second episode, and on that occasion . . .

NK   What gave you the indication that he was slipping into something?

Mrs X   The fact that he became drowsy, was unable to initiate conversation, he would answer questions that were put to him by these friends, but then as the evening progressed I was worried about him socially.

NK   Yes, and he was showing then roughly the same type of behaviour he was showing on the evening of the concert?

Mrs X   I would say he was worse on that occasion.

NK   OK, yes go on, what happened next?

Mrs X   Then I indicated to our friend that I was concerned about him so it was agreed that they would drive us back home and he went into a deep sleep in the car and I had to get him to bed. I had to physically help him undress.

NK   On Sunday morning was he OK?

Mrs X   Sunday morning he was OK, but not as bright as he had been.

Third amnesic episode: interview with Dr X

NK   So what about the next one?

Dr X   The next one was described by my family as partial, there was an evening when we were on holiday in Germany in August and we were guests of some people who lived near the river Rhine and it was a taxing evening because there was little food and it was late. Essentially, we missed our meal and the family says I went into the same state of asking the same questions over again and of appearing glazed.

NK   OK, right and what's your last memory before that one?

Dr X   Well that I can remember arriving at these friends' house by the Rhine . . .

NK   In the morning or in the evening?

Dr X   In the evening. I can remember much of the walk that we went on.

NK   So the episode happened in the evening then did it?

Dr X   Yes.

NK   Your next memory, was that the next day or the day after?

Dr X   It was the next day.

Mrs X's account of the third amnesic episode

NK   Let's go on to the third one then please?

Mrs X   The third one was when we were away on holiday and that would have been in August. It was not as dramatic as the previous two.

NK   How did it start then?

Mrs X   It started when we'd had quite a full day with some German people. We then went out in the evening. There'd been confusion so we weren't actually fed that evening. I just noticed him becoming more and more tired, not in tune with what was happening around him, and not himself.

NK   OK, was he saying the right words or saying the wrong things?

Mrs X   He was finding difficulty in initiating conversations and his speech was becoming slower. It was almost as though he was drunk.

NK   But during this evening there was no repeating the same question again and again like there was before?

Mrs X   There was a little of that, but not as pronounced as on the very first occasion.

NK   And the next day he was OK?

Mrs X   The next day he was OK.

NK   OK. Is it fair to say then that for the first two episodes he had a total memory loss for that day and for the one and a half days in which he wasn't quite right but for this episode he has a patchy memory loss for that evening?

Mrs X Yes.

COMMENTARY

Dr X's case is of interest from several points of view. From the neuropsychological angle, a major feature of his condition was the occurrence of transient amnesic episodes in the context of normal pressure hydrocephalus, which arose due to a midbrain tumour. I will, however, first consider the non-amnesic symptoms.

According to Dr X, the classical triad of symptoms associated with normal pressure hydrocephalus (NPH)—cognitive dysfunction, ataxia, and urinary incontinence—did not appear till quite late in the illness. His first symptom was several months earlier—falling asleep on the shoulders of a dinner guest! It is difficult to be sure if this was related to tiredness as a general symptom, or to a sleep disorder related to hypothalamic dysfunction. In either case, it suggests that more subtle symptoms may in some cases precede the traditional symptom triad associated with NPH. The fact that Dr X was initially considered to have a psychiatric condition was all the more stressful (Dr X himself worked as a consultant psychiatrist), and in a sense it came as a relief when a cerebral basis to his symptoms was discovered.

One of Dr X's memory symptoms prior to surgery was that of forgetting his credit card PIN number and the phone numbers of old friends—such loss of 'semantic memory' or 'general knowledge memory' would seem rather unusual, since episodic memory symptoms tend to predominate in acute neurological conditions such as NPH. Certainly, his report should make clinical neuropsychologists and doctors more alert to the possibility of such symptoms accompanying more common 'short-term memory' complaints, and even in some cases being predominant. It is rare to see cases of 'reversible semantic memory loss', and Dr X's loss and then recovery of such memories comes close to such a condition.

The first indication of Dr X's ataxia was a difficulty in moving forward out of chairs, although other motor symptoms had also been observed, including a high-step gait and a deterioration in his handwriting. Once he was given a neurological diagnosis, Dr X also noted a relative lack of concern and anxiety about his condition, and one wonders if this was due to direct or indirect frontal lobe dysfunction, as Dr X himself speculates. Such dysfunction may also have been related to his further comments that 'zest and spontaneity' took some time to return.

Following surgery, Dr X suffered three episodes of transient amnesia. It is difficult to be certain about the basis for his amnesic episodes. They were too long to be characteristic of most episodes of transient global amnesia, which generally last around 4 to 6 hours (one episode appeared to last 12 hours, and on a second occasion two successive episodes covered a period of one and half days). The occurrence of two amnesic episodes after a period of sleep is suggestive of a possible epileptic basis, although there were few other features that more confidently suggested an epileptic origin (see Kapur 1993). A further unusual feature was the occurrence, prior to the first episode, of a semi-confusional state during the previous evening. During the first episode, which took place during a hospital visit to have a CT scan, there is an interesting dissociation between marked anterograde memory loss and the ability of Dr X to recall an occasion five years previously when he had met the radiologist who was performing the scan. This dissociation is rather unusual for a typical case of transient global amnesia.

Transient amnesic attacks have been reported in association with hydrocephalus (Giroud *et al.* 1987). The number of such reports is too few to produce any characteristic profile, although it seems that in some cases long-standing hydrocephalus, combined with an acute insult such as a head injury, may result in a transient amnesic episode. The mechanism of such amnesic attacks is open to conjecture—it is possible that the hydrocephalus itself may have exerted pressure on basal arteries that fed into the temporal lobe arterial system, or that an expanded third ventricle may have affected normal physiological functioning in limbic-diencephalic structures. In Dr X's case, there is the remote possibility that the midbrain tumour itself may have been exerting pressure on relevant arteries or limbic-diencephalic structures. A further point to note is that during the neurosurgical procedure to insert a shunt, the surgeon reported that he may have grazed the right thalamus—since thalamic lesions have been associated with transient amnesic episodes (e.g. Moonis *et al.* 1988), this too needs to be borne in mind.

REFERENCES

Giroud, M., Guard, O., and Dumas, R. (1987). Transient global amnesia associated with hydrocephalus. *Journal of Neurology*, **235**, 118–19.

Kapur, N. (1993). Transient epileptic amnesia: An update and a reformulation. *Journal of Neurology, Neurosurgery and Psychiatry*, **56**, 1184–90.

Moonis, M., Jain, S., Prasad, K., Mishra, N. K., Goulatia, R. K., and Maheshwari, M. C. (1988). Left thalamic hypertensive haemorrhage presenting as transient global amnesia. *Acta Neurologica Scandinavica*, **77**, 331–4.

GENERAL COMMENTARY

Although the two articles relating to transient amnesia (**Klawans** and **Dr X**) are quite unique, even in the context of other personal accounts of brain dysfunction, it is worth remembering the celebrated case of the pioneering 18th-century British surgeon, Sir John Hunter, who suffered a transient amnesic episode in December 1789. There is a record (Brain 1952, p. 1372) that while Hunter 'was at the house of a friend on a visit, he was attacked with a total loss of memory; he did not know in what part of the town he was, not even the name of the street when told it nor where his own house was; he had not a conception of any place existing beyond the room he was in, yet was perfectly conscious of his loss of memory. He was sensible of impressions of all kinds from the senses, and therefore looked out of the window, although rather dark, to see if he could be made sensible of the situation of the house; this loss of memory gradually went off, and in less than half an hour his memory was perfectly recovered'. The rather short duration of Hunter's attack, and the major loss of knowledge, with the apparent absence of symptoms of anterograde amnesia, such as repeating the same question many times, suggests that his attack may not have been TGA, but some other form of transient amnesic attack, possibly transient epileptic amnesia. Hunter suffered other attacks that were interpreted by Brain as reflecting the occurrence of sensory epilepsy, and a post-mortem examination showed evidence of both cerebral and coronary atheroma. While topographical disorientation is generally associated with dysfunction in the right posterior neocortex (De Renzi 1982), and while Hunter's amnesia probably reflected epileptiform activity from the right parietal region, it should be remembered that transient topographical amnesia has also been reported as a relatively benign condition in the normal elderly (Stracciari *et al.* 1994).

All four case studies in this chapter bring home the distinction between procedural memory on the one hand and declarative/episodic memory on the other, with the case study described by **Klawans** perhaps providing the most dramatic demonstration of such a distinction—during his attack the patient could recall how to perform the surgical procedures required to complete the operation, but he could not recall whether he had carried out parts of the procedure a few minutes before. One could perhaps also consider the distinction as one between two forms of knowledge—knowledge that is over-learned and well-established in relevant storage areas of the brain, as compared to knowledge that has been gained in a fleeting few moments as a result of temporary activation of limbic-diencephalic and cortical structures.

The importance of family support comes across in all four articles. A less well-recognized aspect of such support is the role of the family in providing the patient with feedback on his performance in everyday situations. Where there is lack of insight, or loss of cognitive functions—such as memory—that contribute to such insight, then regular feedback on performance is all the more important from support structures such as family and close friends.

Meltzer's account is notable for the good recovery he made from the global amnesia that characterized the initial stages of his illness. Some of the distinctive features of recovery of memory function, both within a patient and across patients, may be explicable by postulating different neural 'modules' or 'networks' that are responsible for distinctive memory functions. At a more general level, it is possible to postulate a number of functional variables that may play a part in determining the severity of memory loss that occurs after a particular brain insult (more general clinical, anatomical, and physiological variables relating to recovery of function are discussed in the final chapter, p. 408). Such functional variables include:

1. The time since acquisition of the memory (so as to allow long-term consolidation processes to operate).
2. The duration of exposure to the relevant stimuli and learning experiences (e.g. the number of times the skill has been practised).
3. The meaningfulness of the original learning experiences (e.g. whether they were novel, interesting, etc.).
4. The emotional valence of the stimuli (e.g. whether they were life-threatening).
5. The pattern of temporal distribution of any repetition of the experience or similar experiences—it is possible that the spaced versus massed distribution that has been well established in the domain of experimental psychology also holds at the level of everyday retention of more complex events (i.e. 'spaced' learning

generally results in better consolidation of learning than learning where the practice trials are 'massed').

6. The number of modalities in which the experience was represented at time of acquisition.
7. The number and distribution pattern of retrievals of the experience.
8. The 'richness' of the encoding experience at the times of presentation and retrieval.
9. The methods used to test recovery of memory function.

REFERENCES

Brain, R. (1952). The neurology of Sir John Hunter's last illness. *British Medical Journal*, December, 1371–3.
De Renzi, E. (1982). *Disorders of space exploration and cognition*. Wiley, Chichester.
Stracciari, A., Lorusso, S., and Pazzaglia, P. (1994). Transient topographical amnesia. *Journal of Neurology, Neurosurgery and Psychiatry*, **57**, 1423–5.

Language disorders   2

INTRODUCTION

In the United Kingdom, with a population of around 60 million, there are estimated to be more than 200 000 people living with the effects of language disorder ('aphasia'/'dysphasia') as the result of a stroke or a head injury.

It is customary to divide language functions into a number of component parts. These include: spontaneous speech, comprehension of spoken language, repetition of speech, naming ability, reading aloud, reading comprehension, and writing skill. One or more of the component functions may be affected by a brain lesion. In most right-handed individuals, language functioning is controlled by the left hemisphere. A good deal of research has been carried out into documenting the types of language disturbance that result from left hemisphere damage, and to relate sites of damage within the left hemisphere to particular forms of language disorder.

Spontaneous speech is disrupted after most instances of damage to language areas in the left hemisphere, although in a small number of cases a patient may be able to have a normal conversation with a clinician, and the impairment of language may only be apparent on formal tests of naming, reading, or writing. Traditionally, disturbances of spontaneous speech are divided into two types, fluent and non-fluent. In *non-fluent* dysphasic speech, there is a limited amount of speech produced, it appears to require considerable effort on the part of the patient with only one or two words at a time being produced. In non-fluent speech, articulation of the words may be impaired, sentences may be agrammatical with 'function' words (e.g. but, because, etc.) omitted, and much of the person's speech will consist of nouns. Non-fluent dysphasic speech is usually found after lesions in the left frontal lobe, and in particular the posterior part of the inferior frontal gyrus. In *fluent* dysphasic speech, conversational ability may appear to be normal, with no abnormality in the amount of speech, effort, or articulation. However, nouns will often be omitted, and there will be frequent word substitutions or 'paraphasias'. Fluent dysphasic speech is usually associated with lesions in the temporal lobe, and in particular the posterior part of the superior temporal gyrus.

Comprehension of speech involves a range of abilities, including the ability to decode speech sounds into meaningful signals, the ability to understand the meaning of words such as nouns ('semantic processing'), the ability to understand the grammatical components of speech including words such as prepositions ('syntactic processing'), and the ability to hold the information in a short-term memory system so that sentences can be readily understood. Impairment of speech comprehension usually follows damage to the left temporo-parietal region. The combination of non-fluent speech and relatively intact speech comprehension is usually associated with the term 'Broca's aphasia', and a left inferior frontal lesion locus. The combination of fluent speech and rather impaired speech comprehension is usually associated with the term 'Wernicke's aphasia' and a left posterior temporal lesion locus. These aphasias are named after two nineteenth-century neurologists, Paul Broca and Carl Wernicke.

Speech repetition, which is usually assessed by asking the patient to repeat numbers, letters or sentences, is generally affected after left hemisphere lesions that affect areas bordering the sylvian fissure or an area in the anterior part of the inferior parietal lobe known as the supramarginal gyrus.

Naming ability involves a number of prerequisites, including the presence of a normal stored vocabulary, the ability to select the appropriate word from that vocabulary, and the ability to generate the appropriate speech sounds that correspond to the particular word in question. A number of left hemisphere lesion sites may contribute to naming difficulties, though it seems that the temporal lobe plays a particularly critical role in disorders of naming.

Reading is also a relatively complex language function that involves a number of separate processes—the ability to carry out the visual processing of letters and words, the ability to generate sounds that correspond to these visual units, and the derivation of meaning—either directly from the visual forms themselves, or indirectly from the speech sounds. Usually, reading difficulties are present in the context of other language disturbance, and can therefore occur after lesions to frontal or temporal lobe language areas, but in some cases they may occur in isolation. In such cases, the lesion is usually in the posterior parts of the left hemisphere, in the parietal or occipital lobes.

Writing ability can be seen to mirror reading ability in terms of the distinct processes that are involved, and the extent to which a relatively pure impairment may exist in isolation from other language difficulties. Writing shares with spontaneous speech the ability to produce a sequence of words, such that semantic and grammatical constrains are correctly followed, and disturbances in writing may therefore parallel those that occur in the speech output of the patient. However, there are some processes specific to writing, and these include the ability to retrieve the correct pattern of motor movements for individual letters of the alphabet, and the ability to spell a word correctly. Isolated disturbances of writing ability are relatively rare, and tend to be associated with lesions in the left parietal lobe.

It is, of course, something of a paradox to read a detailed account of what it is like to be a dysphasic patient by someone who has suffered a significant language disorder. This achievement in itself could be seen to point to some degree of independence between written and oral output mechanisms, and also between thought and language. However, it is worth bearing in mind that there is probably a selectivity in those brain injured dysphasic patients who have been able put down their thoughts in print. Although in the acute stages their dysphasia may have been quite severe, their residual dysphasia may well have been milder than that of other dysphasic patients. Thus, the cases of aphasia that are reprinted in this book may have made unusually good recoveries from their loss of language, compared to the more general population of aphasic patients.

Keeping such provisos in mind, the accounts that have been written in these papers provide an interesting reflection on some of the long-standing distinctions that have been made in the aphasia literature. Four of the cases reprinted in this book, those of **Andrewes, Rose, Moss,** and **Ashcraft,** approximate the clinical classification of 'Broca's aphasia'/'anterior aphasia' (Benson 1994). In general, except for complex grammar and abstract thoughts, comprehension deficits in these cases were relatively mild or were mainly confined to the early stages of recovery. **Moss'** case was one of an initial global aphasia, with most language modalities being severely affected, but he later recovered to the stage where he primarily had a mild anomia and a slowness of thinking. From the point of view of a patient's perspective on the recovery of a neuropsychological function, **Moss'** case is quite unique in the amount of detailed information that has been recorded. The fact that he made such a good recovery from his stroke, and the fact that his wife kept a diary of events during his early recovery period, meant that **Moss** was provided with an ideal retrospective opportunity to provide a commentary on his thoughts and feelings during the various stages of recovery. I have therefore reprinted both a summary article that he wrote seven years after his stroke, and three chapters from the book that he published four years earlier (and which is no longer in print). The case of **Lordat** is rather different from the other four, and comes closer to an example of Wernicke's aphasia.

In addition to the specific commentaries that follow each article, I have also included a general commentary at the end of this chapter.

REFERENCE

Benson, D. F. (1994). *The neurology of thinking.* Oxford University Press, New York.

FURTHER READING

Goodglass, H. (1993). *Understanding aphasia.* Academic Press, New York.
Ellis, A. W. and Young, A. W. (1988). *Human cognitive neuropsychology.* Lawrence Erlbaum, Hove, UK.
Parkin, A. J. (1996). *Explorations in cognitive neuropsychology.* Blackwell, Oxford.

On being bereft of speech

By a patient

The author of this article, Sir Frederick Andrewes (born 1859, died 1932), was an eminent physician at St. Bartholomew's Hospital, London (where a ward is named in his honour). He was elected a Fellow of the Royal Society in 1915, and he was Professor of Pathology at St. Barts' Medical School.

Our medicine is too objective; a doctor who has himself suffered from a complaint is by so much the more knowledgeable in dealing with that disease in others. Readers of this journal may be interested, therefore, in a short account of the experiences of a patient from a purely subjective point of view.

Being myself a doctor, things naturally meant more to me than to a layman, and I cannot help this fact sticking out now and then, but I will strive to be as pure a patient as I can. I must, however, first state the nature of my disease. It was a 'cerebral accident' involving the cortex of Broca's convolution on the left side, but I must leave the doctors to settle whether it was due to embolism, thrombosis or sub-arachnoid haemorrhage—all of which opinions were expressed. The effect was complete paralysis of pharynx, right half of tongue and face, interference with the movements of the right vocal cord and also impairment of the finer movements of the right thumb and index finger, which made writing clumsy and laborious for a long time. For the first few days there was numbness of the right arm and hand, which soon passed off everywhere except in the ring finger. I am told that the above combination of symptoms is characteristic of block of the anterior branch of the left middle cerebral artery. The lesion, devastating as it was to me, was only an incident in an illness associated with broncho-pneumonia, lasting nearly three weeks, for which I was being treated by the kindness of Dr. T. M. Rivers in the Hospital of the Rockefeller Institute in New York. It occurred on the tenth day of the illness, and in describing my experiences I will confine myself to the aphasia and the associated motor symptoms.

The onset can be timed very closely. At a given moment I was talking naturally to the nurses. Five minutes later an orderly thought I was speaking queerly and was clumsy with one hand. Five minutes later still, aphasia was complete. Dr. Rivers came in waving a cable from a member of my family, with which he expected me to be pleased. But I gazed upon it with lack-lustre eye, and he then held it out to me. I missed it with my right hand and then similarly missed my spectacles. He then asked me if I understood the cable and I nodded. He noticed that my face was on one side, and I saw an expression of alarm come over him. He ran off for his colleagues, who soon gathered round me and made fuller examination.

I can affirm positively that I had not the slightest subjective sensation in my head at the time the incident occurred, or before or after. I may have felt a little dull and stupid, but I quite appreciated the situation. My notions of hemiplegia and aphasia were, however, somewhat archaic, and mostly derived from the P.M. room, so that my first thoughts were 'It's me for the New Jerusalem this trip, and what a rotten way to go out, away from home like this!' My first ray of comfort came from hearing Dr. Rufus Cole say, 'Oh well, it must be a very small one because the neighbouring centres are all right', so I then began to think I might not die immediately, but live for a time as a useless burden on people, communicating by signs, for the idea of recovering effective speech was still far from my thoughts.

A few days after my seizure, Dr. Tilney, the head of the Neurological Department of Columbia University, was called in in consultation. I could now write feebly, and I asked him the prognosis as regards speech. I had been rather dreading his answer, but to

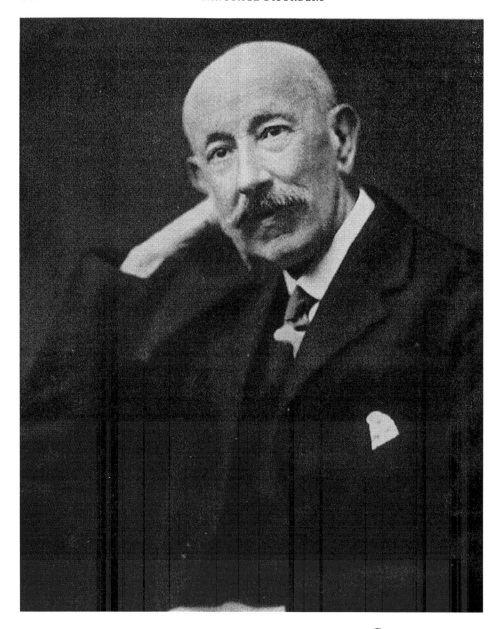

Figure 4. Sir Frederick Andrewes.

my amazement he said I should speak as well as ever and fairly soon too. I shook hands with him, and I am not ashamed to confess to a tear or two of joy and thankfulness.

My first reaction was almost grotesque. I at once abandoned all thought of growing a beard, and summoned an orderly to come and shave me as a symbol of my new hopes.

I was now confronted with the problem of a man, in full possession of his faculties, but cut off from his fellows by a barrier which it seemed hopeless to pass. True, I could nod my head or shake it or point to anything I wanted, but I found people very slow in the uptake. It was a pure motor aphasia. I had all the words ready, but the machinery for uttering them was gone and I could not make a sound. However, I could manage to write feebly and incredibly badly, at first better with my left hand. I once knowingly tried mirror-writing with the left hand, but it was no improvement. In two or three days I could write equally well with the right hand and this slowly improved with practice—though I found it very tiring for a long while.

Suddenly there occurred to me the idea of a box of letters which I could arrange on a board. It so happened that this was at a moment when a niece of mine was spending a week-end in New York, and she kindly made for me what proved to be better than detached letters, namely an alphabet with thick letters an inch high, well spaced on a card, twelve inches by ten. This was easily and quickly handled, and proved a priceless engine of communication with the outside world. Indeed, I am told that the first use I made of the card was to spell out 'Communications re-established'. My forefinger became so nimble with use that others found it difficult to keep up with me; moreover, I developed a certain mental agility in deciding in how small a number of letters I could express a given idea. With this alphabet I found it possible to be laboriously chatty and even waggish, and for two or three weeks, as speech gradually returned, I used little else.

The man whose pharynx is paralysed has disabilities other than that of speechlessness. He cannot suck through a tube and has to be fed by spoon. The nurse duly places between his lips a spoonful of milk or soup but the Lord alone knows where it goes. With luck much of it doubtless reaches its destination, but much may splash around in the flaccid pharynx, perhaps to be rejected with vehemence a little later, and I remember the desiccated remains of yesterday's egg-nogg being once cleaned off the back of my pharynx with a spatula.

About three weeks from the first onset of my illness my temperature became normal and my physical recovery was now uninterrupted. The return of speech, which began in about a week from the onset of the aphasia, was really a process of thrilling interest, and left on my mind no shadow of doubt that it was one of the rehabilitation of the old cortical centres as a collateral circulation was established. How else could one explain the fact that I regained the power of counting the numerals up to 10 simultaneously in English, French, and German?

The return of speech was in a sense independent of my own volition. I did not have to learn de novo, but rather resumed the power as fast as the palsied muscles enabled me to exercise it. That of course is a crude way of putting it; a truer way would be to say 'as fast as the recovering cortical nerve-cells became able to stir the still intact lower motor sectors into action.' Doctors would come and stand over me trying to teach me to speak, urging me to put my mouth into such and such a position. This was uniformly futile. What actually happened was that each day, when I woke, I was able to say more and more, the power having miraculously descended upon me from on High during the night. Thus every morning the nurses used to gather round my bed to hear what new parlour tricks I had acquired.

In my diary I entered the progress I made. The larynx recovered first, enabling me to try vowel sounds. For the first week or so I was totally silent; then I became able to make miscellaneous farm-yard noises and then a low 'Ah,' followed soon by more high-pitched notes, and during the second week from onset progress was very rapid, as the lips and cheek began to regain power. I could soon repeat the alphabet and count the numerals. By the way, I found German and French words to slide out of the mouth more easily than English. English is certainly a very difficult language for foreigners to speak.

Exactly a fortnight after the onset of my aphasia I found myself one morning able to utter the untrue and irrelevant remark, 'I have no need', and this was regarded as a great achievement. A day or two later I was able to repeat what in my own esteem was the first verse of 'Mary had a little lamb'. Early in the morning, when I was fresh, my auditors agreed that it was this poem, but in the afternoon, when I was tired, there was a good deal of doubt about it.

Somehow poetry came easier than prose, and sentences I knew well easier than extemporaneous remarks. Singing came most readily of all, so that in three weeks from onset I could sing the Doxology with power and conviction. When Dr. Tilney came again to see how I was getting on and told me I had improved even faster than he had expected, he was astonished, as he left the room, to hear me break forth loudly with 'Praise God, from whom all blessings flow', but he quite saw the point.

Up to this time my progress in speaking had been rapid. It continued, but now at a slower pace. As a matter of fact a conversation of any length must have been as boring to the auditor as it was fatiguing to me, for much that I endeavoured to say was unintelligible, and I often had to spell aloud the word which had proved too much for me. With one cheek still paralysed it was difficult to get one's mouth into the right shape, and I found, too, that false teeth were a mixed blessing. It was hard enough to learn to articulate anew, but to do so with your mouth full of dominoes aggravated the hardship. However, I persevered, and was assured by all that progress was real. Before I left the hospital, rather more than seven weeks after the onset of the aphasia, I could say almost any word if you gave me time, but I had to dissect the difficult ones into syllables, so that speech was slow, staccato, and monotonous. I remember that the word 'bacteriology' presented peculiar difficulties.

The presence of complete facial paralysis— and this persisted till after I had got back to England—was a great vexation in eating,

for, when I came to sit up and feed myself, the previous mouthful tended to fall out when I opened my mouth for the next. The first time I sat up to lunch I used up three table napkins, and on board the boat, coming home, I had to eat in private owing to my deplorable table manners.

My time in hospital was not rendered the more exhilarating by the heat-wave which afflicted New York during June and July, the temperature remaining usually in the eighties (once 93°), with pretty complete aqueous saturation. However, if you slept immediately under an open window, with only a sheet over you, and kicked off your pyjamas while the night nurse wasn't looking, you sometimes left off sweating just before dawn. This was the reason why I was allowed to come home at the earliest safe moment, to convalesce under cooler skies. But first I had to learn to walk. After seven weeks of absolute bed my back and legs were useless, owing to atrophy from disuse. But ten days' vigorous massage improved matters, and whereas I couldn't offer at standing alone when I first tried, five days later I walked 20 steps without any support.

And so, nearly eight weeks after entering the hospital of the Rockefeller Institute, I was transported in an ambulance to the R.M.S. 'Mauretania', full of thanks and gratitude for the skill and care with which I had been treated and the kindness with which I had been nursed.

On board the boat I learned to walk further each day, until finally my legs joined up with my back and I could walk alone. Once back in England my improvement continued, and even the facial palsy began to clear up under massage and Faradic electricity, much improving both speech and table manners. But here again let the patient drop a hint of what is unknown to many a doctor. If you are having the Faradic current to your face, shave afterwards and not before, or every tiny abrasion will burn like fire.

At the time of writing this article, just three months after the aphasia occurred, my speech still leaves much to be desired, but I can conduct an ordinary conversation without much difficulty, though still rather slowly.

(Andrewes 1931)

COMMENTARY

Andrewes' speech disorder appeared to be a pure motor aphasia, and would probably be classified as an 'aphemia' or 'pure word dumbness' (Benson 1994). It is usually associated with a lesion in the part of the left inferior frontal gyrus known as the frontal operculum.

It is fortuitous that Andrewes had his stroke while he was in hospital for treatment of another condition, and the observations relating to his acute state are all the more interesting for this reason. Andrewes himself observed that the rate of recovery from his loss of speech appeared to slow down after two weeks, and this observation is confirmed by recent data on the pattern of recovery of function in milder forms of aphasia following stroke (Pedersen et al. 1995).

Andrewes found that reciting poetry, using sentences he knew well, and singing, were relatively easy for him compared to other forms of speech (see also the self-report by Rose in this chapter). Most aphasiologists and speech therapists are aware of this pattern of sparing of speech output, but it is a fact that could perhaps be used more often by ward staff, and patients' families, to help encourage the patient in the early stages of recovery from a motor aphasia and to help build up self-confidence when the patient may understandably have feelings of despair.

It is interesting that Andrewes found German and French easier to speak than English. The so-called Pitres' rule, named after the French aphasiologist Pitres, stipulates that in bilingual patients recovery of the primary language usually occurs before languages that are less well-learned. However, there are many exceptions to this rule (Paradis 1989), and it is possible that Andrewes was correct in implying that articulatory fluency was easier in the two foreign languages, due to the simple mechanics of German and French speech sounds compared to English phonemes. An alternative yet intriguing possibility, suggested by recent functional brain imaging data, is that different areas of the brain are involved in the performance of different languages. In a recent study, the putamen was shown to be active when subjects spoke a second language (French) but not when they spoke their native language (English)—see Barinaga (1995) for a preliminary report of these data.

An important point that Andrewes brings up is one that relates to timing and speech—after a few weeks, he could say 'almost any word if you gave me the time' (p. 56), and after a few months, he 'could conduct an ordinary conversation without much difficulty, although still rather slowly' (p. 56). It would seem that in this type of speech disturbance, and perhaps also in some other language disorders, there may be a basic slowing down of processes rather than their abolition, and that it is possible for the patient either to use existing mechanisms successfully if given the time, or to compensate by recruiting other cognitive mechanisms, which also takes time. Perhaps it is the case that general information-processing speed/speed of neural transmission is lost after most brain lesions, and that this will affect a specific cortical function by producing a general slowing down in encoding or in retrieval activities. Where this change in information-processing speed is the only significant change brought about by the cerebral pathology, with the capacity to perform particular cognitive operations being unaffected, then a deficit in timing may be the only behavioural manifestation of the brain lesion in question.

REFERENCES

Barinaga, M. (1995). Brain researchers speak a common language. *Science*, **270**, 1437–8.

Benson, D. F. (1994) *The neurology of thinking*. Oxford University Press, New York.

Paradis, M. (1989). Bilingual and polyglot aphasia. In *Handbook of neuropsychology*, Vol. 2 (ed. F. Boller and J. Grafman), pp. 117–40. Elsevier, Amsterdam.

Pedersen, P. M., Jorgensen, H. S., Nakayama, H., Raaschou, H. O., and Olsen, T. S. (1995). Aphasia in acute stroke: Incidence, determinants, and recovery. *Annals of Neurology*, **38**, 659–66.

A physician's account of his own aphasia

Robert H. Rose

Robert Rose appears to have been a practising physician in New York City at the time of his stroke, although no further information is available.

EDITOR'S FOREWORD

In the spring of 1947, Professor G. W. Stewart of the Department of Physics, University of Iowa, called to my attention a document which he had received from his friend, Robert H. Rose, M.D., of New York City. The document (see Item No. 8, below) was a letter describing the effects, particularly the language disturbances, of a 'stroke' which he had suffered. It was Professor Stewart's perceptive thought that Dr. Rose might be able to provide significant personal observations concerning his recent aphasic disturbances and his ingenius and persistent efforts to regain his language functions.

In September, 1943, Dr. Rose had been admitted to the Neurological Institute, New York City, where a diagnosis of 'thrombosis of the left middle cerebral artery' was made. At that time his age was 67 years, 8 months (birthdate 1–24–1876). The resulting language difficulties and subsequent improvement are described by Dr. Rose in the documents presented below.

A minimum of selecting and editing has been done; Dr. Rose's own statements are presented just as he wrote them, with all errors preserved. Essential correspondence is included.

A validating statement was graciously prepared at the editor's request by Theodore B. Russell, M.D., who has been in contact with Dr. Rose since March, 1944.

I am deeply pleased to express to Dr. Rose the gratitude of all professional students of language disorders for his unselfish and scientific spirit in making his personal and intimate observations of his own difficulties available to the *Journal of Speech and Hearing Disorders*. Professor Stewart is deserving of special thanks for bringing the matter to the attention of the *Journal* editor, for obtaining for him a copy of the phonograph record made by Dr. Rose which is described below, and for cooperating generously throughout the study. Everyone concerned is also appreciative of Dr. Russell's indispensible assistance in supplying essential medical confirmation of Dr. Rose's account.

The letters and documents are presented in chronological order, except for certain modifications made in the interests of overall integration of the material.—Wendell Johnson

1.   FIRST LETTER TO DR. ROSE, 4–14–47

Dear Dr. Rose:

Professor G. W. Stewart of the University of Iowa Department of Physics has been kind enough to tell me something about you. I am writing you in my capacity as the editor of the *Journal of Speech Disorders*, which is the official publication of the American Speech Correction Association. I hope that what I have to propose will strike you not only as appropriate from a scientific point of view, but also as of personal interest to you.

I feel that you would be able to make a valuable contribution to the study of the difficulty with which you are now contending if you would write a personal account of the details of your experiences with aphasia. I realize that you might prefer to take considerable time to do this if it is agreeable with you to do it at all, and I shall of course be happy to wait as long as necessary, because I am convinced that you will be of considerable value to speech pathologists. At your convenience, I would appreciate very much having your reaction to this proposal.

Yours very sincerely,
Wendell Johnson

2. FIRST LETTER FROM DR. ROSE, 4–27–47

Dear Dr. Johnson:

When first I thought this over, I was rather timid about the offer. Dr. J. M. Nielsen, when I learned he wanted the original copies which I did in pencil, Rather puts a new light the work. (You see I could not spell original. I looked it up in Thorndike)

A former patient, Hon. Ralph W. Gwinn said my writing was the same. I wrote him it will be the same when, and, if I recover—the spelling.

I can trace this thing from the beginning, when I could not spell the names of my two books, nor think of their Titles.

I think I can see that what you want is there.

Yours very sincerely,
Dr. Robert H. Rose

3. LETTER FROM DR. ROSE, 6–21–47

Dear Dr. Johnson:

After writing this over three times and correcting a lot of mistakes in spelling and otherwise, I am sending it on to you without typewriting, to make any further corrections you may see.

It is largely confined to in *Memorization* in Aphasia.[1] What it has done for me is beyond compare and *quickly*.

I wrote my sisters every week. Now I have all in my position. There interest is in the writing, mistakes and corrections from time to time—improvement every week. I will

look these over to see what there is, now that I have written Memorization In Aphasia.

My mind is not clear, nor is my memory, what Ideas I have are a product of mulling over my thought and giving them time germinate.

Yours very sincerely,
Dr. Robert Hugh Rose

My boy said he would get me the mechinism for making a record of my voice. I think he saw an advertisement in some paper. It is substantially normal. It wouldn't show in Hamlet's Soliloquy. If he gets it soon, I will send it on to you.[2]

Dr. Robert Hugh Rose

This is typical now, because I seldom think of things when I want to say them. When I write a letter I often send another the next day, to make up for the messages I missed.

Dr. Robert Hugh Rose
I can't fold a paper.
Dr. RHR.

4. LETTER FROM DR. ROSE, 6–25–47

Dear Dr. Johnson:

I am starting right away to suppliment my ideas with others. I think it would add to the text if I added, 'This Memorization serves as an aid in the Treatment of Aphasia.' (Last sentence.)

Page 2, following could not spell, for the stroke area in part was missing.

I received a letter from Dr. G. W. Stewart in which he explained why he wanted my letters in print. Having just finished the paper on Aphasia, I want to look that over before I do anything else. (I received Dr. G. W. Stewart's letter Monday.) I wrote him late Saturday and our letters crossed. I think I might get some ideas if I use my head—though they come slowly.

Sincerely,
Dr. Robert H Rose

---

[1] See Item No. 6. The statement presented under 6, as explained in Dr. Rose's letter of July 16, 1947 (Item No. 5), is a later revision of the document referred to here.

[2] The recording was made on September 23, 1947, and is discussed below under Item No. 11.

5.   LETTER FROM DR. ROSE, 7–16–47

Dear Dr. Johnson:

I have found my speech immeasurely improved by memorization, frequently repeated. I have formed a habit of doing Thanatopsis three times daily to get the maximum effect. My speech took a forward spurt when I started Thanatopsis, Hamlet's Soliloquy. She Was a Phantom of Delight, Tell Me Not in Mournful Numbers and other Poetry. In fact it occurred quickly in 2 or 3 days, there-after.

Now I realize what I have accomplished by using the Radio and Movies so frequently. The first two years I was at the Radio almost constantly. Then I started memorization. This was without pain or discomfort.

I have learned to talk easily and quickly by the use of Poetry and so far as I know the use of Memorization in the Treatment of Aphasia has not been done. The thought came to me to try such treatment.

I was thinking about your saying the article on Aphasia would be more valuable just as it is, but I could add some emphasis as, headlines etc., etc. Perhaps to settle what I mean, the only thing I can do it to send another copy.[3]

Cordially,
Dr. Robert H Rose

6.   STATEMENT WRITTEN BY DR. ROSE, 7–16–47

Memorization in aphasia

On September 12th, 1943, I was seized with a Broca's Stroke. *Speechlessness lasted about three weeks.*[4]

I will try to relate some of my experiences and tell how by memorizing poetry I was enabled *to talk freely. Thus memorization served as an aid in Treatment of Aphasia.*

---

[3] This copy follows. An earlier copy, written by Dr. Rose June 21, 1947, is not included here. It resembles the July 16 copy very closely, but is not quite as detailed.

[4] All italics are Dr. Rose's.

I was in more or less of a haze, when I went to the Medical Center. I was conscious could eat, went to the Xray, followed directions, as to position, etc. Made another visit in a week and received the report that all was improved. Toward the end of this time I went out on the veranda on several occasions and listened to the radio. I understood every sentense, but could not say a single word. At the same time there was some improvement in my general condition.

I then transferred to the Lutheran Hospital where I had an endowed room at my disposal. I gradually acquired the ability to say a few words. One thing which I remember is that when a doctor tried me on the famous phraze *'Fifth Cavalry Brigade,'* I said it several times. I said it for a number of doctors who were at a board meeting. *But the next day I failed utterly to recall the phraze.* Later I thought of it, off and on, and it came and went alternately. The speech gradually improved as I was gaining through resolution. This was a mere part of aphasia.

In the middle of *November 1943,* I practiced my name and address, *since I could not spell,* for the stroke area in part was missing. I kept weekly records, *started them after 3 months.* When I refere to them, I see that I spelled Hospital this way, *'Hospeten',* at first and other spelling on a par with this. I have many of my records in the form of letters which I sent every week to my sisters. In turn they kept them and when I wanted them later they sent them all to me. This is an *especially good statistical* record for the writing, as it shows the mistakes I made from time to time, and *the improvement, both weekly and yearly.* The study of these records will give much information.

When I left the Lutheran, I went to a Nurse Home in Brooklyn for two mounths. I realized that I *had to learn* the *Alphabet,* the *Days of the Week,* the *Months,* of the *Year,* and many other simple things all over again.

Aphasia

Showing how Aphasia haunts me with loss of memory. In January 1944, I thought about my two books, 'Eat Your Way to Health' and 'How to Stay Young' and *I had to ask my sister to tell me what their* names were. I had only a hazy remembrance.

I spent the Spring, Summer and Fall at the YMCA and then came to the Episcopal Home where I am continueing my re-education. It is like being born over again. I have done many things of value and profit, such as the following:—reading papers, learning to write, the use of Thorndike's word book of 20,000 of the most commonly used words, which I have gone over four times, used the radio for practice in speech, regular attendence on the movies and such talking as I could do without a deffinite plan. I am impelled to do something all the time.

Radio a God Send

In the early stages, except for the first 3 or 4 weeks, *I used the radio all day*, as it was the only means which I could use in my re-education. These four years show how slow that was. I listened to *all the stories*, and *news* and *music* and *thus kept my mind occupied. I could use the radio without pain* or discomfort. I used adds for script and spelling practice.

I had trouble spelling *such simple words* as *Tuesday and Wednesday* even after two years. I am still wrestling with the d's, g's, f's, n's, etc. The only thing I can find to do for these is to use Thorndike for spelling practice. I have been writing 'Ready for the Holidays,' 'Here's My Newest Picture' and 'These Things We Hold Dear' for practice and *I am just able to recall them*. I could not use more than 100 words a day, or it would cause pain. That is my experience. It impinges upon the stroke area.

Memory Gone

In late August, 1946, I went down to the chapel to try myself on the Ritual. I could go through all in concert, but when I came up stairs, *I failed to recall even a few lines*—of the *Lord's Prayer*. For some reason I could say, 'Now I lay me down to sleep, etc.' I resolved to re-learn the 'Lord's Prayer,' 'The 23 Psalm,' and 'Crossing the Bar' and build from that point, if possible. I realized that if I could not make progress with such tasks, I would indeed be up against a brick wall. *I used repetition* and could see some headway but it

was very, very slow.[5] My records show that *by the end of November, I Knew these three pieces*. I spent an immence amount of time on them—mostly in repetition.

Now I wanted to continue memorizing such poems—hoping[6] to make the progress real and decisive. I thought of more Psalms, The Beatitudes and other poetry with which I was formerly familiar. I was trying for such as would be easy to memorize. Poe's Bells seemed good but I gave that up for an easier one. The most familiar seem best.

Thanatopsis in Aphasia

Toward the end of February, I found what I had been looking for in *Thanatopsis*. At one time I could almost say it in my sleep. I started to read Thanatopsis and it seemed very easy to me. I went over it a number of times and snatches came back to me and it seemed that I could far more easily re-learn it than the Bells.

The next day when I awoke, I was almost saying it. After breakfast when I lay down, I could say most of it entirely. *It was just a matter of a few days* to clinch it.

I was then resolved to take advantage of *Thanatopsis* and make my speech whole again. I resolved to do *Thanatopsis three times a day* and see what it would do for me. I was not disappointed. My speech took a great forward spurt. The progress was almost unbelievable. I was getting along slowly before, but thereafter I seemed to gain as much in one week as I had previously in three months.

Memorization Opens the Way

When I saw the result I was getting from my excursions in Thanatopsis I went down to show the Superintendent and Secretary how I could talk. The speechless one was talking freely. I could say the words in *Thanatopsis without hessitation*[7] in what might be called

---

[5] Dr. Rose originally wrote this as 'show.' He corrected the typed copy, making the word 'slow.' Other errors in this document that were detected and corrected on the typed copy are so indicated.
[6] Originally written 'hopping'; corrected on typed copy.
[7] On typed copy Dr. Rose put a question mark under 'hessitation'.

perfect speech. This was about 500 new words, quite enough vocabulary for ordinary talking.

There is a wonderful difference in my talking since I started Thanatopsis. I talk almost the same as I did before I was taken sick. Now I am becoming quite facile in speech. *The more I practice Thanatopsis, Hamlet's Soliloquy, She was a Phantom of Delight, Tell me not in Mournful Numbers*; the more quickly I gain. I learn the poetry which I formerly knew very quickly. And it adds to the variety of my vocabulary.

I did not have *Hamlet's Soliloquy* with me; it was among my books in Mount Vernon. *I thought about it for two days* and without a copy, *I remembered it entirely.* So I do that almost as often as I do Thanatopsis. It seems to me that I am getting these former quotations back in memory. While it was hard to learn the first words of the Lord's Prayer last Fall, now it seems easy. Easy also to *re-learn that old* poetry *which I used to know.* It seems to be quite accumulative, more so all the time.

Gray's Elegy

Read often aloud and you will come close to memorizing, but not entirely, you are to become familiar only with new words. This is the treatment you should apply to Gray's Elegy in the Country Churchyard, along with similar poetry and prose, as (and)[8] such prose as Victor Hugo On Immortality. I am sure that you will profit immesely if you carry out these directions consciously. Read them over and over again.

Four Hours at the Movies

Yesterday I went to a movie and remained four hours. This I consider very important since *it did not tire me at all.* The use of my eyes and other faculties involved was entirely comfortable. But it was entirely another matter with the writing, for it hurt me, the *Thorndike word book hurt me,* when I used *it for more than 100 words,* and *most forms of writing hurt me.* In other words I can[9] spend time *using the radio* or at the *movies with entire*

comfort. But not so when I use my writing area *as it impinges upon the stroke area.*

Memorization ideal for talking

Learning to talk by memorization has the advantage that it is free from pain and can be used to your hearts content. (Postmarked New York City, July 16, 1947)

7. LETTER FROM DR. ROSE, 7-1-47

Dear Dr. Johnson:

Thank you for your letter, contents duely noted.

As for the P.S., it is harder for me to say what is the answer, but I shall try.[10] This case is almost 4 years old and I took it up and monopolized it entirely. I met Dr Amill on the elevator and recited Thanatopsis—thus showing him how a could talk. That is the extent to which any one else has taken part in the process, Dr. Amill just resigned, to be succeeded by Dr. F. A. Smith . . . , Dr. T. B. Russell has six months of the service in the Fall.

Dr. Louis Casamajor had me in charge the first 3 weeks. It was there that I had the two Xrays. I had a couple of letters from him in 1946. November 22nd 'I was interested in reading of your experience in the recovery of aphasia. The data you gave me is very interesting and I'm very glad to have it'.

Dr. Louis Casamajor, The Neurological Institute
168th Street and Ft. Washington Avenue
New York 32 N.Y.

I was about 2 months at Lutheran Hospital, Dr. J. Stanleiy Kenney, 924 West End avenue New York City, had me in charge there.

Then I went to a Nurses Home in Brooklyn. Where *Dr. H. F. McChesney* had me for two months. Now he has retired on account of a heart attack, but his address 60 Greenway North

Forest Hills Garden
New York

---

[8]Dr. Rose deleted 'and' from the typed copy.
[9] This word was changed by Dr. Rose on the typed copy from 'cen' to 'can'.

[10] The P.S. contained an inquiry as to Dr. Rose's physicians.

I don't think he answers any letters.

I am enclosing a letter which I wrote last Fall.[11] That gives quite a little history of the case.

I might find some of the M.D.'s away at this time. Otherwise I might go to the various offices[12] and show them how I can talk. That is a possibility.

Sincerely yours,
Dr. Robert H Rose

8. ORIGINAL STATEMENT, DATED 10–5–46[13]

At the request of Dr. Robert H. Rose this copy of a letter is being sent to you. The original was written by him to a Phi Kappa Psi brother, who in turn sent copies to more than twenty others. That gave Dr. Rose an idea: to send copies to some of his friends.

He has consistently maintained an amazing interest in devising procedures for teaching himself to speak, read, and write. From the first he has known what he wished to say; and has been able to read with his *ears*. Radio a godsend.

I have had in mind for a long time, when I reached the point at which I was reasonably able, to answer all the letters which you and your friends so thoughtfully sent. Since there are so many and since you have been one of the prime movers in carrying on this good work, I think it would be better to make a complete history of the case as I see it today. In this way I shall run less risk of making it my last case.

I can't say that I was particularly uncomfortable at any time. I ate every meal as they came to me. I just did not know what was

going on all the time. One of the first things[14] I recall is going to the X-ray to have my skull radiated. I took the chair. I did not have loss of power in muscles. I could get on the table without trouble. I had pictures of the cella tursica. I went back again in two weeks to see how they were doing.

You see I could not say a word. I had trouble making myself understood even for the simpler things. It seemed the attendants were dumb. Before I left Medical Center I can't remember whether I could say a few words. I don't know how long I was at Medical Center—I think about three weeks. I went out on the veranda and listened to the radio. I could hear perfectly. When I went to the Lutheran Hospital I got a radio in my room and listened to it from morning to night—the trash as well as the opera. I had to do something all the time. I could not stand it otherwise. I think my sister was very nervous when she could not understand that I wanted a knife to clean my finger nails. There was a chance that it might be useful for other purposes. Dr. Bauer thought of suicide. I surely did not have that in mind at any time. I only wanted to spruce up. This idea of not being able to communicate one's thoughts is not easy to stand. Dr. Bauer gave me electrical treatments while I was in Luthern Hospital. He was an old friend of mine. Unfortunately he died last Fall at the age of 82.

This is an easy place, the cella tursica, to get a view of the picture desired to show the arteries in that region. After I had some examinations and rest and treatments I moved to the Lutheran Hospital. As I remember I was at Presbyterian Hospital three weeks. (I shall give you this side-light on my condition. I had to look up 'Presbyterian' to see how to spell it. This is one of my greatest difficulties after three years. I can't spell anything without looking it up. Of course I am getting some things settled, but it is just as if I started life all over again. There are three points: spelling, figuring and talking.)

The next chapter is my stay at Lutheran Hospital until about Christmas. I can date

---

[11] This letter follows.
[12] Dr. Rose changed 'affices' to 'offices' on typed copy.
[13] This is the original document which Professor G. W. Stewart called to the editor's attention. It may be assumed that this statement was probably edited somewhat by a person other than Dr. Rose; the first two paragraphs were not written by him. Further changes were made by Dr. Rose later when a copy was returned to him for checking. These later corrections are noted.

[14] This word was written in by Dr. Rose in re-checking the manuscript.

events easily in this way. I began to get a few words and they increased quite rapidly, but the spelling was very slow. In fact it was just as if I were a newborn babe. I had a lesion in my brain, a stroke which blotted out my speech, my ability to figure, to write and to talk. I had to learn the alphabet, to spell, to figure (addition, subtraction, etc.)

I spent six weeks in a Nurse's Home. This reminds me that I had spilled my food on the right side at first. When I went to the Nurse's Home I had a table to myself. I was getting so I could take things pretty well. I took one or two-mile walks. I made a practice of taking two walks a day.

Then I found a nearby movie. From that time I went twice a week to movies except when something interfered. You see I can get everything on the radio—nothing is blocked out there. All things have gradually gotten better.

I was not lacking in muscular power. The fact that I was able to move about without limping kept me from attracting attention. The trouble was in my speech, writing and figuring. I could not add a column of figures. When I left the Nurse's Home I went to the YMCA. I could get along pretty well because I told everyone I lost my speech—I could not say a word for a time. I could select food pretty easily at the cafeteria. When I was at a loss for a word I pointed. I took the change they gave me, asking no questions. I was at YMCA from first of March to November. Then I went to the Episcopal Home opposite the Cathedral of St. John the Divine, where I am for life, or until I get enough better so that I can finish my book which I started (This institution was started in) before I was taken sick.[15] It is all that can be desired in every way.

Now I am improving every week in all ways. I will give you some details of my

record: I started a record once a week. It consisted of the alphabet, the small letters, the capitals, and digits, some figures, some suitable adds from the papers which I repeated just the same every week. This gave me practice in learning these things. Now the condition is the following: I can *talk* more from week to week. I get practice from reading, from the radio, from the movies. I get some practice talking at the table. I can *write* with difficulty. I can figure with the greatest difficulty. I have aphasia, that is loss of memory for letters, words, etc. I have loss of ability to *read*.

Some side-lights on the loss of memory are interesting. I went to a movie. I came back and tried to tell the people at my table what it was. I could remember La Traviata but I could not remember the other piece. All I could think of was 'The Merchant of Venice'. It was 'The Carnival of Venice'. The next day I went down to 104th Street to look at the sign. I thought I could remember then. When I got four blocks away all I could think of was 'The Merchant of Venice.' Then I tried some mnemonics. I started the a, b, c's and it came to me—'The Carnival of Venice'. That way I can get the clue.

I have been working on this letter two months. My eyes get tired when I work more than so much. That is the reason I could not answer your letters before. Three years is a long time, but I will make it sometime in the future. I could not undertake to use a pen. I have learned to sign my name. That is practice.

All my friends who have written me I wish to thank very much. I certainly appreciate the thoughtfulness of their messages.

(Signed) Dr. Robert H. Rose
October 5th, 1946

9.   LETTER FROM DR. ROSE, 8–25–47

Dear Dr. Johnson

Some of my mistakes in Spelling—phrase, (the same), hoping, hesitation. My speech took a great forward spurt.

When I was at the Y.M.C.A. 4 months

---

[15] In the typed copy sent to Dr. Rose a line had inadvertently been left out at this point, so that it read, 'my book which I started in 1872.' Dr. Rose wrote in the missing words 'before I was taken sick.' However, he crossed out 'in 1872' and changed 'It' to 'The time.' The original read: '. . . my book which was started before I was taken sick. This institution was started in 1872. It is all that can be desired in any way'.

after I was taken sick, I spent 9 months, a period in which I thought of what I was to do to regain my speech. Every week we had a sing. When I could talk very little, I could sing all the old songs almost perfectly. This gave me the idea of memorization eventually and I tried it and found that I soon learned to talk. I found my singing speech was clear, that I could say the words when singing them. That was the solution of[16] learning to talk. The conclusion is that the brain pathes for singing takes a course further from the stroke area and there-fore this also holds for memorization. This fact is recognized by M.D.'s The fact that Poetry, music and singing come in. It should be recognized that Poetry, music, singing, and[17] *memorization* comes in—the singing—talking brain pathes are[18] nearer than the the the talking talking, otherwise how could you say in singing what you could not say in plain speech. If this is not clear. think it over, it will come to you.[19] I am trying to work out a thought—bear with me.

My best wishes,
Dr. Robert H Rose

10.   LETTER FROM DR. ROSE, 9-2-47

Dear Dr. Johnson:

I feel that I should give you the news as to my condition—that is keep you up to date. Unfortunately your 500 page book, 'People in Quandaries' was almost my Nemesis. What I found was that my trouble centered in the writing and reading. When I tried to read the book, from the library, in two weeks,[20] I bit off more than I could chew. I certainly would have risked another stroke or some vascular accident if I had followed through. I did not realize that my trouble was

confined so deffinitely in the reading and writing areas. Three mounths after I was taken sick, I read the paper every day and gradually increased the amount but evidently did not get the stress so much concentrated over the writing and reading areas. I shall try it again latter.[21] I see my limit is very deffinite. I find it very interesting[22] but it is too early for me. I could take it in a little time—but a long time from now.

I read considerable in Dr. J. M. Niclsen's book on Agnosia, Apraxia and[23] Aphasia. I could not understand why it was so difficult—now I know.

I think memorization might have a place along with your ideas about stuttering. I have read this part and like it very much.

Cordially and sincerelly
Dr. Robert H. Rose

11.   NOTES ON A PHONOGRAPH RECORDING MADE BY DR. ROSE

The recording begins with the following introduction, spoken by a woman's voice:

'This recording of *Hamlet's Soliloquy* from memory, on the 23rd day of September, 1947, has been made by Dr. Robert Hugh Rose, who suffered a Broca stroke four years ago, and for some weeks lost all power of speech. Thereafter Dr. Rose gradually regained a limited use of the spoken word, but it was not until some months ago when he started on a self-imposed course of memorizing and constantly repeating poetry that he began to recapture greater facility of speech, and incidentally to enlarge his vocabulary. This recording was made as a partial demonstration of results from such a course to date.'

There follows a recital by Dr. Rose, in a well controlled and expressive voice, of the complete 'Soliloquy' from *Hamlet*. According to my count, Dr. Rose spoke 276 words at a

---

[16] Dr. Rose changed 'to' to 'of' on typed copy.
[17] Dr. Rose inserted 'and' on typed copy; he also underlined 'memorization'.
[18] On typed copy Dr. Rose changed 'is' to 'are'.
[19] On typed copy Dr. Rose changed his original wording, 'it will bear elucidation,' to 'Think it over, it will come to you'.
[20] 'Week' changed to 'weeks' on typed copy.

[21] Dr. Rose apparently meant to change 'latter' to 'later;' but instead of crossing one of the t's he crossed out the a and wrote another a above it.
[22] n (interenting) changed to s on typed copy.
[23] The word 'and' was added by Dr. Rose on typed copy.

rate of approximately 150 words per minute. He made only two errors (if they were errors—I do not know how he learned the passage), omitting 'the law's delay,' and substituting 'in' for 'with' in 'with this regard'. The performance as recorded was generally excellent, in my judgment. Professor G. W. Stewart made the recording available to me.—Wendell Johnson

12. LETTER FROM DR. ROSE, 10-28-47

Dear Dr. Johnson:

I wish to make a change in my paper, 'Memorization In Aphasia'.

Gray's Elegy

Since I have found that learning to talk is made far easier through the use of Memorization, I feel the need of enlarging my vocubulary. In addition to the selections mentioned, I find Gray's Elegy serves to supplement admirably and used it in the following manner. Repetition will do you a world of good. Read over and over again. Thus you may become familiar with 1000 more words. Read twice daily, for ten days and repeat as often as you like. Now you can pursue this plan for other poems and make that your pattern. I am sure that you will profit immencely if you carry out this plan consciously.

Yours very sincerely,
Dr. Robert H. Rose

13. LETTER FROM DR. ROSE, 2-26-48

Dear Dr. Johnson:

When Dr. Stewart was here at Christmas Season there seemed to be some doubt about who was to write the introduction to my paper on, 'Memorization In Aphasia'.

It came about as a result of the years which had elapsed in more than four years of my sickness and the changes following to war.

Recently I visited Dr. J. B. Russell, the Physician at the Home, 1060 Amsterdam Avenue, whom I have learned to know intimately and favorably, and who has all my history in his (. . .) and all data of my case from the beginning. Copies of most of the records were sent from Presbyterian and Lutheran Hospital and are there for reference.

The past week I had several talks with Dr. Russell. He is enthusiastic about writing the introduction to my paper. He even regards the subject as having enough material for a book.

Dr. Russell has had me in charge since he came back from the Navy more than a year ago. Needless to say he likes the way I have improved, especially in in speech, doubtless through Memorization.

I am sorry that I did not do this before. But it is very laborious for me. It consumes quantities of time and effort and I thought that when I wrote the paper it was enough— especially for an Aphasiac who is not supposed to be able to do things.

Yours very sincerely,
Dr. Robert H Rose.

14. LETTER TO DR. ROSE, 3-4-48

Dear Dr. Rose:

On October 7, 1947, I sent copies of the enclosed to Dr. Louis Casamajor and to Dr. J. Stanley Kenney. I have had no reply from either of these men. After receiving your letter of February 26, I have decided to send the enclosed direct to you with the hope that you might deliver it personally to Dr. T. B. Russell. I am sending a carbon of this letter to Dr. Russell also, so that he will understand what I need.

The enclosed manuscript is made up of copies of the various letters and statements which you have written to me. I should like to publish these in the *Journal of Speech and Hearing Disorders* because of the value they would have to speech pathologists. In order to do this, I need to have from a responsible physician who knows your problem at first hand an introductory statement which will authenticate your own personal account. You will recognize this, of course, as standard procedure in scientific publication. From what you tell me about Dr. Russell, he should be in a position to write such a statement very satisfactorily. The main thing he should say is that the account as written by you is accurate in essential detail in his judgment as a medical man familiar with your problem. To this he may add, of course, anything that he might desire to say.

I realize that I am asking a great deal of you, but I feel that you will agree with me that this is the best way to proceed. I know that when this material is published you will have a deep satisfaction in the realization that you will have performed a valuable scientific and humanitarian service. I am grateful for the opportunity to cooperate with you in this.

> Yours very sincerely,
> Wendell Johnson, Editor

15. LETTER FROM DR. ROSE, 3–15–48

Dear Dr. Johnson:

I turned over the script on my paper to Dr. Russell. He says he will get it back in a week or ten days. In the meantime I have some points I want to make.

Here is a partial list of the Poems which I have committed.

Thanatopsis, Hamlit's Sol., The Psalm of Life, She Was a Phantom of Delight, Oft in the Stilly Night, Light (the night has a thousand eyes), The Rainy Day, The Beatitudes, Trees, and Crossing the Bar.

The ones I have near-memorized.

The Bridge. The Day Is Done, The Children's Hour, The Village Blacksmith, Gray's Elegy, My Heart Leaps Up, Indian Serenade, Hymn to the Night, Break, Break, Break, The Raven, The Bells, The Man With The Hoe, Rabbi Ben Ezra, Shakespeare (by Arnold).

Near-memorization is very important in that it serves to enlarge the vocabulary. It takes a long time to memorize, but not very long to near-memorize. Hence many of the latter list contains longer poems. I have appended this list, which is enough to show the logic of the process as I conceive it.

I have memorized Thanatopsis (500 words), Hamlet's Sol., The Psalm of Life, Crossing the Bar and others. Then, in order to further increase my vocabulary, I have used Gray's Elegy and all of those in the list of near-memorization.

You can see what I am driving at in making this classifications, how readily they fit into each other. Gray's Elegy is about 1000 words and they would soon use up a lot of words. The illustration makes the point clear, I think.

I shall send you the introduction by Dr. Russell and my paper[24] when both are ready.

16. STATEMENT FROM DR. ROSE, 3–15–48

I think I have improved this somewhat
Use your judgment

Near-Memorization

An added term which is useful. Since I have found that learning to talk is made far easier through the use of memorization, I feel the need of more vocabulary and other aids. Near-Memorization is the connecting link with Memorization. This is the term I have used and I find it very convenient. You dont go to the full length of committing to memory but do a partial job. It is quicker, covers more ground, gives you more vocabulary in a given space of time. You read over and over again until snatches are very familiar. You get some advantages of both methods—a two in one method.

Gray's Elegy, a little more than 1000 words, and familiar to many, is one of the best selections I recall. I have addopted this plan for near-memorization; read twice daily for ten days, and repeat two or three times, according to your individual familiarity with each poem. In this way you can enlarge your vocabulary to any extent you may wish. Next take some of Longfellows or one of your own selection.

I have also provided some poems, which are more difficult—among these are Poe's

---

[24] See Item No. 16.

Raven, The Bells and Markham's The Man With The Hoe. Now with these selections you can carry your vocabulary as far as you desire.

Thus you have the privilege of—

1. Memorizing some poetry, and
2. Near-Memorizing others.

Now one more thing is called to your attention, that is, the possibility of learning by heart many of the selections you are working on. If you wish at any time, you may change, Near-Memorized ones into fully Memorized ones. This was shown me when I found that many passages of Gray's Elegy were half committed by me almost before I knew it. Therefore it is a sort of progressive process.

17. LETTER FROM DR. ROSE, 3-16-48

Dear Dr. Johnson:

I had no longer affixed my stamp to letter until I remembered the Poetry which I learned at about 18 years of age. I wanted to tell you about it as it is the best example I now recall of long forgotten lines. I have no book of Meredith and had to work it out time by line. That is one point I wished to make

The Poetry
You can live without Poetry,
    Music and Art.
You can live without Conscience,
    live without Heart
You can live without Friends, live
    without Books.
But civilized man can not live
    without Cooks.

You can easily see why I have learned to talk after 3 weeks of steechlessness and at first slow return of speech.

Cordially yours,
Dr. Robert H. Rose.

18. DR. RUSSELL'S CONFIRMING STATEMENT, MARCH, 1948

On March 13th, 1944, Dr. Robert Hugh Rose (the author of the preceding article)

applied for admission to the home where I was one of the attending physicians. We had known from the hospital records of Neurological Institute (New York City) of his admission in September, 1943, for a three-week period of observation where a diagnosis of thrombosis of the left middle cerebral artery had been made. As this home takes only people who are healthy and able to take care of themselves it was with considerable hesitancy that his application was reviewed. At that time he told of his sudden loss of speech and of the fact that he had been in several institutions since then and at the time of admission was living alone at the YMCA.

His speech was extremely slow, and it was obvious that it was very difficult for him to express himself. He chose his words slowly and carefully but would often forget them and forget episodes he had mentioned. This obvious frustration in his expression was accompanied by some mild irritability and he would often stop and shake his head, irritated by the fact that he could not find the words he wished to express and which he knew.

He was not admitted definitely to the home for five months, after which time his general condition seemed better and his speech had improved.

In the intervening years his progress has been continuous but slow. He appeared at the infirmary only infrequently and early in his stay would usually bring up his requests in writing, which he labored over as a rule for a good many hours. He frequently used a long word list, which he would attempt to memorize and then write over and over again. His progress in this respect was painfully slow, but there was distinct improvement.

At one time there seemed to have been a very rapid decrease in his difficulty for a short period. This, as he describes in his article, was when he first started to read 'Thanatopsis'.

At the present time Dr. Rose is able to carry on a very intelligent conversation in as steady a flow as most men his age. He occasionally gropes for his words, but his progress has certainly been most remarkable. Although this might have occurred without his extreme effort, certainly his tremendous desire to overcome what seemed to be a hopeless situation, and his persistence and perseverence working alone with a self-taught method, have been a great inspiration to those who have been associated with him.—Theodore B. Russell, M.D.

(Rose 1948)

COMMENTARY

Rose himself indicated that he 'was seized with a Broca's stroke' (p. 61), and from his self-report it would appear that his language disorder probably did resemble a Broca's aphasia. Rose made a number of observations of spelling errors—many of these appeared to be substitutions that were visually similar to the target word. The pattern of Rose's spelling errors has tended to be associated with a particular form of writing disorder, 'phonological agraphia', where the patient is partially or wholly reliant on using an established spelling vocabulary and cannot spell by using sound-based spelling rules (Shallice 1981). Note, for example, that two years after the onset of his aphasia, Rose still had difficulty in spelling *Tuesday* and *Wednesday*, words that do not have a close correspondence between grapheme and phoneme. Rose would, therefore, probably have had particular difficulty in spelling nonsense syllables, if this had been formally assessed.

REFERENCE

Shallice, T. (1981). Phonological agraphia and the lexical route in writing. *Brain*, **104**, 413–29.

Auto-observation of aphasia reported by an eminent nineteenth century medical scientist

Walther Riese

On the following pages an account of an incidence of 'alalia' as reported by the patient himself, and a medical and historical interpretation of the case, are presented. The patient was Jacques Lordat (1773–1870), an eminent member of the medical school of Montpellier (see Biographical Note at the end of this article).

THE LORDAT CASE[1]
(A SCIENTIST'S AUTO-OBSERVATION OF 'ALALIA')

. . . I noticed that when I wanted to speak I could not find the right expressions: this symptom, which came as a surprise, made me wonder. I tried to make myself believe that this impediment had been no more than a temporary distraction and that, with better concentration, my power of speech would be as good as before. In the midst of these reflections I was informed that a person who had come to the house to enquire about my health had refrained from paying me a visit for fear of disturbing me. I tried to utter a few words to acknowledge this courtesy. My thoughts were ready, but the sounds that should convey them to my informant were no longer at my disposal. Turning away in dismay, I said to myself: *So it's true that I can no longer speak!*

My impediment increased rapidly: within twenty-four hours all but a few words eluded my grasp. Those that did remain proved to be nearly useless, for I could no longer recall the way in which they had to be coordinated for the communication of ideas.

I was therefore suffering from an incomplete Alalia.

I was no longer able to grasp the ideas of others, for the very amnesia that prevented me from speaking made me incapable of understanding the sounds I heard quickly enough to grasp their meaning. The effort of remembering each sound would have taken too much time, and conversation is far too cursive to permit the understanding of a sufficient number of words . . .

. . . Inwardly, I felt the same as ever. This mental isolation which I mention, my sadness, my impediment and the appearance of stupidity which it gave rise to, led many to believe that my intellectual faculties were weakened . . .

It was a long while before I became fully aware of my condition. When I was alone and wide awake, I used to discuss within myself my life work and the studies I loved. Thinking caused me no difficulty whatever.

Accustomed as I was to pedagogical duties, I felt fortunate in this ability to arrange in my mind the principal propositions of a lecture, without encountering any difficulty in making whatever added changes I deemed propitious in the sequence of my ideas. My memory for facts, principles, dogmas, abstract ideas, was the same as when I enjoyed good health. Therefore I could not believe myself ill; the impediments under which I suffered seemed to be no more than dreams.

For a long period I had been content to fix the boundaries of thought, to develop it, to set rules for the subordination of ideas: expressions would fall into place without effort.

---

[1] From: *Analyse de la parole pour servir à la théorie de divers cas d'Alalie et de Paralalie (de Mutisme et d'Imperfection du parler) que les nosologistes ont mal connus.* Leçons tirées du Cours de Physiologie de l'année scolaire 1812–1813, par le professeur Lordat. Montpellier, Louis Castel, Libraire-Editeur, Grand'-Rue 32; Paris, J. B. Baillière, Germer-Baillière, Fortin Masson et Cie., 1843.

I did not make any progress in my reflections on my morbid state, each day telling myself that no symptom whatever remained; but as soon as anyone came to see me, I again became aware of my illness by my complete inability to say: 'Good day, how are you?'

I had to realize that the inner workings of the mind could dispense with words; that the embodiment of ideas was entirely different from the process of forming and combining them. Thus, while recognizing the instrumentality of language in conserving ideas, in preserving them for future reference, and in transmitting them, I was unable to accept completely Condillac's theory that verbal signs are necessary, even indispensable, for thought. Yes, I apprehended that of that total *logos* which I previously discussed with you, I was in full possession only of the inner aspect, having lost its external manifestations . . .

. . . If you have not given much thought to the extent of this amnesia, you might expect that I could have solaced myself by reading, but of this there was no possibility at first. In losing my memory of the meaning of articulating words, I also lost that of their visible signs. Syntax had disappeared along with words; the alphabet alone remained, but the junction of letters to form words was a study I would have to undertake.

When I wanted to glance at the book I had been reading when my disease declared itself, I found it impossible to read its title. I will not allude to my despair—you yourself can best imagine it. I was forced to spell out nearly every word, and I must confess, incidentally, this gave me the chance to realize the complete absurdity of French orthography. Then after several weeks of deep melancholy and resignation, it dawned on me that in looking from far away at an in-folio in my library I could read exactly the title *Hippocratis opera*. This discovery made tears of joy come to my eyes. I made use of this faculty to re-educate myself in speaking and in writing.

This re-education was a slow process, but every fortnight I was aware of appreciable progress . . .

Thus it becomes evident that nervous Ataxia, produced by several debilitating factors, had temporarily manifested its disorders in various areas and, locating itself in the brain, had arrested the function of retaining verbal sounds and their oral use, without in the least involving any of the other intellectual functions.

To this disease I have given the name of verbal amnesia . . .

My illness did not consist only in forgetting words and in not recalling the meaning of those I could still remember, but also in an instinctive suggestion of the words I knew but which I used incorrectly. It was not only a condition of amnesia, but a condition I should like to term *paramnesia*, that is, a faulty use of known and remembered sounds. Thus, when I wanted to ask for a *book*, I pronounced the words for *handkerchief*. However, immediately after having uttered this word, I retracted it, feeling that another was indicated. In other instances of disease of this type, I can mention patients who found themselves in a worse plight and who did not even realize that the word they used was not the correct one.

Another manifestation of my paramnesia consisted in an inversion of the letters of syllables in the polysyllabic words that I had just rediscovered; for instance, instead of *raisin*, I asked for *sairin*; for *musulman* I tended to say *sumulman*.

(Translated by Judd Hubert, Ph.D.,
Harvard University)

INTERPRETATION

Since the age of 10 years Lordat suffered from repeated tonsillar abscesses. On the fifteenth day of an attack which appeared on July 17, 1825, after long intellectual work and inner unrest, speech defects occurred, in modern terms, a transient mixed aphasia. In fact, he suddenly became unable to express his thought by the symbols of spoken language (motor aphasia). In his retrospective analysis, he used the term amnesia which was intended to express not only the lack of 'coordination'[2] of movements needed for

---

[2] In this respect it is significant that he shifted the syndrome to the class 'nervous ataxia'.

speech, but also the simultaneous defect of understanding (sensory aphasia). He immediately realized the integrity of thought and ideas which he was perfectly able to arrange and even to modify, in accordance with teaching purposes: 'My memory for facts, principles, dogmas, abstract ideas, was the same as when I enjoyed good health'. At the initial stage, there was also alexia. Moreover, the grammatical structure was lost (syntactical defect). After several weeks, his reading and writing abilities were regained; he then reeducated his speech; but he did not describe the methods used in this reeducation. He called the whole condition 'verbal amnesia', though the faulty use of words (verbal paraphasia) and letters (literal paraphasia) seemed to justify the term 'paramnesia'. That, generally speaking, he thought in terms of loss of memory (evocation) was, I submit, due to his insight into the *transient* nature of the whole condition.

HISTORICAL SIGNIFICANCE

Lordat's auto-observation ranks high among all contributions to the early history of aphasia.[3] Not only does it convey a description of the major defects seen and described much later in aphasics; it owes its specific and unique importance to the fact that it was made at this very initial stage of our knowledge of speech defects resulting from brain lesions, by a person of highest intellectual standing, endowed with a keen sense of self-analysis. But the problem involved, and a problem of greatest scope even to-day, is that of *interrelation of thought and language.*

The problem has been answered by two schools of thought. Humboldt[4] may be cited as a most eminent representative of one of them. Language, he taught, is the organ of *thought.* Intellectual activity passing without leaving any traces, as it were, through *speech* becomes perceptible to the senses. He asserted that intellect and speech are one and inseparable. The former is bound to be related to sound, otherwise thought attains no clarity and images do not ripen to concepts. The inseparable link of *vocal instruments, thought,* and *hearing* with speech has its irrevocable and unexplainable origin in human nature, he concluded.

Contemporary students of *aphasia* reached the conclusion that thought and language are neither identical nor parallel, though closely related to one another. According to Pick,[5] verbalization is, as a rule, preceded by a scheme or design of pure thought. But these two stages, leading from thought to speech, are not always sharply demarcated; at times verbalization taking place, while thought is still being organized. Therefore, the more verbalized thought, the greater the effect of aphasia on thought. 'Inner speech,' one of the most involved concepts, still lacking a unanimous definition, plays an important role in the formulation of thought, particularly, abstract thought. Goldstein called inner speech 'the totality of processes and experiences which occur when we are going to express our thoughts etc. in external speech, and when we perceive heard sounds as language'.[6] Pick believed that aphasia

---

[3] Lordat's influence in the history of aphasia was significant, though only indirect. His interpretation of loss of spoken language without paralysis of the tongue was adopted by the older Dax, who, too, believed in a disorder of the *synergy* of the muscles, needed for pronunciation. Most patients, he said, talk though they use wrong words. One of his own patients was able to move his tongue though he was completely mute. Dax was able to refer to similar observations made by Schenkius in the 16th century. Dax was the first to stress the importance of the left-sidedness of brain lesions in aphasics, though he did not bring it into relation to right-handedness. Nor was his son, who edited and completed the observations of his father, able to answer the question why just the left half of the brain was the site of lesions in patients losing their memories of words. But he ascertained, as Lordat did, their perfect 'intelligence'. (*L'aphasie* by G. Dax. Montepellier, C. Coulet, Paris, V.-A. Delahave, 1878.) See also: W. Riese, The early history of aphasia. *Bull. Hist. Med.,* 21: 322–334, 1947.

[4] W. v. Humboldt: *Ueber die Verschiedenheit des menschlichen Sprachbaues und ihren Einfluss auf die geistige Entwicklung des Menschengeschlechts.* Berlin, 1836, 511 pp.
[5] Aphasie. In: *Handbuch der normalen und pathologischen Physiologie.* Herausgegeben von A. Bethe, G. v. Bergmann, G. Embden, and A. Ellinger. 15. Band; Zweite Haelfte. Berlin, J. Springer, 1931.
[6] *Language and Language Disturbances.* New York, Grune & Stratton, 1948.

may have but little effect on mental behavior and thought in those instances in which only lower levels of receptive and expressive language are involved; it is different, however, as soon as inner speech is affected. But verbalization affects clearness, differentiation, and logical sequence of thought in different individuals in different ways.

Lordat's auto-observation was made a century before insight into the interrelation of thought and language was obtained from the study of aphasia. While his observation displays mastery of *description*, it still lacks the essential prerequisites to an *analysis* of the finer processes involved in disordered speech. More specifically, the extent to which Lordat's thought was verbalized normally, remains undisclosed. Nor are we informed about changes in the inner structure of his thought, once aphasia became manifest. This much, however, can be said, that he would hardly have been able to plan lectures and to organize the material needed, had his inner speech and his thought been affected to any major degree. At any rate, the problem was raised and discussed by Lordat for the first time in the history of aphasia.[7]

BIOGRAPHICAL NOTE[8]

Lordat was born in Tournay, near Tarbes, the 21st of February 1773. He began to study medicine in 1793, in Montpellier, and graduated from that school in 1797. It was

then that his friendship with Barthez began, who at the time of death bequeathed to Lordat his manuscripts. Lordat's teaching career which lasted for about 60 years, began at that time. He taught anatomy, physiology, and various subjects of medicine and surgery. In 1813, he succeeded Dumat as Professor of Physiology. He was a brilliant teacher and remained up to the 87th year of his life the most recognized representative of the famous Montpellier school of medical thought. He died in his 98th year.

List of Lordat's major writings:

1. Observations sur quelques points de l'anatomie du singe vert, 1804,
2. Traité des hémorrhagies, 1808,
3. Conseils sue la manière d'étudier la physiologie de l'homme, 1813,
4. Nouvelles remarques sur les hernies abdominales, 1811,
5. Exposition de la doctrine médicale de Barthez, 1818,
6. Du dialogisme oral dans l'enseignement public de la médecine, 1828,
7. Leçons extraites du cours de physiologie, rédigées par M. Kuehnholtz, 1830,
8. Deux leçons de physiologie rédigées par le même, 1832,
9. Essai sur l'iconologie médicale, ou sur les rapports d'utilité qui existent entre l'art du dessin et l'étude de la médecine, 1833,
10. Deux leçons de physiologie faites en 1832, 1833,

---

[7] One may cite as a counterpart the case of an outstanding figure in literature, Jonathan Swift, who died in the 78th year of his life, whose intelligence was severely disturbed in the last years of his life, and who also suffered from aphasia. This diagnosis was made for the first time by Craik in 1882, who judiciously drew attention to 'the automatic utterance of words ungoverned by intention'. In fact, Swift, though silent (mute) for a whole year, but evidently understanding everything that was said to him, was reported to have replied to his housekeeper who told him on his birthday that bonfires and illuminations were being prepared to celebrate it as usual: 'It is folly, they had better let it alone'. On another occasion, he repeated several times: 'I am what I am'; on still another occasion: 'I am a fool'. Once afterwards, as his servant was taking away his watch, he said: 'Bring it here' and. when the same servant was breaking a large hard

coal, he said: 'That is a stone, you blockhead.' Through Hughlings Jackson's masterly analysis of the 'speechless man' we have become acquainted with the 'recurrent utterances' of the aphasic and the preservation of his inferior or emotional speech. Both these criteria of aphasic behavior were very obvious in the Swift case; they were well described by those surrounding him almost 150 years before they were made the clue for a better understanding of aphasia by the eminent British clinician. (See: John Hawkesworth, *The Works of Dr. Jonathan Swift*, London, 1766; Leslie Stephen, *English Men of Letters*, New York, Macmillan & Co., pp. 186–209, 1882; and: Henry Craik, *The Life of Jonathan Swift*, London, John Murray, 1882, p. 561.)

---

[8] Adapted from the obituary published by the *Gazette des Hôpitaux*, **43**: 203–204, 1870.

11. Douze leçons de physiologie sur les fonctions privées du système musculaire chez l'homme, 1835,
12. De la perpétuité de la médecine ou de l'identité des principes fondamentaux de cette science, depuis son établissement jusqu'à présent, 1837,
13. Ière leçon du cours de physiologie faite en 1840–1841,
14. Deux leçons du cours de 1841 et 1842 sur les lois de l'hérédité physiologique comparée chez les bêtes et chez l'homme, 1842,
15. Sur la philosophie médicale de Montpellier, 1842,
16. Ebauche du plan d'un traité complet de physiologie humaine, 1841,
17. De l'insénescence de l'esprit de l'homme,
18. Sur la nécessité d'étudier les cas rares, 1842,
19. Rappel des principes doctrinaux de la constitution de l'homme, énoncés par Hippocrate, démontré par Barthez et développés par son école, 1857.

(Riese/Lordat 1954)

COMMENTARY

The paper written by Riese/Lordat includes a personal account by Lordat who was a distinguished professor of physiology in the early nineteenth century, having previously also taught medicine and surgery. Additional accounts of Lordat's aphasia have been provided by Alajouanine and Lhermitte (1964) and by Henderson (1989). It is difficult to be certain of the aetiology of Lordat's aphasia, which lasted for several weeks, but which left him with persistent word-finding difficulties for several years afterwards. He apparently had been susceptible to peritonsillar abscesses, and it therefore remains possible that he may have had a cerebral abscess or that he suffered a mild stroke.

Lordat's case is probably one of Wernicke's aphasia, although it could also be classified as 'transcortical sensory aphasia', in view of the intact repetition ability. Lordat himself described his aphasia as one of 'verbal amnesia', an amnesia both for words he spoke and for words that were spoken to him. He commented upon the many situations where he said the wrong word, was aware of this, and then retracted it. He called this 'paraphasia'. He also notes instances of getting phonemes within a word mixed up (e.g. saying 'sairin' for 'raisin').

Lordat's account of his aphasia predated the writings of Paul Broca and Carl Wernicke, and in some respects Lordat anticipated a number of issues that were to arise in their writings. It is a reflection on the sharpness of his intellect and the relative sparing of his thought processes that he was able to make specific observations relating to issues such as spelling errors, loss of meaning for word sounds, paraphasias, intactness of repetition, and the relationship between thought and language.

REFERENCES

Alajouanine, Th. and Lhermitte, F. (1964). Essai d'introspection de l'aphasie (l'aphasie vue par les aphasiques). *Revue Neurologique*, **110**, 609–21.

Henderson, V. W. (1989). Jacques Lordat's contributions to aphasiology. In *Neuroscience across the centuries* (ed. F. C. Rose), pp 177–84. Smith-Gordon, London.

Notes from an aphasic psychologist, or different strokes for different folks
(Overview article)

Scott Moss

Scott Moss was a clinical psychologist at the time of his stroke, having worked as a mental health consultant. He had just taken up a post as Professor of Clinical Psychology at the University of Illinois.

In contrast to other participants in this conference, let me say at the beginning that I am not a learned expert on aphasia—it is simply that I can talk about it from personal experience, that is, from an insider position, if you will. My stroke occurred over seven years ago, and the novelty and the trauma have long since worn off. It is as if it happened in another life or to another person, except that I am constantly reminded even now that talking or, to be explicit, thinking no longer comes easily as it did once. The value of my story is that I was originally trained as a psychologist.

My stroke took place when I was 43. I had just gone to the University of Illinois to inaugurate a program on community mental health. I had no preceding symptoms of which I was aware—in fact, just that day I had undergone a rather rigorous physical examination for admission to faculty status. Ten hours later I was flat on the family room floor, paralyzed on the dominant side of my body. This points out the fallacy of an annual physical exam, unless you have fairly specific symptoms. I had suffered a permanent blockage of the left internal carotid artery (but the meaning of this didn't really penetrate until two years later). I was semiconscious throughout the stroke.

When I awoke the next morning in the hospital, I was totally (globally) aphasic. I could understand vaguely what others said to me if it was spoken slowly and represented a very concrete form of action; otherwise, it was a language deficit which crossed all language modalities. I had lost completely the ability to talk, to read and to write. I even lost for the first two months the ability to use words internally, that is, in my thinking.

Another thing of interest, I had also lost the ability to dream. So, for a matter of eight to nine weeks, I lived in a total vacuum of self-produced concepts, i.e., during the daytime I had absolutely no words to express what was happening to me, not even to myself, and at night I had no dreams. My wife and I have written a book on the experience and the three years of what it was like recovering the lost thinking and language abilities (Moss, 1972).

At the outset, may I say that I have always thought it was most ironic that a psychologist, who had always listed a primary interest in communication in the APA Directory, and who 17 years before performed the first clinical dissertation for Charles Osgood (on a semantic differential study on dreams in psychotherapy), would be the victim of a stroke and resulting aphasia.

So, what is it like to be suddenly transformed from a 'therapist' to a brain-injured patient, one who suddenly cannot talk—one who was cutoff from all the ordinary ways of interpersonal communications? The very first thing to state was the growing awareness that medicine—like psychology—still remains an art rather than a science, despite the fact that there are over 400 000 stroke cases in the United States alone each year. For example, in spite of the fact of the abrupt onset of symptoms, for several days, they were uncertain of whether I had cancer of the lungs or a primary brain tumor. The result was that my wife in desperation had me transferred to a large hospital in Chicago, where they had the proper equipment and trained neurosurgeons, and there, with the aid of an angiogram and a vascular team they finally made the definite diagnosis.

Then, having performed the diagnostic function, we were simply thrown back into the home, totally on our own resources—without consultation, direction, or even medication. My wife must have been out of her wit's end, but she hid it from me, or rather, I was too far out of it to care. The explanation is, that, automatically, I had made the transition from an alive, energetic, enthusiastic husband and father, teacher and professional person to one that was resigned to the approach of death. Hazily, in my addled brain, I really believed that the next breath might be my last—and amazingly, it did not bother me. Even today, seven years later, I plan only for the foreseeable future. The omniscience and omnipotent illusions that surround the young had been penetrated and in one fell swoop I had learned that I was vulnerable. It was as if, in some ways, I was transformed in an instant into an aged old man, one who has constant difficulty in recollecting and putting his thoughts into words. As my wife stated in the book, during the first few months, I was simply the 'star boarder'. I made no demands upon anyone. I got out of bed, climbed into my robe and sat on the sofa, trying to make sense out of some programs on TV. I watched a great deal of TV—as a passive observer, relieved of demands that I interact in any way.

As I stated, we were simply thrown back into the home without any advice, and for some period of time we were completely bewildered, but then at my own insistence we began to take the initial steps at rehabilitation. Another marked feature was that I was rendered *concrete* in terms of my thinking. I retained only the most automatic functions. Thus, there seemed to be a relationship between the loss of language and abstraction. Bette and I began to combat the 'brain paralysis' by simple trial and error. For example, in the months after the stroke, my wife and I went painfully about completing five papers which I had obligated myself to write *before* the accident. I couldn't read and so she would read passages to me, and with her great assistance, she managed to write down what she thought I would have said before I had lost the use of language.

For the first time I began to feel anxious again. We went around and around on each sentence—every single word—on every single abstraction. Time and again I would say something unintelligible—a nonsense syllable as it were—and end up hitting my head with my hand, trying to drive lost words out of me. We were fortunate if we completed three or four paragraphs in a week. Our objective was one paragraph in a day—which in the beginning was a highly idealized and unrealistic goal. However, my wife, who was a former crackerjack secretary, by this stage in our marriage knew more or less the way I phrased things, so it ended up being partly my rendition and largely her understanding, in which she edited freely. The reinforcement came about when one by one every article was accepted for publication. Our old friend, Martin Scheer (of Goldstein-Scheer fame—God rest his soul!) would have been proud of us.

In February (three short months after the stroke) I volunteered to take my first graduate class and the head of clinical psychology was gracious enough to allow me to do so. I was partly motivated just to keep my hand in, and largely because we had no other source of income. It was in no way at the behest of my wife. I took responsibility for supervision in behavioral counseling where I had six students to monitor in the fundamentals of psychotherapy. So each week I would have at least six tapes to listen to in private and followup with consulting with each student about the pros and cons of the interaction. All during the first semester my wife listened with me to the tapes and then typed in my reactions to it. In my contact, I would refer back to the typed notes, more or less privately, I hoped, trying not to be too obvious that there was little, often no spontaneity. To give you some idea of my mental state at this time—I had to sit in my office for ten to fifteen minutes trying to think of how one goes out to the secretary's office and ask for, say, a pencil. The ability to read words had begun coming back to me, but still not the ability to comprehend them. At this juncture, I was still largely dependent on Bette's reading.

A third example, and this was after about

18 months. I still had a problem in auditing what I said, if at the same time, I had to conjure up any response. I could do *one* but not *both* of them. As a result I frequently judged that I did a terrible job talking. Finally, at Christmas time of 1969, I prevailed upon my wife to purchase me a secret tape recorder which I lugged about with me and recorded every lengthy transaction. (It was a briefcase in which one of the locks automatically triggered the recorder, with the mike being in the handle.) In time this did convince me that I did a fairly competent job speaking—all of this was pre-Watergate, of course. This points up that again and again we had to assume the initiative. In retrospect, we lived a daring life—always transversing a very thin line of what I could do and avoiding those things which I could not.

In terms of formal therapy, I had to take the initiative with respect to hypnotherapy, speech therapy and behavior modification. First, in January and February of the year following my stroke—about the same time as I began 'teaching' again—I had my wife call and make an appointment to see a world respected authority on aphasia. We travelled back to Chicago twice where I was tested both times and eventually saw Dr. X. In his opinion only time was required before I regained my former language–thinking facilities. The only difficulty was that the judgment was given without consulting my medical chart (he had assumed that a bit of fat was given off by my heart and had *temporarily* blocked an artery—which was not the case); secondly, he did indicate that speech therapy would do me no good— nevertheless, when we returned home, I promptly had my wife schedule me for speech therapy; third, when I eventually informed him that I was attempting to write an article about my stroke and asked him for the original test data, he indicated with some chagrin that it had been lost. Yet, to be absolutely fair, in retrospect, it was undoubtedly best that Dr. X shared his optimism with us, because we were looking desperately for some ray of hope. But this is about par for professional consultation—at least as we experienced it in the anxiety-filled, frustrating months immediately after the stroke.

Five months after the stroke, and again at my own initiative, I went for a five-day stay at a private psychiatric hospital, again in Chicago. I went for hypnotherapy since this was a technique which I had practiced successfully for 20 years. To say the least, it was a strange experience to be on the other side of the fence—as a psychiatric patient. Before I went, my entire existence was focused exclusively on the here-and-now. The stroke had abolished my memory of the past and projection of the future had absolutely no meaning for me. Even the names of our next-door neighbors in San Francisco, with whom we had been associated for over six years, was obliterated and every-day my wife would sit down to talk to me about past acquaintances and try to get me to remember and verbalize about it. Anyway, I came away depressed from the experience for the treatment had penetrated my intellectualized defenses, but shortly therefore, my life became unified again—the past and future became attuned with the present. In retrospect, this could have been due to the catharsis released under hypnosis—the alternative is simply ascribing it to the effect of 'spontaneous recovery'.

For a year and a half, I was in speech therapy with three successive speech students. In the book I do not treat speech therapists too kindly. I do feel very frankly that they did not know how to treat the higher-ordered difficulties that I presented. They really were corrupted by having to treat aphasic clients who had severe speech disorders—they simply did not know how to 'move upstream' and handle the massive memory deficits and the concreteness of thought. (On the other hand, in the midst of speech therapy, when I took a course on psycholinguistics from a former student of Schuell, it was very intellectually enlightening, but not at all helpful. The professor insisted that not enough was known about the nature of aphasia to plan any form of treatment.) Coming back to speech therapy: I shall always be grateful that they were willing to accept me, that they gave my wife some richly deserved relief, and the generally accepting-supportive type of counseling, even though it was primarily nondirective or self-directed therapy. And if I may say so again, I still feel badly that the head of the speech clinic, with whom I had established a rather close relationship, never acknowledged any of my letters, including two Christmas cards, *after* I sent him a galley of our joint chapter for review.

When I went to Illinois I knew full well that the clinical faculty was steeped in behavior modification. I went with the intention of incorporating behavioral methodology into my specialty, community psychology. Naively, I thought I was being brought aboard to leaven (dilute) the strong behavioral trend. Only much, much later did it become apparent that this was the intention of the other experimental faculty members, not of the militant clinicians. During the period of my recovery it became obvious that if anyone was to change, it had to be me. In reaction, the first course I finally instituted 16 months after the accident was on hypno-symbolism (self-analysis of dreams using hypnosis to circumvent the interpretations of the therapist). This was because I had a large supply of audiotapes which partially relieved me from the duress of talking and partly based on frank rebellion. The point is that even though the clinical services were modeled on behavioral theory and practice, it was a scene that for me was lacking in reinforcement. In fairness, however, let me state that the relationship between myself and the other clinical faculty members was quite good, and again I will always be grateful that the University was willing to carry me on during this period of personalized turmoil.

However, it eventually dawned on me that I would be foolish not to make use of behavioral modification. I searched around among the staff and eventually found a person willing to take me on for behavioral therapy. Once we began behavior therapy, I was very pleasantly surprised to find that the therapist, while following social learning dictates, was also intelligent, flexible and pragmatic, and as a result we got along very well. He began with progressive relaxation and rapidly it developed into systematic desensitization. I went along with his attempt to rid me of a host of anxieties related to speaking. But most of all, I enjoyed the opportunity just to sit down with a peer and discuss my current and pending adjustment. The one thing that I felt was totally lacking was that I still wanted to go back to the trauma (and I stated it at the time to the therapist) to relieve the experience, to cathart and to ventilate, to work through my intellectualized defenses, a need that was only partially taken care of in my brief brush with hypnotherapy. On the basis of his theoretical predilections, of course, he was unwilling to go back. In retrospect, I think his reluctance gave added impetus to writing the book.

Please forgive me if we detour briefly to say a few words about my *self-concept*. I was oriented as to place, time and persons, except I could deal only with the immediate present in terms of very concrete actions. The part of myself that was missing was intellectual aspect—the sine qua non of my personality—those essential elements most important to being a unique individual, rather than being relegated to being a mere cipher lost in the system. After I got over the initial shock of the stroke, this more than anything else spurred me on to the degree of recovery which I made. For a long period of time I looked upon myself as only half a man but each time that I tried to apply myself intellectually, I would be confronted by the absolute inability to do what I had done such a short time before. To spell it out very concretely, four years after the accident, when confronted by an intelligence test, it still took me ten times as long to solve an arithmetic problem as it had earlier, commensurate with my intellectual level. But the most impressive thing was that, given unlimited time, I still was able to solve it.

A lot of emphasis is placed in the book on the term *perfectionism*. Perfectionism, like any other human trait, is a two-sided coin. It undoubtedly grew out of the inferiority that every child experiences, however, the tools to combat it I gathered along the way, specifically in college and in the study of psychology. It may be a gross oversimplification but to borrow from Adler, all of my life has been a struggle to combat the feelings of inferiority by compensation and overcompensation.

Thus, when the stroke hit, I again tried to fight the impairment every way that I knew how. This is the reason why in the book, an autobiographical chapter has been written on my upbringing and the reason why the book was dedicated to my mother.

Seven years after the stroke I am still bothered by residuals. However, whether they are motoric, intellectual, in terms of memory of speaking, I take great pride in compensating for them. Three years after the stroke we moved back to California. The publication of the book on aphasia laid it all out for everyone to see. I took some delight in pointing out to selected new acquaintances the various ways that I compensated. For instance, that I seldom handwrite anything (cursive handwriting still eludes me), or that I am now perpetually confused as to which is 'left' and which is 'right', or that I am very circumspect about carrying on an extended conversation in any context (I still have difficulty in selecting words and my verbal attention span is still limited—thus this paper), or that ever since the stroke my sleeping time has been cut to approximately five hours. This makes me a natural experiment in dream deprivation; e.g., instead of culminating with two hours of dream time, I awaken about 4 or 5 a.m., get up and begin to think about resolving problems for that day.

I have confidence in my ability to keep my handicaps under control, as long as I have the option to plan ahead about my involvement. I still must walk a line between what I can do and what I cannot do. When I came as a psychologist to the prison, my thought was of retirement. Since that time I have been promoted to the Mental Health Coordinator's position and recently I spent seven months as the Western Region Mental Administrator—overseeing mental health activities in all federal prisons west of the Mississippi—a job from which I have since resigned, when it became necessary to move elsewhere.

I have no question that I profited from each formal type of therapy, however, each kind had to be made consistent to my already established life-style. I can say without question that my wife was the primary therapist.

The book, all the way through, is an eloquent testimony to her role as a wife, mother and an untrained paraprofessional worker. It was her love and devotion, her persistence and patience, her willingness to put up with all sorts of problems for which she was totally untrained. In the first three years she spent every waking minute with me, outside of meeting the demands of our three young children.

In recent years my wife and I have attended numerous stroke seminars as joint speakers. I know if she were up here with me that she would emphasize several things:

1. Persistently try and try again whatever treatment methods that are available to you for nobody has *the* answer—but also, as the spouse gets better, feel free to innovate.

2. Remember that the patient (client) does not go through this by himself, he needs the continuous support of his spouse and other family members—which is another way of saying that in the three years of rehabilitation, not once, not a single time was she invited in by any of my therapists. So, she would say, 'make therapy a family affair' because it is an illness that affects every family member.

3. If I may quote from one of her recent talks, 'You work with him, you learn with him, you try to understand him, you praise him and try to maintain a sense of humor, and, of course, most of all, let him know you care'.

She would also state how fortunate she was to have a patient-psychologist as a consultant. Perhaps, in addition to her ever present T.L.C. (tender-loving-care) was the information provided by my professional training and knowledge, plus my determination and the trait of high perfectionism, plus the fact that I was not brain injured enough to lose the potentiality of recovering. This last point is the reason for the title of my paper: It reflects that we still do not know nearly enough about human brain injury to allow us to make many generalized statements. (There is also a hidden reason: If the title still seems inconsistent to the serious body of my talk, I had always taken great pride in my pre-accident sense of humor. After the stroke I could no longer move incisively into a conversation and at the exact split moment render a humorous comment. I still lament this loss.)

Anyway, I would firmly acquiesce in my wife's suggestions and finally make the following suggestion as well: In time I came to realize that every single interaction of mine had at least two implications: It was partly altrustic (as a father, husband and clinician I was *still* busy doing things for others) but in larger part it was very much self-service. That is, every interaction was unabashedly therapy or rehabilitation for me.

In the last analysis, the stroke-afflicted individual (like every other human affliction) must take the responsibility of assisting himself, no one else can do it for you; at the same time, I would say that clinicians should not be so hesitant to take some responsibility for help or assistance to brain injured people. It sounds trite, because all of us are taught this in introductory courses, but then we apparently forget it: Remember that behavior or function always stems from the body or the soma and you can't treat one without the other if you wish to treat the *whole individual.*

In summary, what can I say from this single case presentation? Logically, an aphasic is a person who has total or partial loss of understanding or use of words, caused by brain injury. There is absolutely no doubt that for at least six months I was aphasic, and in the beginning weeks, totally. I did suffer from both an internal and external loss of speech in the beginning. My accident confirms that aphasia presents an overall psychological and physiological syndrome that far outreaches the loss of language skills. (a) Intelligence and memory most affected in my case; e.g., input as well as output, as exemplified by the loss of my total inability to deal with abstract concepts or my inability to conjour up a lost word or sentence. (b) The *psychological trauma* that occurs when the stroke patient discovers that he has not only lost his ability to communicate effectively and to think concisely, but his ability to resume meaningful and challenging work or to function as the head family member. In many ways you become a child again. (c) The factor of *fatigue* was not evident in my case, once I got over the initial impact, except for the *anxiety-fatigue* which accompanied any effort to deal abstractly with my colleagues or students; but the majority of aphasic-stroke patients apparently have little vitality. (d) Motor paralysis is the most apparent symptom of a stroke. Mine disappeared within hours, except for facial paralysis which continued to linger for a couple of days. Yet, there were many times during the three years when I secretly wished I had a white cane to symbolize that something had happened—why I could not speak—why I couldn't think too well.

The presentation dealt mainly with the factors which I believe led to my recovery. One final comment: In my particular brand of aphasia, the key seems to reside much more in deficiencies of memory and/or concreteness in thinking, rather than in rehabilitation in the speech area per se. I never needed to be retaught things—like the a, b, c's—instead, I was always in a tip-of-the-tongue state, where I badly needed constant companionship to remind me of past learning and to put the memory tapes back into some sort of usable order. The memory banks were out of order and the ability to abstract were in total disarray.

(Moss 1976)

The accident and the ensuing six months
(Chapter 1 from the original book)

In September, 1967, I left a position as mental health consultant for the National Institute of Mental Health in San Francisco, where I had enjoyed six years of productive service in promoting the National Mental Health Program in the western region of the U.S. Public Health Service, and took a job as professor of clinical psychology at the University of Illinois. I was returning to the university where I had originally taken my graduate training, and I considered it a distinct honor to be invited back to teach at my alma mater. I was slated to initiate a program in community mental health. The move back to the Midwest did not proceed too smoothly, however; my son Joel fell and broke his arm on the first day of school while we were still in San Carlos. He required surgery and it was decided that the family should remain while I went on ahead.

I lodged in the apartment of my mother, who had preceded us from San Carlos. She had dumped her many cartons into an apartment and departed for Madison, Wisconsin, our original home. I was thankful that at least I had a bed on which to sleep. In the first week of October, I took a flight back to San Francisco, my family met me at the airport with the car fully loaded, and we began immediately the long drive back to Urbana. I had already found a house to rent and shortly thereafter the moving van appeared with the furniture. In the next week we got both the Moss households settled.

The week following I departed for a symposium on the 'New Biology of Dreaming' at the University of Cincinnati Medical School. It was a very cold day and the train from Champaign to Chicago had no heat. I began to develop what seemed to be a bad cold that continued to plague me for the next two weeks. Of course, during all this time I was undergoing a general orientation to university life, there were courses to prepare, and I was beginning to meet the many demands of my graduate students. Just before departing for Cincinnati, for instance, I gave a large group of graduate students and faculty a colloquium address on the scope of things to come in the nationally developing community mental health program. So while things were hectic, I would say that they were no more so than the usual pace of my professional and personal life for the last twenty years. I had no impending awareness at all of any catastrophe.

On Monday, October 30, I was working in my office at about four o'clock when a colleague of mine, Len Ullmann, came in. It was during this session that I experienced an abrupt coughing spell which I attributed to his cigarette smoke. I excused myself and went to the drinking fountain, and after a few minutes the coughing subsided. However, I noticed then that vision in my right eye had become askewed. Also, the thumb on my right hand had become numb. I attempted to continue working, but my vision prevented concentration on the written material. So at a few minutes before five I decided to go home. I commented to my wife on my peculiar symptoms, but actually regarded them as only minor, though troublesome, afflictions that I hoped would soon pass.

After dinner I again attempted to read the newspaper, but couldn't, and I began to experience a sharp pain that was at first in the back of my head and then moved to the left side of my temple. I have never been bothered by headaches and I suppose this should have alerted me that something was terribly amiss, but it didn't. My wife fixed a hot water bottle and I held it to the side of my head. By about ten o'clock the pain had somewhat subsided though my eyesight had not improved, and I settled down to try to watch a replay of a recent Green Bay–Bears game.

At about eleven o'clock I experienced another coughing spell, and this one would not stop. My wife became frightened and, wishing to believe that I was teasing her, turned off the TV. Despite my coughing I made a move toward the TV, only to find myself on the floor. Though I did not realize it at the time, the right side of my body had become paralyzed. Bette thought for a moment that I was malingering; however, as she explained to me much later, she knew something had happened when I tried to smile at her and only the left side of my face lit up. I heard her go to the phone and summon an ambulance. She then came back beside me and attempted to subdue my further efforts to rise.

I was conscious or at least semiconscious the whole time. I vaguely remember seeing the ambulance drivers coming in, being rolled onto a cot, feeling rain fall on my face, hearing the sound of the distant siren, and being taken to the emergency room at a local hospital. There was a nurse and also an attendant there who tried to speak with me. Things were hazy but I was in no pain, although I could not talk back to them. Eventually my wife arrived, having called the director of the clinical psychology division, Don Peterson, who came and stayed with the children while Bette came to the hospital. At about one o'clock the doctor in charge of the emergency calls arrived. I then did in retrospect an amazing thing: the paralysis had largely left me and I shifted over on my side and proceeded to engage in an appropriate conversation, experiencing only one or two blocks.

I was then wheeled upstairs to the pediatrics ward, since there were no beds on the adult wards. Bette stayed with me until almost three o'clock. For some reason I remember feeling very depressed. One could call it a premonition of things to come. Just that morning I had taken and passed my physical exam for incoming faculty members. Thinking about it months later, it became obvious to me that such examinations are limited in value in the absence of specific symptoms, since a few hours after the exam I was to suffer a debilitating stroke.

The next morning when I awoke, I was completely and totally aphasic. I was given a neurological examination, an EEG, and later a chest X-ray. As I learned later, the hospital simply lacked skilled clinicians to diagnose my case, though obviously I was a severely brain-damaged patient. On the fourth day, at the insistence of my wife, I was transferred by ambulance to Presbyterian–St. Luke's Hospital in Chicago. My wife and my mother accompanied me in the ambulance. For eight days the staff there pried and prodded me: a brain scan, spinal tap, skull films, and an angiogram were among the techniques utilized.

My life as a patient was uneventful. I was still in no pain. For the most part, I simply slept or dozed. I did comprehend somewhat vaguely what was said to me, but I could not answer except in gestures or by neologisms. I knew the language I used was not correct but I was quite unable to select the appropriate words. I recollect trying to read the headlines of the Chicago Tribune but they didn't make any sense to me at all. I didn't have any difficulty focusing; it was simply that the words, individually or in combination, didn't have meaning, and even more amazing, I was only a trifle bothered by that fact.

My wife and my mother were with me and they helped comfort me, feeding me at mealtime and keeping me company. My appetite was largely delinquent, and in the next couple of weeks my weight fell twenty pounds. I did not have a bowel movement during the week I was hospitalized, and fortunately or otherwise no one thought to check on it. I did feel critical (and still do) about the way I was handled by the two surgical residents assigned to my case. Quite unintentionally they imparted the feeling that they were only interested in my *neurological* impairment, and didn't respond to me as a whole human being, one filled with *psychological* reactions at having suffered a catastrophic accident. I attributed this initially to the fact that I couldn't communicate with them and therefore was not sensitive to their interactions with me. Now I realize that this was standard procedure for neurosurgeons, but I still think it is a shame not to treat the patient as a whole personality.

As I look back on it now, I had relatively little concern for the children, my wife, or the home—I was too far out of it to care. I had come so very close to death that I more or less welcomed it. It was indeed, as I experienced it, a very painless way to go. In fact, for a long time afterwards I was confident that I was living on borrowed time, and I expected it to expire at any moment. It was as if the stroke had benumbed any emotional investment in the future and I simply shrugged at my perception of my imminent demise.

At the end of a full week, and again at the behest of my wife, I was discharged. A student and his wife drove our car to Chicago and I recall that I was slightly chagrined that I could not converse with them on the drive home. A colleague and his wife had stayed at the house with the children and apparently they all got along very well. It was nice to be in familiar surroundings again.

For a month I stayed in bed or lounged about the house in my bathrobe. A few words of halting, limited speech began to come back to me. Eventually it was time to go to the office again. My wife transported me to and from campus for the next three weeks. They were only token visits and I would stay for about half an hour. Later, when I began driving myself, it was at first strange. It was as if I were learning to coordinate the visual-motor function all over again. The members of the staff seemed glad to see me, and it was nice to be back again, but the difference was simply enormous. I was unable to engage in even normal conversation, let alone deal with more elaborate conceptions. For instance, despite my best efforts I would block even on the most minimal words. Holding a minor conversation of even a few words would be quite taxing for me. I could never tell if what I had to say would come out right—even asking for a pencil from the secretary had to be elaborately planned and painfully carried out.

The second week I ran into a colleague who happened to mention that it must be very frustrating for me to be aphasic since prior to that I had been so verbally facile. I assured him that it was not upsetting and then later found myself wondering why it was not. I think part of the explanation was relatively simple. If I had lost the ability to

converse with others, I had also lost the ability even to engage in self-talk. In other words, I did not have the ability to think about the future—to worry, to anticipate or perceive it—at least not with words. Thus, for the first five or six weeks after hospitalization I simply existed. So the fact that I could not use words even internally was, in fact, a safeguard. I imagine it was somewhat similar to undergoing a lobotomy or lobectomy in the dissociation from the future. It was as if without words I could not be concerned about tomorrow.

In the period of January 9 to January 23, I had two meetings in Chicago with Dr. Joseph Wepman, a psychological expert in aphasia. Bette accompanied me by train on the 125–mile trip. I was given a series of tests, and while my performance was of a high level compared to the average brain-damaged patient, nevertheless I was aware of some impairment on the items. I had extreme difficulty in following abstractions of a professional nature (I could follow the meaning of a single sentence but I had difficulty in comprehending the whole). Similarly, I had difficulty in following a digit span for more than five or six numbers (less backwards) and also in defining proverbs (I could still define them at an abstract level but now I had to work around to the answer rather than going directly to it as I had done before). I also had decided deficits in memory. Immediately upon my return from Presbyterian–St. Luke's, I sat down with my wife and tried to remember the names of people we had known in San Carlos; while I was able to picture them, I was completely unable to recall their names, even those of our two next-door neighbors.

It was with regard to a summary meeting with Dr. Wepman in about the middle of January that I found myself while in the bathtub actually beginning to anticipate the rudiments of a discussion that I would have with him.[1]

---

[1] I used to love hot baths during this period. I liked to soak for 45 minutes to an hour, two or even three times a day. Lest the psychodynamically inclined be tempted to overinterpret, this was because the house we had rented turned out to be incompletely insulated.

Thus, for the first time I was aware that my inner speech was returning. It is difficult to explain what it was like to be entirely without internal verbalizations. I bathed, shaved, and selected my clothing with appropriateness, for instance, on the few occasions when I got dressed, but without words to express what I was doing, even to myself. It was as though I could perform the automatic habits that I had learned through a lifetime, but would be lost once the demands were made for increasing abstractness.

At this meeting on the 23rd, Dr. Wepman reported that I had improved greatly in the three-week interim, and that in several more months I should be largely restored. He did not have knowledge of what had actually happened to me, because he had not had access to the medical report. He assumed that fat had been given off from the heart, had blocked the carotid artery temporarily, and then had been dissolved. He stated that if the block had remained lodged for even four or five minutes, I would have become a 'vegetable'. He also said I would continue to manifest organic symptoms for the next several months, but he saw no reason to continue seeing me since I would readily improve. He would be happy to see me in the spring when I was recovered! He concluded that since I had absolutely no premorbid signs this was a 'one-time' thing for me.

Finally, he stated that I would benefit little from seeing a speech therapist. From his point of view, time was the primary factor in my recovery, and this was a physiological rather a psychological factor. It was in this conversation that he happened to remark that Dr. Erika Fromm (also at the University of Chicago) had worked for the past couple of years with hypnosis in simulating organic symptoms in normal subjects. I at once replied that I knew Erika and it would be interesting to provide her a brain-injured patient, myself, and see what she could do about restoring normality through hypnosis and age regression. Hypnosis and hypnotherapy had been an interest of mine throughout my professional career.

From that date until early in March I continued to improve. I could exchange pleasantries with a person as long as it was not expected that I would initiate topics or provide much information. I still was unable to handle the abstractions involved in clinical work. I could not read literature or really talk with my colleagues about professional issues. My wife and I nevertheless worked as hard as we were able to recapture my facility with professional jargon and to renew my acquaintance with abstract conceptions. Around the time that I began to visit my office again, we sat down to work on five papers which I had committed myself to complete. The first paper was a survey on the 'Experimental Induction of Dreams'. Fortunately, I had progressed considerably on the paper before my accident, but it still had to be finished, tidied up, and typed.

I cannot begin to describe how immensely difficult it was to read and summarize the various passages that still remained. It was an unholy, tortuous business. I attempted to dictate to Bette what I wanted to say, and not being able to do this, I reacted strongly at times, sometimes pounding my fists or simply repeating the same gibberish over and over. The normal anxiety over my immediate performance was obviously beginning to return. It seemed so much easier to have my wife read the passages and have me somehow, with her great assistance, manage to indicate what should be done with them. I would stumble about, trying somehow to voice the meaning, my wife would listen to me for some period of time, and then attempt to repeat the gist of what I had to say. Often we would go round and round on certain issues. The result was that the paper ended up half mine and half her own translation of what she thought I had meant to convey. The editors' acceptance of the paper a few weeks later greatly buoyed our spirits (Moss, 1968). Gradually, over some months, as I did a better job of dictating, these extremely difficult periods tended to subside, although I have always been critical about my performance without really being able to do much about it.

On February 1 I volunteered to take on a section of eight students, monitoring them in psychotherapy. Don Peterson was delighted, but I did this with considerable hesitance. It was again a matter of my walking a narrow line between what I was able to do and what I could not yet afford to do. I could not speak with the students at all in the way that I formerly had, being unable to discuss the therapy recordings in detail or their ramifications. Nevertheless, I could deal with questions in a sort of nondirective fashion, as long as too copious an answer wasn't demanded. I also listened to the student-client recordings between sessions and directed Bette to transcribe selected responses while trying not to rob the sessions of all their spontaneity in the process. I managed to complete the course in June, and the students were most generous in their ratings of my performance, though I felt much less than adequate.

It was of interest to me how in a day or even an hour I could feel relatively good and the next moment regress. This matter of recovery is an uncertain thing—it is an uphill struggle of a most uneven character. When I responded to external demands, I could marshal unusual effort for a limited time; for example, when talking on the telephone with the friends and acquaintances who called us I was probably at my optimum. It reminded me of having heard of stutterers who lose their speech defect on the phone. It may have had some relationship to the restricted number of stimuli which I was forced to cope with on the phone. But given time to sit around the house and dwell on my symptoms, or in any type of direct interpersonal relationship and every contact extended me, I was immediately reminded of my glaring deficiencies.

I also found that I was easily distracted; for example, I was not too restrained with the children. Before, I had been able to select what I wanted to watch on TV and noises had not bothered me. But now I found that any distraction was quite upsetting, and I reacted by removing the offender or turning up the volume on the TV until the noise became intolerable to others. On the other side, the TV was a great pacifier: I could vicariously enjoy the human interactions without being called upon to participate.

In February, 1968, I began therapy with the university speech department. I felt that there was virtue in giving my wife some respite from my many demands on her. I met twice a week with a young graduate trainee who was unstructured in her demands but who gave me her undivided attention for an hour each week. On February 27 I reported that for the first time since my accident I remembered a dream. It was of interest to me that for the four-month period I did not recall a single dream. This struck me as a curious state of affairs since for years I had been interested in the study and meaning of dreams; however, my stroke apparently impaired either the ability to have dreams or my capacity to remember them. I lay down each night for seven or eight hours of uninterrupted sleep. It was as if during the daytime I had no words to express what was happening and at night I had no dreams—it was a complete and total vacuum of self-speech for me.

Perhaps Greenberg and Dewan (1968) are correct in saying that in aphasia dreaming serves to integrate new information into existing past information stores. I tended to dream in pictures, of course, but without words the memory of these nocturnal images was lost. Since my big white boxer dog 'dreams' every evening without words, for example, this leads to the speculation that perhaps I didn't dream during the recovery period from my accident. How else would one account for the fact that even today I hold many waking memories from my period of hospitalization and the first few months when I had no words to describe these events even to myself, but at the same time do not remember having dreamed at all during these four months. Further evidence is that as I recovered my internal verbalizations, the memory of nocturnal mentation began to recur.

When I entered into ordinary conversation after five or six months, I had progressed sufficiently to talk more or less normally until I came to a word on which I might block. Unlike former times at that juncture, *absolutely nothing* came to mind—it was an absolute zero—there were no alternatives from which to choose. I purchased a crossword puzzle book to give me facility in learning synonyms. The problem of dealing with abstractions also continued to plague me during this period. It took a great deal of effort for me to keep an abstraction in mind. For example, in talking with the speech therapist I would begin to give a definition of an abstract concern, but as I held it in mind it would sort of fade, and chances were that I'd end up giving a simplified version rather than one at the original level of conception. It was as though giving an abstraction required so much of my addled intelligence that halfway through the definition I would run out of the energy available to me and regress to a more concrete answer. Something like this happened again and again.

It was also fascinating to me how completely and totally fixed I was on the 'here and now'. Even former events just prior to my accident had faded. In regard to my professional work, I recognized the terms that were used, but in a sense they had receded into the distant past rather than being immediately in my awareness. And in the same vein, thought about the future was most difficult. So both the past and the future had faded for me, and I existed almost exclusively in the present. In working with my speech therapist, for instance, I had been attempting to explain the general conceptions of community health. As long as I stuck to the paper or an outline, I did relatively well. But without the outline I rapidly floundered, although I could answer specific questions that were asked. In essence, then, I was unable to keep in mind a verbal outline of what I had to say. This in broader perspective is what happened to me generally. I was unable to generate a gestalt of either my previous life or the future, and therefore life beyond the immediate situation was meaningless. This restriction held not only for my work but for all personal life as well. For example, five months after the accident I was able to recall occasionally the names of some people who were our San Carlos neighbors, but I could not embroider them with associations as I had formerly.

From March 14 through March 18 I was a patient at Michael Reese Hospital, where I had volunteered as an experimental subject for Dr. Doris Gruenewald, a colleague of Erika Fromm whom I had also met previously. I traveled to Chicago without my wife, which indicates that I was making some progress. It was Dr. Gruenewald's job, if possible, to induce me into hypnosis, cause me to regress beyond the time when I had suffered my stroke, and determine whether I had recovered, to any appreciable extent, my normal method of speaking and thinking. It was at best a far-out experimental effort which reflected my desperation that hypnotheraphy might help.

I was admitted to a locked psychiatric ward in which most of the patients had partial 'open-door privileges'. It was a peculiar and unique personal experience for anyone, especially for a clinical psychologist who often had wondered what the experience would be like behind locked doors. I was treated exactly the same as all the other patients; for instance, the nurses immediately went through my suitcase and took my medicine and my razor. Prior to any attempts at hypnosis, I was given a complete physical and neurological examination. I passed the examination in excellent shape. I also had a prehypnotic EEG taken while I was in a drugged sleep. The reason for this phase of the study was a report by Kupper in 1945. Through hypnotic age-regression he had supposedly transported an epileptic patient back beyond the period of traumatic injury and what had previously been very morbid then turned into a normal-appearing electro-encephalogram. I was extremely skeptical of this experiment; no one had replicated the study to my knowledge.

During the examination with Doris Gruenewald, it occurred to me to tell her of an experience which I had suffered twenty-two years before. I was stationed for the last year of military service in World War II with a B-29 group on Guam. When we were not busy with the planes, we used to play a great deal of bridge, often three to five hours a day. In the middle of February, 1946, I was transported back to the United States and in a couple of days was separated from service. Sometime that summer, a group of us were sitting around when I suggested that perhaps we could play bridge. None of the rest knew the game so I volunteered to teach them. I took a pack of cards, shuffled them, and then found I couldn't remember a thing about how to play bridge, that is, I couldn't remember how many cards were dealt, if you drew for some cards—in short, absolutely nothing. I had to buy a book to recapture how to play bridge. I attributed this experience to essentially two factors: (1) a complete change of setting so that past associations with bridge had been completely cut off, and (2) the repression with which I dealt with my combat experiences. During the period of military service, I had kept rather complete records of what I did. Later, in going through these diaries, I recalled the things that had happened to me, but in a very real sense I had intellectualized and isolated them from the associated affect. It was in a way as if I had never been in service at all. I recalled this as a way of explaining my sense of distance from things both of a personal and professional nature prior to my accident.

Dr. Gruenewald, of course, suspected that perhaps I had an ulterior motive in telling her of this episode. It became increasingly clear to me as we talked that I had never really experienced any real affective discharge toward this stroke. For the first six or seven weeks I had experienced no emotion at all, then later, until now, I had experienced momentary frustrations toward internal or external obstacles, but again, no ventilation regarding my disability. I had in a sense treated my whole accident as if I were sort of an experimental subject, an 'object' for investigation rather than a person who had experienced a terrible trauma. It was a defense consistent with my identity as a professional person interested in research. Each person adapts to his organicity with his inbuilt psychological mechanisms.

The first session brought home to me the degree to which I had suppressed the situation. I was not a good hypnotic subject, as I might have suspected from studies having to do with the susceptibility of other operators. Nevertheless, I listened to Doris's induction procedures on hypnosis and tried to follow them, although it was very difficult not to intellectualize the situation. I succeeded in going into a very modest trance or at least a hypnoidal state. During this initial session,

Doris asked me to go back to San Carlos and, through a projective hypnotic technique, inquired what I was doing. I thought of the house and pictured Bette and me working outside, planting flowers. I was immediately caught up in what it had meant for Bette and the children to move to Illinois. It was quite a concession for her to have to cut herself off from her friends and her home there. Very soon the tears were flowing. Bette and the children had given up so much to come here, primarily for the furthering of my professional career, which had now been cut short.

In the second session, Doris relinquished her attempts at hypnosis and placed the responsibility directly on me. Again, I have the feeling that I was partially successful in inducing self-hypnosis, although we spoke mostly of my professional activities with NIMH. I recalled that the night before I had had what might be called a posthypnotic dream. I was back working for NIMH and was busy looking through a list of research-approved grants, attempting to find out what happened to the grant of a colleague at the university. Then the scene was transformed and I was engaged in giving research consultation. I don't remember the details, but we were having an excellent time and I performed most adequately. This recalled in turn the first dream that I had had on February 27. In that dream I had accepted the fact that I was limited because of my stroke and had gone back to work at Fulton State Hospital (in Missouri). I was in charge of the psychology training program. Since I was unable to train people directly, because of my accident, I was looking through a file drawer of previous tapes that might be utilized for that purpose. We felt that the dream about NIMH was relatively positive in contrast to the earlier dream, which featured my acceptance of my disability.

Dr. Gruenewald had prepared a series of psychological tests based on my description of the areas in which I still suffered some deficit. On the day of my admission, I took a test battery in the waking condition and repeated it under hypnosis; but I do not think it was really successful. On Monday afternoon, prior to my departure from the hospital, I had a postexperimental battery. We tried hetero- and auto-hypnosis in relation to the test battery, but the effect, if any, soon wore off. In the EEG laboratory I attempted autohypnosis in lieu of drugs and surprisingly seemed to go to sleep without any medication. The lab technician at the time reported that I had been deeply asleep, but later in her written report of the examination stated that I was awake during the procedure, apparently because no medication was given to induce physiological sleep. The second EEG was essentially similar to the first. Six weeks later, a report from Doris on the psychological tests stated that there was no difference between the pre- and post-tests other than a slight positive finding on the post-test which could be attributable to a practice effect.

There is one other important event that bears mention in this brief period of hospitalization. I was interviewed by the ward psychiatrist, and in going over what had happened to me I recounted how the past and the future seemed to have lost all meaning for me. He dismissed this symptom as a variation of retrograde amnesia, although he admitted he had never heard a patient discuss the symptom quite as I had. In retrospect, I doubt very much that his conception could have been an explanation of what I had experienced. As I understand it, the victim either organically blots out or represses the specific circumstances surrounding the time of his accident and the immediate

events leading up to it. My problem was exactly the opposite: I remembered in great detail the situation leading up to my accident and the trauma surrounding it. It was, in effect, an event that I remembered *too well* (even though I had no words to describe much of it at the time). The stroke acted as some sort of massive retroactive inhibition[2] which caused the gross dilution of all other experiences in my life.

Anyway, I came home from the hospital and for the next three weeks was deeply depressed. It was a most unusual depression for me since formerly I had tended to bounce back quickly from adversity. Bette was coming down with a cold and I did not tell her what had transpired except in very general terms. But when the depression lifted, the sense of distance from my past and future life was also gone. My life had become unified again! Somehow I connect my perception of the concept of *time* with this event. When I came to Illinois, I had an infinite amount of time to continue my professional career; after the accident, every minute was at a premium. It was as though in the instant of the accident I had been transformed from a very much alive, striving, professional person to a patient in a state of complete acceptance of death. Six months after the accident I still felt that if I could just interact in the next brief interpersonal exchange I would be thankful. I counted my objectives as measured by the hour, day, or, at most, a week.

---

[2] This is a psychological-experimental term which in learning theory means the intervention of a strident stimulus that causes preceding learned stimuli to be forgotten or repressed. Much later, I ran across the term 'cultural shock' which seemed to me to capture at least part of the original sharp constriction. Cultural shock refers to a world that one can no longer make sense of nor understand. It designates the massive psychic reaction which takes place within the individual plunged into a culture vastly different from his own. It seemed that this to me is what a brain-injured person also goes through in attempting to make sense of his former (now foreign) life.

REFERENCES

Greenberg, R. and Dewan, E. (1968). Aphasia and dreaming: a test of the P-hypothesis. *Psychophysiology*, 5, 203–4.

Jones, L. V. and Wepman, J. M. (1965). Aphasia research opens new insights into brain mechanisms. In *Research projects summaries*, No. 2, pp. 69–77. NIMH, Bethesda.

Kupper, H. I. (1945). Psychic concomitants in wartime injuries. *Psychosomatic Medicine*, 7, 15–21.

Moss, C. S. (1968). Experimental manipulation of dreams. In *Progress in clinical psychology* (ed. L. E. Abt and B. F. Reiss), pp. 114–35. Grune & Stratton, New York.

(Moss 1972)

Recovery at twelve months
(Chapter 3 from the original book)

In November of 1968 I summarized the daily log on my progress to date in the following way.

It has been a year since my accident. My family and I agree that I still continue to progress, although the improvement has gradually slackened. What residuals of my stroke am I aware of?

I used to be more or less continually happy. In the morning, I usually awoke humming a little tune and generally the adverse events of the day did not bother me for long. That optimistic edge was taken away by my stroke, or, more precisely, rightly or not I attributed this partially to my medication. Presbyterian—St. Luke's prescribed nothing for me when I left the hospital; however, a neurologist whom I saw for a single visit two months later prescribed a recently developed anticoagulant, which I began taking twice a day. I took the pills for over eight months, never realizing that I should see any physician about possible side effects. One consequence was that during this entire period I was relatively depressed. On the other hand, let me be fair and admit that the confounding factor was that this was the period of my greatest readjustment. When I gave up the anticoagulant my mood seemed to brighten somewhat, so I can render this only as a highly subjective judgment.[1]

I still find it difficult to write (agraphia)— after a few words or a sentence or two, my handwriting deteriorates rapidly. Similarly, my typing became abominable after the accident, but now is slowly improving, more than my handwriting. The trouble is that my writing is very labored and my thoughts soon outstrip it. As I fall further behind, I try to speed up the handwriting and thus it becomes completely illegible. The typewriter does a better job, although I notice that I have difficulty sustaining adequate pressure with right-hand keys. I end up with the left-hand letters being firmly imprinted, and the right-hand letters serving as sort of 'shadows' to them. The most familiar analogy that I can give is that it is vaguely similar to the experience of writer's cramp. My difficulty in writing and typing is naturally a holdover from the original paralysis. In contrast, my ability to play ping-pong has not suffered the same disability—which testifies to the exquisite visual-motor coordination in writing.

Where I suffer in writing the most is in making mnemonic notes to myself in formal group settings. For years I had the habit of making cryptic little notes to speak from; now I can't do this, which, in combination

---

[1] Bette writes: We were advised to get in touch with a local neurologist and we went down to see him one day. He had made the original diagnosis, and he of course didn't say anything about that, but he did apologize to us for not having run these tests himself ('We have all of the equipment here but not anybody to run them'). I can't be convinced that even had the tests been run that he would have known how to read them. He prescribed an anticoagulant for Scott and while on it Scott seemed to be depressed. His days had been 'ups' and 'downs'; some days were good, but on other days he would start out feeling good but almost as quickly as you could snap your fingers he'd go into a depression. But when he was on the anticoagulant he seemed depressed most of the time, although we didn't realize what was causing it.

Our social life was nil, or almost so, but a couple of times we would go to some gathering of the psychology faculty. Scott would go if there was a large group of people, which meant he wouldn't be required to talk much. You can pretty much just listen when you're around a big group of people, especially if the group has had a bit to drink, because everyone wants to talk. That's when we ran into one of the psychology wives who had had some heart problems causing her to go into the hospital. Her physician advised her to take this same anticoagulant, but she refused because of all the side effects. When she told us this, Scott took it upon himself to discontinue taking the anticoagulant; immediately he began to feel better and the depression was lifted. This is just another example of the frustration we felt from lack of reliable medical knowledge.

with my spotty memory, makes speaking a hazardous affair at best. (I have toyed around with the idea of taking some kind of simplified shorthand.) Also I still have some difficulty in reading (alexia). I read the newspaper or magazines such as *Time* or *Life* now without any appreciable difficulty, at least the shorter articles, but textbooks or journal articles are much more time-consuming than formerly. High-level conceptions take more time and I rather quickly tire of that level of reading or communication.

Most mention here has been of my problems in expressive speaking or writing, and I presume that this part of my communication system suffered the most; however, I also suffer difficulties in receptive intake or comprehension of what is said or written. This was most apparent immediately following the stroke, especially where the messages were multiple and/or came at too fast a rate. When I returned to the clinic, for example, I attended all of the weekly staff meetings religiously, and I tried hard to listen carefully and make sense out of what was being said, but so many people's verbalizations invariably stupefied me. Trying to follow each person's contribution, to integrate the various topics, and also attempting to formalize what I might say in response was just too taxing, and after a while I inevitably lapsed back into a semiconscious reverie.

Fortunately, this situation has greatly improved; at least now I can follow most of what is said, only I still cannot make any sort of rejoinder, because by the time that I have put my thoughts into words, the conversation has drifted well beyond that point. This is somehow related to the fact that I feel most confident on the phone, or in individual conversations, where I have only one person to relate to. It is reminiscent of the feelings that I still have when I go to any of the shopping centers. I become rapidly inundated by the plethora of incoming stimuli—it is almost more than I can assimilate—I actually get to feeling dizzy after a few minutes. There is nothing wrong with my vision, I might add. I recently had a complete eye examination, including an eye field scan, and nothing unusual could be detected.

One other thing while I think of it—if I don't stop to think before I give directions, I am quite likely to confuse myself or other people by getting left mixed up with right or vice versa. In close-order drill I would really be a Gomer Pile. This indicates some damage to the *parietal lobe*, which again may or may not be related to a common error in writing. More often than not I now interchange letters or occasionally words. Similarly, if I miss a word in typing and later discover it, there is a definite tendency in replacing the missing word to put it slightly earlier than it should occur. All such errors occur automatically. If I stop and think I can usually catch such mistakes even before they happen, but this makes it very difficult to function spontaneously.

Basically, the main problem is that I block on words and I am still 'shocked' into silence by my inability to find appropriate words. I often fall silent rather than say what I know will be an inappropriate word. I still stumble on even the most pedestrian words. In fantasy I sometimes pretend that my accident never happened or that if it did, I am fully recovered, but I am brought back to reality by the very next relationship. To put it another way, my 'inner speech' seems to have made a partial recovery, and when I block on a word this reflects that I am still blocked internally, that is, the instant I know a word, then I can say it. This points up another thing, that thinking is not speech or vice versa. They are distantly related cousins but for the most part my perception is that I am more capable of thinking things than in explaining them in words. They are decidedly not the same thing.

My ability to capture appropriate words seems affected by either anxiety or fatigue. In connection with the former, I do find interpersonal relationships extremely tiring, particularly with professional contacts. With my colleagues, I am frequently at a loss to specify a necessary conception, while at the same time I feel that I must measure each word precisely to make certain that it communicates the exact meaning that I intend it to have. The upshot is that the process of searching for words defeats me, and I then have the definite tendency to withdraw from professional and even social contacts.[2]

With my own children, where I am relatively relaxed, the opposite is true. I am liable to slur my speech or even to engage in word-finding difficulty or occasional neologisms (i.e. I frequently call one of them by the other's name or ask them if they want to go to the Antifreeze rather than the Dairy Queen, or request them to get into their BVD's when I mean swimming suits, or, when hurried, may actually use a term which is a nonword—a nonsense syllable). My children seem to take it in stride, laughing in good nature at a particularly peculiar mal-use of words.

Actually, my work day spans more or less the same length of time as formerly—about sixteen to seventeen hours. I do not tire easily doing physical chores, and I am relieved to know that at least I still have much of the physical stamina that I had formerly. I swim, wrestle with the children, bowl, and play ping-pong—and I am apparently in excellent physical health. I took a policy with an insurance company about three months ago, and

the examining physician could detect no physical or psychological deficiencies at all (I gauged my conversation with the doctor very carefully, of course). The company did increase my rate by 25 percent for the next eight years, so I infer that actually I am not on my actuarial deathbed yet. My overriding objective is to make my family's life financially secure, not in the event of death but in the event of another totally disabling 'accident'.

I felt it was extremely important to reestablish and strengthen the emotional ties with my family. In the summer of 1968 we purchased a home in a newly developed subdivision and in many ways it has been highly therapeutic for me to have to attend to so many household duties. Joel, our ten-year-old son, has made Little League again this summer, and my wife and I attended each of his games. All three of the children were enrolled in summer school. Their schedules varied and this necessitated a more or less continuous taxi service. My wife's observation is that I now enjoy the children as much or more than I ever did.

Through the past ten years (long before my stroke), I held to the fantasy that someday, happily, I might develop some sort of an innocuous illness, like a mild case of t.b., that would force me to bed for a year or so, and give me the time to catch up on all of the professional journals and books which attracted my attention, but for which I simply had no time. Instead, I ended up with a health complication that prohibits me from indulging in most intellectual pursuits.

Consciously, I vaguely feared a heart attack as I approached a very active middle age, but at the same time I suspect that I actually feared damage to my intelligence. I had no trouble sleeping, but once in a great while I had what could be considered a nightmare, and three or four of these had a common theme. In 1952, for example, I had had a dream in which I was a patient in a psychiatric hospital. I was sitting in the canteen with some of my friends, but due to the fact that I had received a series of convulsive shocks, I was completely unable to converse with them. I awoke from the dream feeling

[2] Bette again writes: We had done a lot of entertaining when we were in California and enjoyed it, and knowing that university people make their own entertainment more or less, we looked forward to this, too. All of this was drastically curtailed with the accident. We went over to Don and Jean's one night and they had the Weirs over, too. Cecelia wanted us to come over for dinner, so with some reluctance Scott agreed to go. It turned out to be one other couple and us, and Scott was extremely quiet while there and this bothered him. I'm sure he felt ill at ease the whole time and I felt bad because of him. Then as soon as we had eaten dinner we sat down in the living room to talk. It couldn't have been more than five minutes later when Scott indicated to me that he wanted to go home. I felt bad for having eaten and then immediately left. I felt they would understand but from then on we didn't go to any more gatherings like that, because I realized what a horrible strain it was on Scott. People at the university knew what had happened to him and we didn't get invitations after a while, and if we did get invited to a party, we usually turned it down. After being used to an active social life it is hard to get adjusted to being alone, but any attempt to socialize was simply not worth it. For a while I had the urge to have someone in for dinner or the evening, but the strain on Scott simply made it not worth doing. I think we've become partly acclimated and I really don't miss it much any more.

panicky but was immensely relieved to find that it was only fantasy. In my wildest imagination I have wondered, these days, could there be a homunculus who directed that the clot would end up in my head rather than my heart, and thus deprive me of the time that I would devote to reading and thinking?

Actually it has rather astonished me that I have withstood the acute and later the non-flagging stress of severe brain damage as well as I did, without resorting to various neurotic defenses or to depression or even worse. Perhaps it is only because I was sensitized to numerous cases of acute and chronic brain syndromes in persons who had developed psychiatric symptoms that I was predisposed to expect that I too would develop a more morbid disorder. For example, I found my memory drawn back to a patient that I had seen almost fifteen years earlier, whom I must have unconsciously partially identified with. The patient was middle aged at the time, married, and formerly employed as a professor of mechanical engineering, who had undergone numerous deleterious personality changes since removal of a tumor from the right frontal lobe five years before. Whereas formerly he had been reported as exceedingly capable, industrious, and sociable, he had become irascible, garrulous, and captious—behavior which confounded every one of his interpersonal relationships, and finally resulted in his confinement at a hospital.

I remember attempting to work with the patient in psychotherapy for some months, but he was without insight into the seriousness of his condition, and I couldn't breach his absolute denial. The patient lacked entirely any sensitivity in his interpersonal relationships, his tolerance for frustration was extremely low, and when exceeded (as it was several times a session) he would react in an agitated and rigid manner, although he was not physically assaultive. He made frequent defensive protests of his own personal superiority and was hypercritical and tactless in dealing with others; for example, he was very verbal about the ignorance and deceit of the members of the staff who kept him hospitalized, and he wrote dozens of letters to local, state, and even national officials excoriating them over his unjust imprisonment. The point is that I was worried about such cases on the basis of possible self-reactions to my own disorder, but apparently this was a gross misconception on my part.

I am aware that with some frequency a stroke patient suffers a severe denial of disability associated with his illness or of some residual defect. As I learned, the term *anosognosia* is generally used to refer to an unawareness of some aspect of a disease process, including even a complete denial of a hemiplegia. There is as yet no general agreement concerning the etiology and significance of this defense. It seems that it is not so much the site or even the side of the lesion as much as it is a common and even characteristic feature of cerebral disease in general, and that certain types of personality traits existing before the neurological damage may well play some part in determining the patient's attitude toward his disability (Ullman, 1962). I have sometimes thought that in terms of my reaction toward the remaining deficits I would be better off if I could summon some denial rather than always being supersensitive to the residual manifestations of my disability, but apparently one doesn't have a choice in this matter.

Despite my emphasis on pathology, I like to believe that I appear to have remained largely the same person that I was before. I have no difficulty in physical or motor activities (outside of typing or especially writing) and no perceptual disturbances, and I think my judgment is unimpaired. Even the first morning when I awoke aphasic, my wife said clever little things to me and I attempted to respond with a smile (Bette told me later that it was a one-sided smile since the paralysis did not leave my face for several days). The main effect of the stroke on my personality has been twofold: generally, as I have mentioned, I have the tendency to withdraw or avoid most social contacts; and specifically, aphasia has played hob with my humor since I can no longer make spontaneous remarks with the superb sense of timing that I am sure I previously displayed!

During the summer term in 1968 I helped

assess potential clients to be seen by students in the fall at the clinic. This was one of the first times that I felt exposed, since there is absolutely no way to plan for the highly individualistic problems presented to me. However, I drew upon my years of diagnostic experience and only occasionally goofed, e.g., once I persistently called a young child Kevin when his name was Scott; his parents were so overawed by the formalities that they never corrected me and I only caught it when I listened to the tape. Considering everything, I felt that I did an adequate job in interviewing and wrote some reasonably good diagnostic reports. In the fall I continued to teach a psychotherapy laboratory and also began instruction in a course designed to teach students an awareness of the hypnosymbolic use of dreams and fantasy. In this course I attempted a change of pace from my former teaching technique, giving a didactic lecture during the first hour, followed by the playing of relevant tapes illustrative of the points that I had stressed. It occurred to me later that my very first dream after the cerebral insult was predictive of the way that I structured the course.

I still have real difficulty in composing and delivering my lectures. I tend to compensate by writing them down in complete and highly exact detail before delivering a lecture. I continue to tell myself that I can write or lecture or conduct research—it is only that it takes longer. I guess I haven't resigned myself yet to the fact that I am no longer as verbally fluent as I was earlier. This is a tremendous step for a person who throughout his lifetime could count on his ability to persuade others to his point of view and in effect sell his ideas through his ability to communicate.

Although I have undergone numerous diagnostic procedures we really have no real knowledge of either the precipitating or the predisposing factors in my illness. The experts vaguely refer to the fact that perhaps at some time earlier—even twenty years ago—I sustained damage to the artery which became apparent when I suffered my stroke. The physicians will not admit that my cold had anything whatsoever to do with my stroke, and I am about ready to agree with them. Probably the hard cough which I suffered for the two weeks before my accident was really due to the fact that the artery was being slowly closed; at the moment of the stroke the cough completely disappeared, and rather surprisingly I haven't had a cold since. The single period that I had been hospitalized earlier was when I spent a part of a month in a military hospital for a combination of a left mastoid infection, a tonsillectomy, and measles. At that time, for the one and only period in my life, I suffered excruciating headaches. When discharged from the service at the age of twenty-one, I applied for a disability allowance due to the fact that I was prone to develop episodes involving a very painful and stiff neck, but it was disallowed. I continued to experience this stiffness periodically for eight to ten years, but it gradually disappeared.

I have maintained that I had no premorbid symptoms, which is technically true, but two years before we left San Francisco I was bothered by two temporary yet troublesome afflictions. I began developing leg cramps while sleeping. When I happened to complain of this development, the regional mental health director spoke knowingly, and said that it was probably due to my growing older, since he had experienced the same condition for some years. It may be of some significance that I suffered no cramps once I came to the university.

A year before we left, I took charge of the mental health program in the western region when the associate mental health director took leave for six months to conduct a tour of mental health conditions in the new and developing countries of Africa and Asia. During this period my other symptom developed. It was more serious and prompted me to seek the medical advice of an internist (i.e., 'Uncle George'). For several months, usually immediately after lunch, I would develop a condition where the periphery of both eyes was surrounded by an aura of bright color and I would find 'holes' in my field of vision, about where I imagined the nerve would enter the back of the retina. After a series of tests the internist came to the conclusion that possibly

I was a borderline diabetic. He prescribed a diet for me which I held to for a couple of months. In thinking back, this may have been the first neurophysiological sign of the coming stroke. The condition cleared up over time and I promptly forgot about it.

Let me also mention, while I am on the matter, two other potential health hazards. Even before graduation from high school my weight fluctuated by fifteen to twenty pounds yearly. I tended to gain in the winter and take it off in the spring. As time and age mounted, I found it increasingly more difficult to shed the weight each year and was overweight by twenty-five pounds at the time of the stroke. The other thing has to do with a peculiar condition of my veins and arteries. In tenth grade I volunteered to give blood for a classmate who had leukemia. The doctor had to puncture six or seven veins *in each arm* because the veins would collapse and the flow of blood would stop. I had forged my mother's signature to the permission slip; later she was shocked when I assisted her in hanging up some wet clothes and I inadvertently revealed my coal black arms. Who knows whether any or all or none of these were related to my cerebral accident.

About four months after the stroke, I began laboriously to keep notes on my condition, and now I have begun writing an account of my personal experience for possible journal publication, basically for three reasons. First, because this is a unique experience for anyone of my age and particular professional background to suffer, and I am sufficiently pleased about my recovery and compulsive enough to want to document it; second, for whatever insights this record may contribute to professional people who have an interest in gaining knowledge of cerebral pathology and what they might do to partially alleviate it; and third, to attempt to give some understanding to my friends and colleagues who often, in their contact with me, maintain, to me at least, that they do not have the perception of any dramatic deficiency in my speech and writing.

This experience is a lonely one for an aphasic and his family. Even though I am at a major university and a member of an outstanding psychology department, I have reluctantly come to the conclusion that no one really knows much about how to treat my brand of aphasia. We have conferred with a number of authorities and all of them say that this sort of thing takes time and they can do nothing specifically to assist me. Joe Wepman is doubtlessly correct when he estimates that only 30 percent of aphasics get treated (Jones & Wepman, 1964). There are, of course, numerous treatment centers for patients who have suffered massive strokes and attempts are made in physical therapy for their gross deficiencies. My residual disability isn't with speech per se, but rather is with a disorganization in the brain which gives rise to difficulties primarily in word-finding signs or what some experts have termed *nominal aphasia*. I have maintained that my residual disability is no more than 10 percent—I simply fail to recall highly significant and special words that I would like to use. I know what I want to say, but cannot get at the words at that particular moment. This is a problem in selecting the precise informational words needed to communicate my thoughts accurately in either external communication or even internal speech.

There are two alternative explanations for this situation: I possess an organic deficit with an overlay of anxiety or I suffer a basic lack of self-confidence due to my accident, with some residual organic component. It is more hopeful for me to stress the second alternative—it leaves me something that I can continue to work on. My progress will in part be affected by the continued tolerance of my colleagues and the good will of my speech therapist, but in large measure my further recovery from my disability will eventually come about through the passage of time, through continued hard work with my wife, and through remaining highly motivated and not becoming too discouraged to continue working on the problem.

While I have not been overly preoccupied with thoughts of self-destruction, the idea of suicide does occasionally cross my mind. I am reminded that almost twenty-five years ago I attended a course given by Professor Harry Harlow in physiological psychology.

He was a compulsive, though witty and sometimes cynical, teacher. I recall the essence of a story which he told, to wit, that God had made the porpoise in a fit of malicious wrath. Next to man and the apes, the porpoise supposedly had the highest intelligence of any mammal, but it had been given no mechanism for expressing its creative thoughts. Harlow maintained that he could think of nothing more damaging to the ego than to have an intelligent brain but no equipment for expressing it. Nor can I.

REFERENCES

Jones, L. V. and Wepman, J. M. (1965). Aphasia research opens new insights into brain mechanisms. In *Research project summaries*, No. 2, pp. 69–77. NIMH, Bethesda.
Ullman, M. (1962). *Behavioral changes in patients following strokes*, pp. 69–93. C. C. Thomas, IL.

(Moss 1972)

Two years later
(Chapter 5 from the original book)

By November of 1969 I could sum up my progress in the following way.

Underlying my difficulties in speaking, it seems to be that my filing system for the selection of words has become slightly out of kilter. Objectively, I speak normally now, except for occasionally floundering on a word or two. It is, most times, a slight semantic or meaning distortion. I haven't lost any language, I still have all the words that I ever had, but I no longer have the ability to recapture them as quickly as before. At such times I have to rely on the input of other people in conversation to lead me to them. Subjectively, I never had the impression that I had to reeducate myself in the language. There was never the sense of the speech therapist teaching me new (or forgotten) words. Therapy only stimulates the aphasic to produce the words that he still knows at some level. Psychologically this seems to be a matter of concentration; it takes far longer for me to develop an idea fully, and I still have difficulty in carrying a conception through to its completion.

If you are looking for difficulties in word-finding, as Bob Simpson put it, then you are bound to find them—even in normal people. I have also become very much aware that my frantic searching for words is not always reflected in my external appearance. People are often quite surprised if I confess to them the difficulty that I am experiencing in word-finding. Talking is something that the average individual takes for granted (unless he is confronted with having to give a formal speech), and I seldom gave it a second thought before my accident.

During the past year the technique which probably has served me best is a concealed tape recorder housed in an attaché case which can be triggered by closing one of the clasps. My wife got it for me at Christmas, 1968, at my request, and I secretly collected a large number of tapes of various interactions which I participated in, ranging from highly informal contacts to classroom lectures and even speech therapy. This led to an astonishing discovery for me: where I thought my speech was poorly formed and suffering from chaotic lapses as I frantically searched for words, I discovered that except for occasional pauses, it sounded perfectly normal. I was amazed!

Bette states: 'What he wanted was a little tape recorder that he could put in his pocket—a little tiny thing like a pack of cigarettes, and he could have the microphone on his tie clasp or pen. That was fine for Dick Tracy or Mickey Spillane, but when you get down to trying to find them. you can't, or if they do make them the microphone isn't very sensitive. But finally I went to a hi-fi place and discovered that you could take a small tape recorder (cassette) and put it in a special attaché case which had a microphone in the handle. This was great because Scott could carry the case with him, and whenever he wanted to record, he only had to touch the handle and it would immediately start to record inside. It was sensitive and would pick up for some distance. It has been a marvelous instrument for him because he has been able to get conversations down without making notes. More than that, I have attempted to point out to him time and time again that in listening to his conversations you cannot tell who the aphasic is. If you stop and listen to some other person, there are pauses and hesitations while that person is gathering his thoughts. Nobody speaks as though he is reading off a sheet of paper, but this is what Scott wants to do and this is the way he used to do. He used to prepare lectures ahead of time, study them, then simply make notes and follow his outline when he actually gave the talk. He gave marvelous addresses; people were always commenting on his ability to speak. But he took a lot of time in his preparation. He has always done that, but it paid off. Anyway, the recording of his conversations with other people should really convince him that he doesn't block the way he thinks he does any more. Perhaps it is only his fear that he might block that causes him such anxiety. Of course, nobody can get inside his brain and know exactly how to change his own feelings. People whom we know now, who didn't know that he had had a stroke, are always amazed; they would never dream that anything like this had ever happened to him.'

If I sounded normal, what then accounted for the tremendous rise in anxiety and the distorted perception during speaking? I have come to the conclusion that my reaction is actually related to my subjective effort to conjure up continually the words which I need to speak, and much of the tension is not evident to the other party. To help the reader empathize, it is as if an American were suddenly transported to a France where everyone speaks only French. Our hypothetical American had a couple of semesters of French in college, but now finds that all of his communications must be translated into the foreign language before he can make his needs, wishes, and thoughts known. In addition, he projects onto the situation the belief that he will suffer admonishment for each error he makes. (Everyone knows the attitude of many Frenchmen toward any foreigner who speaks their language less than perfectly.) The analogy begins to break down if you imagine that in thinking of concepts the American must first begin with the English equivalent; in my case, often I had no English words even to begin the translation, at least in the months following my stroke. Even now, two years later, the finding of words is at times most tenuous.

Despite this knowledge provided by the tapes, I am still prone to make misjudgments about my speaking ability—which shows that 'insight' alone doesn't effect a cure. For example, Julie came to lunch the other day and asked if I could say 'toy boat' three times. When I responded and became all mixed up in my pronunciation, the very first thing that came into my mind was a condemnation of my brain-addled tongue. Fortunately, I subsequently came to witness the fact that the other members of the family were similarly afflicted, but in a very real way this intropunitive obsession influences all of my dealings.

Anyone who has had a severe physical trauma—like the loss of a limb or eyesight or coordination—has a similar reaction, I'm sure, but I have no readily apparent disability, not even a partial paralysis, on which I can blame my incompetence. Despite Wepman's prediction that in time I would forget my stroke, the effects have always continued to plague me. Even the very fact that I feel compelled to write this autobiographical sketch reflects that I don't ever forget it for long.

Perhaps it would be well to spell out very concretely some of the types of memory difficulties that still concern me. I awaken each morning about 6:00 or 6:30 by my inner-alarm clock, get up, let out and feed the dog, and then listen to the 7 o'clock news on the 'Today' show. It so happened that on a typical weekday morning recently I could not remember the master of ceremonies, even though the name seemed to be on the tip of my tongue. Finally, after worrying about it for twenty minutes or so, I turned to my wife, who had then awakened. She replied, 'Think of UP'—at which I immediately provided 'DOWNS'. A few minutes later I was unable to come up with the name of the woman who cohosts the show with him. I again turned to my wife, who said (you can see by her responses that she is well used to this need to jog my memory): 'What does a man do when he needs a HAIRCUT?' I at once answered, 'He goes to see the hairdresser' (perseverating on the woman whose identity I sought). When I was told, 'No, he sees the BARBER,' I was then able to supply my wife with both the first and last names of Barbara Walters. These sorts of cues almost always sufficed since I was in a typical TOT (tip of the tongue) state. In quite a similar vein, I am always getting Johnny Carson of the 'Tonight' show mixed up with the former star, Jack Paar. This happens to me now all the time in every field, not just in show business.

To continue a bit further with the 'Today' show, here is an actual sample of my thought processes just as I attempted to write them down not long ago: 'A couple of months ago they had on an olympic star, no, a decathalon winner . . . Nope! She was an award-winning movie star . . . What's it called? What is her name? . . . An Empy, huh uh! Emmy, yes, but that's an award for TV . . . A gold statue (then a long pause, searching for the correct title, trying to picture an award-winning ceremony) . . . I'm really stumped . . . (then comes insight) AN OSCAR-WINNING STAR and her name is Patricia Neal . . . But now I can't remember the book which she said will depict her struggle against brain damage'. At this point I gave it up since the very real possibility existed that the name of the book never registered.

Or to make it more public, less subjective, bringing it much closer to home: for several weeks recently, I developed a habit of calling Mary Jo (my present secretary) by the name of Jo Ann (my former secretary), or of getting the names reversed and calling a colleague by his last name, 'Paul', rather than his first name, 'Gordie'. (This is the price of having two first names, just as people upon first acquaintance tend to call me Moss for Scott or Dr. Scott or occasionally Dr. Moss Scott.)

When I used to complain about the ambiguousness of my memory, the response almost always elicited was, 'Why, this happens to me all the time' (followed by a recitation of the last time that it happened). In time one gets turned off by this type of response. It is somewhat like a schizophrenic who tries to tell a behavior therapist about his delusions. The therapist ignores them and at some juncture the patient quits talking about them, in which case the symptom is rated cured. This habitual response to me indicates that most people try to deny the seriousness of what you are saying by relating it to something that occurs fairly frequently in the normal, everyday course of events. The loss of memory is familiar especially as we grow older, but it is a relative matter. It bothers me much, much more now than it did two years ago. The stroke suddenly aged me overnight both in memory and speaking. Reflectively, a conversation with me now reminds me of speaking with an elderly gentleman, say Bette's father—except that he often appears much more mentally agile than I. For someone who still cannot get his own children's names correct, the business of conducting professional affairs is a hazardous undertaking indeed.

In the spring of 1969 I entered into correspondence with the chief psychologist at a large V.A. hospital in the western part of the country about a possible position. I knew him casually and he was very responsive to my inquiry, in spite of the fact that he knew that I had suffered a stroke. I assured him of my almost complete recovery, which was in a sense the truth—I had recovered in excellent fashion, everything considered. In applying for any job I was faced with a peculiar dilemma. If I confronted a potential employer with what I perceived as my residuals, it might very well forestall any thoughts of hiring me (countless people had told me by this time that I grossly exaggerated my disabilities); on the other hand, I felt a failure to do so was a misrepresentation of myself with consequent guilt about the duplicity and the fact that I would soon be found out. I tried to stipulate that I was interested in a clinical-type position, one which I felt competent to handle, but when the offer came it was for a job as the chief program evaluator of the hospital, with the promise that in a short time I would be promoted to the vacant chief research psychologist's position.

Because of my abiding interests in research, I almost accepted that position in spite of the many doubts that it immediately raised; however, there were other factors that made me hesitate. I felt loyalty to the director of clinical psychology at Illinois and he was currently on a six-month sabbatical and would not return until fall. During his absence I held down several fairly responsible duties. Then my mother underwent another heart failure just at the time of the final decision. She was hospitalized for a month and her physician informed us that more than likely her illness would be terminal (fortunately it wasn't). But in the final analysis, my many doubts about myself persisted and I was simply unconvinced that I could accept such a responsible position. I eventually turned it down.

So in the fall of 1969 I again entered into my academic job, even though I had many reservations about continuing it. It soon became apparent that I could not promote the community mental health (community psychology) program in the way that I had been hired to do. Even though I was convinced of a strong public service orientation and believed that psychologists, among other professionals, should be responsible to meet the problems growing out of great social needs, it was impossible to make and sustain the numerous contacts which would be required in promoting an expanding community program. As the first semester neared its end, I forfeited the leadership to another staff member. In discussion of my future role with the director and the chairman of the department, it was decided that in the coming year,

1970–71, I would give up entirely attempting to teach community psychology and substitute instead two successive sections of abnormal psychology, while still keeping a laboratory on psychotherapy. It was some small consolation knowing that probably I could handle large didactic courses in abnormal much better than the less structured seminar courses with bright graduate students.

My primary reason for coming to the university was to teach clinical graduate students some of the things that I had learned over the past seventeen years, particularly what I had been doing in relation to community mental health in the previous six years. There was no way of knowing that even without a stroke much of what I knew (or thought I knew) would be discounted because in my orientation I was considered to be a representative of the 'old school; in contrast to the new militant behaviorism (see Chapter 7).

However, a strong, secondary reason for my having chosen Illinois was that it would bring me once again into contact with Charlie Osgood and the possibility that we could collaborate on a book that I had in mind. We had had a half-dozen contacts in the first few weeks after I arrived, and had already come to the conclusion that the majority of writing must be left to me, since he was (as usual) tremendously overcommitted. After the accident and the resulting aphasia, the possibility of my doing any writing seemed remote. But eight months later, out of desperation and seeking yet another form of self-help, I began to dictate to my wife the beginning outline of the book.

The book gradually took on a structure and form somewhat different from what I had originally intended, since I was no longer capable of writing with nearly the style or spontaneity that I had two years earlier. However, when one gets to the point of writing a book, much of the material is already on hand in thought and on paper. The book as it was transformed became a casebook composed of a dozen previously handled cases selected from among those in my files, some of which had already been reported in various professional journals. All that was really left for me to do was to put the cases in some sort of logical order, and to write three chapters: an introduction and two other integrative chapters, one on the experimental and one on the clinical aspects of exploring dream symbolism with hypnosis. After all, this had been part of my clinical practice for twenty years and I should have been thoroughly familiar with it. On the other hand, absolutely nothing came to me as easily as it had two years before—neither the thoughts nor how to unify them nor how to translate them from my head into written language. But my wife and I plugged away, having plenty of time since my professional activities and our social activities were greatly curtailed.

At the appropriate time, Charlie sat down and prepared a critique of the book for me and then wrote a foreword to it. We decided that I should approach the University of Illinois Press, both because it had published Osgood's initial text on the semantic differential (*The Measurement of Meaning*, 1957), and because I had neither the energy nor the poise to enter into protracted negotiations with other publishers. As it turned out, the editors of the press were very receptive to the book, and accepted it for publication (*Dreams, Images and Fantasy: A Semantic Differential Casebook*, 1970). They also wished to publish a supplemental paperback book prepared on the treatment of an illustrative phobic case (*Black Rover, Come Over*), written largely by the patient herself, along with an accompanying tape of selected episodes from the actual psychotherapeutic sessions.[1] In my judgment the two books were reasonably well written, but the content often had to be rather painfully dredged from my reduced intellectual and language capacity. Incidentally, I again played a little game with myself and the publishers and never mentioned my brain damage to them.

So two years after my stroke I am beginning to work as hard at my professional duties as I was earlier, but accomplishing less. Although I now do much of my work at

---

[1] The *Black Rover* tape, by the way, is a reasonably good sample of my premorbid personality and the accompanying patterns of thought and speech.

home rather than in the office, I nevertheless am busy at my typewriter or listening to tapes or composing lectures four or five hours each day, including Saturday and Sunday. I am amused at my halfhearted attempts to 'take it easy' in the face of the habits of a professional lifetime. Even though I still toy with the idea of retiring to a tropical beachside hut, I don't think I will ever make it. The demands for a full-time and active life are impossible to avoid within the constraints of a slight impairment. In recent months, I have become aware that my physical tempo has begun to pick up and at times bears a resemblance to the hectic manner in which I used to balance at least a half-dozen tasks at once. This increased activity still feels strange and rather uncomfortable and as soon as I am aware of what I am doing I attempt to slow down, but little by little I seem to be getting back into the old acrobatic mold.

Quite by chance, it was pointed out to me by one of my students that I had 'unconsciously' learned to compensate partially for my handwriting disability. By this time I had learned to sign my name without embarrassing halts and jerks and without the last letters disintegrating into inconspicuous marks. But what was pointed out to me when I was signing a curriculum card was that the index finger of my left hand seemingly steadied (actually it pushed against) the right hand which held the pen. I was amazed when this was pointed out; I had no realization that I was doing this to compensate for the loss of power and mobility in the afflicted hand. Later I noticed that I did this habitually. However, at the time it happened, I took some hidden pride in the fact that I immediately came forth with the rationalization that this was the way I had learned in early childhood to write across a page without lines, and then we laughed at the odd ways children learn to write. In the time ahead, with a little practice, I learned to sign my name without the extra effort supplied by the member of the opposite hand, thus doing away with another sign that might give me away. This works fine as long as I don't have to sign my name several times in a row. If it is required that a sentence or two be written, I almost always, on some pretext, give the pencil and pad to another person.

Having been sensitized to the automatic way that my body compensated for my right hand, I then looked at other related features, and discovered that in my gardening I now made adjustments so that the left hand would take on most of the more intricate or demanding tasks, and in driving the car I now tended to steer with the left hand. The right hand was still functional in most activities but quite involuntarily the other hand had begun to replace it in the more arduous or complicated jobs.

In some ways I was extremely fortunate that the stroke occurred in the university setting, since the faculty had been so tolerant of my limitations during my recovery. On the other hand, I was suddenly very impressed with the limited financial resources that are available to a severely handicapped person in this society. I had slowly built up a private life insurance program which would modestly protect my wife and family in the event of my death, but it never occurred to me that I should take out some form of wage insurance as well, since I had never been hospitalized in my life except for a short episode in the service.

I had given up my disability retirement based on more than sixteen years of federal employment and my federal health insurance when I came to Illinois. I had the foresight to take out a fairly expensive family health insurance which covered about 80 percent of my hospital bills (which came to almost $1000 for less than two weeks' hospitalization). Inadvertently, I had skipped the group insurance policy, but thought that I would pick it up at the next eligibility period; however, when I tried to obtain coverage after my accident, I was politely but firmly turned down.

In terms of the university's retirement system, during the first five years of employ-ment, rather than receiving a disability annuity, employees are provided with a lump-sum cash benefit equal to half the salary received during the term of employment. For me this meant that if I were declared disabled after two full years I could receive approximately $20,000 paid over two following years. In the back of my mind was the concern that I really was worth much more dead than permanently disabled. My Social Security was paid up (44 quarters) but there was the qualification there that in cases of disability you had to be covered in five of the last ten years. I was covered for 1959–60–61 before I returned to federal service, so I had to sweat out paying two additional years from the small income that I derived from my two earlier books, which I did in the early springs of 1969 and 1970. This made me eligible for a small stipend in case of permanent and total disability. This is why I wanted to return to federal service and to complete at least my twenty years, which would qualify me for a part-time pension if I had another accident. Security for my family was my overwhelming objective.

My experience brought home to me the wisdom of having a federally sponsored national health and disability insurance program which everyone would be required to join. After all, I am a living example of the fact that absolutely no one can tell that he might not, today or tomorrow, suffer from an accident that would partially or totally disable him, with a catastrophic result in most cases, both for the individual and most or all of the people who are dependent upon him. On the other side of the coin, insecurity can be a prime motivating factor. One never knows how much he can do until he is forced by circumstances to do it.

(Moss 1972)

COMMENTARY

Overview article (1976). Moss initially suffered from a global aphasia, with an associated right hemiplegia, but this clinical picture changed significantly over the first few months of his recovery. Moss' comment (p. 81), that in his particular type of aphasia the deficiencies in thinking and memory were more prominent than impairments in speech articulation, points to the involvement of posterior temporal regions rather than frontal regions. A further clue in this respect is the excellent recovery of motor function—Moss' right-sided paralysis recovered quickly and largely disappeared after a few hours, suggesting the absence of major damage to frontal or parietal areas associated with motor or sensory functioning. Moss' recovery of physical deficits left him with the paradoxical predicament whereby he did not appear to be visibly disabled and he secretly wished that he had a white cane to symbolize that something had happened to him, and to alert others that there was a reason for the impairments in his speech and in his thinking! Moss reports that 'the ability to read words had begun coming back to me, but still not the ability to comprehend them' (p. 77). It is possible that at this stage of his recovery he had a form of reading difficulty that could be characterized as a 'central alexia' (Benson 1994)—this is associated with the presence of Wernicke's aphasia and with lesions in the inferior part of the left parietal lobe/posterior part of the superior temporal gyrus.

Book, chapter 1 (1972) (The accident and the ensuing six months).   When Moss started to drive again after his stroke, it 'was as if I were learning to coordinate the visual-motor function all over again' (p. 84). At one level, it is rather surprising that a well-established skill such as driving appeared to be lost. However, if one sees this loss as a form of apraxia—a loss of complex motor behaviours that cannot be explained by primary sensory or motor loss, or by loss of language or motivation— then it could be conceived within the framework of disorders that may accompany significant left hemisphere pathology. One might hypothesize that the association between left hemisphere disease and apraxia is due to the fact that these motor actions were initially encoded in a verbal fashion, and that human beings end up with a form of motor vocabulary, with discrete motor 'scripts' that are in many ways automatic and unconscious but still retain some vestigial element of verbal coding.

   Moss also indicates (p. 84) that in these early stages he could never tell if what he was going to say would come out right. Such meta-language skills, knowledge about one's knowledge, appears for understandable reasons to have been somewhat neglected in aphasia research. It is possible that, as he became more familiar with his limitations in the use of language, Moss became more knowledgeable about what he was likely to say correctly and what he was unable to say. In Moss' initial observations, there is certainly a contrast with the self-reports of stutterers (e.g. Petrie 1994), who are often able to predict with great precision whether a word will be spoken fluently.

Book, chapter 3 (1972) (Recovery at twelve months).   Moss' report of comprehension difficulties in certain situations probably reflected in part auditory-verbal episodic memory impairment and also semantic retrieval impairments—'trying to follow each person's contribution, to integrate the various topics, and also attempting to formalise what I might say in response was just too taxing, and after a while I inevitably lapsed back into a semiconscious reverie' (p. 91). He had to comprehend, hold and manipulate items in memory, relate them to existing concepts and then retrieve and collate the words necessary for a response. His report that he now limits his reading to short articles may also reflect an impairment of memory, although his symptom of difficulty with 'higher-level conceptions' (p. 91) suggests an additional comprehension difficulty with some words or phrases.

Moss' comment (p. 95), that it was the 'precise informational words' which gave him most trouble with regard to his word-finding difficulty, mirrors reports in the literature relating to the retrieval of proper names, such as names of people (Shallice and Kartsounis 1993; Hittmair-Delazer *et al.* 1994). Perhaps such deficits simply reflect an impaired access for words with the fewest associations, rather than necessarily being a form of category-specific retrieval difficulty.

Book, Chapter 5 (1972) (Two years later).   Moss decries the oft-mentioned reassurance by his friends that they frequently suffer the same word-finding and memory symptoms of which he himself complains. He gives a good description (p. 98) of being in a tip-of-the-tongue state, and how semantic and acoustic cues help him retrieve the word in question.

Moss describes a number of fascinating examples where he unconsciously initiated new sets of motor behaviours (e.g. using his left hand to steady his right hand when signing his name, using his left hand in particular ways when gardening or steering his car). At the perceptual and encoding phases of cognition, information can be processed, even up to semantic levels, without awareness by the individual (Weiskrantz 1991). Moss' report suggests that at the level of motor behaviour the 'executive system' can, without reference to any conscious awareness, initiate new ways of responding that help the individual to cope more effectively with the demands of a particular task.

REFERENCES

Benson, D. F. (1994). *The neurology of thinking.* Oxford University Press, New York.

Hittmair-Delazer, M., Denes, G., Semenza, C., and Mantovan, M. C. (1994). Anomia for people's names. *Neuropsychologia*, **32**, 465–76.

Petrie, R. X. A. (1994). The luxury of fluency. *British Medical Journal*, **309**, 547.

Shallice, T. and Kartsounis, L. D. (1993). Selective impairment of retrieving people's names: a category specific disorder? *Cortex*, **29**, 281–91.

Weiskrantz, L. (1991). Disconnected awareness for detecting, processing, and remembering in neurological patients. *Journal of the Royal Society of Medicine*, **84**, 466–70.

A personal case history of transient anomia

Mark H. Ashcraft

Mark Ashcraft was an associate Professor of Psychology at the time of the onset of his illness, having specialized in cognitive psychology.

What is it like to lose one's language abilities? What is the inner experience, both cognitive and emotional, of an individual whose language or memory abilities are disrupted? Research on aphasic and amnesic syndromes has provided an impressive catalog of evidence about the behavioral consequences of brain abnormalities and damage, and there is no need to repeat or review these consequences here. But what of the mental consequences, as experienced subjectively by the affected individual?

Two reasons for inquiring into the subjective experience of language dysfunction may be offered. The first is basic curiosity about the nature and extent of an individual's disruption. For example, a neuropsychologist may attempt to draw inferences about a patient's subjective experience based on whatever evidence is available, often the fragmented language a patient can generate or the apparent emotional reaction displayed by the patient. Second, it is not uncommon to marshall additional evidence about a patient's cognitive status from the individual's apparent subjective state or emotional reaction; for example, Kertesz (1982) described the neologisms of a Wernicke's aphasic by adding 'There is a rather curious cool and calm manner about her speech as if she did not realize her deficit . . . a very characteristic feature of this disturbance' (p. 42). However difficult it is to devise thorough assessments in such a case, the patient suffers a double disadvantage, being unable to communicate fluently or precisely and naive about the cognitive and linguistic processes that have been disrupted. Our inferences about preserved and disrupted functions, therefore, generally remain somewhat uncertain and tentative.

In this paper, I offer a detailed recollection of inner mental experience during an episode characterized by anomia or word-finding difficulty. Because my recollection is not subject to the typical double disadvantage, the analysis may shed some light on the nature of thought in the absence of fluent language ability. While I do not claim that my experience is to be taken as universally true for all such language disruptions, it is quite similar to at least one reported case (Kay & Ellis, 1987; see Part 3 below). As such, it may be useful in corroborating inferences drawn by these investigators and in devising assessments in future research.

For organizational purposes, I have divided this case history into three parts. The first part is background, which describes relevant demographic, setting, and diagnostic information. In the second part, I relate the several events that occurred during the 45-min episode, including my thoughts and reactions to those events. The two individuals I spoke with during the episode have corroborated the observable events and behaviors I describe in this account. My assistant and I independently wrote diary-like accounts of the episode, hers within 2 weeks, mine within a month. These agree with my current recollections, which can still be described as indelible. Finally, in the third part I attempt to identify general characteristics of the episode that may be of interest to the study of cognition and the neurosciences.

PART 1—BACKGROUND

At the time of the seizure, 14 September, 1988, I was 38 years old, an Associate Professor of Psychology, with a 1975 Ph.D. in Experimental Psychology. My specialty is cognitive psychology, and my research is in the area of cognitive arithmetic. I had taught Cognitive Psychology for approximately 12 years, and Psychology of Language for 3 years. The only noteworthy exception to general good health was a single grand mal seizure at age 18, my sophomore year in college, diagnosed at the time as due to overwork and fatigue.

On the date of the episode, some 2 weeks before the beginning of Fall term classes, my research assistant, Machelle, and I had spent several hours at professional 'housekeeping', selecting which printouts, many of which were at least 10 years old, to keep for archival purposes and which to discard. While my assistant continued this activity, I spent the last few hours of the day reading and doing paperwork, sitting at the desk in my office. The episode began at approximately 4:45 PM, and was over at 5:30 PM.

The episode was tentatively diagnosed by the attending emergency room physician that evening as a transient ischemic attack, with instructions to see my regular doctor the following day. Eight days later, angiography revealed an arterio-venous malformation (AVM) in the anterior left temporal lobe. Two neurosurgeons independently diagnosed the 45-min episode as a seizure caused by the 'steal effect'; i.e., blood is 'stolen' from brain tissue by the AVM, triggering a seizure. There was no evidence of prior hemorrhage in any diagnostic test. Some 10 weeks later, the AVM was surgically removed with no complications and no short- or long-term sequelae.

PART 2—THE EPISODE

For clarity, I adopt the following notational conventions in Part 2. Explanatory information about the settings and activities surrounding the six events of the episode appears in normal typeface. My verbatim overt speech appears in double quotations. I note paraphrases of overt speech, mine as well as Machelle's and my wife Mary's, in single quotations; not surprisingly, I cannot quote these two people verbatim, nor myself in the lengthy conversations of events 5 and 6.

My thoughts during the 45-min episode are described in italics and set off in brackets [*as shown here*]. It is critical to this account that the following point be clear. My inner thoughts, stated in the present tense to convey the stream of consciousness, are described as if they consisted of straightforward, syntactically and semantically fluent sentences. They were not simply inner or subvocal speech, however. The most powerful realization I had during the episode, and the most intriguing aspect to me since then, was the dissociation between a thought and the word or phrase that expresses the thought. The subjective experience consisted of knowing with complete certainty the idea or concept that I was trying to express and being completely unable to find and utter the word that expressed the idea or concept. The thoughts can only be described in sentence-like form, because they were as complex, detailed, and lengthy as a typical sentence. They were not sentences, however. The experience was not one of merely being unable to articulate a word currently held in consciousness. Instead, it was one of being fully aware of the target *idea* yet totally unable to accomplish what normally feels like the single act of finding-and-saying-the-word.

Event 1, 4:45 PM

I was looking at a printout from a study on math anxiety, unable to tell if it was one of the old analyses, in which we analyzed three levels of anxiety, or a newer one, with four levels. It vaguely seemed like too much trouble to figure out which analysis I was examining, although looking at the degrees of freedom would have answered this question. Machelle came into my office with a computer printout, put it in front of me on my desk, and said 'I don't know if you want to keep this one or not, or what label to put on it if you do want to keep it'.

[*This is the ANOVA printout from Ben's experiment, the study on 3rd, 4th, and 6th graders. We always call it DevCogArith.*]

I said 'Oh, that's . . . uh . . .' After a few seconds, I tried again. 'It's the . . .' [*That's sort of funny; I can't remember DevCogArith, or the words printout or experiment.*]

I recognized the printout immediately. The abbreviation stood for Developmental Cognitive Arithmetic, since it was the first developmental study on arithmetic that we had conducted, in school year 1978–1979 (Ashcraft & Fierman, 1982). Handwritten on the printout was G-3 4 6, indicating that the factor labeled G was for those three grades.

I chuckled audibly at my inability to label the printout, then said 'We'll have to do this tomorrow'. Machelle returned to her office and I remained at my desk. Her written recollection 2 weeks later says: 'He seemed distracted. He said something about not being able to find the words, laughed a little, and continued to stare at the printout'. She later explained that she assumed I had been engrossed in what I was doing and was unable or unwilling to shift to a different topic.

Event 2, 4:55 PM

Machelle came into my office again. [*I've been sitting at my desk for about 10 min, staring at the desk lamp, with nothing on my mind; I'm not even daydreaming.*] Machelle asked me another question about some printouts, and I was again unable to respond with anything more than sentence fragments. [*I know exactly what I'm trying to say, why won't the words come to me?*]

Event 3, 4.56 PM

As Machelle left, I turned to the computer on the table opposite my desk. The message on the screen indicated that I was still logged onto the mainframe computer. [*It's late, I have to log off so I can go home.*] As I positioned my hands at the keyboard, I realized I could not remember the command to log off—the command, of course, is simply *logoff*, a command I issue with great regularity. I stared at the screen for a few moments, still could not remember the command, and at that point realized that something unusual was happening.

Event 4, 5:00 PM

[*This is weird, something is wrong. I wonder if I'm ok. I'll test myself, I'll walk to the restroom and see if I'm weaving down the hall, or if my vision is distorted.*] I had no difficulties walking to the restroom and returned to my office satisfied that I was physically all right.

Event 5, 5:10 PM

Although it was not unusually late for me to be at the office, I decided to phone home anyway to say I'd be leaving shortly. I was sitting at the computer again, still unable to remember the logoff command. I reached for the phone next to the computer, pressed the line button for a dial tone, pressed 8 for an outside line, and dialed my home phone number with no difficulty or hesitation.

Mary answered, and I said 'I'm coming home'. Mary was immediately aware that something was wrong, given that I was speaking quite hesitantly, and said 'Are you all right—you sound funny'. I responded 'I guess I'm confused'. 'Confused about what?' Mary asked. [*Well, we were cleaning out the cabinets, going through printouts of old experiments, and I couldn't remember the words printout or experiment—but I still can't remember those words. I can't even remember the word cabinet. How can I explain what I'm confused about when I still can't think of the words to say it?*]

I attempted several times to start a sentence that explained my inability to remember these words, but each one trailed off after 'well, we were' and the like. Mary said, roughly. 'Stay there, I'm calling Steve to come get you'. I knew, however, that this colleague had already left for the day, having seen his darkened office during Event 4. I said 'No, I'll just come home'. Mary insisted 'Something is wrong, and you have to go to the emergency room'. I became very stubborn about driving myself home. [*I have to sound very calm and firm; I don't want to leave my car here overnight, so I have to persuade Mary I can drive home.*] Mary said 'Stay there' and then hung up. The line was busy when I phoned again.

Machelle came into the office again, and I told her 'Mary is worried about me'. I do not recall mentioning the computer problems, but Machelle's written record indicates that I also mentioned that I could not remember how to logoff from the computer.

Event 6, 5:20 PM

I reached my wife by phone again and once again insisted that I drive myself home. I said 'I'm leaving for home now. If I'm not there in half an hour, or if I have problems, I'll stop at a phone booth and call you'. [*I just want to get home. And I don't want to leave my car here overnight.*] Mary insisted that I not drive and then asked to speak to Machelle, asking her to drive me to the hospital; I gave up on driving myself home. Machelle hung up, said she was going to get her car and would be back in 5 minutes. She left the office.

At approximately 5:25, I looked at my computer again and with no difficulty at all remembered the logoff command; I typed the command, logged off successfully, and turned off the computer. As I waited for Machelle, I remembered the words I had had difficulty with and said them out loud to myself; 'printout, data, experiment, results'. When Machelle returned, I said 'I'm fine now. I can drive myself, but I'd like you to follow me just in case'. She agreed reluctantly, and we left the office. As we walked down the hall, I looked at my watch—it was 5:30—and I realized that whatever had happened was now over. I repeated this to Machelle. I forced myself to concentrate on driving, not letting myself think about what had just happened.

PART 3—ISSUES

There are several interesting facets of this experience that deserve mention. Given my involvement, however, I would offer only three; even now, these seem completely certain to me.

(a) Emotional Reaction

It seemed mildly amusing to me, to the point of chuckling, that I was unable to think of those words, for the most part my ordinary and routine 'professional vocabulary' (but I was also unable to retrieve 'cabinet', which is not plausibly described as part of 'professional vocabulary'). The feeling was similar to a tip-of-the-tongue (TOT) experience,

except that no synonyms, word initial letters or sounds, or alternate ways of expressing the idea came to me either. I responded to the retrieval difficulty by slowing my rate of speech, hesitating, and stopping when the next word was unavailable ('fumbling for words', in my wife's description). Stated differently, I did not substitute general words (e.g., 'thing', 'stuff'), i.e., did not invent the circumlocutions typical of more permanent anomia. Event 3, however, represented a memory failure that made me aware of a genuine disorder. In response, I tested myself by walking down the hall, careful to note physical balance, vision, and so forth.

There was never a sense of panic or desperation during the episode, which I attribute to the nature of the disruption. I imagine that sudden pain or physical inability might easily generate panic; see, for instance, Kolb's (1990) reaction upon discovering that his visual field defect was binocular, hence central rather than retinal. Furthermore, my reaction would very likely have changed to concern or desperation if the episode had lasted substantially longer. But the largely mental nature of my disruption seems to have yielded a slightly bemused and puzzled reaction. Normally, we do not become overly concerned if we momentarily 'block' on remembering a word, the name of a film. etc., and this is how the experience seemed to me at the time.

(b) 'Train of Thought'

Event 4 is a clear demonstration, in my opinion, of how a relatively complex sequence of thought proceeded without disruption during the seizure. I realized that something was wrong, devised an assessment of my coordination and perception, collected data by self-observation, and then drew a conclusion from those data; the sequence seems quite similar to Kolb's (1990) self-test of visual functioning. In my interpretation, this activity represents a straightforward instance of conscious (i.e., not automatic) cognitive processing and problem solving, which was conceived, devised, and accomplished during the seizure itself. (Note also that it was during

Event 4 when I noticed that my colleague Steve had left for the day, a fact I then retrieved during Event 5.)

Nonetheless, I cannot say how the undeniable stubbornness at Events 5 and 6 should be judged, a disruption of logical thought or an overriding (yet subdued) emotional reaction. I clearly felt competent to drive, wanted to be at home, and tried to be persuasive enough to win the argument. On the one hand, the motivation for this, not leaving my car in a downtown University parking lot, strikes me as understandable, and the ensuing 'phone booth plan' was rather complex. On the other hand, it also seems irrational; objectively, people should not drive during a seizure (but of course I did not self-diagnose the seizure). In some ways, there was no gross disruption of ongoing thought. Being unaware of the potential gravity of the episode, however, may be evidence of a greater disruption of thought than I suspect, or of the overruling of rational thought by emotional reaction.

Ironically, it did not occur to me to test any other mental capacities during the seizure; as the 'subject' in an unplanned study of temporary brain dysfunction, I failed to act as an 'experimenter' in testing other mental functioning. Awareness of the word-finding problem could have prompted me to determine if other nonprofessional words besides 'cabinet' were also blocked. I could have tested my ability to do arithmetic or math problems, given my involvement in a project on acalculia among brain-damaged children. In retrospect, a major disappointment is that my assistant did not refer to the printouts by name; my guess is that I would have correctly recognized that word even though it was blocked from retrieval (see below).

I infer that sensory–motor processes, short-term memory, and a good deal of long-term memory were unaffected by the seizure (e.g., vision, physical balance, etc. were intact; I maintained the topic in the conversations with my wife, I recognized the need to logoff in Event 3, and I retrieved my home phone number in Events 5 and 6). I conclude that attention/awareness, short-term memory, and problem solving processes

requiring a sustained 'train of thought' were relatively unaffected by the seizure. Based on preserved functions, the language retrieval deficit that was apparent, and the location of the AVM, I assume that the seizure was restricted largely to the left temporal lobe and those nearby regions that could have been affected by the steal effect. If this assumption is correct, then the preserved cognitive functions apparently do not depend in any major way on these left temporal regions, or, alternatively, they can be accomplished by other regions if need be. In either case, and regardless of the localization of the seizure, the preserved cognitive processes and functions do not seem to depend on fluent and undisrupted word retrieval.

(c) Thought and Language

I reiterate the conclusion—problem solving and cognition accomplished during the seizure—with one addition; the problem solving and cognition were *thoughts without language*. I was not saying sentences to myself mentally as I planned to assess my coordination and perception, or as I attempted to converse with my wife. The idea, expressed in Event 4 as [*I'll test myself; I'll walk to the restroom . . .*] was as complete and full as any idea one might have normally, but was not an unspoken mental sentence.

James (1890, p. 651) described the experience of recalling a memory as occurring 'in one integral pulse of consciousness'. I understand this to refer to an immediacy of awareness, the sense that an idea comes into awareness *right now*, as it were. Such a description is a completely apt expression of my experience during the seizure, in terms of accessing concepts and ideas. It is also an introspectively appealing description of the normal operation of memory and recall. When a student asks a question during my lecture, I know—in a seeming instant—what idea to express in answering the question. I then proceed to verbalize my answer, occasionally laboring over a word or phrase, but more usually generating the sentence quite automatically. It was the unusual 'gap' in this usually seamless process, a process taken completely for granted in normal circumstances, that amazes me and requires expression here.

Throughout the seizure, I was completely aware of the concepts and meanings I wished to express. This was not merely awareness of a general meaning or some vague approximate idea. It was, to use standard terminology, complete and successful semantic access to (retrieval of) the precise target concept. In several cases (e.g., the specific experiment in Event 1), there was also successful retrieval of exact episodic concepts of memories. But for those 'professional' words, *no words or labels accompanied the retrieval*.

I think of the events that occurred in terms of three sequential steps, with a disruption in the second step of the normal sequence; see the Post Script below, where a strikingly similar explanation by Kay and Ellis (1987) is described. Step 1 is semantic retrieval, which yields access to and awareness of the idea to be expressed. Step 2 is the process of accessing the word or phrase that names this retrieved idea, essentially lexical access. Finally, the fluent articulation of the retrieved word name is Step 3. Typically, the three steps occur quite rapidly and automatically, as in James' 'integral pulse'. And needless to say, we are not introspectively aware of the three-part separation. During my seizure, however, the seamless operation of the sequence broke down, because of a disruption in Step 2.

Note three points about the proposed Step 2. First, it was not tied uniquely to articulation; beyond the inaccessible words 'printout', 'experiment', 'cabinet', etc., I could not access the logoff command to be typed at the computer keyboard. Second, word retrieval was not totally disrupted, in that retrieval and articulation of 'confused' and 'phone booth', along with more common, everyday words, was successful. It is tempting to cast my distinction between 'professional' and everyday vocabulary in other terms, for instance the abstract/concrete dimension, or in terms of word frequency (e.g., Ellis, 1985), and to claim that the mental lexicon or the process that accesses the lexicon is sensitive to that dimension. On the other hand, my claim about 'professional' words may simply be the result of not having attempted to converse about other substantive topics.

Third, the specific retrieval failures in Step 2, although possibly not surprising in anomia, are peculiar from the perspective of memory and cognition. There is a wealth of information concerning retrieval cues, context, and the effects of encoding specificity (e.g., Schacter, 1989; Tulving, 1983, chap. 9). As a rule, the more similar a retrieval attempt is to original encoding of information, the more successful retrieval will be. As such, it is odd that those particular words were inaccessible in the very location where they are normally most common, my office.

POST SCRIPT

Since drafting this paper, I have discovered a fascinating report by Kay and Ellis (1987), discussing patient EST's permanent anomia. In most respects, and with the obvious exception of the permanence of the anomia, the cases seem quite similar, even down to EST's awareness of his deficit, apparent in several of his verbatim remarks (e.g., 'I should know this', 'I jumped at the wrong thing'). I comment here on two points raised in that paper.

First, EST's performance led Kay and Ellis to conclude that EST suffered little or no semantic impairment, but instead that he suffered a phonologically based anomia. In particular, their explanation of EST's anomia suggests a partial disconnection between the semantic system and the phonological lexicon, realized as 'weak or fluctuating levels of activation between corresponding representations' in the two systems. If my failure to retrieve the logoff command for *motor* output can be attributed to the same phonological lexicon that failed for 'printout', 'data', and so forth, then the explanation fits my anomia extremely well. Alternatively, the lexicon may be described as phonological merely because its output is normally in spoken form, as is output in our typical assessments.

Second, Kay and Ellis discuss the observation that 'anomic patients, in some sense, "know" the word that they are trying to find'

(p. 614), i.e., that semantic access may be preserved in some anomias. Two citations they provide, however, have apparently argued against this TOT view (Geschwind, 1967; Goodglass, Kaplan, Weintraub, & Ackerman, 1976). In those reports, patients did not show the classic TOT pattern to pictures they were unable to name to confrontation, i.e., they were unable to demonstrate even partial access to phonological and morphological information about the lexical target (respectively, word initial sounds and number of syllables). My experience suggests that classic, partial access to the target may be only a coincidental part of the TOT experience. If the typical TOT state can be described as *informed* by partial access, then my anomic TOT state was *uninformed*. I had no sense at all of knowing word length or initial sounds, nor did I retrieve similar sounding words. Yet I 'knew' the words I was looking for at the time and said them aloud after the seizure was over. I am confident that I would have

recognized 'printout' as the target word in Event 1 if my assistant had said 'printout' instead of 'this one' and 'it', just as patient EST correctly recognized picture names with 94% accuracy (Kay & Ellis, 1987).

An outside investigator might have mistaken my word finding problems, and my lack of knowledge for word length and initial sounds, as evidence for a semantic based anomia. Instead, I argue that the pattern described by Kay and Ellis, complete semantic retrieval *and* partial, word-specific blocking of lexical access, is indeed possible in anomia. The feeling is difficult even for me to describe and is no doubt more difficult for someone to imagine without having experienced it. The description that anomics 'in some sense, "know" the word' may be to blame. I did not 'know' the word, at least in its articulation or output sense. I did 'know' the word in its semantic, 'idea' or 'concept' sense, without a hint as to the verbal name for the idea.

REFERENCES

Ashcraft, M. H. and Fierman, B. A. (1982). Mental addition in third, fourth, and sixth graders. *Journal of Experimental Child Psychology*, **33**, 216–35.

Ellis, A. W. (1985). The production of spoken words: A cognitive neuropsychological perspective. In *Progress in the psychology of language*, Vol. 2 (ed. A. W. Ellis). Lawrence Erlbaum, London.

Geschwind, N. (1967). The varieties of naming errors. *Cortex*, **3**, 97–112.

Goodglass, H., Kaplan, E., Weintraub, S., and Ackerman, N. (1976). The 'tip-of-the-tongue' phenomenon in aphasia. *Cortex*, **12**, 145–53.

James, W. (1890). *The principles of psychology*. Dover, New York.

Kay, J. and Ellis, A. (1987). A cognitive neuropsychological case study of anomia: Implications for psychological models of word retrieval. *Brain*, **110**, 613–29.

Kertesz, A. (1982). Two case studies: Broca's and Wernicke's aphasia. In *Neural models of language processes* (ed. M. A. Arbib, D. Caplin, and J. C. Marshall), pp. 25–44. Academic Press, New York.

Kolb, B. (1990). Recovery from occipital stroke: A self-report and an inquiry into visual processes. *Canadian Journal of Psychology*, **44**, 130–47.

Schacter, D. L. (1989). Memory. In *Foundations of cognitive science* (ed. M. I. Posner), pp. 683–725. MIT Press, Cambridge, MA.

Tulving, E. (1983). *Elements of episodic memory*. Oxford University Press, New York.

(Ashcraft 1993)

COMMENTARY

Although Ashcraft has classified his attack as a seizure, it could equally well be seen as a transient ischaemic attack. Ashcraft's continual staring, 'with nothing on my mind' (p. 106), is suggestive of an epileptic event, but unlike most epileptic states he did appear to be aware of external stimuli and of his attempts to respond to these. The range of difficulties experienced by Ashcraft (naming problems, memory difficulty, difficulty in reading, writing impairment) were rather limited in extent and could be interpreted by some clinicians as reflecting an 'acute confusional state' following an epileptic episode.

Ashcraft's very specific naming difficulty, with apparently intact semantics, points to the presence of a 'word selection anomia' (Benson 1979)—such a pure anomia has tended to be associated with lesions in the posterior portion of the inferior temporal gyrus of the left hemisphere.

In addition to being unable to express thoughts into sentences (e.g. explaining to his wife the problem he was encountering), he could not recall a single word—'logoff'—that had to be applied in a specific context, namely terminating his computer link at the end of his day's work. Other words that he could not retrieve were 'printout', 'data', 'experiment', and 'results'. These were probably all rather low-frequency, abstract words in Ashcraft's vocabulary. While his overall recollection of the experience appeared to be quite clear, Ashcraft did appear to have a limited memory deficit for a few items, such as his inability to remember mentioning his computer problems to his research assistant. Ashcraft's main concern was for his physical well-being, and his sense of bemusement did not become one of panic as long as the event remained a cognitive one. It is possible that someone with a different professional background to Ashcraft, in a different setting, where there was no necessity to recall low-frequency, abstract words, might have dismissed the episode without regarding it as pathological.

REFERENCE

Benson, D. F. (1979). Neurological correlates of anomia. In *Studies in neurolinguistics*, Vol. 4 (ed. H. Whitaker and H. A. Whitaker), pp. 298–328. Academic Press, New York.

GENERAL COMMENTARY

1. Language and thought

Views on the relationship between thought and language have a long history. On the one hand, writers such as Immanuel Kant in the eighteenth century, and in more recent times Noam Chomsky, emphasized the close relationship between thought and language. On the other hand, protagonists such as John Locke in the seventeenth century and Jean Piaget in the twentieth century put greater weight on the independence of language from thinking. The evidence from the personal accounts of aphasia presented in this book demonstrate that in some forms of aphasia thinking may be significantly altered as a result of language deficits, while in other types of aphasia thinking may be completely unaffected. The data in the self-reports suggest that the degree to which there is memory loss, in the form of impaired memory for specific sets of knowledge that were readily accessible prior to the brain illness/injury, may play a role in determining whether 'thinking ability' is disturbed, and this may in turn relate to the degree of temporal lobe damage that is present.

Some of the aphasia self-reports in this section point to an impressive dissociation between speech production ability/verbal fluency on the one hand, and cognition on the other hand, and they provide as good an illustration as any on how these two facets of brain activity can be functionally separated. It would seem that much of **Andrewes**' thought processes were relatively preserved—he considered himself to be a man 'in full possession of his faculties' (p. 55), and with his communication device he was able to develop 'a certain mental agility in deciding in how small a number of letters I could express a given idea' (p. 55).

Lordat found that his thought processes were untouched by his dysphasia. **Lordat** commented, 'Inwardly, I felt the same as ever. This mental isolation which I mention, my sadness, my impediment and the appearance of stupidity which it gave rise to, led many to believe that my intellectual faculties were weakened . . . My memory for facts, principles, dogmas, abstract ideas, was the same as when I enjoyed good health . . . Thus, while recognizing the instrumentality of language in conserving ideas, in preserving them for future reference, and in transmitting them, I was unable to accept completely Condillac's theory that verbal signs are necessary, even indispensable, for thought' (pp. 71–2). This observation was made despite the fact that **Lordat** admitted losing his 'memory of the meaning of articulated words'.

Ashcraft's major symptom was a dissociation between the *thought* that was clearly represented in his mind, and the inability to find and therefore articulate the correct *words* that would enable him to translate that thought into speech. 'The most powerful realization I had during the episode, and the most intriguing aspect to me since then, was the dissociation between a thought and the word or phrase that expresses the thought' (p. 105). The relatively benign nature of his lesion, an anteriovenous malformation, may have played a part in the quite focal language deficits that he displayed and in the integrity of his concomitant thought processes.

Ashcraft was able to initiate and entertain thought processes (e.g. generate and test hypotheses as to how ill he really was), while at the same time having a significant nominal dysphasia. His 'train of thought' was relatively intact, implying that attention/awareness, short-term memory and problem-solving processes were not markedly affected. Whether he was totally aware of all aspects of his episode and his limitations remains in doubt, in view of his insistence that he should be allowed to drive home. As **Ashcraft** himself points out, this could have also been partly due to a heightened emotional reaction to his situation.

In contrast with the above observations, even seven years after his stroke, **Moss** noted slight but significant difficulties that impinged on his thinking ability: 'thinking no longer comes as easily as it did once' (p. 76). Although, two years after his stroke, **Moss** did go back to many of his former academic duties, he found that he could not fulfil these to quite the same level as was required. He thus gave up trying to teach community psychology, some of which involved less structured seminar courses with bright postgraduate students, and he concentrated on more didactic courses in abnormal psychology. It could be argued that the latter courses did not involve the same level of speed or abstraction in thinking, further confirming his observations of some impact of his dysphasia on his thinking ability.

2. Memory

Most of the authors of the self-reports had little in the way of 'pre-traumatic' amnesia for events prior to the onset of their aphasia, and authors such as **Andrewes** and **Ashcraft** were also able to offer quite vivid memories of events that occurred in the hours and days afterwards. These sets of data highlight the sparing of retrograde and anterograde memory functioning in such cases of discrete pathology, and one suspects that the greatest sparing occurred in cases of Broca's aphasia following focal lesions in the frontal region. There is an obvious contrast with cases of closed head injury, where even a relatively minor injury can result in loss of memory for pre- and post-traumatic events.

Moss talks about existing, for a period of time, only in the present, without having a detailed awareness of the past or thoughts about the future: 'I was unable to generate a gestalt of either my previous life or the future' (p. 87). Up to five months after the accident, **Moss** could recall the names of former neighbours but he 'could not embroider them with associations' as he had formerly. **Moss'** psychiatrist regarded this to be a form of retrograde amnesia. If one takes retrograde amnesia as representing loss of knowledge for any information that was readily available prior to the illness, then one could indeed say that **Moss** had a form of retrograde amnesia. Even **Moss'** difficulty in recalling how to drive his car could, in this sense, be seen as a retrograde amnesia. All dysphasics who have lost the ability to use language after a brain insult could equally be seen to have suffered a form of retrograde amnesia. However, the latter term tends to be used more often for loss of memory for specific, personally experienced events. Loss of factual knowledge, whether it be about things or people, tends to come under the rubric of impaired 'semantic memory'.

Moss' possible interpretation of his loss of past memories (which proved to be a temporary loss) is that it may have been due to a 'massive retroactive inhibition', such that a shocking event may inhibit other memories neighbouring in time to the critical event. While such an explanation is attractive, and has some plausibility, it is more likely that his brain lesion resulted in a true disruption of those neural networks that related to the storage or ready access of facts or events, and the various associations to these facts and events.

For **Moss** (p. 81), his 'memory banks were out of order' and he 'needed constant companionship to remind me of past learning and to put the memory tapes back into some sort of usable order'. In another part of the chapter (p. 78), he describes how 'the stroke had abolished my memory of the past'. **Moss** also reports that he never felt he was learning a new language during his recovery period, simply improving his retrieval mechanisms. The fact that many of his lost memories did eventually return, and the fact that **Moss** refers to a lack of order in his memories, suggests that the stored representations of memories were not damaged but that some form of access/retrieval deficits lay behind his difficulties. (cf. Warrington and Cipolotti (1996))

It is of interest that **Ashcraft**'s initial symptoms appeared to consist of a loss of familiarity of material—he was unable to say if a particular computer printout was one of an old data analysis or of a new data analysis. These symptoms are similar to a report of transient partial amnesia, possibly due to a seizure-related phenomenon, where the individual could not recognize names in her diary as being familiar (Damasio *et al.* 1983).

3. Social and emotional sequelae

It is tempting to view language deficits in isolation from the social and emotional roles played by verbal communication skills. The articles in this section provide a welcome reminder of the relationship between language ability, social adjustment, and emotional stability, although the exact nature of this relationship is often difficult to delineate.

Moss' observation that he suffered from deep depression for about three weeks after he came home, and that when this resolved his sense of loss for past events also resolved, may well be coincidence rather than pointing to a psychological basis to his memory symptoms. It is worth pointing out that depression has been associated with left hemisphere damage (Robinson and Szetela 1981), and that in positron emission tomography studies left frontal hypometabolism has been associated with primary depression (Bench *et al.* 1992).

Moss' eloquent analogy with the mind of a porpoise, being unable to express intelligent thoughts through language, highlights the frustration and feelings of depression that **Moss** reports, and which he signals with his admission to having occasional suicidal thoughts [cf. Ireland (1990) and Oswin (1992) where aphasia was misdiagnosed as reflecting a psychiatric condition!].

Interestingly, **Moss** sees 'denial' as a compensatory and supportive mechanism, and he contrasts this with his own supersensitivity to his residual difficulties. **Moss** notes two changes in his personality—a withdrawal from social interactions, and a loss of his sense of humour. In the case of social withdrawal, **Moss**' observations bring home the fundamental point that language is our major means of handling relationships with other people, of expressing emotions and aspirations, etc. and that a language disorder will therefore inevitably lead to some difficulties in social settings. His loss of sense of humour appears to relate to a difficulty in producing appropriate timing into his spontaneous remarks. The latter feature is very important for a good sense of humour. His wife later reported (p. 175 of the original book) that about four years post-injury his sense of humour appeared to come back in his utterances, although notes that he did display glimpses of a sense of humour even in the early stages of recovery (p. 26 of the original book).

4. Management/rehabilitation

Rose describes how memorizing large amounts of text and poetry appeared to improve his language fluency. **Rose** also contends that 'near memorization', as opposed to complete committal to memory, was beneficial for his speech, and he pointed to the increase in vocabulary that resulted from either procedure. His technique included reading material twice daily for ten days. and repeating this two or three times. Amongst the items he memorized was Hamlet's soliloquy. It is interesting that he thought of the idea of 'memorisation' as a treatment strategy after finding that. even though his speech was limited. he could sing old songs almost perfectly. He himself commented (**Rose**'s writing errors have been retained): 'The brain pathes for singing takes a course further from the stroke area and there-fore this also holds for memorisation' (p. 66). A form of speech therapy. melodic intonation therapy. whereby the individual intones a melody for simple statements (Sparks *et al.* 1974). has in fact been tried with dysphasic patients. but it has had limited success in producing major improvements in everyday speech.

Moss. in his 1976 article (p. 78). bemoans the inability of speech therapists to 'move upstream' and do something about 'massive memory deficits' and 'concreteness of thought'. as opposed to speech articulation and other more typical foci of speech therapy. This aspect of language and cognitive functioning lies in a grey area that borders the province of speech therapy and neuropsychology. and it is perhaps an area where cognitive rehabilitation could fruitfully be applied.

Neurological patients with language difficulties perhaps need more understanding and consideration than other neurological patients due to the nature of their disability. and the myths that surround aphasic patients. These myths were cogently summarized in a self-report account written by Wulf (1979. p. 165):

Myth 1 If the patient appears comatose. he will not hear anything. and if he should hear he will not understand. and if he should understand he will not remember.

Myth 2 The patient does not understand anything that is said to him. so it is all right to talk about him. Even say he is never going to be any better than he is right now.

Myth 3 The aphasic will not remember. so it is OK to say almost anything in his presence. Tactless words? He will not remember them.

Myth 4 All aphasics are sorta kooky anyway.

Myth 5 Speak loud. The patient cannot talk and does not seem to understand so he must be hard of hearing. (Truth is. sounds often become the most horrendous kind of noise and can be very distressing to the aphasic.)

Myth 6 He said that word yesterday. There is no reason why he cannot say it today.

Myth 7 Aphasia destroys the thinking. whole person. (And that is probably the unkindest cut of all.)

REFERENCES

Bench. C. H.. Friston. K. J.. Brown. R. G.. Scott. L. C. Frackowiak. R. S. J.. and Dolan. R. J. (1992). The anatomy of melancholia—focal abnormalities of cerebral blood flow in major depression. *Psychological Medicine.* **22.** 607–15.

Damasio, A. R., Graff-Radford, N. R., and Damasio, H. (1983). Transient partial amnesia. *Archives of Neurology*, **40**, 656–7.

Ireland, C. (1990). I'm not mad—I'm angry. *Nursing Times*, **86**, 45–7.

Oswin, M. (1992). The quiet menace. *Nursing Times*, **88**, 40–1.

Robinson, R. G. and Szetela, B. (1981). Mood changes following left hemisphere brain injury. *Annals of Neurology*, **9**, 447–53.

Sparks, R., Helm, N., and Albert, M. (1974). Aphasia rehabilitation resulting from melodic intonation therapy. *Cortex*, **10**, 303–16.

Warrington, E. K. and Cipolotti, L. (1966). World Comprehension. The distinction between refractory and storage impairments. *Brain*, **119**, 611–25.

Wulf, H. H. (1979). *Aphasia, my world alone*. Wayne University Press, Detroit.

Visual disorders 3

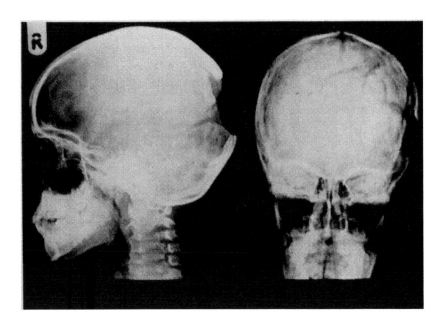

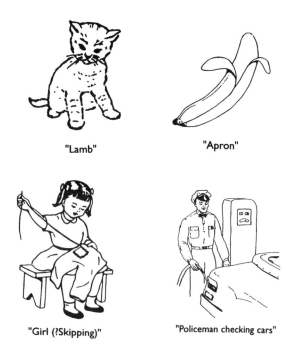

"Lamb"

"Apron"

"Girl (?Skipping)"

"Policeman checking cars"

Figure 5. Nine-year-old girl who sustained a penetrating missile injury, caused by a bomb explosion, that fractured her skull and caused massive damage to both occipital lobes. This resulted in blindness for the first few months, and an apperceptive visual agnosia after this period. One year after her injury, she was asked to name these pictures, and her responses are shown.

INTRODUCTION

Disturbances of visual function are more commonly associated with damage to posterior rather than to anterior parts of the brain, and to the right rather than to the left hemisphere. Visual disorders may take a number of forms:

(1) *Visual field defect.*   This reflects the inability to be consciously aware of stimuli in a certain part of one's visual field. Such a deficit usually follows discrete lesions in one or other of the occipital lobes or in pathways leading from the retina to the occipital lobes. Where there is massive damage to both occipital lobes, then 'cortical blindness' may follow. One of the major themes of the articles in this section of the book relates to the ability to be unconsciously aware of stimuli that are presented in the area of a visual field defect ('blindsight').

(2) *Visuospatial deficits.*   This refers to deficits in the ability to make spatial judgements—these may include the inability to localize an object or one's own body in space and to make related judgements such as directionality, distance, movement, etc. Visuospatial deficits may also encompass impairments in attending to and responding appropriately to objects in certain parts of the visual field ('visual neglect'), even when there is no visual field defect.

(3) *Visuoperceptual deficits.*   At an elementary level, visuoperceptual deficits refer to impairments in the accurate perception of a figure, in the absence of any significant visual field defect. They may encompass impairments in the ability to see an object as a whole, or even to see more than two stimuli at once, however small they may be. At a further stage of processing, there may be an inability to analyse and synthesize the parts of a complex visual figure into a visual representation that accurately reflects the figure. The patient may be unable to make a copy of the figure or to make specific visual judgements about the stimulus (e.g. identify the same figure when viewed from a different angle). A deficit may occur at a relatively late stage of processing, and reflect an impairment in the ability to derive meaning from the visual stimulus, even when the stimulus can be accurately perceived—such a deficit is known as a 'visual agnosia' (a 'percept stripped of its meaning' is a useful way of thinking of it). Visual agnosias may be specific to particular types of stimuli—one that is specific to the ability to identify faces is called 'prosopagnosia'.

(4) *Visuoconstructive deficits.*   With these types of impairments, there is an inability to perform tasks which have both a visual and a motor component. These may include assembly-type tasks, such as putting a jigsaw puzzle together, or skills such as writing.
   The four self-report articles reprinted in this chapter deal with quite specific forms of visual dysfunction, mainly ones of a transient rather than a chronic nature. In two cases (**Lashley 1941; Boles 1993**), there is a description of transient visual disturbance related to migraine attacks. In one case (**Mize 1980**), there is a description of visual hallucinations, and in the remaining case (**Kolb 1990**) there is an account of recovery from a right occipital stroke. Of these four cases, the one by **Kolb** is more closely related to classical neurological syndromes.

Other articles in this book, such as the one by **Medawar** in Chapter 6, also touch on visual disorders such as unilateral neglect.

FURTHER READING

Ellis, A. W. and Young, A. W. (1988). *Human cognitive neuropsychology*. Lawrence Erlbaum, Hove.

Farah, M. J. and Ratcliff, G. (ed.) (1994). *The neuropsychology of high-level vision*. Lawrence Erlbaum, Hove.

Parkin, A. J. (1996). *Explorations in cognitive neuropsychology*. Blackwell, Oxford.

Patterns of cerebral integration indicated by the scotomas of migraine

K. S. Lashley

Karl Lashley was one of the outstanding neuropsychologists of this century, and for a while he was Professor of Psychology at Harvard University.

The scotomas characteristic of ophthalmic migraine have been described by a number of investigators.[1] The visual disturbance precedes or accompanies other symptoms of migraine and is usually of short duration. It is generally restricted to one half of the visual field, the right or the left, and ranges in size from a scarcely noticeable blindspot to total hemianopia. A great variety of forms have been mentioned in the literature, but those which have been described in detail are of much the same type. The scotoma starts as a disturbance of vision limited to the neighborhood of the macula and spreads rapidly toward the temporal field. With increase in size the disturbed area moves or 'drifts' across the visual field, so that its central margin withdraws from the macular region as its peripheral margin invades the temporal. Spread from the temporal toward the macular region has also been described and is apparently more frequent when complete hemianopia develops. The area may be totally blind (negative scotoma), amblyopic or outlined by scintillations. A scotoma of the last type takes the form of 'fortification figures', so called from the suggestion of a map of the bastions of a fortified town. They appear as series of parallel, white or colored scintillating lines, forming angles or polygons along the margins of the scotomatous area. The scotomas are symmetric for the two eyes and so are almost certainly the result of a cortical disturbance.

Two characteristics of the scotomas have not previously been reported and are of some interest as suggesting the nature of the inherent organization of cortical activity. These are (1) the maintenance of the characteristic shape of the scotoma during its drift across the visual field and (2) the 'completion of figure' described by Gelb and by Poppelreuter as occurring in scotomas of traumatic origin.

Over a period of years I have had opportunity to observe and map a large number of such scotomas, uncomplicated by any other symptoms of migraine. The scotoma usually occurs first as a small blind or scintillating spot, subtending less than 1 degree, in or immediately adjacent to the foveal field. This spot rapidly increases in size and drifts away from the fovea toward the temporal field of one side. Usually both quadrants of one side only are involved, the right and the left being affected with about equal frequency. Occasionally the scotoma is confined to one quadrant. Rarely, there is complete hemianopia, and in 1 instance, in more than 100, there was complete blindness in both lower quadrants, with sparing of the macula.

RATE OF DRIFT

The outline of the scotoma is readily charted by fixating a mark on a sheet of paper, moving a pencil toward the blind area along different radiuses and marking the places at which the point of the pencil disappears—the usual method for crude demonstration of the blindspot. When this is done, each scotomatous area is found to have a distinct shape, and when the charting is repeated at brief intervals, this specific shape is roughly

---

[1] For an account of the symptomatology of ophthalmic migraine, with references, see H. Richter (in Bumke, O., and Foerster, O.: Handbuch der Neurologie, Berlin, Julius Springer, 1935, vol. 17, pp. 166–345). The most detailed description of scotomas is that of F. Jolly (Ueber Flimmerskotom und Migräne, Berl. klin. Wechnschr. 39:973–976, 1902).

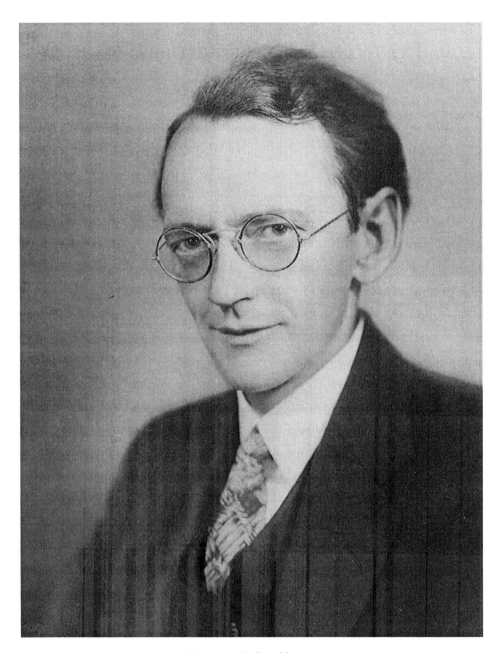

Figure 6. Karl Lashley.

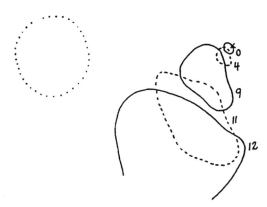

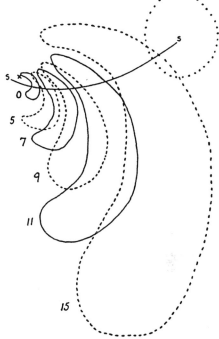

Figure. 1. Maps of a negative scotoma confined to the lower left quadrant. The successive sketches were made at intervals of no, four, nine, eleven and twelve minutes after the area was first noted. Alternate sketches are outlined with broken lines to avoid confusion. The fixation point is marked by X. The dotted circle is an outline of the blindspot of the homolateral eye, to indicate the size of the visual field. In this instance the form was not well maintained.

Figure 2. Maps of a scintillating scotoma sketched at the intervals, expressed in minutes, shown at the left. Scintillations were confined to the region above the line s-s. Arrangement as in figure 1.

preserved as the area drifts across the visual field. Figures 1, 2, 3 and 4 show the successive positions and shapes of four such areas charted at intervals of from two to five minutes. Occasionally the shape is not well preserved, as in the area shown in figure 1. Generally, however, within the region between the macula and the optic disk[2] the form is maintained, as shown in figures 2 and 4, and occasionally, as in figure 3, successive charting reveals almost perfect correspondence of forms. As the scotoma drifts to the temporal field accurate mapping becomes impossible, since the pencil point can no longer be clearly seen.

Not only does the form of the scotomatous area remain constant as it drifts across the visual field, but when there are fortification figures, these also maintain their characteristic pattern in each part of the area. The size of the fortification figures does not increase

with increase in the size of the scotoma, but additional figures are added as the area grows. It is not possible to sketch the figures accurately. The rate of scintillation is near 10 per second[3] and the form changes rapidly, but small figures can be distinguished from large and simple angles from polygonal figures. Differences of the sort indicated in figure 5 are unmistakably present and persist while the area drifts for considerable distances across the field. I have the impression, without adequate data to confirm it, that the size and shape of the fortification figures are constant for each radius of the field. That is, the pattern is finer and less complicated in the upper quadrants than in the lower, as indicated in figures 4 and 5. If true, this suggests that the pattern is a function of the

_____

[2] The blindspots do not, of course, interfere with binocular charting of the scotoma. In the figures the outline of the blindspot of the homolateral eye is inserted to indicate the position and size of the scotoma in relation to the visual field.

[3] This rate is above the maximum for counting but well below the flicker fusion point. The rate may be related to the alpha rhythm.

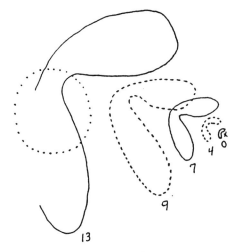

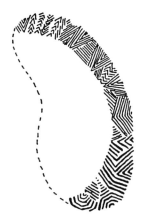

Figure 3. Successive maps of a negative scotoma, arranged as figure 1.

Figure 5. Sketch to show apparent differences in fortification figures. The coarser and more complicated figures are generally in the lower part of the field.

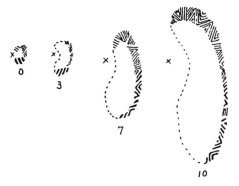

Figure 4. Successive maps of a scintillating scotoma to show characteristic distribution of the fortification figures. The X in each case indicates the fixation point.

anatomic substratum, rather than of the nature of the propagated disturbance. More certainly, when the fortification figures are limited to one part of the area, they continue in that part only throughout the entire drift, as shown in figure 2.

Whatever the precipitating cause of the disturbance, these facts indicate that an inhibitory process, in the case of blind areas, or an excitatory process, in the case of scintillations, is initiated in one part of the visual cortex and spreads over an additional area. As the process spreads, activity at the point where it was initiated is extinguished, and

the process of extinction also spreads over the same area at about the same rate as does the active process.

The increase in size of the scotoma as it passes toward the peripheral areas does not necessarily mean that the disturbance starts from a point and spreads to larger areas. Apparent size in the visual field is not related to the size of the excited region of the striate cortex, since the cortical field of the macula is probably as large as that of all the remaining retina.[4] Apparent size must be determined at a later stage of integration, and in the case of smaller scotomas the actual extent of cortical area involved in the disturbance is probably constant as the disturbance drifts.

The drift of the scotomatous area is what might be expected from the spread of excitation across a succession of reverberatory circuits, as described by Lorente de Nó,[5] with the activity of the circuits extinguished at the inner margin of the blind area at the same rate as it is propagated to new circuits at the advancing margin. The rate of propagation may eventually have some significance. For a

[4] Poliak, S. (1932). The main afferent fiber system of the cerebral cortex in primates, Univ. California Publ. Anat. 2, 1.

[5] Lorente de Nó, R. (1938). Analysis of the activity of the chains of internuncial neurons, J. Neurophysiol., 1, 207–44.

number of observations the rate is fairly uniform. Ten to twelve minutes is required for spread of the outer margin from the region of the macula to the blindspot of the homolateral eye. The rate beyond this point is rapid and difficult to estimate, but the total time required for the disturbance to spread from the macular area to the temporal field is approximately twenty minutes. A negative area of the size shown in figure 2 is determined by an inhibitory phase lasting for about five minutes. The development and the recovery of complete hemianopia each requires about fifteen to twenty minutes, indicating a propagation of the disturbance at about the same rate, with a longer period of inhibition, sometimes lasting half an hour.

The anteroposterior length of the striate area is about 67 mm.[6] The disturbance starts very near the midline of the visual field, which is probably projected near the occipital pole; propagation to the temporal margin requires about twenty minutes. These figures give a rate of 3 mm. per minute or less for the propagation of the disturbance.

In each attack the disturbance seems to spread with different characteristics along different radiuses of the visual field. Thus, in the scotoma sketched in figure 2 scintillations were confined to the upper quadrant and the duration of the inhibited phase was apparently greater in the lower part of the field than in the upper, as measured by the width of the band. The constriction in the band, shown in figure 3, indicates a negative phase of short duration, passing out along a definite radius above the margin of the lower quadrant. Poppelreuter[7] has pointed out that in scotomas of traumatic origin there are indications of dynamic organization of the visual field such that effects of fatigue, etc., tend to spread along the radiuses of the field, and the evidence from the scotomas of migraine leads to a similar conclusion. No anatomic basis for such phenomena is

known at present, but some anteroposterior polarization of the striate cortex is indicated.

The scintillations must represent a phase of intense excitation. The lines are of dazzling brightness, subjectively of the order of direct sunlight reflected from a white surface. They occur along the advancing margin of the area,[8] followed by the blind region, as if a wave of strong excitation were followed by a phase of total inhibition (fig. 4). However, part or all of the area may show no signs of excitation, yet advance at the same rate (fig. 2, lower part). From this it seems that the inhibitory phase may spread without a preliminary phase of excitation, and at the same rate. Occasionally the negative phase fails to develop, and objects may be seen in the field immediately behind, or even between, the fortification figures, as shown in the sketches of Jolly.[1] The propagation of the excitatory phase with or without a subsequent protracted inhibitory phase and the propagation of the inhibitory phase without evidence of previous excitation raise an important problem of the interrelations of these processes.

LIMITATION OF SPREAD

The definite limitation of symptoms to those of primary visual disturbance argues for a sharp functional separation of the striate areas from adjacent regions of the cortex. The disturbance, spreading as a scintillating or negative scotoma, is evidently intense, or at least dominant over other cortical activities; yet it appears to be blotted out completely at the margin of the striate cortex. Except for a very slight torticollis associated with complete hemianopia. I have been unable to detect any additional symptoms during or after the scotoma. It seems to move off the side of the visual field and leave no after-effects whatever. The absence of any symptoms associated with the peristriate

[6] Filimonoff, I. N. (1932). Ueber die Variabiltät der Grosshirnrindenstruktur. J. f. Psychol. u. Neurol., 44, 1–96.
[7] Poppelreuter, W. (1917). Die psychischen Schädigungen durch Kopfschuss im Kriege 1914–1917. L. Voss, Leipzig.

[8] In the early stages, when the area is near the macula, it may be entirely filled with scintillations, but later these form a band of varying width along the advancing margins. Circular bands radiating from a point have been reported.

areas indicates that the disturbance does not spread beyond the margin of the primary visual cortex. The interconnections between architectonic areas must therefore be of a very different nature from those of a single area.

In experiments with animals I have been unable to demonstrate any symptoms of visual disturbance after knife cuts which partially sever the striate cortex from surrounding areas, even when difficult problems of visual generalization are used in the tests.[9] The complete blocking of the excitatory wave of the scotoma suggests that in man also there may be a greater autonomy of function in the different architectonic areas than is generally assumed to be the case.

REPETITIVE PATTERNS

The activity within the scintillating area is perhaps of some theoretic interest. The scintillations have the form of distinct parallel lines, which cannot be counted but give the impression of groups of five or more. These seem to sweep across the figure toward the advancing margin and are constantly renewed at the inner margin, like the illusion of movement of a revolving screw. The pattern of lines and angles is much the same in the experience of all persons who have reported them. Its significance is in the reduplication of activity throughout a considerable area. Repetitive patterns of activity have been reported in other cases of pathologic cortical activity. They are frequently mentioned as characteristic of the visual hallucinations following mescal poisoning,[10] and perhaps are represented on the motor side by the convulsive movements of an epileptic attack.

Such repetitive patterns should be predicted from the free spread of excitation through a uniform neural field having the structural arrangement of reverberatory cir-

cuits described by Lorente de Nó.[11] Although nothing is known of the actual nervous activity during the migraine, the picture suggests that the propagated disturbance is so intense as to be independent of the afferent supply of the cortex and that the patterning represents the type of organization into which the cortical activity falls as a result of inherent properties of the architectonic structure. I have elsewhere outlined briefly a theory of cortical integration based on interference of spreading waves of excitation,[12] and the patterning shown in the migraine scotomas is consistent with that theory.

COMPLETION OF FIGURE

The 'principle of completion' in visual organization was first pointed out by Fuchs[13] and confirmed by Poppelreuter.[7] It states that certain simple geometric patterns (square, circle, triangle, stripes) when exposed so that a part falls within the blind field of a patient with hemianopia of traumatic origin are always perceived as complete figures, although it is certain that the part falling within the scotomatous area is not actually seen. When the migraine scotoma is without scintillations the same phenomenon may be observed. Two examples stand out in my experience in which there was opportunity for careful observation.

A negative scotoma may completely escape observation, even when it is just off the macula, unless it obscures some object to which attention is directed. Talking with a friend, I glanced just to the right of his face, whereon his head disappeared. His shoulders and necktie were still visible, but the vertical stripes in the wallpaper behind him seemed

[9] Lashley, K. S. The mechanism of vision: XVII. Autonomy of the visual cortex. J. Genet. Psychol., to be published.
[10] Klüver, H. (1928). Mescal, pp. 1–116. Kegan Paul, trench, Trubner & Company, London.

[11] Lorente de Nó, R. (1934). Studies on the structure of the cerebral cortex: II. Continuation of the study of the ammonic System. J. f. Psychol. u. Neurol., 46, 113–77.
[12] Lashley, K. S. (1931). Mass action in cerebral function. Science, 73, 245–54.
[13] Fuchs, W. (1920). Untersuchungen über das Sehen der Hemianopiker und Hemiamblyopiker: II. Die totalisierende Gestaltauffasung. In Psychologische Analysen hirnpathologischer Falle, (ed. A. Gelb and K. Goldstein), pp. 419–561. J. A. Barth, Leipzig.

to extend right down to the necktie. Quick mapping revealed an area of total blindness covering about 30 degrees, just off the macula. It was quite impossible to see this as a blank area when projected on the striped wall or other uniformly patterned surface, although any intervening object failed to be seen.

On another occasion, with complete hemianopia, including the macula, it was possible to divide a complex object on any line of fixation. A human face was sharply divided by fixating the tip of the nose, so that half, including one nostril only, was visible. At the same time it was impossible so to fixate a circular object that only half was seen. Fixating a chalk mark on the middle of a billiard ball failed to make any part of the ball invisible, although the ball was considerably larger than the readily divided nose.

These observations are of interest as showing that filling in the blindspot and the completion of figures in scotomatous areas are not the result of habits of disregarding blind areas or of identifying part figures. The phenomena appear immediately with new blind areas. They must, then, represent some intrinsic organizing function of the cortex. The figures completed are reduplicated patterns or very simple symmetric figures. The relation of this fact to the tendency to reduplication in fortification figures and other patterns of 'spontaneous' activity of the visual areas is suggestive of a common mechanism.

Such phenomena can be made intelligible by the assumption that the integrative mechanism of the striate cortex tends to reproduce a pattern of excitation, aroused in one region, in any other region also if the latter is not dominated by different afferent patterns. Such a reduplication of patterns should result from the spreading of waves of excitation from points of initial stimulation, by analogy with the transmission of wave patterns on the surface of a liquid. Recent work on the histology of the cortex reveals an anatomic basis for radiation of such waves, in that the interconnections are so numerous as to constitute virtually a homogeneous conducting mechanism.

SUMMARY

Maps of the scotomas of ophthalmic migraine sketched at brief intervals during an attack suggest that a wave of intense excitation is propagated at a rate of about 3 mm. per minute across the visual cortex. This wave is followed by complete inhibition of activity, with recovery progressing at the same rate. Sometimes the inhibition spreads without the preceding excitatory wave. Limitation of the disturbance to the primary visual cortex raises questions as to the nature of the interconnections between architectonic fields. The observations are interpreted in relation to the possible integrative effects of radiating waves of excitation in the cortex.

(Lashley 1941)

COMMENTARY

Lashley reported that his migraine attack brought about blind spots, elementary visual hallucinations that included scintillating scotoma, and visual completion effects—these observations are strongly suggestive of occipital lobe involvement (Silberstein and Young 1995). Scintillations in themselves have been shown to occur after stimulation of the occipital lobe in man (Brindley and Lewin 1968). Lashley interpreted his visual symptoms as supporting a theory of 'cortical integration based on interference of spreading waves of excitation' (p. 126). While this particular view is not precise enough to have been substantiated by subsequent research, there would be general support for his further comment that the limitation of spread of the visual disturbances suggests significant autonomy of function in different architectonic areas, at least in occipital areas of the brain. The slow migration of Lashley's scintillating scotoma could be seen to support a mechanism of 'spreading depression' of neuronal activity that results in reduced blood flow during the migraine attack (Pearce 1985). The interesting point with regard to Lashley's visual aura, which itself is representative of other self-reports of visual aura experienced by migraine sufferers (Airy 1870), is the co-occurrence of an excitatory phenomenon (scintillations) and an inhibitory phenomenon (scotoma).

Lashley's comment (p. 126) that a negative scotoma may completely escape observation, unless it obscures some object to which attention is directed, adds to the growing list of clinical phenomena where a subtle brain abnormality may be present, but may not result in a change in conscious awareness by the subject—these can be seen most clearly in subclinical epileptiform cognitive changes (e.g. Rugland 1990). Lashley's anatomical speculations were mostly general ones that pointed to possible mechanisms in the striate and extrastriate areas of visual cortex. Recent brain-imaging studies of subjects, carried out while they have been experiencing a migraine attack, have similarly implicated association areas of the visual cortex, but have also pointed to involvement of the anterior cingulate region, auditory association areas, and the brainstem. Indeed, activation persisted in the brainstem after resolution of the migraine attack (Weiller *et al.* 1995).

REFERENCES

Airy, H. (1870). On a distinct form of transient hemiopsia. *Philosophical Transactions of the Royal Society*, **160**, 247–64.

Brindley, G. S. and Lewin, W. S. (1968). The sensations produced by electrical stimulation of the visual cortex. *Journal of Physiology*, **196**, 479–93.

Pearce, J. (1985). Is migraine explained by Leao's spreading depression? *Lancet*, 2, October 5, 764–6.

Rugland, A. L. (1990). 'Subclinical' epileptogenic activity. In *Paediatric epilepsy* (ed. M. Sillanpaa *et al*), pp. 217–24. Wrightson Biomedical, Petersfield, UK.

Silberstein, S. D. and Young, W. B. (1995). Migraine aura and prodrome. *Seminars in Neurology*, **15**, 175–82.

Weiller, C., May, A., Limmroth, V., Juptner, M., Kaube, H., v. Schayck, R., *et al.* (1995). Brain stem activation in spontaneous human migraine attacks. *Nature Medicine*, **1**, 658–60.

Visual hallucinations following viral encephalitis: a self report

Kathryn Mize

Kathryn Mize was a medical student at the time of her illness.

I. INTRODUCTION

Visual hallucinations may accompany a gamut of metabolic, neurologic or psychologic conditions. In a descriptive stage, the visual hallucinations of physiologic and drug-induced circumstances have been found to have characteristic qualities remarkably similar from person to person. Clinical categories of visual hallucinations have been outlined. This paper is evidence that visual hallucinations produced during a disease state are characteristic of those described in other hallucinatory conditions.

The phenomenology of visual aberrations and hallucinations has attracted many investigators. Klüver was the first really to distill a categorization of mescaline-induced imagery. This drug-induced hallucinosis consisted of two stages. In the first stage Klüver[1] described four categories of form constants: (1) *grating, lattice, honeycomb, chessboard*, fretwork, filigree; (2) cobweb; (3) tunnel, funnel, alley, *cone*, vessel; (4) *spiral*. In the second stage the form constants elaborated into intricate arabesques, filigrees, Persian carpet patterns, tapestries and finally into the visualization of scenes, faces and objects. Klüver observed that this phenomenon occurred in a variety of hallucinatory conditions, with the eyes open or closed, and was beyond conscious control. In addition to constants of form, Klüver additionally suggested constants in multiplication and deformation and in modification of temporospatial relationships of hallucinations.

Smythies[2-4] undertook a detailed categorization and analysis of the complex visual perceptions produced by looking at a uniform flickering field. Brown and Gebhard[5] had previously categorized these stroboscopic patterns into two phases: the dark phase, a function of the externally dark eye, and the bright phase, a function of the externally simulated eye. Smythies categorized the dark phase patterns into seven types. A particular type of dark phase pattern was found to remain constant for one individual for many months. Smythies further classified the bright phase patterns into seven classes and three grades. Patterns of movement, interrelationship of pattern and movement and mode of change of movement could also be classified. Again, the bright phase patterns had individual but classifiable variations and remained constant for the subject for many years. Smythies made the additional observation that many stroboscopic patterns were common to the form constants described by Klüver in the first stage of a mescaline-induced hallucinosis (these are the italicized items in the listing of Klüver's form constants above).

Siegel[6] had described the second stage of mescaline-induced hallucinosis. This complex imagery was found to consist of form constants, similar complex imagery, religious symbols and images. Small animals and people were seen and described as friendly and often represented as cartoons or caricatures against a geometric background. Improbable views such as aerial or underwater scenes were described. Like the form constants of the first stage in the intoxication and the stroboscopic patterns, these complex images showed a remarkable similarity from person to person.

Hécan and Albert[7] have proposed an outline of clinical varieties of visual hallucinations with subsequent attempt at clinicoanatomic correlation. They suggest two categories:

elementary and complex hallucinations. Complex hallucinations are then subdivided into esthesic, associated with dreamy states, oneirism, and associated with ophthalmologic lesions. By combining clinical reports, anatomicoclinical studies and cortical stimulation studies, they suggest that visual hallucinations have a unity of causation with diverse but categorizable clinical manifestations.

The purpose of this paper is to document my hallucinatory experiences following a viral encephalopathy. In doing so I have developed a chronological staging of my behavior and reaction to this phenomenon as well as a categorization of the hallucinations themselves. I describe stages in which I seek to emphasize the circumstances under which I experienced hallucinations. A more thorough classification of the hallucinations as to form, movement, color and content follows the description of stages.

Seven months ago I was admitted to University Hospital for sudden onset of a *grand mal* seizure. I remained unarousable for approximately 40 hr. I am 25 yr old and have no previous history of a seizure disorder. Ten to twelve days prior to admission I was ill with influenza. By history, physical and EEG findings, I had post-infectious viral encephalopathy. The resultant seizure disorder was treated with phenobarbital and phenytoin. In 2 weeks I returned to the classroom to complete my second year of medical school. Such is the preface for the extraordinary hallucinatory experiences that beset me about 6 weeks following my initial seizure.

Chronological staging of my hallucinations

Stage I (6 *weeks*). (All time periods date from my initial hospitalization.) The first vivid hallucinatory experience occurred approximately 6 weeks following my hospitalization. Upon closing my eyes while seated during a lecture, red shimmering geometric forms appeared in the blackness. This startled me, but the shapes were captivating so I watched them in absolute wonder. What I saw with my eyes closed was fantastic. Vague circles

and rectangles would coalesce into beautiful symmetric geometric forms. There was a constant expansion, reabsorption and expansion again about these forms. I remember what seemed like an explosion of black dots in my right field of vision. The dots gracefully floated outward from their origin and were superimposed upon a red scintillating backdrop. Two red rectangular planes appeared and moved in opposite directions. A red ball on a stick moved in a circular fashion beside these planes. Then a red shimmering rippling wave appeared in the lower field of my vision. It moved upward as if I were going under water with my eyes open. I felt like I was floating and my mind was dissociated from my body. It was a beautiful feeling. While at home that day, I began to see incredible forms crystalize when I would close my eyes.

The next morning I sketched out about a dozen patterns that I had seen. Within an hour after completing this, I was walking across a plaza on my way to the school library. The buildings surrounding the plaza were very geometrical in design, emphasizing horizontal and vertical lines, cuboidal and rectangular spaces. Suddenly, the building bowed out as if I were looking through a fish-eye lens.

By this time I began to see images at will, but I had learned there were a few rules about calling them up and maintaining them. At any chosen time or place I had only to close my eyes, relax and concentrate on the darkness. When forms began to appear I had to concentrate only on the center of my apparent field of vision and not allow myself to concentrate on the periphery to absorb some detail of pattern or movement; otherwise the image would dissolve.

It was at this time that my hallucinations were most enjoyable and fascinating. I seemed to have acquired a sixth sense. I knew how to bring images on and turn them off. The images themselves were most aesthetic. The forms would make a very simple beginning and gracefully elaborate in form and movement. I was fascinated not only by the form and movement of the images, but also by their dimensions and space. Red shimmering forms existed in a blackness where gravity and time seemed not to exist. I became very cautious about whom I spoke with concerning this phenomenon by now.

Stage II (8 *weeks*). I was awakened about 3.00 a.m. by the most brilliant and elaborate images I had yet seen. Every time I closed my eyes and tried to fall asleep, I was overwhelmed by elaborate images. The image began as if my face were pressed directly against the pattern and then I seemed to recede from it seeing greater intricacy and detail. Now it seemed as though I could tumble into the images as if thrown into a rotating house of mirrors.

This hallucinatory experience developed a different character for me. The images had become much more complex. I had no control over the images and at times actually felt part of them. They haunted me most when I tried to read. This would frustrate me and I would become very angry. The angrier I became, the more intense the images were. Finally I would give in and stretch out on my sofa thinking I would watch them carry on and then return to my studies. This usually resulted in my becoming engrossed in watching the images and then falling into a deep sleep for several hours.

Stage III (10 *weeks*). Whenever I closed my eyes. I saw hallucinations. Even if I had conscious thoughts running through my mind, they did not seem to interrupt the forms but developed almost into rivalry, like having two thoughts in my mind at once. Overwhelmed by images, often frustrated and angry with them, I found the best way to endure them was to stretch out, relax and watch them until I fell asleep.

Stage IV (11 *weeks*). I continually saw hallucinations when I closed my eyes. The images were brilliant and beautiful but they had exhausted me. I considered them now something to be endured and preliminary to a complete serenity of mind, for if I could relax and endure the initial barrage of images, I would experience a mind out of body sensation that was transcendent. The hallucinations progressed from forms to scenes. I was plagued at this time by rapid mood swings, especially anger and depression. Usually the stimulus for anger was appropri-

ate, but my response exceeded it. The depression would follow when I considered how irritable I had become. I would cry because I had no better control of myself. I often saw scenes during such depressions and I began to experience vivid hypnopompic imagery.

Stage V (16 *weeks*). The trance-like stage of hallucinating I have described began to be interrupted by myoclonic jerking of my head and terrific headaches. It seemed that I could not even progress beyond the preliminary stage of geometric forms before my head was jerking and the darkness and forms became very viscous and caused a great headache with their churning. The hypnopompic imagery subsided and I began to experience very vivid hypnogogic images which kept me awake and caused terrific headaches.

Stage VI (20 *weeks*). The hallucinations gradually died away. I no longer see form constants whenever I close my eyes nor am I bothered by the onset of vivid scenes. I occasionally experience vivid hypnogogic imagery during periods of anxiety. Recovery has set in.

II. CATEGORIZATION AND DESCRIPTION OF HALLUCINATIONS

I have categorized my hallucinations as follows: (1) form constants, (2) intermediate images of form constants and body parts, (3) complex scenes, e.g. visualization of myself, Christ figures, cartoon characters and symbolic scenes. The form constants have been further categorized as to pattern and movement. Peculiar features of the complex scenes are noted.

(1) *Form constants*

In my case these form constants consisted mainly of stars, swirls, chessboard, mosaic, crosses, ellipse, grecian scrolls, and tunnels. Figure 1 illustrates examples of these form constants and is characteristic of the imagery seen in Stage I. Figure 1(a) demonstrates the lack of fusion of apparent uniocular fields observed with several patterns on different

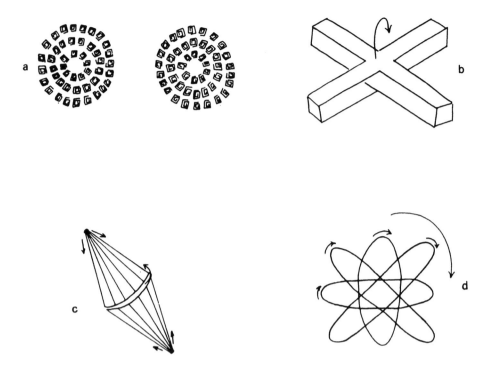

Figure 1. Types of mosaic form constant: (a) both patterns visualized simultaneously; (b) cross flipping over; (c) spindle-streaming movement; (d) multiple rotating ellipses.

occasions during Stage I. All form constants were brilliant shimmering red on a jet black background.

By Stage II the simple form constants elaborated into very complex imagery. Many of the forms were characterized by exquisite geometry and symmetry. The form constants of Stage I still existed but seemed to have acquired another dimension. Figure 2 depicts examples of this period. By this stage I was disturbed by brilliant hypnopompic imagery (Fig. 2c). Perhaps Fig. 3 could serve as a representative image in terms of increasing complexity. There is the basic perspective of a tunnel walled by a chessboard design. When I saw this tunnel I had to look at what was to me the center, approximately where I have drawn the x (not part of the image). If I concentrated on the periphery, the entire vision would dissolve. The right side of the drawing is incomplete because it was peripheral and I was unable to absorb any of the detail. If I looked at the center, however, the vision would become clearer and approach me. The squares were shimmering red and black and eventually exhausted me to look at them, especially when the entire tunnel began to rotate. The small insert was a plane more forward than the rest of the vision. In addition to increasing dimension, geometry and symmetry, superimposition of planes was a common method for visions to become more complex.

(2) Intermediate images of form constants and body parts

The few intermediate scenes of form constants and body parts were seen only in Stage III. These scenes always followed an elaborate display of form constants, filigrees and Persian carpet patterns. The scene itself originated in a very hazy fashion superimposed upon the form constants, until only the scene was visualized. A clear image was only instantaneous, then it drifted away intact like a tissue floating in water with form constants

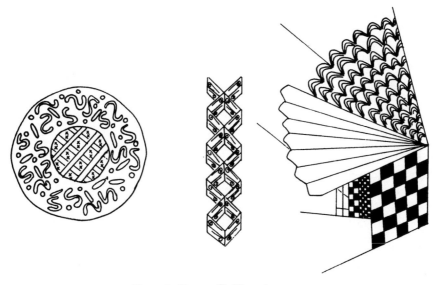

Figure 2. Types of brilliant imagery.

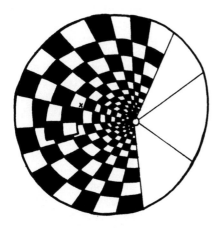

Figure 3. More complex image (see text).

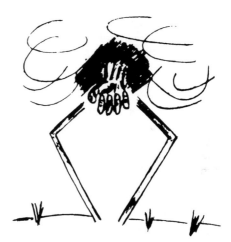

Figure 4. Example of combination of form constant and body parts.

again visible. Figure 4 is the best example of these intermediate scenes. In this image, there is the symmetry of geometric forms and a human hand in the context of a landscape. The scene was in full color, primary and intermediate colors, but seemed muted like a pastel drawing. There was a rolling green grassland and a jet black sky illuminated by an area of golden light from which the hand emanated.

(3) Complex scenes

Out of the great number of scenes, I have grouped them into categories by subject con-

tent and included a discussion of color. (a) Form constants designed with objects: I can recall only one vision of this type but it was very impressive and occurred in Stage III. The image began close to my apparent field of vision, then receded. I saw the red outline of primitive animal forms lining the sides of a black spiral like a frieze. (b) Elaborate geometric forms in primary colors: This occurred during a period of rapid mood swings described in Stage IV. I saw a cascade of cubes and circles. Only one or two faces of the cubes were colored either red, green, yellow or blue. The other face or faces would be white. There was a preponderance of yellow where the cubes were largest. The circles were muted red. (c) Visualization of myself: I saw a great variety of this type of hallucination. They occurred in Stage IV but not necessarily always during mood swings. Examples include a primitive outline of a body form dividing at the waist with the two divisions floating off in opposite directions or a profile of my head in a recumbent position with a canvas stretched over my face and tacked to the ground. These particular images were red outlined on black. I saw these images and felt that I was looking at myself, not that what was represented physically occurred. (d) Religious scenes: Many of these scenes are combinations of other categories, e.g. cartoon figures or improbable views. These hallucinations occurred during Stage IV and Stage V and were muted pastel colors. For instance, I saw a pastoral scene with a shepherd tending his flock. This scene, especially the sheep, was very childish or cartoonish in form. I saw a monk facing a golden light against a rugged mountainside. The most impressive scene was an aerial view of the crucifixion with Christ looking up to the heavens in agony while three cartoonish characters stood at the base of the cross. (e) Symbolic scenes: I have chosen an hallucination which occurred during Stage IV to describe. In the image, the characters were aligned in a tunnel-like prospective and in a 13th century setting. From the outer view of the tunnel inward, a knight in armor faced a skeleton dressed in a robe and seated before a wall. The wall was illuminated by a golden light and beyond it stately figures gathered around a table or perhaps a coffin. In these types of scenes I felt as though I had landed in the midst of activity or a story and would begin assigning roles to the characters and evaluating my reaction to them. (f) Improbable views: I saw many aerial views. The viewpoint was never stationary but constantly moving as if I were flying. Some of these views were described in the religious and symbolic scenes. (g) Animated cartoon characters: The animated characters I saw were always friendly and interesting. As I described in the symbolic scenes, it seemed as if I had suddenly landed in the midst of a fairy tale and would immediately react to the personality of the characters and the activities in which they were involved. I saw a character with the mop hair running along looking over his shoulder. He was then seen springing from a chair with very deep red upholstery and golden embroidery.

III. CLASSIFICATION OF MOVEMENT

(1) Simple movement of form constants or geometric shapes:
   (a) *Rotational movement*—Fig. 1b.
   (b) *Epicyclic*—movement of wheels and ellipses, Fig. 1d.
   (c) *Clockwise movement of the center and counterclockwise movement of the periphery*—catherine wheels.
   (d) Downward flutter of a paddlewheel seen at a constant frequency.
   (e) Revolving movement of wheels, cylinders and cones around a central axis.
   (f) Snake-like—approaching or retreating as if watching a train go by if all the cars were identical.
   (g) Two superimposed planes moving in opposite directions. Figure 5a demonstrates this type of movement. Originally I saw only red planes that moved slowly, fascinating to watch. The type of pattern I have drawn in the figure is associated with a very rapid movement. The most forward plane (1) appears first, then the plane behind it (2). Both planes move rapidly and it quickly makes my head hurt to watch them. Planes (1) and (2) are equally florid.
   (h) Constant transition of form pattern—Fig. 5b.
   (i) Movement in alternate directions either away from or toward a central axis (a star waving its arms)—Fig. 5c, and various complex circular movements.

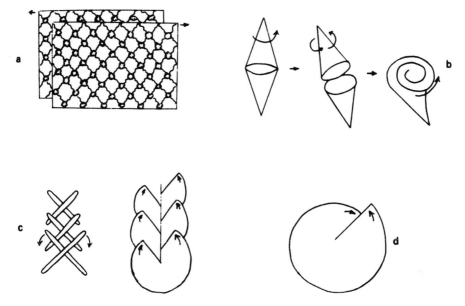

Figure 5. Types of movement visualized (see text).

The italicized movements are common to the stroboscopic form constants described by Smythies.

(2) Movements associated with a physical sensation:
    (a) Sudden reversal of direction in movement of superimposed planes—vertigo.
    (b) Planes swirling in opposite directions around a central point—vertigo, Fig. 5d.
    (c) Sweeping viewpoint or complicated transition of form—floating, flying or dissociated from my body (movement and sensation common to mescaline intoxication).
(3) Complicated movements of form constants and geometric forms:
    (a) Rotation of cylinder in background with approaching snake-like movement in foreground.
    (b) *Whole pattern approach or retreat from visual field* with a particular region of the design appearing central and "immediately pressed against my eyes" at one point during the movement (italicized movement common to the stroboscopic patterns).

    (c) Rapid elaboration of geometric forms from a single point (Fig. 1c).
    (d) Rapid peripheral movement of tunnel walls as if I were falling down the tunnel (common to mescaline intoxication).
(4) Movements characteristic of scenes:
    (a) Sweeping viewpoint as if flying over the scene.
    (b) Animated movement—figures animated as if many stationary views were moving in rapid sequence.
    (c) Approach or retreat of image.
    (d) Slow, deliberate, seemingly timeless movements of simple objects suspended by a wire in space.
    (e) Combinations of all of the above movements occurring when viewing a scene.

Movements (a) and (b) are common to mescaline intoxication.

IV. DISCUSSION

My hallucinations are intermediate between the stroboscopic form constants described by Smythies and the complex scenes described

in the height of a mescaline-induced hallucinosis.[6] Many of the hallucinations I experienced are comparable to the dark phase of
the stroboscopic patterns,[2] that is, occurring
in the externally dark adapted eye. The pattern and movements, however, are reminiscent of those described for both the bright
and dark phase[2,3] and cannot be related to a
uniform flickering field. With the chronologic
progression in complexity, the images take
on more the character of a mescaline intoxication. The form constants become more em-
bellished, symmetrical and common to the
four categories originally described by Klüver.
The scenes transiently visualized are remarkably similar to the second stage of a mescaline
intoxication as evidenced by their surrealistic
quality and content of caricatures, improbable views and religious scenes.

In considering the clinical categories of
visual hallucinations outlined by Hécaen and
Albert[7], I find I do not fit into any of these.
The lack of significant affective components,
visual rememorizations, temporal spatial disorientation and externalization of possible
perceptual choices among real stimuli are
significant negatives in my experience that
do not result in easy placement within the
categories described. Brilliance of phantasmic
images, movement, animation and scintillation effects described in hallucinations associated with ophthalmologic lesions are
simplistic elements common to my experience. However, the chronologic complexity
of my hallucinations goes beyond this category of hallucination.

Hécaen and Albert[7] suggest a functional or
pathological activation of the visual system

underlying all forms of visual hallucinations.
They propose that visual hallucinations
result when spontaneous activity of the
visual system is liberated from normal inhibitions. The hallucinatory categories are then
grouped into cortical, primarily temporal and
occipital lobe, and subcortical or peripheral
lesions, i.e. geniculostriate and ophthalmologic lesions. Definitive focal action of hallu-
cinogenic drugs remains a question.

The disease which I suffered was a diffuse
cerebral insult. The resulting hallucinations
are remarkable in that they more closely
resemble a drug-induced hallucinosis than a
focal lesion and contain elements of form
constants and patterns of movement that are
basic and similar from person to person. It is
unlikely that these hallucinations could be
attributed to anticonvulsant medication, since
their onset was 6 weeks following initial
dosage and the images have resolved while
maintenance doses of medications continue.
The cortical irritability of a viral encephalopathy in my case resulted in a selected interference with normal visual inhibitions producing
a subacute exacerbation of hallucinations
individual but categorizable with those described in drug-induced circumstances.

This is my account of visual hallucinations
produced during a disease process. It is my
hope to provide insight into the world of perceptual aberrations in which I suddenly found
myself. Such insight on the part of my physician was of much therapeutic value for me.

I would like to record my sincere gratitude
to Dr. John R. Smythies for his guidance
throughout the course of this illness and his
support, review and criticism of this paper.

REFERENCES

1. Klüver, H. (1942). Mechanisms of hallucinations. In *Studies in personality*. McGraw-Hill, New York.
2. Smythies, J. R. (1959a). The stroboscopic patterns. I. The dark phase. *British Journal of Psychology*, 50, 106–16.
3. Smythies, J. R. (1959b). The stroboscopic patterns. II. The phenomenology of the bright phase and after images. 50, 305–24.
4. Smythies, J. R. (1960). The stroboscopic patterns. III. Further experiments and discussion. *British Journal of Psychology*, 51, 247–55.
5. Brown, C. R. and Gebhard, J. W. (1948). Visual field articulation in the absence of spatial stimulus gradients. *Journal of Experimental Psychology*, 38, 188–200.

6. Siegel, R. K. (1977). *Scientific American*, Hallucinations. **234**, 142–40.
7. Hécaen, H. and Albert, M. (1978). Disorders of visual perception. In *Human Neuropsychology*. Wiley, New York.

(Mize 1980)

COMMENTARY

Mize's report is unique and, to my knowledge, has rarely if ever been reported following focal cerebral pathology. It is a pity that there was no report of specific brain-localizing signs. Mize appeared to have some control over the onset and cessation of her hallucinations. She had only to close her eyes, relax, and concentrate on the darkness and they would appear. A further unusual factor was the delayed onset of the symptoms (6 weeks from time of admission), the limited duration of symptoms (14 weeks), and no clear indication as to what precipitated their onset and their cessation. There is no evidence in this paper to exclude or substantiate the possible role of psychological factors in the aetiology of her hallucinations. Mize does note that at one point in time, when she was having hallucinations that were 'brilliant and beautiful', she was plagued by rapid mood swings, especially anger and depression.

Instances of focal pathology associated with visual hallucinations have tended to involve the right temporo-occipital region (e.g. Cummings *et al.* 1982), though other structures such as the frontal lobes or diencephalic areas have also been implicated (Hécaen and Albert 1978). Mize's report suggests that it was the presence of occipital seizure activity which was responsible for the 'form constants' such as stars, swirls, crosses, etc. It would seem that the presence of right temporal lobe seizure activity may have determined her experience of more complex images such as scenes and cartoon characters.

Mize reports that hallucinations involving visual movement were a major part of her experience. Recent evidence from positron emission tomography suggests that there is a specific extrastriate region (region V5) that specializes in the visual perception of movement (Zeki 1991).

REFERENCES

Cummings, J. L., Syndulko, K., Goldberg, Z., and Treiman, D. (1982). Palinopsia reconsidered. *Neurology*, **32**, 444–7.
Hécaen, H. and Albert, M. L. (1978) *Human neuropsychology*. Wiley, New York.
Zeki, S. (1991). A thought experiment with positron emission tomography. In *Exploring brain functional anatomy with positron emission tomography*. Ciba Foundation Symposium No. 163. Wiley, Chichester.

Recovery from occipital stroke: a self-report and an inquiry into visual processes

Bryan Kolb

Bryon Kolb is a neuropsychologist, and is the co-author of a standard textbook in neuropsychology (Kolb and Whishaw 1996).

Damage to the visual systems is manifested in a great variety of symptoms. Thus, although complete central blindness is possible, damage to neocortical regions produces only relative blindness such that form perception, for example, is lost but light detection is maintained. Similarly, the relative blindness may be for a single feature of visual perception, such as colour, or may be manifested as an inability to know or understand the meaning of visual stimuli, as in an agnosia. (For a review of visual perceptual symptoms see Kolb & Whishaw, 1990, chap. 12).

Although the principal means of studying visual organization in the first part of this century was the study of clinical cases with anatomical verification (for a review see Polyak, 1957), the last 50 years has seen an emphasis upon laboratory investigations of the effects of surgical ablations and the activity of single units in different cortical regions. Nonetheless, the investigation of clinical disturbances of vision remains a powerful tool in understanding the nature of visual disturbances and especially in understanding the changes in visual symptoms after a cerebral injury, which I shall refer to as *recovery*. One difficulty in studying human cases with damage to the visual cortex, however, is that in view of the location of this tissue, which is buried deep within a sulcus on the medial surface of each hemisphere, it is rare to have access to patients whose damage is restricted to just the primary visual region. Hence, when such patients become available it is significant and worth studying in some detail (e.g., Weiskrantz, 1986).

SYMPTOMS OF DAMAGE TO THE PRIMARY VISUAL CORTEX

Although the effects of damage to the striate cortex have been studied for well over 100 years, there is still uncertainty over the nature of the visual loss. Studies of the effects of striate lesions in nonhuman primates have shown that animals can still respond to light, and indeed, monkeys show evidence of some ability to discriminate between both relatively fine gratings (11 cycles/degree) and a difference in orientation of lines of as little as 8° (Pasik & Pasik, 1980). What is curious, however, is that most clinical reports of visual capacities of humans with striate lesions refer to regions of hemianopia or scotoma, with the clear implication that the affected region is 'blind'. For example, after his careful studies of field defects in patients with occipital lesions, Holmes (1918) concluded that the visual defect was frequently complete as shown by an absence of response to white light, colour, or movement. Not all reports confirm this conclusion, however, as it appears that at least some patients do have some type of visual responsiveness within scotomata (e.g., Riddoch, 1917; Weiskrantz, 1986).

The apparent discrepancy between the laboratory animal and human reports is likely due in large part to the difference in the questions being asked. Thus, in the animal work the experiment is designed to determine if the animal is able to use certain visual information to obtain reward; in the human studies the investigation focusses upon what the patient says or how they perform different tasks. In each type of work inferences are subsequently made regarding the nature of the visual disturbance, but the data base is clearly different in the human and nonhuman studies.

A particular difficulty with case studies of humans is that if patients do not spontaneously report peculiar visual phenomena, the clinician may not know what to ask, and the description of the effects of visual lesions may be overly influenced by descriptions of a small sample of patients. For example, there is a general folklore regarding scotomata, in that they are visually silent and are usually 'filled in'. Although there is some evidence of this in the literature, systematic studies have not shown this to be ubiquitous (e.g., Warrington, 1962, 1965). Furthermore, as one reads the literature on field defects, it is difficult to gain any flavour for what the patient's perception of the visual loss is, and it is hard to imagine what the patients are experiencing. Hence, as both a neuroscientist and a patient, I was led to write this account of the subjective experience of the effects of visual cortex damage as well as to collect quantitative data on the defect and its evolution over time. Indeed, I was unable to find a single description of the changes in the visual phenomena that began its report from the onset of the damage. The principal goal of this paper, therefore, is to describe the effects of primary visual cortex injury in myself, consider whether there are any changes in the symptoms observed over the subsequent 4 years, and describe details of visual events that were produced by the lesion. I will conclude with a more general discussion of issues surrounding recovery and visual perception.

THE POSTERIOR CEREBRAL ARTERY, MIGRAINE, AND VISION

The posterior cerebral artery originates from the basilar artery at the level of the rostral portion of the pons. As the artery progresses, it gives off a series of small branches that supply the substantia nigra, red, nucleus, part of the midbrain, and parts of the thalamus (e.g., medial geniculate, dorsomedial, pulvinar). Larger branches later go to the hippocampal formation and other medial temporal regions, posterior cingulate cortex, the occipital cortex, and portions of the inferior posterior temporal cortex (see Polyak, 1957, for details). The branches into the calcarine cortex are of particular interest here, since interruption of this source of blood will compromise the striate cortex.

In recent years there has been increasing interest in the events associated with disturbance of the occipital branches of the posterior cerebral artery. One common reversible neurological symptom associated with altered blood flow of the posterior cerebral artery is classic migraine, which is characterized by severe headache and preceded or accompanied by focal neurological symptoms, which are usually referred to as *auras*. It is generally believed that visual auras are the most common neuropsychic correlates of migraine, and a systematic prospective examination of aura symptoms confirmed this: It revealed visual aura in 94% of cases, somatosensory aura in 40%, motor disturbances in 18%, and speech disturbances in 20% (Jensen, Tfelt-Hansen, Lauritzen, & Olesen, 1986). Curiously, 20% of the patients reported no headache following the aura. Although visual auras could be noncortical in origin, cortical origin is likely, since the aura is usually present in both fields (e.g., Lashley 1941).

Until recently the etiology of the neurological symptoms was assumed to be vascular, an assumption that has now been confirmed with blood flow studies (e.g., Olesen, Larsen, & Lauritzen, 1981). Furthermore, it has now become clear that stroke is occasionally associated with migraine; that is, it appears that in some cases the migrainous event is sufficiently severe to produce cortical ischemia leading to permanent brain damage (i.e., an infarct). The incidence of migraine-related stroke is quite rare, but incidence of migraine is estimated at 15–25% of the population (Waters & O'Connor, 1975). Nonetheless, there are now a number of papers documenting migrainous stroke in well over 100 cases, most of which involve the posterior cerebral artery (e.g., Bogousslavsky & Regli, 1987; Bogousslavsky, Regli, Van Melle, Payot, &

Uske, 1988; Broderick & Swanson, 1987; Fisher, 1986; Henrich, Sandercock, Warlow, & Jones, 1986; Rothrock, Walicke, Swenson, Lyden, & Logan, 1988; Spaccavento & Solomon, 1984). The majority of these cases are female, with the mean age across different studies tending to be in the mid-thirties. The most common putative causes of the cerebral ischemia in these cases is either vasospasm or embolism associated with mitral valve prolapse. However, Bogousslavsky et al, studied a group of patients with ischemic stroke during an attack of classic migraine and concluded, on the basis of cardiological and cerebral angiographical studies, that mitral valve prolapse, arterioral dissection, and vasospasm were not likely to be significant causes of the stroke during the migraine. A similar conclusion was reached by Lauritzen (1987), who suggested that some sort of neuronal depression may trigger the event, with subsequent local changes in blood flow, which in turn leads to the ischemia and infarct.

The symptoms of migraine-associated stroke vary considerably, but most cases have permanent field defects and some motor symptoms, the latter possibly related to damage to the thalamus. There has been no systematic study of neuropsychological consequences of migraine-associated stroke, but it is likely that those patients with damage to the medial temporal regions have memory deficits as well, especially if the hippocampal formation is damaged (for a review of such symptoms, see Kolb & Whishaw, 1990, chap. 22). The occurrence of migraine-related stroke is especially relevant to the current report, since the author had a 15–year history of classic migraine, which was characterized by scotomata virtually identical to those described by Lashley (1941). The incidence has been about one attack per year, and most, if not all, of the scotomata were in the left visual field.

CASE BK

I will begin this account with a general description of the evidence surrounding the stroke, including a description of the neurological evidence. I will then give a subjective account of the changes in the field defect over time, followed by a quantitative description of the field changes.

History

At the time of the stroke, I was a 38–year-old professor of psychology. On the night of Jan. 8, 1986, I went to bed about 11:00 pm after having consumed about 8 oz of red wine and some 'odd tasting' Dutch chocolate. (Both red wine and chocolate are commonly reported to be associated with migraine.) I arose early on the morning of Jan. 9 in order to prepare a lecture. Upon rising, I walked to the kitchen in the dark and turned the lights on. My first reaction was the lighting was rather dim and that one of the kitchen lights must have burned out. I proceeded to open a can of cat food, and, in doing so, I was startled to discover that I could not see my left hand. My initial assumption was that I must have had a retinal detachment. When I tested my visual fields independently, however, using a kitchen knife that I brought across the visual field from the left, I was shaken to discover that the field defect was binocular, indicating that the disorder was central and involved most of the left visual field, including all of the upper quadrant and the upper part of the lower quadrant. I immediately examined my motor and somatosensory abilities and was quickly satisfied that I could not detect any difference in sensitivity or movement between the left and right hands. I turned on the radio and appeared to have no difficulty in understanding the newscast, and I seemed able to speak and write. I could not read, however, as the field defect was far too distracting. I proceeded to shower and then tried to shave but had great difficulty, again because of the field defect. The lighting still seemed generally dim to me, and the affected part of the left visual field appeared to be dark, which, of course, is quite unlike the normal experience of regions beyond the visual fields. It became apparent to me that I would have to cancel my lecture, and I arranged to be taken to the emergency room at a local hospital.

Upon arriving at the hospital, I had considerable difficulty convincing the internist that I had had a stroke, as he was certain I must have had something wrong with my eyes; in spite of my objections, I was forced to wait to see a retinal specialist. Upon explaining my situation to the ophthalmologist, however, he immediately agreed that the problem must be central, and I was returned to emergency. By noon, I eventually despaired at getting the appropriate referral (there is no neurologist in Lethbridge, which is a city of 60 000 located about 200 km south of Calgary, Alberta, Canada). I left the hospital and, with my colleague Ian Whishaw's help, tried to contact friends at the Clinical Neurosciences Department at the University of Calgary. By about 2:00 pm, I talked to Dr. Robert Lee, Head of Clinical Neurosciences at the University of Calgary, and he agreed that the likely diagnosis was occipital stroke, possibly of migrainous origin. Since my condition was not liable to change quickly, it was agreed that I would come to Calgary the following morning for a neurological examination, including a CT-scan.

By this time I had begun to experience an incredible headache. Although I had a history of visual aura characteristic of classic migraine, I had never had a migraine headache. By evening the headache was excruciating, and even Tylenol 3, with 30 mg of codeine and 15 mg of caffeine, did little to change that. I tried to sleep and, at one point, awoke from a dream in which somebody was driving spikes into my head in order to get me to sign some sort of statement! The dream ended, but the spikes remained. There was no relief from the headache the next day, and moving around was very difficult indeed. Upon arrival at the hospital, Dr. Lee gave me a neurological exam, the results of which seemed normal, although curiously I did have some difficulty coming up with the names of objects placed in my left hand. I recognized the objects immediately, but I seemed slightly anomic for this hand. The field defect was now clearly restricted to the left upper quadrant, which was still dark. The CT-scan, which was done the morning of Friday, Jan. 10, showed an infarct of roughly 4 cm^2 in the right occipital cortex, as shown in Figure 1. I was admitted to hospital and stayed over night. I agreed, reluctantly, to have an angiogram and various cardiological tests beginning on Jan. 13, and I was discharged to my parents' home in Calgary for the weekend. My headache, which was unilateral and centred on my right eye, forehead, and temple, had not subsided. Since I had read that caffeine sometimes aborts migraine headaches, I asked my mother to make me some very strong black coffee. She did, and I drank two cups, to no avail. An hour later she asked me if it made a difference that the coffee was decaffeinated! We tried the experiment again, and the headache began to clear within minutes. Although I was left with a slight headache for a couple of days, it was clear that it was largely gone within an hour

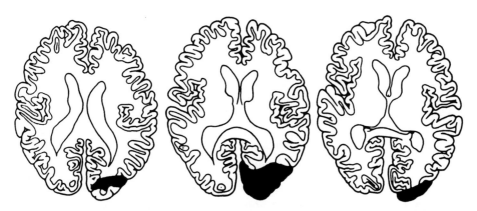

Figure 1. Schematic illustration of BK's CT-scan showing the infarct in the right occipital area.

of drinking the caffeinated coffee, which likely contained in excess of 100 mg of caffeine per cup.

The angiogram was clear, and there was apparently no evidence of mitral valve prolapse. I was discharged on Jan. 16 and returned to Lethbridge. I attempted to teach Jan. 21 but I still had great difficulty reading, and I found it extremely stressful. After my class, I had chest pains (presumably stress related) and experienced a visual aura in the left visual field. This aura took the form of a very bright jagged line, much like lightning, that scintillated. It began in the foveal representation of the lower left quadrant and slowly enlarged and moved laterally over a period of about 5 minutes before vanishing. The aura did not extend into the field defect. It was decided that I would not be able to teach, and I was placed on sick leave for the remainder of the semester. On Jan. 22 I had another aura, which had two components. The first was identical to the previous day, except that it extended into the field defect by about 3°. The other component was also a jagged bright white line, but it was far more jagged and looked rather like the teeth of a comb. This line appeared to extend about a degree into the field defect, although this was difficult to establish. Both lines were gone in about 5 minutes. There has been only one additional aura in the subsequent 4 years, occurring in 1988. It was entirely in the left lower quadrant and was similar to the premorbid auras, which were virtually identical to those described by Lashley (1941) and illustrated in Figure 2.

I was determined to return in my previous lifestyle as quickly as possible and attended the Winter Conference on Brain Research in the last week of January. I had real difficulty in reading slides at talks, however, and had to sit well back in the audience in order to follow them. Presumably, this allowed me to get most of the information into my right visual field. I also decided to try skiing that week. I was able to ski without difficulty, although I tended to overcompensate for my field defect and actually ran into a tree in my good field whilst trying to avoid a bush several meters away on the left!

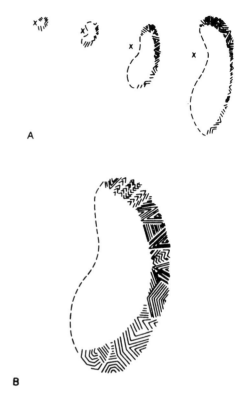

Figure 2. Successive maps of a scintillating scotoma showing the characteristic increase in the size of the scotoma and the location of the so-called fortification figures. (After Lashley, 1941)

Emotional Effects

There have been suggestions that right posterior strokes might be associated with depressive symptoms (Robinson et al., 1984). As one might expect, I had some difficulties coming to terms with a cortical injury, both because of my profession and because of the confrontation with a serious illness that is supposed to happen to 'old people.' Once it became clear that I could not simply return to my previous life I did suffer periods of depression, which were characterized by considerable lability in affect. I could be happy one moment and in tears the next—for no apparent reason. While the affective experiences were clearly related to the stroke, they did not appear to be any different than one normally experiences with other traumatic experiences. On one occasion about 4 weeks after the stroke, I had a 'panic attack' as I attempted to go shopping for groceries in a large supermarket. The store was crowded, and I was having a great difficulty in reading the labels on items. I simply bolted from the store, leaving my basket in the aisle. Having never experienced such an event before, I was quite shaken by it. After sitting down for about 20 min, I returned to the store, found my basket still in place, and quickly completed my shopping. No similar episode occurred again, although I continued to experience periods of emotional lability for at least a year.

Evolution of the Field Defect: Subjective Changes

Beginning on Jan. 10 I kept a diary of my subjective impressions of the field defect. Over the ensuing 4 years I also routinely and systematically tested my field defect with the goal of charting any changes in its extent over time. I shall summarize the subjective changes by summarizing my diary entries over the first 60 days after the stroke. I have made occasional editorial comments in square brackets and have kept the narrative in the present tense.

Jan. 9, 1986. The entire left upper quadrant appears dark grey, as though I am looking through smoked glass. I can see no movement or changes in light. I have real difficulty in recognizing faces, especially of people who appear from my left.

Jan. 10, 1986. As I am driven to Calgary, I am continually surprised by automobiles and buildings suddenly appearing in my good field when I look to the left. I have no idea that they are there. By evening the bad field appears less grey, and I can detect large things moving in the field, although I only seem aware of them once they are visible in the good field.

Jan. 11, 1986, 11:20 am. I notice that I can detect cars going by on a highway visible from the hospital window. It seems like some sort of wave moves across the field, and when it gets to the edge of the defect, a car pops out. The wave is much larger than the car, how-

ever, as the cars appear to be about 5° in size, but the wave includes the entire left upper quadrant. I also seem to be able to keep track of two or three waves moving across the field at a time.

Jan. 11, 1986, 1:00pm. I am suddenly aware of new symptoms. I am starting to get double vision. Visual information from the edge of the good field seems to move over into the bad field. Is this an analogue of allesthesia observed in patients recovering from contralateral neglect? [It is probably not. I suspect now that it was my attempt to understand the visual noise that later became a permanent feature of the scotoma.]

Jan. 12, 1986. The double vision is still there. I had an idea that the equivalence of simultaneous extinction should occur. I covered the good field with a piece of cardboard and was under the impression that the vision in the bad field improved as the double vision stopped. When I covered the bad field, there was clear improvement in the rest of field, suggesting that there may be some interference. While towelling down after showering I noticed that the mirror was steamed. It struck me that I could see movement in the mirror in the good field, but I could not determine what anything was; I am struck by the similarity with my bad field. I think the best analogy I have now is that my bad field is like a mirror fogged with steam.

Jan. 12, 1986, 6:00 pm. I have another analogy for the bad field. It reminds me of the experience of wearing a pair of glasses with one lens missing. It makes me feel queasy in the same way. The double vision seems different. It seems to be flashing on and off, much like auras do. [From here on I used the terms *visual noise* and *scintillating scotoma* to describe this.]

Jan. 12, 1986, 8:30 pm. The field defect appears to have a very sharp boundary down the midline and across the horizontal meridian. It looks like a perfect right angle in the centre of the fovea. The scintillating scotoma now seems to be made of little squares, much like a quilt, which begin at the fovea and extend out to include about 25% of the field. It reminds me of 'snow' in a coloured television set (see Fig. 3).

Jan. 13, 1986. I am aware that I can see in

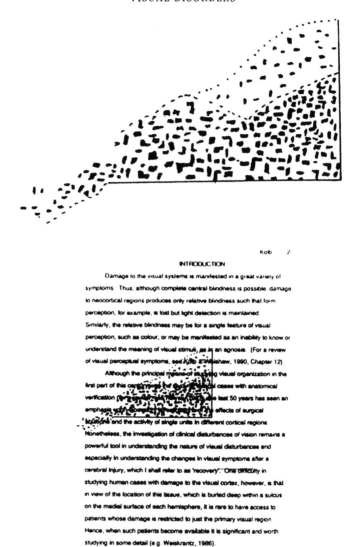

Figure 3. Top: Schematic illustration of the pattern of BK's scintillating scotoma. The dark areas assume the colour of objects in that portion of the field. The white areas are always 'whiter than white'. Bottom: Illustration of the scotoma relative to an 8.5″ × 11″ sheet of paper viewed at normal reading distance. The centre of the visual field is at the 90° angle of the scotoma.

the lateral regions of the bad field. I think it is absolutely normal. [I was wrong!] Formal perimetry was done for the first time. It strikes me that although I cannot 'see' the lights as they move about the field defect, once they enter the good field I am immediately aware that I had seen them. Further, I can indicate roughly where they entered the field. This must certainly be what Larry Weiskrantz means when he talks of 'blindsight in hindsight'. Curiously, I cannot force myself to report the light any sooner, even though I try. In discussing this with the perimetrist, she indicates that other people have mentioned this, although she seemed to think they were being unco-operative.

Jan. 14, 1986. The illusions [i.e. the visual noise] in the bad field are a real nuisance, as they make me feel dizzy. It is far better in the dark because the scintillation is not present. It returns as soon as the lights are turned on, however. When I close my eyes in the light, the image stays.

Jan. 15, 1986. My impression is that the scintillation is more stable. It doesn't seem to move as much.

Jan. 16, 1986. As I am driven back to Lethbridge, I am impressed with the difference from the drive up a week ago. There are not so many surprises. I am cheered that I may be able to drive again one day. It is still my impression that when the bad field is blocked off, my vision is improved in the good field, which still suggests some sort of interference.

Jan. 17, 1986. I tried using my computer and discovered to my surprise that the screen is far more difficult to read than the printed page. It is very difficult to find the cursor if it is on the left side of the screen.

Jan. 18, 1986. I can clearly see my pen (held at arm's length) move through the scintillation, although I have no idea what it might be.

Jan. 19, 1986. I am now aware of colour in the bad field; that is, it takes on the hue of things under it, such as blue for the sky and brown for the hills visible from my office window.

Jan. 23, 1986. My subjective impression is that the field defect, but not the area of scintillation, is getting smaller.

Jan. 26, 1986. I tried skiing. I had no problem at all because I failed to notice the field defect. Reading graphs of people's data (from 35 mm slides on a screen) is a real nuisance, however.

Jan. 27, 1986. I entered a room looking for a colleague, scanned the room, and saw nobody. It turns out that he was on my left talking on the telephone, and I apparently 'looked right at him'. I was totally unaware that he was there. [This apparent 'neglect' of people is a constant problem as I scan from right to left. I must overscan to the left to ensure that nothing is ignored.]

Jan. 30, 1986. The area beyond the scintillation continues to improve. This morning as I attended a session I could 'see' the pointer arrow in the scintillating area move. This is the first time I could see something so small move. It seemed to have some shape to it, too. Presumably, the very high contrast helped.

Feb. 3, 1986. I took 10 mg Ritalin and did a variety of field tests [see data]. My impression is that colours are much brighter and that the field defect is smaller. [It wasn't.]

Feb. 5, 1986. My impression is that the visual noise worsens as the amount of visual information increases. Sitting alone in my office the scintillation is not bothersome. As visual input goes up (as in walking in the hall among others), however, the noise increasingly distracts me, and I feel far more stressed.

Feb. 7, 1986. Shopping was very stressful. [See above.]

Feb. 8, 1986. I am beginning to get depressed since the field does not seem to be improving any more. I've lost my appetite, and I'm beginning to feel sorry for myself.

Feb. 10, 1986. I took 10 mg Ritalin again. I had the subjective impression that my vision was better, even though quantitative testing did not show that on the first test.

Feb. 16, 1986. I played squash. I had to watch the ball very closely, and if I lost it in the scotoma, I had no idea where it was. The visual noise was very distracting in the bright white court. [This problem continues. When I first step into the court the noise seems overwhelming and is 'whiter than white'.]

Mar. 12, 1986. The fields seem the same, and the noise is clearly unchanged. However, it doesn't seem as bothersome reading, although I still 'lose' capital letters.

June, 1989. There is no change in the vision, but I am aware that my fixation point has moved. Thus, if I look at a point, I am clearly looking about 1.5° up and 1.5° to the left. I have to really force myself to line up the field defect on the fixation point. [It seems likely that this may account for some case reports of people recovering from field defects involving the fovea; that is, they learn to shift the fixation point slightly, thus placing it into the intact region of the fovea.]

Dec. 3, 1989. I still have more difficulty with faces than I used to and occasionally will walk past people on my left without noticing who they are. I still miss capital letters when reading text. I have difficulty reading signs that I come upon suddenly, since I seem to assume that I can see the entire sign when I first look at it; I frequently cannot, and I am puzzled by the odd spellings or messages. For example, a sign stating *Women* can be misread as *Men* or one saying *telephone* may be misread as *lephone*. I still continually lose things in front of me, such as keys, pencils, and so on. I am aware of movement in the scotoma, especially things like birds or insects, although I have no idea what they might be. Driving is no problem, although I am very careful to scan back and forth at intersections. The scintillating scotoma is still present, although most of the time it does not bother me. It still assumes the colour of objects in its field, and I remain blind to objects in the scotoma. I have tested for negative colour afterimage in the scotoma on several occasions, but it does not occur. I have no difficulty catching balls or playing tennis, squash, or badminton, although I do occasionally lose the goal object. I find it very difficult to follow the flight of golf balls, however. Finally, I am unaware of any nonvisual symptoms and have no reason to suspect that my nonverbal memory has suffered as a result of hippocampal injury related to the ischemia. Formal testing on the Corsi block span in February, 1986 revealed a span of 8 and a normal learning curve on the Corsi span of + 1 (e.g., Milner, 1974), both of which suggest that my nonverbal memory has not suffered. I cannot do most other standardized tests of visual memory because I am not naive to their contents.

Evolution of Field Defect: Quantitative Changes

Formal perimetry was done on two occasions (Jan. 13, 1986, and Feb. 27, 1986). In addition, I designed two simple field tests that are easy to administer, that yield data similar to the perimetry, and that can be repeated over time without prejudice to the data. The procedure is that I stand leaning over a table, which is covered in white cardboard, so that my eyes are 81 cm from the table. On the first test (red dot perimetry) I fixate on the bisection point of two bold red lines (10' of visual angle in width), and a Q-tip that has had the cotton tip soaked in red ink is moved across the visual field. The red tip is about 1° by 20' of visual angle in size. I indicate when I can either begin to detect, or fail to detect, the stimulus. Direct comparison of these results with the results of the perimetry reveals a virtually identical area of inability to detect the stimulus. On the second test (colour and pointing) my eyes are closed, and a plastic token (one of the small square tokens from the Token Test of aphasia, which measures 1.74° by 1.74°) is placed at different points spaced about 3° apart in left or right upper quadrant. The task upon opening my eyes and fixating upon a red dot is to point (and touch) the token and to indicate its colour, which can be red, green, or blue. In view of the putative role of noradrenaline in recovery from stroke (e.g., Feeney & Sutton, 1986), I was administered 10 mg of Ritalin on February 3 and 10, 1987, and the red dot perimetry and colour and pointing tests were done before, during, and after the drug.

Formal Perimetry: The chronic results of the formal perimetry are shown in Figure 4. On the original test the scotoma extended about 10° upwards and 20° laterally from the fixation point. Six weeks later, this was reduced to about 7° by 12°. In addition, whereas the field defect extended into the lower quadrant on the first test, it had completely cleared 6 weeks later.

Red Dot Perimetry: The results of the red dot perimetry was analyzed in three ways. Thus, the area of scotoma was calculated first by using a computerized graphics tablet upon which the scotoma was traced. Then, the vertical and horizontal extents of the defect were measured in degrees. All three measures were made repeatedly over nearly 4 years, and the results for representative tests are plotted in Figure 5. It is immediately apparent that the total area of scotoma decreased over the first 50 poststroke days and then remained stable until present.

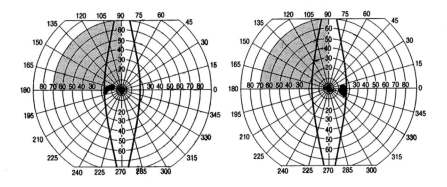

Figure 4. Illustration of the visual fields of BK 6 months poststroke. The dark region shows the area of densest scotoma. The lighter region shows the area of reduced acuity. The normal blind spot, which is also marked in black, is shown for each eye. It merges with the scotoma in the field of the left eye.

Moreover, a similar pattern was observed for both the horizontal and vertical changes in the field defect. There would seem to be little reason to expect further reductions.

One striking feature observed in the red dot test is the contrast between the normal blind spot, which is apparent on monocular testing, and the scotoma. In the blind spot there is absolutely no visual experience, whereas even in the densest region of the scotoma I am aware of something. This contrast between the blind spot and the field defect has been used in other clinical studies (e.g., Weiskrantz, 1986), and it may be a useful routine test to examine residual visual capacities in other patients.

Colour and Pointing: The colour and pointing data were analyzed by calculating the mean number of errors (max = 30) over five repetitions of the test in February, 1986 and comparing it to a single test in November, 1989. On the initial testing I had difficulty in identifying the colour accurately throughout the scotoma; I could point relatively accurately, with exception of the region of the scotoma (Fig. 6). nearly 4 years later there was marked improvement in both functions, and all errors were in that portion of the scotoma in the fovea. The best score in February, 1986 still had more than twice as many errors as the November, 1989 test.

Ritalin: Ritalin had virtually no effect upon test performance either during or after the drug. There was a 15% increase in the area of the field defect during both drug tests, but this was absent the following day in the post-drug test. Furthermore, the Ritalin did not appear to have any effect on the slope of the recovery curve. Similarly, on the colour and pointing tests, there did not appear to be any significant effect on performance, in spite of my subjective impression that colours in the environment were far brighter.

DISCUSSION

I have described the effects of a localized infarct of the occipital cortex that is likely to have resulted from migraine associated ischemia. There was a large left-visual field scotoma that shrank over the first 50 days and has remained stable since then. There are several particularly interesting features of the scotoma, some of which appear to be previously unreported. First, the scotoma was initially dark and quite unlike the psychological experience of visual information outside the normal visual field, such as our experience of visual information behind us. Second, I soon became aware of the movement of large objects in the visual field, which were perceived as travelling waves. Third, within a

REDUCTION IN FIELD DEFECT

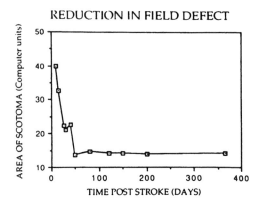

POINTING

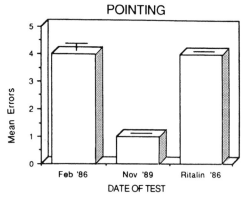

REDUCTION IN VERTICAL DEFECT

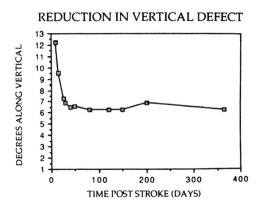

COLOR PERCEPTION

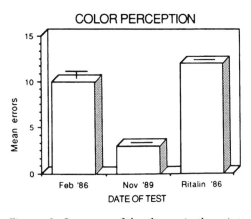

Figure. 6. Summary of the change in the pointing and colour perception errors over nearly 4 years. The Ritalin test is the effect of 10 mg of Ritalin on 2 different days in February, 1986.

REDUCTION IN HORIZONTAL DEFECT

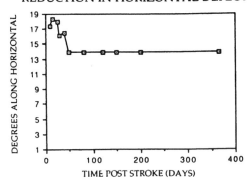

Figure 5. Summary of the change in the size of the field defect over time. The top figure shows the total area of the scotoma, and the lower figures show the vertical and horizontal extents along the meridia.

few days of the stroke the darkness cleared and was replaced by a scintillating scotoma that has continued to this day. Fourth, within a few more days colour perception returned. Fifth, beginning by the fourth post-stroke day I was able to see objects in hindsight, much as Weiskrantz has described in some detail for Case D.B. (Weiskrantz, 1986). The frequency of this phenomenon was markedly reduced as the vision improved, but in those rare instances that something moving appears in the area of scotoma I am still taken by surprise with the blindsight in hindsight. Sixth, the area beyond the scintillation has considerably better vision than the area within the scotoma, but it is not normal. This is difficult to quantify, however, since it is outside the fovea, which makes it a challenge to test; subjectively, at least, there is little doubt that acuity is less sharp, much as though my correction for myopia (which is about -9.5 diopters) is off by a couple of diopters. (This could be likened to the experience of wearing an old pair of eye glasses with a correction that is too weak.) Seventh, there is no evidence of macular sparing. Eighth, there is no evidence of visual closure of items in the scotoma. Indeed, I am constantly surprised by what appear to be partial objects or words when the stimulus falls partly into the scotoma. Ninth, I appear to have learned to compensate for the loss of one quarter of the fovea by directing my gaze about 1.5° upwards and lateral from the normal fixation point. Finally, in spite of the continuing visual noise in the scotoma, I am generally unaware of it unless I am asked to concentrate on a particular visual object.

On the whole, these results are consistent with the sparse literature on human cases (e.g., Polyak, 1957; Wieskrantz, 1986). In particular, both my infarct and the size of the associated field defect are remarkably similar to that of Mallory, a case which is described in detail by Polyak. Of note, Polyak remarks that although the field defect began with a left upper quandrantanopia, the region beyond the final scotoma, which was almost identical to my own, slowly returned, but that it never reached the 'normal level possessed before the insult.' This, too, appears to be the same outcome I have experienced.

The results of the current case are also in general accord with the data that implicate the striate cortex of primates in pattern vision but not in other aspects of visual perception, such as colour and movement perception. Hence, the loss of pattern vision in the face of colour and movement perception is further evidence that vision, and visual experience, is not a monolithic thing but, rather, is the summed activity of multiple systems that somehow combine to present to us a single percept (e.g., Livingston & Hubel, 1988). Indeed, in view of the anatomical and physiological evidence of over a dozen distinct visual representations in the nonhuman primate cortex, it seems reasonable to ask what other visual abilities might remain within the scotomata of human patients with occipital cortex lesions.

The return of less than normal vision in the area lateral to the scotoma is possibly explained by suggesting that some cells that were especially sensitive to ischemia died, leaving the vision slightly impaired. A similar explanation was used by Polyak (1957) to account for Mallory's symptoms. However, the one visual effect that is not easily explained is the continuing scintillating scotoma. I can find no reference to any such phenomenon in the literature, although Dr. C.M. Fisher reported to me in a letter that: 'I have looked over my patients with persistent scintillations along the line between the scotoma and the normal seeing field and in several instances they were still present after two months. I think they all ceased eventually or I would have heard about it. The prognosis for their ceasing is probably 100%.' It is possible that Dr. Fisher's patients may not have stopped experiencing the scintillation but, rather, simply stopped complaining, although this is mere conjecture on my part. Nonetheless, it would be worthwhile to do a systematic investigation of patients with field defects to determine the incidence and anatomical correlates of scintillating scotomata. Indeed, if my own experience can be generalized, it seems reasonable to suppose that, contrary to the popular belief that scotomata represent areas of total blindness, scotomata might actually contain considerable visual activity in certain types of patients, even though the activity may appear to be visual noise. A systematic survey of chronic patients with occipital strokes would seem to be in order to determine the incidence of such events.

There have been suggestions that visual field defects contract over time, leading to hope for some sort of recovery (e.g., Zihl & von Cramon, 1985). My own experience suggests that field defects may show some reduction, but there was virtually no recovery after the first 50 days and virtually no improvement at all in the area of the dense scotoma after the first week. Larger studies of groups of patients with visual field defects resulting from cortical injuries are also not optimistic about the likelihood of significant recovery after the immediate injury period. For example, Aldrich, Alessi, Beck, and Gilman (1987) concluded that the prognosis in cortical blindness is poor when caused by stroke and that bioccipital abnormalities are associated with an especially poor prognosis. Similarly, in his study of World War II veterans with field defects resulting from penetrating brain injuries, Teuber (1975) reported that 43% of the cases showed at least some recovery in the field defect, but fully 57% showed no change. In sum, it appears that Polyak's conclusion some 23 years ago is still appropriate: 'In fact, the cortical representation of the fovea and, in general, of the retina is the very antithesis of the idea of "cerebral plasticity"' (Polyak, 1957, p. 747). It seems that most recovery that appears is likely to be related to nonstriate function (e.g., colour, motion) and that, even when some of the visual field returns, vision is not likely to be normal.

In spite of the absence of a reduction in the objective size of the scotoma beyond 2 months poststroke, there is little doubt that my visual abilities continued to improve for some time. In particular, my reading speed, facial recognition ability, and eye-hand coordination have shown considerable improvement over the ensuing years. It seems likely that a major reason for this is the shift in the point of fixation such that the centre of the visual field now falls about 1.5° by 1.5° into the lower right quadrant. The importance of this shift in fixation point in studies of recovery of function cannot be underestimated

because mapping of scotomata is dependent upon fixation on a central point. If the fixation should shift by only a degree of visual angle, the field defect in the foveal region will appear to be smaller. Indeed, there could even appear to be macular sparing. Significantly, I now find it very difficult to fixate directly on objects because I have clearly learned to compensate for the foveal loss by shifting my fixation. This behavioural change argues strongly in favour of the argument that many apparent examples of recovery of function may actually represent behavioural compensation rather than neurological change (e.g., Miller, 1984).

Finally, in recent years there have been suggestions that certain cortical injuries may be associated with affective illness, possibly as a result of neurochemical changes in the cortex following a cortical stroke (e.g., Robinson, Kubos, Starr, Rao, & Price, 1984; Sinyor, Jacques, Kaloupek, Becker, Goldenberg, & Coopersmith, 1986). As has been reported for other patients with right posterior stroke (e.g., Robinson et al., 1984), I too experienced a depression in my normal affect for at least 3–4 months following the stroke. It was difficult for me to determine any particular cause for the depression, but it was my impression that it was not related directly to particular concerns regarding mortality or loss of vision. This may speak to the possibility of neurochemical imbalance following stroke, although this is conjecture on my part. In any event, it is worth recognizing that depression may accompany occipital stroke, and, in some instances, this may be expected to affect the course of recovery.

REFERENCES

Aldrich, M. S., Alessi, A. G., Beck, R. W., and Gilman, S. (1987). Cortical blindness: Etiology, diagnosis and prognosis. *Annals of Neurology*, **21**, 149–58.
Bogousslavsky, J. and Regli, F. (1987). Ischemic stroke in very young adults: Etiology and prognosis. *Archives of Neurology*, **44**, 137–40.
Bogousslavsky, J., regli, F., Van Melle, G., Payot, M., and Uske, A. (1988). Migraine stroke. *Neurology*, **38**, 223–6.
Broderick, J. P. and Swanson, J. W. (1987). Migraine-related strokes: Clinical profile and prognosis in 20 patients. *Archives of Neurology*, **44**, 868–71.
Feeney, D. M., and Sutton, R. L. (1987). Pharmacotherapy for recovery of function after brain injury. *CRC Critical Reviews in Neurobiology*, **3**, 135–97.

Fisher, C. M. (1986). Unusual vascular events in the territory of the posterior cerebral artery. *Canadian Journal of Neurological Science*, **13**, 1–7.

Henrich, J. B., Sandercock, P. A. G., Warlow, C. P., and Jones, L. N. (1986). Stroke and migraine in the Oxfordshire Community Stroke Project. *Journal of Neurology*, **233**, 257–62.

Holmes, G. (1918). Disturbances of vision by cerebral lesions. *British Journal of Ophthalmology*, **2**, 353–84.

Jensen, K., Tfelt-hansen, P., Lauritzen, M., and Olesen, J. (1986). Classic migraine: A prospective recording of symptoms. *Acta Neurologica Scandinavica*, **73**, 359–62.

Kolb, B. and Whishaw, I. Q. (1990). *Fundamentals of human neuropsychology*, (3rd edn.). Freeman, New York.

Lashley, K. H. (1941). Patterns of cerebral integration indicated by the scotomas of migraine. *Archives of Neurology and Psychiatry*, **46**, 331–9.

Lauritzen, M. (1987). Cerebral blood flow in migraine and cortical spreading depression. *Acta Neurologica Scandinavica, Supplementum 113*, **76**, 1–40.

Livingston, M. and Hubel, D. (1988). Segregation of form, colour, movement and depth: Anatomy, physiology, and perception. *Science*, **240**, 740–9.

Miller, E. (1984). *Recovery and management of neurological impairments*. Wiley, London.

Milner, B. (1974). Hemispheric specialization: Scope and limits. In *The neurosciences third study program*, (ed. F. Schmit and F. Wordon). MIT Press, Boston, MA.

Olsen, J., Larsen, B., and Lauritzen, M. (1981). Focal hyperemia followed by spreading oligemia and impaired activation of rCBF in classic migraine. *Annals of Neurology*, **9**, 344–52.

Pasik, T. and Pasik, P. (1980). Extrageniculostriate vision in primates. In *Neuro-ophthalmology*, Vol. 1 (ed. S. Lessell and J. T. W. van Dalen), pp. 95–115. Elsevier, Amsterdam.

Polyak, S. (1957). *The vertebrate visual system*. University of Chicago Press.

Riddoch, G. (1917). Dissociation of visual perceptions due to occipital injuries, with especial reference to appreciation of movement. *Brain*, **40**, 15–57.

Robinson, R. G., Kubos, K. L., Starr, L. B., Rao, K., and Price, T. R. (1984). Mood disorders in stroke patients: Importance of local lesion. *Brain*, **107**, 81–93.

Rothrock, J. F., Walicke, P., Swenson, M. R., Lyden, P. D., and Logan, W. R. (1988). Migraine stroke. *Archives of Neurology*, **45**, 63–67.

Sinyor, D., Jacques, P., Kaloupek, D. G., Becker, R., Goldenberg, M., and Coopersmith, H. (1986). Poststroke depression and lesion location. *Brain*, **109**, 537–46.

Spaccavento, L. J., and Solomon, G. D. (1984). Migraine as an etiology of stroke in young adults. *Headache*, **24**, 19–22.

Teuber, H.-L. (1975). Recovery of function after brain injury in man. In *Outcome of severe damage to the nervous system*, Ciba Foundation Sympsium 34. Elsevier, Amsterdam.

Warrington, E. K. (1962). The completion of visual forms across hemianopic field defects. *Journal of Neurology, Neurosurgery and Psychiatry*, **25**, 208–17.

Warrington, E. K. (1965). The effect of stimulus configuration on the incidence of the completion phenomenon. *British Journal of Psychology*, **56**, 447–54.

Waters, W. E., and O'Connor, P. J. (1975). Prevalence of migraine. *Journal of Neurology, Neurosurgery, and Psychiatry*, **38**, 613–16.

Weiskrantz, L. (1986). *Blindsight: A case study and implications*. Oxford University Press.

Zihl, J., and von Cramon, D. (1985). Visual field recovery from scotoma in patients with postgeniculate damage. *Brain*, **108**, 335–65.

(Kolb 1990)

COMMENTARY

Kolb observed that the main part of the scotoma resulting from his right occipital stroke shrank over the first 50 days, but appeared to remain fairly constant after this. This temporal pattern of recovery would appear to tie in with studies of recovery of function after stroke (Skilbeck *et al.* 1983), where the initial period of two–three months is often considered as the phase where the greatest recovery of function takes place. It should, however, be borne in mind that Kolb's stroke was a moderate rather than severe one, and that a more severe stroke might well have been associated with a longer period of recovery. It is also of note that, inspite of this short recovery period for improvement in his visual field loss, Kolb reported that more general perceptual functions continued to recover for some time after this. These functions included reading speed, faces recognition ability, and eye–hand co-ordination. This would suggest that cognitive adaptation and readjustment have a longer time course than recovery of discrete perceptual or cognitive processes. Kolb's observations during the initial recovery phase are of interest because of the relative paucity of published data from early stages of recovery after brain injury or illness. These observations include—his awareness of the movement of large objects from his area of field loss into his intact visual field, appearing as 'travelling waves'; the replacement of a 'dark scotoma' by a 'scintillating scotoma'; and the early return of colour perception.

Kolb's observations highlight a two-stage process of recovery of function—an initial stage of spontaneous, 'biologically driven' recovery which seems to last for a few months at the most; and a second, adaptive, 'psychologically driven' recovery phase that extends over several years. The former was probably behind the reduction in size of Kolb's scotoma, and the latter may have contributed towards his improvements in functions such as reading and faces recognition. These improvements included specific adaptive changes such as a shift in his fixation point, and more conscious activities such as actively overcompensating for his left-sided visual field defect—during a ski trip, he avoided a bush on the left, only to collide into a tree on the right! Three years after his illness, Kolb still found he had some everyday difficulties, inspite of the recovery outlined above. He might misread words and misidentify faces, and he found it particularly difficult to follow the flight of a golf ball. Perhaps the latter type of task could in some way be incorporated into a diagnostic test of visual perceptual function!

Kolb's report of 'blindsight in hindsight' (in his case, noting the appearance of movement of a stimulus in the area of his scotoma) provides first-hand support for the phenomenon reviewed in detail by authors such as Weiskrantz (1991) and Cowey (1994). There remains some controversy about the actual mechanisms underlying reports of blindsight (Gazzaniga 1994), where the patient is not consciously aware of a visual stimulus presented in a blind part of his/her field, but in some other way (guessing, pattern of response to a related stimulus in the intact field, etc.) shows evidence of having successfully carried out some level of visual processing of the stimulus in the blind field. In order to explain Kolb's subjective experience of movement within his scotoma, it would appear that retinal inputs bypass striate cortex and somehow influence neurones in area V5 (also known as area MT), the area in the extrastriate cortex that appears to be sensitive to visual movement. This influence may be via retino-tectal pathways, with the involvement of structures such as the superior colliculus, or as a result of direct connections from the lateral geniculate nucleus to the extrastriate cortex, or due to both mechanisms. Whatever the precise neural mechanism, it would appear that in such cases of blindsight some form of orienting mechanism remains intact, despite the absence of conscious perception of part of the visual field.

It is also important to emphasize the converse experience reported by Kolb—less than normal vision in an area of the visual field that is outside the area of the scotoma. Rather surprisingly, Kolb does not report visual closure of objects that were partially perceived within his area of scotoma, something that was reported by Lashley during his migraine attacks (see p. 126). Kolb's relative lack of awareness of his scotoma, unless he was asked to concentrate on a particular visual object does, however, mirror Lashley's own experience.

Kolb's pre-stroke clinical history is of interest, in that he suffered from classical migraine for 15 years, with one attack a year. These attacks included transient scotomata in the left visual field that turned out to be identical to the permanent scotoma that he eventually suffered as a result of his stroke. In this case at least, it would seem that the pathophysiological mechanisms underlying his migraine were similar to those that caused his stroke.

Note that, like Ashcraft, Kolb's initial reaction after the onset of his symptoms was to carry out a miniature neurological self-examination to ascertain the range and severity of his difficulties, and to exclude any major problems. Due to their specialized backgrounds, both he and Ashcraft, who were experienced researchers, could do this with a certain degree of expertise, testing and excluding 'mini-hypotheses' about their condition. It is also worth noting that Kolb was able to use his initiative in persuading others as to the correct diagnosis, and even in treating one of the painful symptoms in the early recovery phase—a severe headache that only resolved after drinking lots of caffeinated coffee. Kolb himself, however, made the cardinal error so often seen in recovery from brain injury/illness of returning to work too soon after his stroke (in his case two weeks). He soon found that he had latent deficits which only became apparent in specific, taxing situations.

Like Meltzer, Kolb does refer to emotional side-effects from his brain illness, and in particular to a post-stroke depression that lasted 3–4 months. He considered that these emotional changes were directly, rather than indirectly, related to his brain damage, although it is likely that frustrations related to cognitive and perceptual difficulties may have interacted with other changes to result in episodes of depression or panic.

REFERENCES

Cowey, A. (1994). Cortical visual areas and the neurobiology of higher visual processes. In *The neuropsychology of high-level vision* (ed. M. Farah and G. Ratcliff), pp. 3–31. Lawrence Erlbaum, Hillsdale, NJ.

Gazzaniga, M. (1994). Blindsight reconsidered. *Current Directions in Psychological Science*, **3**, 93–6.

Kolb, B. and Whishaw, I. Q. (1996). *Fundamentals of human neuropsychology*, (4th edn). Freeman, New York.

Skilbeck, C., Wade, D. T., Langton-Hewer, R., and Wood, V. A. (1983). Recovery after stroke. *Journal of Neurology, Neurosurgery and Psychiatry*, **46**, 5–8.

Weiskrantz, L. (1991). Blindsight. In *Handbook of neuropsychology*, Vol. 2 (ed. F. Boller and J. Grafman), pp. 375–85. Elsevier, Amsterdam.

Visual field effects of classical migraine

David B. Boles

David Boles is an experimental psychologist.

INTRODUCTION

Classical migraine is typically characterized by unilateral headache, often alternating sides between successive attacks, preceded by a sensory aura. The aura is usually visual and involves the perception of scintillating lights and characteristic 'fortification' structures, which are zigzag lines that move over time from central vision outward toward the periphery. The aura, like the headache, is usually unilateral and is seen in homologous fields of the eyes (Diamond, Diamond-Falk, & Largen, 1981; Hockaday, 1978; Lauritzen, 1984; Meyer, 1981).

One view of classical migraine that is gaining increasing acceptance is that a physiological mechanism of spreading cortical depression is involved. Such a mechanism was proposed by Karl Lashley, himself a migraineur, who self-timed the spread of fortification structures and inferred a progression of 3 mm per min across the visual cortex. This rate corresponds closely to that of chemically induced spreading cortical depression in animals (Lauritzen, 1984). Lashley's observations have since been confirmed in blood flow studies conducted during migraine attack, finding focally reduced flow that spread at a rate of 2.2 mm per min. The depressed blood flow is independent of arterial distribution in that it generally spreads throughout posterior cortex, an observation that argues against a vasospasm explanation of migraine (Lauritzen, 1984; Oleson, 1985; Oleson & Lauritzen, 1984). However, the trigger for the spreading depression is poorly understood, with some research pointing to roles for blood platelet activity associated with the release of serotonin (Grotemeyer, Viand, & Beykirch, 1985; Kudrow, 1981) and for dietary tyramine (Ghose, Coppen, & Carroll, 1978).

Regardless of the mechanism, the unilateral aspects of classical migraine indicate that it produces a disturbance of neural activity limited to one cerebral hemisphere. Accordingly, classical migraine serves as a 'natural experiment' in which the posterior portion of one hemisphere is made temporarily dysfunctional. One would expect therefore that tasks performed during migraine attack, and requiring lateralized processing, would show behavioral effects consistent with the side of attack. Unfortunately, there appears to be a complete absence of such studies in the literature, perhaps because of the difficulties involved in obtaining and testing patients during the attack phase of the headache. In contrast to this relative absence of research on phasic concomitants of migraine stand a number of behavioral and physiological investigations of possible tonic changes, conducted in the intervals between attacks (Hockaday, 1978; Igarashi, Sakai, Kan, Okada, & Tazaki, 1991; Osborn, Alder, & Mitchell, 1991; Puca, Antonaci, Savarese, Covelli, Tarascio, Bellizi, Lamorgese, Musmeci, & Sorrento, 1985).

The purpose of the present research was to examine the phase effects of lateralized migraine attacks within a single subject who in effect was readily available on a continuous basis for purposes of research (i.e., the experimenter himself). The results should be regarded as preliminary in nature, but may represent the first concerning the effects of classical migraine on lateralized tasks.

In the study, four visually presented tasks were used, requiring a total of about 35 min of testing time per episode. Testing consistently took place well within what is at least a 2– to 3–hr duration of hypoperfusion of cortical tissue, observed following classical migraine attacks (Lauritzen, 1984). Testing was also conducted between attacks to provide a baseline of performance for comparison.

METHOD

Subject

The male experimenter was 36 years old at the time of initial testing (October 1988). Writing is done with the left hand, and a recent administration of the Edinburgh handedness inventory (Oldfield, 1971) revealed an extreme left-handed score of −100. The first known migraine attack was experienced in 1975, but is believed not to have recurred until about 1986, when attacks commenced with some regularity (retrospectively estimated at about once every 3 months). No prophylactic medication was taken until after the data were collected for the study. However, a regimen of 650 (later 375) mg of aspirin per day (Grotemeyer et al., 1985) implemented in October 1991 has produced a complete cessation of attacks through mid-November 1992.

Apparatus and Stimuli

Stimuli were presented using an Apple II Plus computer, an Amdek 300 monitor with a P31 (green) phosphor, and a two-key external keyboard. Testing was carried out in the subject's home under dim room lighting conditions. A chinrest was not used due to the physical location and the wide temporal spacing between migraine attacks, both of which rendered the setup and maintenance of a more formal testing apparatus impractical. Instead, an attempt was made to maintain a fairly constant distance across testings, estimated at about 50 cm. Because of the imprecision of this figure, all measurements of visual angles should be regarded as approximate.

There were four lateralized tasks, called 'words', 'typing', 'bar graphs', and 'locations'. The choice was made in the earliest phase of factor-analytic research that has since clarified the nature of the tasks. Specifically, the words and typing tasks tap into a left hemisphere lateralized visual lexical function; the bar graphs task represents a right hemisphere spatial quantitative function; and the locations task represents a right hemisphere spatial positional function (Boles, 1991, 1992a). Loadings of these tasks on their respective factors are quite comparable, ranging only between + .69 for typing and + .77 for locations, when averaged across several studies (Boles, 1992a).

Words were the word names of the numbers 1 to 8 (e.g., 'ONE'). They were presented in a vertical orientation in capital letters at an eccentricity (to the near edge) of 1.2°, subtending 0.3° horizontally and 1.3° to 2.3° vertically.

Typing stimuli were three-letter words (e.g., 'COD'), with the letters likewise in capitals and stacked vertically at an eccentricity of 2.1°, subtending 0.3° horizontally and 1.3° vertically.

Bar graphs were rectangular boxes representing whole numbers between 1 and 8, extending vertically for variable lengths and plotted against horizontal reference lines at the 0, 4, and 8 levels. Bar graphs were at 1.6° eccentricity and subtended 1.6° horizontally and 3.9° vertically (as measured using the top and bottom reference lines).

Locations stimuli were dots about 0.2° square, presented at one of 12 locations that composed a 3 × 4 (horizontal by vertical) grid in each visual field (VF). The eccentricity from the midline varied between 2.3° and 5.2° depending on the location, with each location having a mirror-image counterpart in the opposite VF. The vertical extent of locations in the grid was 3.1°.

Procedure

All four tasks were administered in a session, using a Latin-square design with corresponding but separate squares for (a) left hemisphere attacks, (b) right hemisphere attacks, and (c) control sessions. As this statement implies, migraine attacks varied between hemispheres, as inferred from the lateralized visual aura and as reflected by the ensuing unilateral headaches (always contralateral to the aura).

Table 1 indicates the dates of the testings,

Table 1 Testing Dates, Inferred Side of Attack, and Temporal Characteristics of the Migraine Attacks. Intervals: 1, beginning of aura to beginning of testing; 2, beginning of testing to beginning of headache; 3, beginning of headache to end of testing

		Duration of interval (min)			
Date	Side	1	2	3	Total
10/28/88	Left hemisphere	33	?	?	?
11/9/88	Right hemisphere	25	?	?	?
12/?/88	(Control)	—	—	—	—
3/3/89	Right hemisphere	27	13	?	?
2/10/90	Right hemisphere	33	5	33	71
3/11/90	(Control)	—	—	—	—
8/20/90	Right hemisphere	29	?	?	?
9/19/90	Left hemisphere	28	22	9	59
11/2/90	(Control)	—	—	—	—
11/6/90	Left hemisphere	28	−14	?	?
11/28/90	Right hemisphere	32	4	29	65
2/19/91	Left hemisphere	26	10	23	59
2/22/91	(Control)	—	—	—	—

which are thought to include nearly all of the migraine attacks (with one known omission when testing could not be performed) during the period of testing (10/28/88–2/22/91). The control sessions were run when there was no unilateral headache, usually several weeks after an attack.

No practice was given on the tasks, as the experiment was highly familiar with each. When an attack occurred, the position of the aura in the VFs was monitored while the apparatus was readied, and testing began just after the aura passed from view in the periphery. Brief notes were also taken during most attacks, which often allowed time intervals to be estimated as shown in Table 1. The mean duration from the beginning of the attack to the beginning of testing was 29.0 min (s.d. = 3.0, $N = 9$). The mean time from the beginning of testing to the beginning of the headache was 6.7 min (s.d. = 12.0, $N = 6$) and from then until the end of testing averaged 23.5 min (s.d. = 10.5, $N, = 4$). It can be seen that in the available data, there was always a brief delay between the end of the aura (beginning of testing) and the beginning of the headache phase, except in one instance when the headache began halfway through the aura. More importantly, it is clear that the total duration (mean = 63.5

min, s.d. = 5.7, $N = 4$) is well within what is at least a 2- to 3-hr lifespan of hypoperfusion of cortical tissue following migraine attacks (Lauritzen, 1984).

In all four tasks, the stimulus to be recognized was presented to one VF at random, accompanied by a randomly selected stimulus of the same kind in the opposite field and an arrowhead at fixation indicating the stimulus to be recognized. Such bilateral displays were used because they have been found to substantially increase the size, significance, and reliability of VF differences relative to unilateral displays (Boles, 1983, 1987, 1990, 1992b).

The words, bar graphs, and locations tasks were similar in that a fixation cross was first presented for 750 msec, followed by a 100–msec blank period and then a 100–msec stimulus display. The words and bar graphs tasks required responses within a deadline of 4 sec from the beginning of the stimulus display, using the two-key external board, with the 'far' key for 'odd' numbers (1, 3, 5, or 7) and the 'near' key for 'even' numbers (2, 4, 6, or 8). The subject pressed one of the keys as quickly and accurately as possible with simultaneous responses of the two forefingers (odd) or thumbs (even), and brief feedback was given as to the speed and accuracy of response.

Responses for the locations task were handled differently, however. Following the stimulus display, a 3 × 4 letter grid appeared in the center of the screen, and a letter had to be typed into the computer console that corresponded to the position of the dot within the grid as it would be transposed to the appropriate VF. This response was untimed, and the grid remained until a response was made.

Responses for the typing task were similarly untimed. A fixation box first appeared in the center of the screen for 750 msec, followed by a 133-msec blank period, a 133-msec stimulus display, a 100-msec blank, and then a 133-msec masking display consisting of X's in the letter positions in both VFs. The subject then typed the three-letter word into the console.

In the words, bar graphs, and locations tasks, 144 trials were given (72 per VF), whereas in the typing task, 72 trials were given (36 per VF).

RESULTS

For each VF, task, and session, percentage errors were calculated and median correct RTs where appropriate. Subsequently, each dependent measure for a task was entered into a VF (left vs. right) by Condition (left hemisphere attack vs. right hemisphere attack vs. control) COANOVA. The covariate was the serial position of the session (1 to 13) and was used to control for any practice effects operating across sessions. The results are described separately for the individual tasks.

Words

The RT measure for the words task showed a significant Condition main effect ($F[2, 9] = 5.24, p < .05$), as well as a VF × Condition interaction ($F[2, 10] = 5.01, p < .05$). Table 2 shows the means and indicates that the interaction was due to contrasting field effects across conditions: right visual field (RVF) advantages were found in the control condition (+21 msec) and in the right-attack condition (+31 msec), but a left visual field (LVF) advantage pertained in the left-attack condition (−23 msec).

Table 2 also shows the mean percentage errors. The only significant effect was the main effect of VF (+3.8%; $F[1, 10] = 10.58, p < .01$), although the Condition term produced a marginally significant effect ($F[2, 9] = 3.71, p = .07$). There was no VF × Condition interaction ($F[2, 10] = .08$).

Typing

The only dependent measure in the typing task was percentage errors. The COANOVA showed a significant Condition main effect ($F[2, 9] = 6.96, p < .02$), as well as a VF × Condition interaction ($F[2, 10] = 7.70, p < .01$). As Table 3 indicates, there was no VF difference in the control condition (−0.7%), a LVF advantage in the left-attack condition (−19.4%), and a RVD advantage in the right-attack condition (+8.3%).

Table 2 RTs (in msec) and Percentage Errors in the Words Task

	Left-attack	Right-attack	Control
RT			
LVF	583	594	566
RVF	606	563	545
Dif	−23	+31	+21
Percentage errors			
LVF	7.8	8.5	11.2
RVF	4.3	4.0	7.8
Dif	+3.5	+4.5	+3.4

Table 3 Percentage Errors in the Typing Task

	Left-attack	Right-attack	Control
LVF	10.5	20.7	11.2
RVF	29.9	12.4	11.9
Dif	−19.4	+8.3	−0.7

Bar Graphs

The RT COANOVA showed no significant effects, although all three terms were marginally significant: Condition ($F[2, 9] = 3.44$, $p = .08$), VF ($F[1, 10] = 4.04$, $p = .07$), and VF × Condition ($F[2, 10] = 3.71$, $p = .06$). The percentage error analysis found only one significant effect, that of VF ($F[1, 10] = 9.30$, $p < .02$). As Table 4 indicates, there was a LVF advantage in errors (−3.9%).

Locations

Percentage errors showed a main effect of VF ($F[1, 10] = 42.78$, $p < .001$), and a VF × Condition interaction ($F[2, 10] = 10.12$, $p < .005$). The Condition main effect was marginally significant ($F[2, 9] = 3.39$, $p = .08$). As Table 5 indicates, an overall LVF advantage was enhanced during left hemisphere attacks (−21.9% vs. −5.7% for the other two conditions).

Symptomatology

The written notes taken during the migraine episodes were subjected to a content analysis to determine whether some symptoms were lateralized.

Several emerged that occurred at least twice during attacks involving one hemisphere, but not during attacks involving the other.

With respect to left hemisphere episodes, alphabetic indistinctiveness was twice noted (on 9/19/90, for words, 'RVF stimuli were indistinct, esp. the bottom half', and for typing, 'stimuli seemed indistinct in RVF'; on 11/6/90, for words, 'letters in RVF seemed dim, indistinct'). Difficulty in maintaining eye fixation was thrice noted (on 11/6/90, for words, 'great effort to maintain fixation due to jitter', and for bar graphs, 'ditto on fixation'; on 11/28/90, for both words and bar graphs, 'difficulty maintaining eye fixation'; on 2/19/91, for words, 'Noticed great difficulty maintaining fixation'). A third left-hemisphere-associated symptom was nausea (on 10.28/88, 'feel mildly nauseous'; on 11/6/90, 'stomach somewhat upset immediately preceeding (sic; preceding) & during attack').

Turning to right hemisphere episodes, spatial disturbances were noted on three occasions (on 11/9/88, '"otherworldly" detachment from space'; on 3/3/89, 'strong feeling of "otherworldliness" and detachment from space, particularly upon walking'; on 2/10/90, ' "otherworldly", spatially disconnected feeling on walking'). The only other right-specific symptom was numbness of the upper extremity (on 8/20/90, 'reduced sensation in L hand & arm'; on 2/10/90, 'Slight

Table 4 RTs (in msec) and Percentage Errors in the Bar Graphs Task

	Left-attack	Right-attack	Control
RT			
LVF	660	681	625
RVF	713	666	648
Dif	−53	+15	−23
Percentage errors			
LVF	7.7	8.0	7.7
RVF	10.5	10.8	12.2
Dif	−2.8	−2.8	−4.5

Table 5 Percentage Errors in the Locations Task

	Left-attack	Right-attack	Control
LVF	28.7	31.8	22.8
RVF	50.6	37.7	28.3
Dif	−21.9	−5.9	−5.5

numbness in L Hand noted'). The numbness was slight and should not have affected responses to the tasks; certainly no motor impairment was noted.

Two other multiply occurring symptoms showed nonexistent or only weak lateralization. These included notations of the presence of color in the visual aura (two left and one right episode, probably substantial undercounts of the true frequencies), and judgments of the predominant direction of movement of fortification lines in the aura (up: three left, one right; down: zero left, two right; horizontally outward: one left, two right). The remaining symptoms were each noted only once: a bitter taste sensation (left attack), reduced hearing (right attack), and "tunnel vision" (right attack).

DISCUSSION

The results of the self-study suggest that classical migraine does produce detectable effects on processes in the affected cerebral hemisphere. With respect to the VF-by-Condition interaction, all four tasks resulted either in significant effects (the words, typing, and locations tasks) or marginally significant effects (the bar graphs task).

However, it is important to distinguish between effects on lower levels of the visual system (e.g., early analytical processes such as those localized to the visual cortex) and those at higher levels (i.e., those more proximal to pattern recognition). Some lower level processes may be lateralized only in the sense that a VF projects to one hemisphere. It may be only at higher levels where true functional differences emerge (Moscovitch & Radzins, 1987). This distinction between levels may

be particularly relevant in the study of classical migraine, because the existence of a visual aura implies lower level effects, specifically within occipital areas (Meyer, 1981; Oleson, 1985). Although in the present case hemianopia was never experienced following an aura, mild depression of visual sensitivity in the affected field was not only possible but probable, and this is encompassed within what is meant by low-level processing.

A purely lower level effect should be limited to the VF projecting to the affected hemisphere. The other VF, projecting to the hemisphere that is unaffected by the migraine attack, should show normal performance. Such a pattern is quite pronounced in the case of the typing task (Table 3). Relative to the control condition, left hemisphere attacks affected only the RVF, and right hemisphere attacks the LFV. The most parsimonious conclusion is that in the typing task, interference due to migraine was at a predominantly low level in the visual system.

It is interesting that no lateralized effect was found for typing in the control condition (Table 3), unlike most subjects performing the identical task (Boles, 1991, 1992a). Perhaps this is a function of familiarity with the task, transforming it into a lower level one. Unlike most subject, who are unfamiliar with the word set, this subject is quite familiar with the stimuli. Therefore, instead of performing the task on a lexical level as is found with naive subjects (Boles, 1991, 1992a), a prelexical strategy may have been used in which an attempt was made to recognize particular letter fragments that were diagnostic of particular words. Such a low-level analysis could result both in an overall lack of lateral differences and in field-specific interference by migraine attacks. It should be noted that the other lexical task, words, produced an asymmetry in the control condition (+21 msec) that is indistinguishable from the mean (+20 msec) over a large number of right-handed subjects (Boles, 1992a). In that speeded, unmasked task, a letter fragment strategy would not be productive of fast RTs. The outcome indicates that the absence of asymmetry in the typing task was not due to an absence of hemispheric asymmetry, an otherwise plausible interpretation due to left-handedness.[1]

In contrast to the typing task, the locations task showed a pattern of results that cannot be characterized as "low level." Specifically, right hemisphere migraine appears to have caused interference in both VFs relative to the control condition (Table 5). Thus the effect seems consistent with interference on a higher level spatial positional function lateralized to the right hemisphere (Boles, 1991, 1992a).

The patterns of results in the remaining tasks (words and bar graphs) cannot be interpreted without ambiguity, because speed-accuracy response biases seem to have confounded comparisons to the control conditions. In both cases, although more pronouncedly in the case of words, the occurrence of a migraine attack on either side appears to have resulted in a response bias that stressed accuracy over speed, lengthening overall RTs but decreasing errors in comparison to the control condition. As a consequence controlled comparisons cannot easily be made to determine whether lower or higher level processes were affected.

In any event the typing and locations tasks illustrate opposing interference patterns in which lower and higher level types of interference, respectively, are implicated. Because responses were made at leisure as accurately as possible in these tasks, they are presumably less sensitive than the RT tasks to speed–accuracy response bias shifts.

A final issue concerns the possible operation of demand characteristics. The subject in this study is knowledgeable of both laterality research and the nature of migraine, and it is conceivable that this knowledge affected the results. Although a demand effect cannot be conclusively ruled out in the absence of naive subjects, two arguments suggest that the effect was minimal in this study. First, the contrasting results of the typing and locations tasks were in no way foreseen, nor was the absence of a lateral difference in the typing task control condition. Indeed, the logic involved in distinguishing lower level from higher level effects was not worked out until all of the data had been collected. The contrasting results suggest that they were not produced as a consequence of familiarity with laterality research and the nature of migraine.

Second, it is clear that in neither task was there a performance tradeoff between VFs. If demand characteristics operated to produce the results, one might expect them to be manifested as an attentional bias to one field, enhancing performance there but at a cost to the other field. Instead, performance was either degraded in one field while the other was unaffected (typing), or it was simultaneously degraded in both fields (locations).

It is hoped that future studies of the lateralized effects of classical migraine can find a way to employ naive subjects, not only in order to definitively rule out the influence of demand characteristics, but also to increase the generalizability of the results. If the logistics involved in transporting subjects to an experimental apparatus in the midst of an attack proves insurmountable, an alternative approach might be to pursue lateralized symptomatology, perhaps by means of questionnaires completed by subjects following each attack. To this subject, left hemisphere attacks appear to make alphabetic characters indistinct, to cause difficulty in maintaining eye fixation, and to promote nausea. Right hemisphere episodes seemed to result in spatial disturbances and in numbness of the contralateral upper extremity. Two of these symptoms, those concerning the perception of alphabetic characters and of space, are well grounded in known hemispheric asymmetries of function (Boles, 1987, 1991, 1992a; Bryden, 1982; Faglioni, Scotti, & Spinnler, 1969; Kolb & Whishaw, 1990). It will be interesting to learn whether they, too, are 'real' effects not due to demand characteristics.

---

[1] With the exception of typing, asymmetries in the control conditions were strikingly similar to those of the average right-handed subject (Boles, 1992a). Thus words produced asymmetries of +21 msec and +3.4%, compared to +20 msec and +0.4% in right-handers; bar graphs −23 msec and −4.5%, compared to −30 msec and −1.3%; and locations −5.5% compared with −5.5%.

REFERENCES

Boles, D. B. (1983). Hemispheric interaction in visual field asymmetry. *Cortex*, **19**, 99–114.

Boles, D. B. (1987). Reaction time asymmetry through bilateral vs. unilateral stimulus presentation. *Brain and Cognition*, **6**, 321–33.

Boles, D. B. (1990). What bilateral displays do. *Brain and Cognition*, **12**, 205–28.

Boles, D. B. (1991). Factor analysis and the cerebral hemispheres: Pilot study and parietal functions. *Neuropsychologia*, **29**, 59–91.

Boles, D. B. (1992a). Factor analysis and the cerebral hemispheres: Temporal, occipital, and frontal functions. *Neuropsychologia*.

Boles, D. B. (1992b). Parameters of the bilateral effect. In *Hemispheric transfer: Data and theory* (ed. F. L. Kitterle). Lawrence Erlbaum, London.

Bryden, M. P. (1982). *Laterality: Functional asymmetry n the intact brain*. Academic Press, New York.

Diamond, S., Diamond-Falk, J., and Largen, J. W. (1981). Update: Biofeedback in the treatment of vascular headache. In *Treatment of migraine: Pharmacological and biofeedback considerations* (ed. R. J. Mathew). SP Medical and Scientific, New York.

Faglioni, P., Scotti, G., and Spinnler, H. (1969). Impaired recognition of written letters following unilateral hemispheric damage. *Cortex*, **5**, 120–33.

Ghose, K., Coppen, A., and Carroll, D. (1978). Studies in the interactions of tyramine in migraine patients. In *Current concepts in migraine research* (ed. R. G. Greene), Raven, New York.

Grotemeyer, K.-H., Viand, R., and Beykirch, K. (1985). Effects of different doses of acetylsalicylic acid on frequency of migraine attack, platelet prostaglandin synthesis, and platelet aggregation. In *Updating in headache*, (ed. V. Pfaffenrath, P.-O. Lundberg, and O. Sjaastad). Springer, Berlin.

Hockaday, J. M. (1978). Late outcome of childhood onset migraine and factors affecting outcome, with particular reference to early and late EEG findings. In *Current concepts in migraine research* (ed. R. G. Greene). Raven, New York.

Igarashi, H., Sakai, F., Kan, S., Okada, J., and Tazaki, Y. (1991). Magnetic resonance imaging of the brain in patients with migraine. *Cephalalgia*, **11**, 69–74.

Kolb, B. and Whishaw, I. Q. (1990). *Fundamentals of human neuropsychology*. Freeman, New York.

Kudrow, L. (1981). Biochemistry of migraine. In *Treatment of migraine: Pharamacological and biofeedback considerations* (ed. R. J. Mathew). SP Medical and Scientific, New York.

Lauritzen, M. (1984). Spreading cortical depression in migraine. In *The pharmacological basis of migraine therapy* (ed. W. K. Amery, J. M. Van Neuten, and A. Wauquier). Pitman, London.

Meyer, J. S. (1981). Measurements of regional cerebral blood flow (rCBF) and their application to migraine research. In *Treatment of migraine: Pharmacological and biofeedback considerations* (ed. R. J. Mathew). SP Medical and Scientific, New York.

Moscovitch, M. and Radzins, M. (1987). Backward masking of lateralized faces by noise, pattern, and spatial frequency. *Brain and Cognition*, **6**, 72–90.

Oldfield, R. C. (1971). The assessment and analysis of handedness: The Edinburgh Inventory. *Neuropsychologia*, **9**, 97–113.

Oleson, J. (1985). Vascular aspects of migraine pathophysiology. In *Migraine: Clinical and research advances* (ed. F. C. Rose). Karger, Basel.

Oleson, J. and Lauritzen, M. (1984). The role of vasoconstriction in the pathogenesis of migraine. In *The pharmacological basis of migraine therapy*, (ed. W. K. Amery, J. M. Van Nueten, and A. Wauquier). Pitman, London.

Osborn, R. E., Alder, D. C., and Mitchell, C. S. (1991). MR imaging of the brain in patients with migraine headaches. *American Journal of Neuroradiology*, **12**, 521–4.

Puca, F. M., Antonaci, F., Savarese, M., Covelli, V., Tarascio, G., Bellizi, M., Lamorgese, C., Musmeci, G. M., and Sorrento, G. (1985). Memory impairment and painful side. In *Migraine: Clinical and research advances* (ed. F. C. Rose). Karger, Basel.

(Boles 1993)

COMMENTARY

The experimental investigation by Boles is a fascinating one, reminiscent of self-inflicted neurophysiological studies carried out by 19th-century neurologists. Research on hemispheric specialization would be concordant with Boles' basic observations, namely, that left hemisphere migraine attacks appeared to make alphabetic characters distinct, while right hemisphere migraine episodes resulted in spatial disturbances. The familiarity of Boles to some of the stimuli used in the experimental tasks, as well as his knowledge of relevant research findings and facts about migraine, need to be borne in mind. Nevertheless, his comments about a 'levels-of-processing' approach to the effects of his migraine on his vision are in tune with most recent studies of the neural basis of vision, where low-level visual processing related to features such as form, location, etc. is in many ways distinct from higher-level processing that subserves visual identification (Zeki 1993).

REFERENCE

Zeki, S. (1993). *A vision of the brain.* Blackwell, Oxford.

PART II

Clinical conditions

Parkinson's disease 4

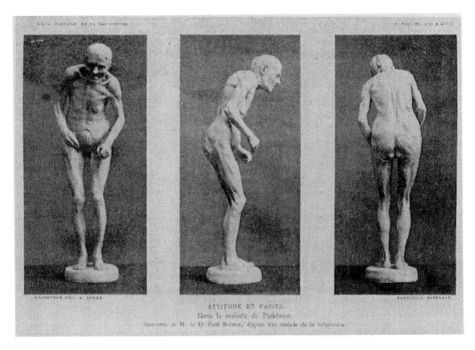

Figure 7. Statuette by Dr Paul Richer, showing the typical posture of a patient with Parkinson's disease.

INTRODUCTION

Parkinson's disease is a progressive disorder of the brain that is estimated to affect around one in every 800 individuals.[1] It owes its name to a description of the condition by James Parkinson in 1817, and the major symptoms of the disease include tremor, muscular rigidity, absence or slowness of movement, and an abnormality of posture. Parkinson's disease patients characteristically have a shuffling gait, and in many cases there is also a notable reduction in size of their handwriting. The usual age of onset of symptoms is between 50 and 59 years, with about 40% of patients having the onset of their disease in this period. Most patients with Parkinson's disease are estimated to survive for around 10–15 years after the onset of symptoms, although a few cases may survive for over 20 years without any major disability.

Parkinson's disease results from degeneration of the *substantia nigra*, neurones that synthesize the neurotransmitter dopamine, and innervate the basal ganglia. The basal ganglia are a collection of subcortical nuclei involved in the regulation of motor function. There are anatomical links between the basal ganglia and structures involved in psychological functioning, such as the thalamus, amygdala, and frontal cortex.

Dopamine replacement therapy has become the major treatment option for Parkinson's disease, though after a number of years there is usually habituation to this medication and also the risk of side-effects. In recent years, attempts have been made to improve Parkinson's disease symptoms by the surgical ablation of discrete structures that make up the basal ganglia, such as parts of the globus pallidus, and there have also been attempts to relieve symptoms by implanting dopamine-rich foetal tissue. It is difficult to be certain at present about the long-term benefits of either treatment, or whether these surgical procedures will benefit a large number of patients.

Cognitive dysfunction, which includes a slowness in thought processes that appears to parallel the slowness in motor responses, and also depression, are present to a varying degree in some patients with Parkinson's disease. It is uncertain at present why certain Parkinson's disease patients and not others develop psychological deficits. The incidence of 'dementia' in Parkinson's disease has tended to vary between 10% and 40%, although this will depend on the stage of the disease at which dementia is assessed, together with the exact criteria used to make a diagnosis of dementia. In some cases, dementia may be due to the co-occurrence of Alzheimer's disease, and this is more likely in the older patient with Parkinson's disease. Some of the cognitive deficits that are found in Parkinson's disease patients are presumed to reflect indirect frontal lobe pathology, and are manifest in test impairments that involve the use of strategies in problem-solving settings, initiating and switching responses according to task demands, and making temporal judgements in memory and other tasks.

---

[1] Unless otherwise stated, the values given in this book for the occurrence of a particular brain disorder are prevalence rather than incidence figures. For further information on the epidemiology of neurological disease, the reader is referred to Anderson, D. W. (ed.) (1991). *Neuroepidemiology: A tribute to Bruce Schoenberg.* CRC Press, Boca Raton, FL; and to Walton, J. (ed.) (1993). *Brain's diseases of the nervous system, (10th edn).* Oxford University Press.

The following articles provide a wide spectrum of the types of difficulties faced by Parkinson's disease patients. Indeed, there appear to be more published articles by doctors who have suffered Parkinson's disease than by doctors with any other neurological condition! Although there is a natural concentration on physical symptoms, such as tremor or motor inco-ordination, most of the authors do refer to the occurrence of cognitive or emotional symptoms. None of the cases, however, report severe cognitive impairment such as might be associated with an Alzheimer-type dementia. Although this is probably an accurate reflection of the degree of cortical involvement in Parkinson's disease in general, it may also be due in part to the stage at which patients wrote their accounts—most appear to have been written in the early or middle stages of the illness. None of the accounts offers the experience of surgical ablation of brain tissue to relieve Parkinsonian symptoms. In a book that was written after his article, **Todes** (**1990**) does refer to the stages involved in undergoing transplantation of neural tissue to improve his condition.

In addition to the specific commentaries that follow each article, I have also included a general commentary at the end of this section.

FURTHER READING

Koller, W. C. (1992). *Handbook of Parkinson's disease*, (2nd edn). Marcel Dekker, New York.

Parkinsonism

The anonymous writer of this article had worked as a naval doctor, and then went into general practice.

Sleepy sickness is perhaps one of the cruellest afflictions to be endured by man. Though myself a doctor, I know little about the pathology of the disease; and indeed I have no knowledge of its clinical course or ultimate end, beyond the sequence of events that have already befallen me. I make no inquiries, nor do I dip into periodicals and books dealing with the complaint; for it is foolish, in my estimation, to anticipate what may never happen.

'Creeping paralysis'—the title already given to another disease—would be an excellent name for this disability, which drags unrelentingly along its laborious course. It is quite impossible to say 'I'm worse than I was a week or a month ago'. It is necessary to look back much further to recall little things that could once be managed but are now impossible or very difficult.

I am supposed to have contracted the disease in 1924, when I was 29. I ran a temperature for a few days and saw double for a week. This diplopia rather alarmed me at the time, but a brother houseman reassured me by saying that this phenomenon indicated only fatigue of the eye muscles, which was to be expected in any febrile condition. Previously the Navy had claimed me for eight years, but now I went into general practice at a seaside town, where I joined the local sailing club.

It was while sailing that I got the first inkling that all was not well with my make-up. Several boats had reached a mark-buoy round which it was necessary to gybe—a tricky moment, which would have disturbed the most hardened seaman, for a general smash-up seemed inevitable. Suddenly my hand started to vibrate on the tiller; it was a most curious sensation though only momentary. I mastered myself, regained my grip, both mental and physical, and steered round the buoy without incident.

Another warning came a few days later at a public luncheon. I was on my feet, proposing a vote of thanks to the speaker, when my right hand started to vibrate again. I havered a bit, rammed my hand into my trouser-pocket, and continued. I don't think anyone else noticed the contretemps. Some time after this I noticed that it was becoming difficult to write, quite a short letter taking a considerable time; and my handwriting, which always had been a bit of a puzzle, became completely illegible. Soon I lost my nerve for the excitement of sailing. There is always a spice of danger in navigating, even in local waters; and competing in the single-handed race—which I myself had instituted—became for me a most alarming affair.

At this stage I consulted my brother, a general practitioner, who arranged for me to see a London neurologist. The three of us rendezvoused at the great man's country house; and, without my knowing, he diagnosed my ailment over the teacups. Afterwards he took me for a stroll in the garden. I remember he asked me if my mouth seemed wetter than usual. I answered No. Little did I realise that as the years went by excessive salivation was to become the greatest tribulation of my life. In the kindest and most gentle way he told me what I was suffering from. In a way it was a relief to know something definite.

Things went from bad to worse, and I had difficulty in memorising my patients' faces and what I had prescribed for them. Deciding to give up my practice and go back to the Navy —my first love—I went to the Admiralty for medical examination, and felt guilty enough at putting my signature to a written statement that I was free from physical disability. In this early stage I could easily have fooled the whole Royal College of Physicians. But life on a submarine depot-ship, spending hour after hour with nothing to do but just sit and think or perhaps listen to Service jargon, proved an impossibility for me. I lasted a couple of months, then collapsed and was invalided out of the Service.

This just about finished me, and I found it beyond my powers even to think of a job of work. In the backwater of a village, with my wife and child, life became happy; and in the winter months I enjoyed rough-shooting, though slow on the trigger. My age was now 34. Then tremor and salivation began to trouble me. The embarrassment of excessive salivation is comprehensible only by those who have suffered it; it is very trying to have one's mouth perpetually full of fluid, waiting to spill over at the slightest relaxation of the facial muscles. My brother put me on a proprietary preparation of scopolamine, which for years acted like a charm, drying up the mouth, reducing tremor, and making me feel fairly well. But as time wore on it lost its almost magical effect, which has never returned. I was now treated with a preparation of stramonium, which still has a remarkably consistent action. Unfortunately it takes an hour to act, and in that time there is an almost overpowering temptation to hurry things up by taking a little more. The result of an overdose is devastating: a bone-dry mouth, a feeble heart-beat, a feeling of distress, and hysteria producing an exaggerated sense of humour, though in the background all the time is a sober awareness. If, on the other hand, I take too little, salivation deluges me. It is remarkably hard to strike a happy mean, for the path between the two extremes is very narrow. Owing to the atropine in stramonium, the pupils dilate, and strong glasses are needed. Before a fire the heat is sufficient to dry up the conjunctivae and the upper lid tends to stick to the eyeball. This is sometimes quite painful. The trouble is alleviated by a kettle steaming on the hob, or a dish of water placed before the fire.

Gradually difficulty in swallowing has manifested itself; it is impossible to get down any food without copious draughts of water, and even this does not always work. I never take a meal with any but my own family, for eating demands my whole attention. Though right-handed, I use a fork in the left hand (the less affected) for almost all varieties of food; a fork is much easier to manipulate than a spoon. Crisp dry food is the most readily masticated; anything that cloys is anathema. 'Ryvita', recrisped in the oven, is ideal. Of a different texture, sponge-cake is also excellent, seeming to dissolve in the mouth. A satisfying meal entails an hour's hard work. One of the greatest irritations is the inability, through being unable to swallow quickly, to join in the conversation, however trite my unspoken comment. By the time I have swallowed, the talk has swung on to some fresh subject.

My speech has become indistinct. Until I got used to it, this caused me great annoyance. How maddening it is to receive a grotesquely irrelevant answer to some simple remark, from someone trying his best to understand. How much better it would be if he said that he did not comprehend. My latest affliction is inability to walk well—the 'festinating gait'. This is much worse indoors, when my way is beset with many corners. Once on an open road I can get along with a certain ease; but there are ominous signs that this will not last. Curiously enough it is easier to walk backwards than forwards.

For the last twenty years I have been writing, punching the typewriter with my left forefinger—the only digit of the ten that will perform this duty. Free-lancing is surely the most disappointing of all occupations. I must have had some two hundred articles rejected; but slowly my name is getting known, for I seem just now to be selling two articles a month, and two plays have been accepted by the B.B.C.

This tremendous interest keeps me going; but a snag—inevitably, I suppose—has recently developed. I can no longer type with any ease or dexterity, my one good finger refusing to function. This is really distressing; but, as nearly always happens, there is a way out. In America they are manufacturing an electric typewriter, which at the softest touch does everything, even rolling on the paper and shifting the keyboard; but naturally it is expensive.

I have to fight my own peculiar demon— the devil of frustration. Everything is difficult to accomplish; little details which come like second nature to the normal person are a series of puzzles to me; and sometimes there is no solution. Putting on clothes, doing up shoe-laces, fastening shirt buttons, holding a cup of tea without its slopping over—all these are obstacles in the routine of life. Some of these things have to be done for me.

So here I am, at the age of 55, with difficulty in walking, talking, eating, writing, and typing, with a whole host of minor ailments; yet a happy man with dozens of compensations. How has this disease affected my character and temperament? All for the better, I think. I can bear the keenest disappointment with almost complete equanimity; this happens two or three times a week when those big buff envelopes, addressed by myself, pass through the letter-box, and also when some new disability asserts itself. I am now much more sympathetic and can better understand other people's foibles, peculiarities, bothers, and ailments.

My belief that man possesses a separate entity apart from his husk of a body has been greatly strengthened by my experiences. I sit, as it were, inside my carapace watching my person behaving in its vile fashion, while my being is a thing apart, held a prisoner for a time. This rather queer sensation of being outside oneself has been exaggerated by my complaint: it is most comforting, and strengthens my faith that there is not complete extinction ahead, but a better deal in a new life.

(Anonymous 1952)

COMMENTARY

The account by the anonymous doctor is of historical interest in that it gives an idea of what it was like to cope with Parkinson's disease before the introduction of L-dopa and related compounds. The report by this doctor of a feeling akin to depersonalization, 'the rather queer sensation of being without oneself', may well have been an indirect reaction to the illness itself rather than reflecting specific cortical or subcortical pathology. Excessive salivation, difficulty swallowing, and impaired articulation all appeared to be more frustrating and depressing to him than tremor or motor inco-ordination. His comment that it was easier for him to walk backwards than forwards is an unusual and interesting observation!

Inside Parkinsonism ... a psychiatrist's personal experience

C. Todes

Cecil Todes initially specialized in dentistry in South Africa, before qualifying in medicine in London. He worked as a consultant child psychiatrist, specializing in psychotherapy.

At the age of 39 I was diagnosed as having idiopathic Parkinson's disease (IPD). Living with the illness over the past 12 years has stimulated thoughts and insights I would like to share. An immediate difficulty emerges, which takes me to the very heart of the condition: I have to be 'on', that is, having a positive reaction to medication, in order to write, and sufficiently free from the fatigue and restrictions of side-effects that my thoughts flow unimpeded. As the illness progresses to involve more and more brain cells, the continuous recall of events is disrupted and thoughts of a conceptual nature become less readily available. Flexibility, both internal and external, is at a premium; by this stage of the illness, there are only 3 or 4 really good hours a day and, hopefully, another 6 mediocre ones with mobility. On/off plays havoc with the predictability of life, and hence erodes continuity and confidence. When the initial symptom of left-arm tremor was diagnosed as IPD, it seemed more acceptable than the fulminating brain tumour I had imagined. At 39, to identify my tremor with that of the shuffling old folk seen in outpatients was inconceivable. Besides, 10–20 years ahead seemed very remote— and who knew what pharmacological discoveries might not alter my future?

After the first shock, the automatic reaction was intellectual acceptance. At a deeper level, however, I was denying the whole experience. After all, I had an active life to lead, family and professional responsibilities, and ambition. I had recently completed my training as a psychoanalyst, and had begun a stimulating consultant appointment in child and family psychiatry. Under the pressure of an increasing workload, the symptom became more persistent, and I began to take levodopa, which had recently come into general use in the treatment of Parkinson's disease. Taking the drug marked my entry into the realm of patienthood. The defect was still, however, predominantly on the left side, and, saturating myself with the high doses then in use, I soldiered on. The advent of 'Sinemet' (carbidopa plus levodopa) eliminated some of the discomfort of nausea and hypotension and enabled me to maintain saturation levels. The hope was that levodopa might halt or slow down the progress of Parkinson's disease.

By 1975, after 5 years' illness, other difficulties began to emerge—growing frustration and fatigue. Sleepiness worsened because of a tendency to overdose myself to mask my tremor. I was depressed: it was the beginning of the summer holidays; an important colleague had suddenly died; my neurologist emigrated; and his replacement distanced himself from any meaningful discussion by proferring a different pill for each and every symptom. Reacting to all of this, I stopped the sinemet, taking on my shoulders the integration of the physical and psychological. I was excited by the thought that Parkinson's disease might, in my case, have had its genesis in early traumatic emotional experience. (My theory of the psychosomatic link between IPD, endogenous depression, and bereavement, entitled IPD and Depression: a Psychosomatic View, is being prepared for publication.) After 4 drug-free days, I experienced withdrawal symptoms of hypomania—a state similar to that induced by amphetamines, followed by 4 sleepless nights. My GP gave me chlorpromazine and I went into a catatonic state from which I was sure there was no return. I felt like a tiny animal curled up in a corner and about to fade away into death. After recovery in hospital, I gave up my bid for a self-cure, and the theory, modelled on hysteria and repression, behind it. If early emotional traumas were precursors of neurological disorder, they were not, in my experience, reversible.

In retrospect, my reaction to the illness, once the quiet, defensive denial was inadequate, had become a hysterical one based on raw fear. This was understandable, considering the erosion of a still-idealised body image, increasing immobility, depression, and diminished life expectation. An attempt to regress might have seemed preferable to facing the dismal future: a good cry might have produced some relief. Yet it seemed that the very nature of the illness inhibited emotional release. The holiday came to an end and the demands of life and work resumed. I went back on to low doses of sinemet, found a new neurologist, and returned to my patients. New zeal as a therapist seemed to emerge from the straitjacket of my former training alongside my experience of illness. I was able to treat my patients in a more active and participating manner.

Beside a putative role in the genesis of the illness, the personality of the patient is vital in determining the response to the established disorder and its therapy. I found that, with psychotherapeutic help, my response to medication improved. In my self-exploration over the years, I had become aware of a deficiency in subtlety of emotional response and modulation through experience. I have concluded that a deep fear of being alive, aggressive, and vulnerable early on had predisposed to a somatic breakdown in the form of Parkinson's disease. I speculate on the link between emotion and motion with the striatum intimately involved in the modulation of movement. Any access of emotion certainly disturbs the body, which is not surprising when it is remembered that the organism responds as a whole at multiple levels simultaneously. Crises in the course of my illness have usually been related to psychological adjustment, that is, when I have relinquished certain aspirations or areas of functioning in

order to carry on within a more limited capacity. It is an exaggeration of the ordinary adjustments made in the face of retirement, but more acute, and begun 10–15 years earlier. A chronic illness at the age of 39 is more difficult than one in later years. Concern over earning a living to maintain the family during what are expected to be prime earning years is considerable. The choice of working flat out and living as actively as possible or living slowly and steadily had to be made. I opted for the former, working half-time in private practice rather than the more secure full-time hospital work.

The on/off syndrome is, without doubt, central to patients with chronic parkinsonism. Earlier, when I experienced the drop towards the end of a dose of medication. I could adjust the timing so as to avoid any lag in the drug relay system. By careful titration according to absorption time, I was able to achieve some continuity, which was later undermined by mid-dose drops. These were not easily managed and led to systematic experimentation with other drugs, including deprenyl, which gave me vice-like headaches, single doses of enkephalin and beta-endorphin, to see if they had any effect, lisuride, bromocriptine, and, over the past 2 years, pergolide. The latter seemed initially to bridge some of the off gaps, but further deterioration diminished its effectiveness. Hope of maintaining a good on, as in the first morning response, remains high, although in reality it is difficult to achieve. Reassurance lies in the quality of on, which may insure against gross dementia—a constant terror. The on capacity, brief though it is in response to medication, supports an assumption of striatal synaptic pathology, rather than any extension to cortical brain cells. It is interesting to compare the on/off of 9 years ago with the present experience, when the whole body is affected: in those days, off revealed a chink in my defensive armour; today, on has come to represent a gift gladly accepted from the Fates. The quality over 24 hours has also changed: in the early days, on would last up to 8 hours, but today I am happy with 4 hours and must often be content with just 2. During the day, I experience small-scale mood swings. Most striking is the depression and hopelessness just prior to coming on with the first dose of the morning. Being on is tinged with excitement and/or fixed orientation. I experience genuine, spontaneous flexibility only during my morning on and after a mid-afternoon nap. Otherwise, the feeling may lie anywhere along the manic-depressive spectrum, without modulation.

Alertness and memory are increasingly affected by the disease. In my experience none of the so-called agonist drugs produce an on unless levodopa is taken as well. I am most alert after a sleep, and I can identify four times (8 AM, 1 PM, 6 PM, and 11 PM) in a 16–hour waking cycle when it would seem that residual dopamine concentrations peak: in between these times concentrations decline. This pattern has become a background rather than a clear demarcation as it was earlier. Recent and medium-term memory is now affected, although, paradoxically, early childhood memories have become more accessible. Overdosage, leading to dyskinesia, also works against both recent and long-term recall. When off, I am preoccupied with my body and its limitations. Bilateral disease has diminished the righting reflexes and compounded the loss of flexibility. Intellectual thrust appears to be directly related to the remaining production of dopamine. The apprehension involved in running to an appointments schedule with the sword of Damocles overhead, is wearing. Fortunately, work as a psychotherapist involves subtle skills as opposed to strenuous activity.

Reserves from training and habit have somehow sustained me in difficult circumstances. It remains something of a mystery just how the ring of the doorbell to admit a patient, can stir me into action.

12 years of the illness have not diminished my fascination with it—when on. There can be no other condition in which the body can be so rapidly and completely transformed as if the gods were breathing fire into it. The contrast when off, and the feebleness of mind and body, is a perpetual reminder of one's decline. In experiencing a two-part existence in one lifetime, I feel like Lear, who in his dotage could say: 'We are not ourselves when nature, being oppressed, commands the mind to suffer with the body'.

(Todes 1983)

Somatopsychic

C. Todes

I continued to strive to make sense of my Parkinson's disease through psychosomatic theory, but had at the same time neglected the converse, somatopsychic which had equal, if not greater, relevance to my condition. The mind's reaction to the changed body and the impact on the body image is considerable and as important as the effects produced by the mind on the body.

In Parkinson's disease this altered body image is experienced through the effects of the illness on posture, gait, handwriting and, ultimately, on self-expression—all the effects of premature ageing. This has to be fought in order to preserve self-esteem and an ego in danger of being fragmented.

I watched the development of the illness from a minor disability to one which now effectively prevents me from carrying on my profession and threatens me with increased immobility. Far from being a linear progression that one might suppose from reading about the illness, it is more of an emotional rollercoaster that one learns to negotiate or rather, one takes the ride knowing there is no alternative. The variation in behaviour is more usefully compared with the development of a musical composition with its highs and lows, repetition and development of themes.

The capacity to respond positively to the medication supports the hope, each time, that one can lead an unrestricted life for part of the time. The elation felt while being On stirs even the most inhibited people into a hopeful and lively existence. It is as if the gods breathing fire into a knotted body free it to feel and think, to show expansion and to live with rhythm. Life is then worthwhile and one evades the sure knowledge of a return to an emptiness.

We all carry within us an image of our functioning in an ideal way. This is made up of memories of ourselves and others we may have seen or heard about. The more *real* an experience one gets, the greater the likelihood that we can live with *our* standards, rather than comparing ourselves unfavourably with the ideal.

This process goes into reverse gear when one is afflicted with a deteriorating movement disorder. One is prone to automatically resurrecting the ideal image of oneself and using this illusion to fight off and deny recognition of increasing physical discomfort or immobility. Further, one may increasingly look for treatments aimed at achieving an ideal state rather than to be content with slight benefits. The search for an ultimate drug or the ideal transplant operation, which would do away with supplementary medication, will make one susceptible to miracle-seeking solutions.

Difficulties with dosing may play a central role, manifest in the side effects and the On-Off. It is in the nature of chronic degenerative disorders that a negative reaction to the illness shows itself. The responsive part of the patient takes the drug control of the illness seriously, hoping, as in ordinary illness, that good behaviour will be rewarded. It is a let-down of magical expectation to discover that one is getting worse not better, and more than that, the doctors can't do anything about it.

In sounding out Parkinsonians, they always complain that they are never given enough time to talk to their doctors. In over-booked clinics, discussion with the neurologist is focused on the minutiae of medication rather than the many newly occurring difficulties the patient is experiencing with the condition. A psychotherapeutic listening attitude is not formally installed in training. The patient's working knowledge, as an expert in

his disease, needs eventually to surpass that of his doctor if he is to maximize his inner psychological independence. It is surprising how enshrouded in mystery this whole relationship with the doctor, and the need to keep the illness secret, can be. It cuts across class and educational boundaries but predominates in the over-fifties who were too late to benefit in their own upbringing from the liberalization of attitudes in our society.

Revealing one's hopes and frustrations, one's aggressive fantasies and loving wishes, has to it something of the aura of coming out of the closet. Many people, especially the elderly, find this unfamiliar and impossible and therefore withdraw, preferring to rely on their religious belief and personal techniques to shield their feelings.

Treatment of PD demands an alliance of doctor and patient directed to modify and maximize the response of a patient made available by drugs.

Psychotherapy is a valuable, but generally neglected, procedure. In skilled hands, it offers stabilizing insights into the mind–body under the pressure of emotional situations. It is particularly helpful in the depressive reaction to the illness, if not to the underlying depressive core that may be fundamental to it. Finally, it can help with the drug-related depression.

Mobility is naturally affected by fatigue and one soon learns that intermittent rest periods are vital to sustain good On periods. In the early stages of the illness, sleep benefit is such that one wakes up On after a good sleep. Accepting this as part of one's body image in action is important, and self-hatred should not be allowed to interfere with rest. In other words, over-ambitious compensatory efforts may be maintained at a considerable price. One develops a parenting attitude towards one's body if it hasn't developed already. This differs from hypochondriacal attitudes and is much more supportive and understanding. It includes optimizing the time On, keeping one's body in good condition, in expectation of improvements that are awaited in the near future.

The sick body carries with it the penalty of an affected ego, as well as diminishing self-esteem and wounded narcissism; in experiencing a two-part existence in one lifetime, I feel like Lear, who in dotage could say: 'We are not ourselves when nature, being oppressed, commands the mind to suffer with the body'.

(Todes 1990)

COMMENTARY

Todes initially feared that he had a brain tumour, a common initial worry expressed by authors in this book, and it was somewhat of a relief to him when he was told he had Parkinson's disease. Since his Parkinson's disease (PD) was a fluctuating one in respect of significant symptoms, Todes therefore had to write about it during his good phases, when his medication was having beneficial effects and minimal adverse effects.

Todes' account is a good illustration of how psychological factors may gradually come to play an increasingly important role in the disability suffered by the PD patient. After five years, by which time he thought his disease might have been slowed down by the drugs, Todes had growing frustration, fatigue, and sleepiness (due to taking large doses of the drug, Sinemet). He developed depression, tried to take himself off all medication in the belief that psychological factors were behind his illness, as a result of early traumatic emotional experiences. This resulted in rather catastrophic sequelae. His reaction to his illness varied from a defensive denial to one based on fear. The latter resulted from his depression, immobility and decreased life expectancy. 'Beside a putative role in the genesis of the illness, the personality of the patient is vital in determining the response to the established disorder and its therapy' (p. 173). In addition to this support, Todes claimed that psychotherapy helped improve his response to medication.

Todes' account is rather unusual in that, compared to other self-reports of PD patients, his illness struck him at a relatively young age and in the midst of his career. He noted that a chronic illness at the age of 39 is different than one at an older age. Earning a living and maintaining a family meant he had to decide between living as active a life as possible for perhaps a short period, or going at a slower, steady pace. He chose the former. His life became one of playing around with 'on' and 'off' periods, trying to maximize the 'on' periods. He found it difficult to have to juggle appointment peaks in his clinical work with the 'high' and 'low' times of his disease. The contrast with 'on' and 'off' states was a stark reminder of the effects of the disease, resulting in a 'two-part existence'.

Todes' later account (Todes 1990) is a useful reminder of the effects that the body can have on the mind, as opposed to the more commonly discussed effects of the mind on the body. Todes rightly points to the ways in which his changes in bodily functions, such as posture, gait, etc., affected his self-image. It is worth pointing out that his overall mental state at any given time in the course of his illness probably reflected a complex interplay between the effects of body on mind, and of mind on body. To the extent that psychotherapy or other forms of psychological counselling may help the Parkinson's disease patient to understand and come to terms with his condition, then it has an important part to play in the overall management of the disease.

Alleviation of severe emotional symptoms by carbidopa–levodopa, MSD, in a Parkinson's patient: a personal report

John Doe, Ph.D.

'John Doe' is the pseudonym of a clinical psychologist who specialized in psychoanalytic psychotherapy.

I am a certified clinical psychologist with postdoctoral training in psychoanalysis, in full-time practice of psychoanalytic psychotherapy. I am 67 years old.

In September, 1982, I was diagnosed as having parkinsonism. At that time, I had the characteristic rigidity of my right side and typical pill-rolling movements of my right hand, as well as tremors of the right leg. My neurologist put me on a regimen of Carbidopalevodopa, MSD (Sinemet; 25–250 mg), three times daily. Within a month or so, my motor disturbances disappeared and continue under control to the present.

Also within a month or so after going on Sinemet, I experienced the rapid ending of severe emotional symptoms that had afflicted me for at least 5 years. I will now detail these symptoms.

The most central symptom was a profound sense of personal or emotional instability—an inability to know from one time to the next how I would be feeling—up, down, anxious, depressed. Something was seriously amiss. There were very intense feelings of self-consciousness—a tense awareness that I was 'empty' and that others would notice this. On a trip to Europe the summer before the diagnosis of Parkinson's disease, I experienced disorientation and inability to accommodate to rapid shifts in place and time. Exhaustion was my constant companion. I had an anxious dread of 'empty time'; the filling of time with naturally sequential activities was absent. Anxiety of a severe type, as well as depressive feelings of despair and futility, was omnipresent. There seemed to be no predictability about my state of being, as though some central "governor" was not operating.

For many years before the appearance of the clinical symptoms of Parkinson's disease, I was in analytic treatment with two different medical analysts as well as taking antidepressive medication, all with very minimal improvement. Subjectively, I had the sense that there was something profoundly wrong with me and was driven to the conclusion that it was something of an organic nature.

Currently, what is so remarkable is the striking freedom from disturbing emotional symptoms—a sense of well-being, absence of anxiety and depression, and even a sense of serenity that I had never experienced before.

I could not help but wonder whether such severe emotional disturbances before the diagnosis of Parkinson's were indeed the earlier manifestations of the slowly developing disease process of Parkinson's. Could it be that, as the dopamine slowly diminishes in cerebral availability, the organism reacts with very unsettling emotional disturbances? I realise how difficult it would be to arrive at a definitive answer in a single, subjective case report. Perhaps the great relief I experienced had to do with finally knowing what the 'enemy' was, *i.e.*, definitive diagnosis is often a relief in itself to the patient.

The reason for this report is twofold:

1. To possibly sensitize the mental health practitioner to the possibility of a presymptomatic syndrome in older patients, which would lead to an earlier diagnosis of Parkinson's. In my own experience, during my analytic treatment I recall experiencing body tremors during sessions, which both the therapist and I assumed were anxiety. Perhaps there could have been inquiry about other organic symptoms—by that time, my right

arm had stopped swinging normally and my handwriting had deteriorated.

2. In reviewing in my own pre- and post-Sinemet experience described above, I would say that I was *not* suffering from a depression per se (in DSM terms) but from a more profound 'emotional instability', which contained elements of anxiety and depression. It felt more global in character; the analogy of a damaged 'governor' comes closest to describing the feeling. I would suggest that researchers in the field of parkinsonism review the presymptomatic period of their patients' lives with this revised perspective in mind.

('J. Doe' 1987)

COMMENTARY

'J. Doe' had severe emotional symptoms for five years prior to the diagnosis of his Parkinson's disease. This was characterized by a profound sense of emotional instability, an inability to know from one time to the next how he would be feeling, as if some central 'governor' was not operating. All of this appeared to result in anxiety and depression, though he did not feel that he suffered from depression *per se*. His medication greatly helped with these symptoms, and he felt much less anxious and depressed. It remains possible that it was the diagnosis itself and the more important motor symptoms, that resulted in J. Doe's mind being taken away from the emotional symptoms to other aspects of his condition.

As well as the practical implications of emotional symptoms in the early diagnosis of PD, the paper raises the more theoretical point that the basal ganglia, directly or via some connection with the frontal lobes, or the chemical dopamine, may have the role of a 'central executive' or 'governor' for the emotional side of adjustment, just as the 'central executive' is assumed to play such a cognitive role in 'working memory'.

From the practical point of view, the paper again raises the issue that our neuropsychological assessment is limited by the procedures that we have available. Some symptoms reported by J. Doe, such as 24/48–hour adjustment to changes in time and place, and 'emotional instability', are not readily assessed in neuropsychological settings.

Parkinson's disease

Donald B. Hackel

Donald Hackel was, at the time of writing the article, a 65–year-old Professor of Pathology at Duke University, North Carolina, USA. One of his major interests was cardiovascular disease.

My feelings about writing this essay on my life with Parkinson's disease are mixed. On the one hand I am afraid that there is nothing especially important or unique in what I have experienced. On the other hand, I feel some enthusiasm in using this opportunity to review my situation, perhaps because of a feeling that in so doing I might discover something about myself.

I had never really been sick until March 1972, when I developed a mild to moderately severe case of infectious hepatitis. I felt lucky, however, that I wasn't as sick as the pro-sector of the autopsy from which we both probably caught the disease. She was unable to return to work for more than six months while I was better after only one month. In September of that year I noticed some awkwardness in writing which disturbed me since I was in the habit of writing the first drafts of my reports and manuscripts in long-hand. This 'writer's cramp', as I thought of it, was noticed by the secretary, who had become used to my old handwriting and was bothered by its deterioration. The letters tended to fade off into smaller and smaller sizes, which is typical of Parkinson's disease and even has a name, 'micrographia', so that if I had been alert enough—or interested enough—I would have been able to make a diagnosis at that point. Shortly after this I became aware that my facial muscles were tense, that I had trouble smiling, and that I was bothered by frequent eye blinking. I had not yet put the two sets of symptoms together and did not worry about them since they had come on so gradually. Furthermore, they did not significantly affect my ability to do my daily work, and I passed them off as merely changes that might be expected with aging.

The symptoms did progress, however, and I began to have some real difficulty in sitting through an hour's lecture (although not in giving one) because of the eye blinking, which was exaggerated by the experience. The eye blinking really got to be embarrassing when it interfered with my ability to talk freely on a one-to-one basis with others, especially since it was made worse by emotional stimulation. When, for example, a problem was brought to me for action or advice, I found that my muscles became more rigid, the eye blinking got worse, and it was difficult to concentrate on the problem at hand. This was so even when I had no real personal involvement or any stake in the problem and would not ordinarily have had any reason to be nervous about the situation. Still, it was embarrassing and it brought out another symptom that I had, until then, pretty much ignored, a slight tremor of my right hand. It started with difficulty using my hand in quick repetitive movements such as brushing my teeth or shaving. I recall it first appeared about a year after the onset of the 'writer's cramp'. The tremor came on only once in a while, and I remember the first time when I was no longer able to ignore it. This occurred while I was a guest speaker in the pathology department at Yale. I was having lunch before the talk and rattled my spoon, but I was able to eat lunch without actually spilling any soup and to present my talk without undue difficulty.

By this time I had, of course, begun to think of the possibility of Parkinson's disease—although I hoped that it might be almost anything else. My dislike of this disease was particularly strong because of my experience with the helplessness it produced in people I knew who had had it, and I certainly did not want to be dependent and a burden to my family. However, the slow course of the symptoms and the minor interference with my professional activities until then encouraged me, and I finally went to see a neurologist. He recommended that I try L-dopa as a diagnostic test, and, with some trepidation, I started taking the drug. I wasn't sure whether I wanted the drug to work— which would confirm my fears that I had this bad disease—or whether it would be better for it to fail—which would mean that I had something that could be worse but might be better! In any case, I was surprised and pleased at how dramatically it relieved my symptoms so that I began to 'feel human' again for a change. Ever since this experience I will admit that I have been less of a therapeutic nihilist and recognize the value of drug treatment when it is specifically indicated.

My reaction to the trial therapy with L-dopa surprised me. It was one of relief! I was partly relieved, of course, at having an answer to the cause of the bothersome symptoms and a drug that would help alleviate those symptoms. However, in retrospect, it seems to me that there were some other considerations which influenced me and which are difficult to describe clearly: (1) I felt some relief at finally hearing that I had Parkinson's disease. (2) This was explained by me at the time as the natural result of finally having an answer to the troublesome symptoms. (3) I did not want to tell my colleagues or even my family (except for my wife) about the diagnosis until the symptoms became so bad that I could not avoid it. (4) I can now see another reason for the feeling of relief as being due to the fact that I would now be released from the expectation (mainly from myself) that I continue to achieve and move upward rather than to keep on with my present work, which was clearly what I most enjoyed doing. (5) My reason for not wanting to talk about the diagnosis—I told myself at the time—was a desire not to be 'labeled', but it was probably also due to a reluctance to use the disease as an excuse to avoid the pressure which I felt was a good and desirable stimulus, and which had served me well in the past.

It is now about 13 years since I first noticed the symptoms of Parkinson's disease, and I really cannot complain very much. I have been able to continue most of my activities, including teaching the pathology course to first-year medical students, continuing as director of the course with responsibility for organizing and overseeing it, and participating actively in teaching a laboratory section of 20 students. In addition, I am the department 'professional advisor', which means that I am responsible for the 17 or so elective courses that we give to third-year medical students, and in addition to which I give an elective on cardiovascular pathology each year. I have been able to continue my experimental research work as before, and my other medical school responsibilities are not much different from what they had been— although I have somewhat curtailed my involvement in committee work. My national consulting activities have been almost completely eliminated. I especially miss the project site visits and study section meetings that I used to participate in frequently for the NIH. I enjoyed them because I made so many good friends through them and felt that they were my one best learning experience.

I end with two comments:

1. The fact that my symptoms were preceded by a bout of infectious hepatitis makes me wonder whether there is a causal relationship between that illness and the subsequent development of Parkinson's disease. As a scientist and a physician, I am alert to sequential phenomena looking for a relationship. Is what I experienced coincidental? After all, neither infectious hepatitis nor Parkinson's disease is rare. Is it causal? There is no scientific evidence for such a relationship. However, I can't help wondering.

2. I would think that my experience with Parkinson's disease should be comforting to other newcomers to the club, since the disease varies greatly in its speed of progression and can respond well to drug therapy. Thus, the only reasonable attitude is one of optimism that your affair with the disease will be as slowly developing as mine has been.

(Hackel 1987)

Parkinson's disease

Louis B. Guss

Louis Guss was 71 years old when he wrote his article, having worked for 30 years in paediatric medicine.

I learned I had Parkinson's disease when I had a daughter in college and two other children preparing to follow her—quite a blow. My family was my first concern, and then there was the realization of all the manifestations of the illness well remembered from my medical texts.

A painful left knee was my first symptom in 1972 when I was 58 years old. I used some simple analgesics and bought an exercise bicycle. Since I stood many hours a day in my office practice, I thought exercise might be beneficial.

In September 1972 my wife and I went to Yugoslavia, where I attended sessions for my CME credits. It was here that I first fell. At the time, I thought, I had merely lost my balance and tripped. A few months later I went to Atlanta, where I took a course in infectious diseases. In the hotel bathroom I noticed that my bare feet stuck to the tile floor. Getting in and out of a car was getting more difficult. Also, my handwriting became smaller and almost illegible.

When my symptoms increased I consulted my friend and internist, Dr. M., who thought I had Parkinson's disease and suggested I consult a neurologist for verification. This must have been difficult for my colleague and friend to tell me.

Dr. P. of the Department of Neurology confirmed the diagnosis. I was disappointed because I felt I had so much that I wanted to do. He was most supportive and encouraging, and I needed that so much. He thought that I would be able to carry on my practice for an indefinite time and do what I had to do (or at least that was what he told me).

Artane mg 2 t.i.d. was my initial medication. After a few doses I was elated because I felt stronger and was able to walk without difficulty. Two days later, however, I developed nausea, and this was a great disappointment. This was badly timed because I was looking forward to driving to Vermont to pick up my daughter, who was attending a summer session at Middlebury College.

The dose of Artane was decreased to mg 1, and this in combination with Symmetrel kept me going. I was able to function fairly well and carry on a practice for another 11 years. My stamina was greatly diminished, however, and I tired easily. It was difficult for me to project my voice, and because of my instability I fell several times. How to get up was something that my wife and I had to figure out. I would have to roll over and get on my knees, place one foot flat on the ground, and have someone pull me by my belt. Something stationary in front of me to hold onto was most helpful.

An area of great concern to me was how my patients would react to having a pediatrician with a condition such as Parkinson's disease care for their children. Would they think that I was incapable? My mind and judgment certainly weren't impaired but I'm sure that there were those who felt that their physician should be not less than perfect. Nevertheless, many still trusted me implicitly and this was rewarding. I'm sure this trust gave me strength.

I did not feel like my old self, and I definitely could feel a change. My wife and I were so disappointed. It was difficult to accept and we could not even call my condition by name. And—most of all—we didn't even want to speak to others about it. At the same time my colleagues and co-workers were considerate and sensitive to my condition. How often the girls in the nursery helped me tie the strings of my gown! The first things I gave up were attending cesarean sections and taking care of newborns.

Even though I would have liked to have felt more limber, Dr. D., the neurologist to whom I was assigned, felt that at this early stage of illness my medication was appropriate. Fortunately, I was, and still am, practically tremor-free. As he explained to me, 'More medication or L-dopa would be like shooting a bird with a cannon'. This philosophy has stayed with me through the years—'Use the least to be the most effective'.

So for another period of time I managed to plod along the best that I could. As a result of the Symmetrel my feet and ankles became edematous and I had to wear larger shoes. I also developed an ulcer on my right foot that was extremely difficult to heal.

Until June 1983 I managed to carry on an office practice on a limited basis. At this time the medications were no longer effective and I was stiff, weak, and unable to walk. I thought that 'the day' had come.

Then I consulted with Dr. R., a local neurologist who had much knowledge and experience with Parkinson's disease. I found him to be compassionate, brilliant, and interested in me not because I was a physician with Parkinson's disease but because I was a patient in distress who needed medical attention. My wife and I were already making adjustment to the almost complete disability when he advised hospitalization. This was to monitor and regulate new medication and to begin physical therapy for me to be ambulatory once again. Needless to say, my wife and I felt that this was a gift of rebirth. He gave us great faith and encouragement. All our negative feelings were dismissed, and we were imbued with the spirit of hope. I will always be grateful to him for his sincere interest. The sparkle of his eyes and facial expression denote the reward he derives when I am functioning well. He is a dedicated physician and a very special person.

The EMT who accompanied me to the hospital in the ambulance was one of my former 'little patients'. He said that it was about time that he did something for me since I had attended him on several occasions for asthmatic attacks. It is comforting to know people, especially in times of distress. Even though it seems strange to be on the receiving end, I have readily accepted the role of being a patient. When one is 'down and out', there certainly is no choice. I recall that I felt very helpless and weak.

In the course of about two weeks I was stabilized on a combination of Artane, Sinemet, and bromocriptine. Physical therapy was used, beginning with passive leg exercises when I was in bed. The therapists helped me to walk again. Never did I think that I would have to learn with a walker. I was apprehensive about getting into the car to be discharged. The therapist accompanied me to our car and showed me what to do with my body and legs. I lacked confidence, and I was fearful of falling. It really takes time to learn how to balance oneself.

For a few months I continued with physical therapy. The rehabilitation staff were interested and supportive. They also used massage for my neck, back, and chest. I enjoyed the massage very much because it relaxed my tight muscles, but unfortunately the effect was only temporary. Nevertheless, the entire therapeutic team is so delightful that visiting them in itself would be therapeutic.

I experienced nausea, probably from the Sinemet, mostly in the early morning. Saltines and cracked ice helped. Flushing and frequent hot flashes from the Sinemet were almost unbearable. Faintness, headache, and lateral numbness of the head came from the bromocriptine. I was functioning, but it was a big price to pay. Tagamet was prescribed for symptoms of hyperacidity. This worked fairly well but I had an intense headache. When I eliminated the Tagamet and changed to Zantac, the headache diminished and the acid control was effective.

Constipation is another drug-related problem. Because of the anticholinergic effect the stool is large in diameter and dry. As a result of passing 'cement', I developed an inguinal hernia. Increased fluid intake, figs, and a Fleet enema every other day really are helpful. Hard peppermint candy helps with the dryness of the mouth.

To complicate the management of my illness, I have a fairly good size hiatus hernia. The anticholinergic drugs used for Parkinson's disease increased the symptoms of the hiatus hernia. The most distressing is abdominal distention. At one time there was absolutely no peristalsis and I must have had an ileus. Nothing was moving and I felt as if I were going to blow up. Reglan was ordered. What a marvelous 'Roto-Rooter'! My GI tract was relieved and I was more comfortable. However, it completely canceled the Parkinson drugs and I was stiff and practically unable to walk.

Bromocriptine also presented other problems. I developed ergotism with hemorrhagic areas on my toes. The thought of gangrene is not a pleasant one. When the medication was eliminated my toes became warm and pink again.

So my present medications are at a minimum. The regime is Artane mg 1 t.i.d., Sinemet 25/100 1 every two hours during the day (this had diminished the hot flashes somewhat), and Zantac b.i.d. I still am able to walk, eat by myself, and get along fairly well, but, of course, my performance is not as good as when I was on the bromocriptine. However, it is best to be able to function fairly well at the least. It's like a balance. For a while I was wearing out the pages of the PDR checking out all my symptoms.

Special commendation is to be given to the staff of the surgical supply company for the many comforts that were given to me. Just to mention a few: straightening out the kinks in the motorized bed, solving the problem with the wheelchair, and suggesting the special mattress for my sore and aching back. The Thermophore moist heat pack was also very helpful for my stiff neck. They made several adjustments to meet my needs and were always courteous and caring. When we moved to our town house apartment a chair lift was promptly installed.

In retrospect I do feel that having the responsibility of my office practice gave me the strength to carry on and a purpose to life. It would have been very easy to have 'given in'.

As you can see, it has not been any one person that has contributed to my functioning *status quo* but a group working as a team.

I now have been retired for two years, and I am trying my best to enjoy it.

I am not happy to be dependent upon others, especially my wife, who anticipates my every need. But I believe that I am now resigned to this fact, and I accept it as graciously as it is offered. To my family, friends, and colleagues I will be ever grateful.

Another one of my disappointments is that I am unable to read as much as I would like because of the atropine effect of the medications. So my day's physical activities are often limited to a walk about 10:00 a.m., when my medication (which I refer to as 'my fix') enables me to take off. I enjoy visiting friends as well as having them visit us. Movies and television have been helpful.

Traveling is not the easiest because there are many adjustments for me to make and a great deal of planning for my wife. This past December we flew to California and visited with our daughter, son-in-law, and two grandchildren, but I am more comfortable at home. I certainly did have the royal treatment—we were given the master bedroom and they had rented a motorized bed for me. No doubt I am insecure being away from my physicians, but it is necessary that I be more courageous.

Since I lose my balance easily and find it difficult to walk in close areas or behind another person in close range, I have a lot of mental programming to perform.

Just the other day my carpenter and friend, Richard, put some ball casters on my chair at the dining room table. This enables me to be comfortably seated. We are still learning to be innovative to make life easier.

I do think that I would prefer having syphilis. At least I would have deserved the risk taken, and the treatment is specific and effective. However, my faithful wife of 41 years might have some reservation in this regard. So, inasmuch as I had no choice in being afflicted as such, I am making the best of it.

(Guss 1987)

COMMENTARY (Hackel, Guss)

Hackel's report highlights the subtle interactions that may exist between physical, cognitive, and emotional factors in the functional deficits of a Parkinson's disease patient—for example, the continuous eye-blinking from which he suffered was worse in emotional settings and then affected his concentration when he was tackling a particular problem. Hackel alludes to an interesting clinical feature of Parkinson's disease—its diagnosis may in part be confirmed by the immediate response to a single treatment, in this case whether the first administration of L-dopa resulted in a reduction of tremor, as it did in his case. Hackel does not report major cognitive limitations that resulted directly from the disease—at the time of writing the article, he had continued for 13 years in an active academic setting. This observation highlights the variability in neuropsychological deficits associated with Parkinson's disease. This variability is perhaps not as often highlighted as it should be in the research literature, where there is a natural tendency to report and concentrate on the cognitive disabilities found in Parkinson's disease patients. Hackel indicates that he developed Parkinson's disease not long after suffering a bout of infectious hepatitis. At the end of his article, he speculates as to whether the hepatitis may have been a contributory factor. I have been able to find one post-mortem case study that suggests a link between the two pathologies (Yoshimura *et al.* 1992).

It is worth noting that all of the authors in this section, and most authors in the book, were leading busy lives prior to the onset of their illness. Guss noted that his work gave him 'the strength to carry on and a purpose to life', a stimulus and an incentive to keep going. On the other hand, with such busy and mentally taxing lives, there was more likelihood that some degree of disruption of everyday activities would take place.

REFERENCE

Yoshimura, N., Hayashi, S., and Fukushima, Y. (1992). Diffuse Mallory bodies in the liver, diffuse Lewy bodies in the brain and diffuse fat replacement (lipomatous pseudohypertrophy) of the pancreas in a patient with juvenile Parkinson's Disease. *Acta Pathologica Japonica*, **42**, 826–31.

On being a Parkinsonian

A. W. S. Thompson

A. W. S. Thompson was a physician who worked as Director of Clinical Services in the New Zealand government from 1955 to 1975. He died in 1987.

1

I find myself in a situation which, as a school-boy, I should have considered extremely romantic.

One afternoon when I was fifteen, I dipped into a book entitled *The Romance of Asiatic Exploration*, which belonged to one of my elder brothers. Idly turning the pages, I came across an account of a party of explorers who were dying of thirst in a wilderness. The muddy hollow which had yielded a meagre supply of water had finally dried up and their last hope had gone.

One member of the party was a doctor, and as I sat there with the book open on my knees I became acutely conscious of the poignancy of his situation. With his knowledge of the human body and how it worked, he would have been able to study the development of his own symptoms, knowing exactly what each of them signified. Yet for all his ability and training, there was nothing he could do about it. He was no better off than his companions, except that he could observe the process of his own dissolution with an expert eye.

A truly romantic predicament, thought I.

How much more fascinating should I have found the position of a medical man suffering from a slowly advancing, mortal disease, which no form of treatment could arrest, characterized by a host of symptoms affecting most of the bodily functions, the nature of which was well known to the patient! Such has been my situation for over ten years.

I have Parkinson's Disease, otherwise known as parkinsonism, or paralysis agitans, or the shaking or creeping palsy. This was the condition which affected the man who was told by Christ to 'take up his bed and walk'. It is not an uncommon disease, occur-

ring as it does in about one person in 1000 of the general population, and in one per cent of those over the age of sixty.

The characteristic features of the fully developed disease are coarse trembling or shaking of the limbs, stiffness of the muscles, and slowness of bodily movement. These symptoms are due to damage to certain cells at the base of the brain and are associated with deficiency of a substance called dopamine. This deficiency can be corrected by drugs, thus relieving the symptoms, but nothing can yet be done to arrest the underlying degenerative processes in the brain. Replacement therapy with the drugs at present available is not the complete answer at any stage, and sooner or later it is liable to break down.

The condition was first described by Dr. James Parkinson in 1817. The cause is still unknown. Some drugs and one or two infections (notably the 'sleepy sickness' which broke out after the First World War and later disappeared) can induce a complex of symptoms of parkinsonian type, but this is not the classical disease described by Parkinson. True parkinsonism mainly affects the elderly and generally pursues a relentless but very slow course, so that it may have been present for twenty years or more before the patient is totally disabled. It is often stated, echoing James Parkinson in his original paper, that throughout the course of the disease 'the senses and the intellect are preserved', but that is not strictly true. There is probably some impairment in all cases, and one patient in four eventually exhibits changes in both intellect and personality.

The course of the disease and the nature of the predominating symptoms vary considerably from patient to patient. Cases occur in both sexes and in all races, but there seems to be no evidence to suggest that the disease is hereditary. My own hunch is that it is due to an inherited predisposition, the condition being triggered by a virus infection of some kind. So far as I know it has not previously been present in my own family.

Although, as already mentioned, no two cases of this disease are identical, it may be of interest if I recount the manner in which the symptoms developed in the early stages of my own particular case. I shall also attempt to indicate my personal reactions to this development.

2

I believe I can pinpoint the day and the hour when I experienced my very first symptom of parkinsonism. It was about four o'clock in the afternoon of Wednesday, 25 July, 1973. My age was sixty-three and a quarter years.

Two American friends, man and wife, were taking me on a motor tour round a number of Civil War sites. At the time in question we had left New Market and were driving north along the beautiful valley of the Shenandoah. We were discussing the part played on the battlefield we had just visited by a group of cadets from the Virginia Military Institute, who had covered themselves with glory in this, their first experience of being under fire. The conversation turned to the young people of today. In their defense I told a story about my youngest daughter and her college friends which I thought did them credit. I had recounted this incident on previous occasions in an admiring but matter of fact manner but this time, to my surprise and embarrassment, in the middle of my tale I was overcome by emotion. As I was seated in the back of the car, my friends could not see my face, but my voice betrayed me and I had difficulty in finishing what I had to say.

I could not understand what had happened. There was nothing in the story to explain my reaction, and I was ashamed to have behaved in so soppy a fashion.

I now consider that this trivial incident was the first symptom of parkinsonism. The emotionalism—or rather, the false

emotionalism—which I experienced on that lovely summer's day has been with me ever since. Two months later I took my second daughter on a motor trip in France and Italy. We had seen very little of each other for several years and we enjoyed ourselves immensely. Yet when we visited the scene of the battle of Marengo I found it impossible to describe the dramatic arrival of the gallant Desaix at the climax of the struggle, without a wholly inappropriate display of emotion. True, this was one of the more moving episodes in the Napoleonic story, but one would hardly expect to lose control of one's voice when speaking about it; and I had dealt with it on previous occasions without difficulty.

The same thing happened again when we were approaching Hyeres, and I recited from memory what Robert Louis Stevenson said about it:

I was happy only once. That was at Hyeres; it came to an end for a variety of reasons, decline of health, change of place, increase of money, age with his stealing steps; since then, as before, I know not what it means. But I know pleasure still; pleasure with a thousand faces, and none of them perfect, a thousand tongues all broken, a thousand hands, and all of them with scratching nails.

Certainly these are moving words; but a normal individual should be able to repeat them aloud without sounding as if he was on the point of dissolving into tears.

I am still subject to this peculiar weakness. The essence of the problem is the falsity of the emotion involved; it comes out in relation to subjects whose emotional content is minimal and which have no particular significance for me. I cannot quote a line of poetry without risk. Sometimes there happens to be a mild element of emotion in the subject, but I tend to react as if it were profound.

To give an example, my wife and I often drive past a house in a neighboring village which was once the home of Nelson's Hardy. On several occasions I have wanted to tell the story of the incident when Nelson risked his ship by heaving to when being pursued by a superior enemy force, in order to pick up Hardy, who was in a boat and in great danger.

'By God', cried Nelson, 'I'll not lose Hardy!' I have never yet related this story, knowing that Nelson's words would be my undoing.

I cannot be sure, but I have a feeling that there is another side to this question. When I was younger, perhaps up to about ten years ago, I was by nature a pugnacious individual, with a quick temper and a marked tendency to react to provocation with a violent display of anger. In recent years I have mellowed considerably. This could, of course, be due to the process of aging; but I suspect there is more to it than that. My impression is that while a bout of false emotion is all too easily triggered off by an unimportant stimulus, my normal emotions are somewhat blunted.

3

Early in September, 1973, about six weeks after the incident in the Shenandoah Valley, I experienced a symptom which I immediately attributed to parkinsonism—drug induced, as I thought. I began waking in the morning to find my pillow wet with saliva, due to drooling while I slept. I had been taking an anti-depressant drug, Tofranil, for eight years (I have been subject to periodic attacks of depression for most of my life), and I was aware that medicines of this class are liable to give rise to certain symptoms of a parkinsonian nature. It did not occur to me that there might be another and more sinister explanation of this symptom.

I cut down my daily dose of Tofranil on 12 September, 1973, and made a further reduction on 14 October. The drooling lessened, and finally disappeared. I again suffered from it about five years later and it has bothered me from time to time ever since.

I finally abandoned the use of Tofranil in May, 1974.

4

One evening about the middle of November, four months after Shenandoah, I was half way through a letter I was writing when I suddenly realized that my handwriting had become very small and crabbed and that I had difficulty in making it larger. I put this down to Writer's Cramp, a condition about which I knew very little; but when I consulted the medical library I quickly discovered that my complaint was not Writer's Cramp but a condition called Micrographia, which is a feature of parkinsonism.

At the outset this symptom bothered me only from time to time. When it did, it generally presented itself when I had completed a certain amount of writing, and then I could finish my task only with difficulty. Gradually it became more troublesome, coming on earlier in a piece of writing, and sometimes at the beginning. It was worst when I was tired.

In the office I had to give up the practice of drawing up a preliminary draft before dictating letters and memoranda, contenting myself with a few jottings. Sometimes, even these brief notes were almost indecipherable; I noticed that this depended to some extent on my interest in the subject in question. I solved the problem of private correspondence by typing all my letters on an electric typewriter.

Micrographia as it affected me at the early stages led me to write words about two-thirds normal size, and they became smaller still as I continued to write. If I hurried, only the first two or three letters in each word were properly formed, the rest consisting of a jerky, wavy line. If I took pains I could still write a large, round script, but this was done slowly and without spontaneity; I felt as if I were "drawing" the letters rather than writing them, like a child copying a piece of copperplate handwriting.

5

These two symptoms, drooling and micrographia, I still believed to be side effects of Tofranil and they did not worry me unduly. It seemed a small price to pay for the benefits conferred by the drug and I felt confident that if I ever managed to give up using it, these symptoms would clear up. The nocturnal drooling had, as already mentioned, responded to a reduction in the dose.

When, following on a new and happy marriage, I finally ceased taking Tofranil in May, 1974, I looked forward to getting relief from my micrographia. To my surprise and chagrin, this did not happen, and as the months passed without improvement I began to wonder how long this symptom would continue.

In January, 1975, fourteen months after the onset of micrographia, and eight months since giving up Tofranil, I seized the opportunity of a visit to my office of a Professor of Clinical Pharmacology, to ask some questions. How long should it take for drug-induced parkinsonism symptoms to clear up once the drug was abandoned?

I have never forgotten the expression which flashed across my visitor's face—startled, and concerned. I realized in that moment that he thought that my symptoms were probably due to the progressive disease, true parkinsonism, and a cold finger touched my heart as it occurred to me, for the first time, that this might well be so. But this idea had hardly crossed my mind before I dismissed it. No member of my family, so far as I knew, had ever suffered from parkinsonism, and my condition had not altered in more than a year.

The professor was unable to give me an immediate answer to my question but promised to look into it. Further enquiries left him no wiser.

And there the matter rested for another seven months.

6

On 27 May, 1975, having reached retirement age (sixty-five) I spent my last day as a civil servant with the New Zealand Department of Health. A week later my wife and I sailed for England, where she owned a house in a seaside hamlet in Dorset.

We had hardly settled into our new home when I was assailed by a severe attack of depression. Several factors had precipitated it: retirement, homesickness for New Zealand where I had lived for 29 years, shock at the high cost of living in England, dismay at the heavy summertime traffic on the roads and the overcrowding in the streets and shops

and on the beaches. This placed me in a quandary. At all costs I was determined not to recommence taking Tofranil; but if the alternative proved to be shock treatment, I wondered how this might affect my parkinsonian symptoms. I still believed them to be drug-related, although they had not improved during the previous fourteen months. (On the other hand, they did not seem to me to be any worse.)

Not long after our return to England some friends from New Zealand paid us a visit. I was in the grip of my depression. The husband was an experienced general practitioner who knew me well, and I was shocked and surprised when he told me that he had been taken aback by my appearance. It was obvious, he said, that my condition had deteriorated in the three months since he last saw me. He mentioned my lack of facial expression, and slow movements. He urged me to arrange for an assessment by a specialist.

Not being familiar with the medical setup in England, I sought advice from a wartime friend in London, who arranged for me to see an eminent psychiatrist at Southampton. I visited him on 18 September. By this time, thanks to the support and understanding of my wife, my depression had completely disappeared. The consultant agreed that no treatment was called for and referred me to a neurologist.

I first saw Dr. Peter Robinson on 1 October, 1975. After a thorough examination, he dismissed out of hand any suggestion that my symptoms might have been drug-induced, indicating firmly but kindly that there could be little doubt that the condition was true parkinsonism. I was a little surprised, but not dismayed; I realized at once that he was right, and that for some time I had, almost unconsciously, been coming round to the same opinion. Dr. Robinson accepted my view that the symptoms were so slight that no treatment was required at that time.

7

For about four years after the diagnosis of true parkinsonism was made, progress of the condition, in so far as it was reflected by symptoms, was so slow that it was almost imperceptible. It reminded me of what Caesar said about the Rhone—that the river was so big and flowed so slowly that one had to throw in a stick to find out which way it was going. It was June, 1980, before I began to feel that the development of symptoms had speeded up, and another year before I realized that other people were aware of this.

The principal symptoms which I experienced up to the end of 1981 (that is to say, during the first eight or nine years of the condition) made their appearance in the following order:

Slow movements. I date the onset of this symptom as August, 1975, although subjectively I was not aware of it at that time. My doctor friend from New Zealand who paid us a visit that month drew my attention to it. It was three or four years before this symptom forced me to take much notice of its presence, and it was 1981 before it became really troublesome. Even then I was not as conscious of it as were other people; what I felt was not so much that I was slow, as that certain things around me had speeded up. What I called 'timing by doing' no longer worked properly; formerly I knew that if I switched on the stove under a saucepan of milk, I could clear the dining table before it boiled, but now I would come back to find the milk boiling over.

Fully developed, this is an exasperating symptom, both for the patient and his family. It is also a very odd one. There seems to be no observable reason why the victim should move about or tackle a simple task so very slowly, and the sight of his slow, clumsy and feeble efforts must tax the patience of the onlooker, however sympathetic he or she may be.

In one textbook the author states that 'the parkinsonian patient appears disinclined to move,' and that is precisely what the patient himself feels about it—disinclination rather than inability. I feel I could move faster if I really wished to do so, but some kind of mental blockage robs me of the will. If I force myself to try to complete some task quickly,

my limbs seem to freeze up and my hands shake violently. But I still have the feeling that the difficulty is mental, not physical—all I need is the will.

Clumsiness. I first became aware of this in October, 1975, shortly after the initial consultation with Dr. Robinson. I noticed that I had some difficulty when I stirred a cup of tea. I found myself taking hold of the extreme end of the handle of the teaspoon, between the tips of my thumb and index finger, instead of grasping it in the normal fashion. When I tried to take more of the handle between finger and thumb, I had to use my other hand to shift the spoon. Then when I commenced stirring I observed that instead of flexing my wrist, I was holding it rigid and stirring from my shoulder, using my forearm like the connecting rod from a piston.

Loss of muscular power. I noticed some general diminution of strength from the beginning of 1976, mainly in my arms and legs. In April, 1977 weakness of the muscles of the right hand and forearm forced me to give up typing with that hand in the usual fashion, and to use one finger instead. This was despite the fact that I was using an electric typewriter, with its relatively light touch. The left hand appeared to be unaffected, and I was able to continue to use all five digits on that side, while prodding the keys with one finger on the right. After I commenced taking the anti-parkinsonism drug Madopar (a combination of L-Dopa and benserazide) in July of that year (1977) an almost immediate effect was the disappearance of this symptom, so that I was able to type again in the usual manner.

In August, 1981 I began to have a little difficulty from time to time in opening my eyes when they had been shut tightly. The lids failed to respond to orders immediately, but after one or two seconds they would snap open, generally one at a time, the left being first.

Loss of self-confidence. In February, 1976, I realized that I had become 'nervy' about meeting people, especially strangers, and was finding it rather difficult to go shopping by myself, because of loss of confidence.

Difficulty in speaking. In July, 1975 I became conscious that my voice tended to sound flat and lacking in expression. About June, 1977 I began to have difficulty in speaking, especially when using the telephone. My voice had become softer and I was unable to enunciate certain words clearly. When answering the telephone or meeting anyone I could, with an effort, speak quite strongly for a few moments, but if I went on talking my voice would fail and I could do no more than whisper. I felt when this happened as if I 'had run out of steam', and if I took a deep breath I could often overcome the difficulty for a short sentence or two. There seemed to be two factors in this problem; first, my vocal chords had become weaker than they had been, and second, I was not controlling my breathing properly. By taking deep breaths and deliberately speaking out strongly—if necessary by almost shouting—I could converse for a little while, but if I persisted in trying to keep my end up, my voice would fail completely. My throat hurt and efforts to force myself resulted in a severe irritable cough.

Seborrhoea. About the middle of 1977 the seborrhoea of the scalp which had troubled me for many years became more active than hitherto, and despite regular treatment it continued to be a problem at this higher level of activity.

Undue tiredness when walking. In September, 1977 I complained to my doctor of tiredness after walking more than a mile. This became troublesome enough to spoil my pleasure in walking about May, 1981.

Stoop. About August, 1979 I noticed that I was walking with a stoop. This has gradually worsened, despite efforts to correct it.

Memory failure. I have always had a good memory. It began to fail, in the form of a general deterioration, about mid-1980. The anti-parkinsonian drug Artane interfered

dramatically with my memory for recent events. When reading a book I would find that when I turned a page I could not recall what was on the bottom of the previous page. When Artane was replaced (after an interval) by Disipal (an antispasmodic), it had a similar effect, but less severe. It was however bad enough to make typing rather difficult, as I found it necessary to keep looking back continually to check what I had just typed. This became less troublesome as I continued to take my daily dose of Disipal.

Difficulty in sitting. In June, 1980 I began to experience a painful stiffness of the thighs and lumbar region whenever I rose from an armchair. If I attempted to move off immediately after rising to my feet, the pain was severe enough to force me to move very slowly for several minutes. The severity of this symptom did not appear to depend to any great extent on the length of time I had spent in the chair; it could be quite troublesome after a brief sitting.

In February, 1981 a feeling of numbness and pain in the gluteal region began to trouble me whenever I sat in a chair for any considerable length of time. This was most pronounced when motoring, whether as driver or passenger. After about an hour in the car seat the trouble would begin, progressing fairly rapidly to a condition which could not be ignored. If I was driving, this painful numbness would pass down into the thighs, making me wonder if it was going to hinder the use of the clutch pedal or brake. On a journey I found it necessary to pull over and walk about until the symptoms disappeared. This generally meant a five-minute halt in every hour, the intervals of comfort gradually becoming shorter. This symptom troubled me for about 18 months and then gradually disappeared.

Sleep problems. About September, 1980 I began to have difficulty in turing in bed. I seemed to have forgotten how to execute this maneuver, and found myself flapping about and raising myself on one elbow in an effort to throw myself into the desired position. About two months later I began to find it difficult to lie on either side, the only comfortable position being flat on my back. There were two reasons for this: first, when I lay on my right side, my hip joint was painful; and second, I could not remember how to dispose my trunk and limbs for ease and comfort when lying on either side. I could no longer relax properly in that position, and had to sleep on my back.

Mouth breathing. This began when I started sleeping on my back. At every awakening my mouth and throat were unpleasantly parched. I assumed that this was caused by my mouth falling open during sleep, but I soon realized that this was only part of the story; for mouth breathing appeared to have become natural to me. There was nothing in the nature of nasal obstruction to account for this. Even when fully awake in bed and conscious of the fact that I should breathe through my nose, I would often catch myself breathing through my mouth, which was almost but not quite closed. When out walking I would often notice that I was breathing through my mouth, and after deliberately correcting it, would find that I was doing the same thing a few minutes later. I suspect that this symptom of mouth breathing in the parkinsonian represents regression to the habits of primitive man: 'mouths were made before noses'. It could be that the nasal passages of our earliest ancestors were habitually choked with mucus, forcing them to breathe through their mouths.

Involuntary arrest of movement. About the middle of 1981 I noticed that occasionally when I was tying a shoelace my fingers would stop moving in the middle of the operation and would refuse to continue for some time—varying from a few seconds to about half a minute. A similar difficulty occurred from time to time with other actions involving a degree of skill or dexterity, such as doing up buttons, especially small ones.

'The shakes'. Sometime in June, 1981 I began to have minor attacks of shaking when I wakened early in the morning. They lasted only for a few seconds and were some-times confined to one hand, sometimes more general. In the latter case it was often difficult to decide whether it was indeed 'the shakes', or merely an attack of shivering, due to cold. Now and then during the daytime my hand would shake violently when I attempted some task such as tying up a parcel or stowing something in a plastic bag. This coarse and irregular shaking of the hands was particularly embarrassing when shopping, if I had to extract paper money from my wallet or put notes into it.

Fortunately this symptom responded quite well to adjustments in my anti-parkinson medication.

8

Table 1 (Development of symptoms) depicts the progress of the disease, as represented by symptoms, up to the end of 1981. I have not included a number of symptoms which may possibly be related to parkinsonism, but are not clearly so: recurrent attacks of pain in the back, involuntary burping associated with achalasia of the cardia, pains in the right shoulder region and wasting of the muscles of the upper arm. (Achalasia is a condition in which the esophagus fails, because of neuromuscular incoordination, to deliver its contents into the stomach as it should.)

9

The most interesting and most disconcerting symptom which I experienced up to the end of 1981 was clumsiness. I shall try to describe how it affects me, and how it developed.

October 1975: *Difficulty in using a teaspoon.* As already mentioned, this was the earliest form of clumsiness of which I became aware. I could see, as an observer, that the difficulty was due to my faulty approach, but this did not help very much. I watched my hand stretch out and take the extreme tip of the handle between the tips of my thumb and index finger, and saw myself waggling the

Table 1. *Development of Symptoms*

1973	July	Emotionalism
	Sept	Drooling
	Nov	Micrographia
1974		
1975	Aug	Lack of facial expression
		Slow movements
	Oct	Clumsiness
1976	Jan	Loss of muscular power
	Feb	Loss of self-confidence
1977	June	Difficulty in speaking
		Seborrhoea troublesome
	(July	Madopar commenced)
	Sept	Undue tiredness when walking
1978		
1979	Aug	Stoop
1980	June	Memory failing
		Sitting problems
	Sept	Difficulty in turning in bed
	Nov	Mouth-breathing
1981	June	Involuntary arrest of movement
		'The shakes'
	Aug	Difficulty in opening eyes

spoon around in a feeble and absurdly in-effectual fashion; but there seemed to be some kind of mental blockage which made it difficult to interfere. In order to shift my grasp on the spoon I had to use my other hand to hold it while I changed the position of my right finger and thumb; but the new grip seemed neither natural nor easy, and when I commenced stirring I noted that I was moving the whole arm and forearm and keeping the wrist stiff, instead of stirring from the hand and wrist.

It was not hard to perceive that the essence of the problem was the failure of the auto-matic control mechanisms to function nor-mally. It is these mechanisms which enable us to carry out simple operations without thinking about them. The healthy individual stirs his tea without giving it a thought, using well-worn neuromuscular pathways established long ago in his early childhood. Some of these pathways are now denied to me—wholly or in part—so when faced with the simple, everyday problem of stirring a cup of tea I find myself reacting like a child who has never done such a thing before.

'How should one do this?' I ask myself. 'How do you grasp the spoon? Why does it feel so awkward whatever way I do it? How can I be so clumsy?'

Similar comments would apply to most, if not all, of the other instances of clumsiness which I shall mention. I had never realized, before I experienced this symptom, how many of our everyday actions are automatic. When I was a student we were taught that in right-handed persons the left side of the cerebral hemispheres initiated and controlled voluntary movement (in cooperation with the right), while the right side looked after those operations which are carried out auto-matically. Assuming there is some truth in this conception—or that some mechanism of a similar nature is involved—it has come as a surprise to me to discover how widely the system is employed in our daily lives. It sur-prises me even more to learn by observing myself in action how badly one carries out a simple task when one is forced to take thought in performing it. When the auto-matic mechanisms pack up, efficiency goes with them. I now know that when, in the past, I stirred my tea, or tied my shoelace, or threw on my jacket, or put it on a coat-hanger, or took a match from a matchbox—and so on, and so on—I was actually carrying out a somewhat complicated operation which I had taught myself as a child to perform so easily that it had become automatic. These trivial tasks involve a degree of dexterity which I had never before suspected; they are skills which the healthy individual masters when very young. Switching them over to the automatic pilot saves him a lot of bother—and time, energy and thought.

December 1975. *Circular motions when washing up.* This difficulty developed fairly suddenly. I noticed one evening when washing the dinner dishes that I was having difficulty in dealing with the inside of a saucepan. I was, as usual, wielding a plastic mop with a handle, but when I tried to sweep the mop round the inner surface of the saucepan my arm displayed a strange reluctance to co-operate. By an effort of will I managed to force my hand to carry out the desired circular motion, but I found it impossible to exert any pressure against the side of the utensil. The mop head simply sailed around, barely touching the deposits which it was intended to remove. I had to overcome the difficulty by placing the saucepan on its side on the draining board and working round the inner surface with a straight up and down application of the mop.

This symptom has troubled me ever since but it varies in intensity; at times I am barely aware of it, at others it is disconcertingly stubborn and unpleasant. When it is bad, efforts to make my hand obey orders are futile, and a peculiarly disturbing pain shoots through the muscles of my forearm—mainly those on the palmar aspect.

Sometimes I have found a partial solution to the problem by grasping the mop handle in my fist and employing it in the manner of a mortar and pestle.

When this symptom is at its worst, it feels as if my hand and forearm were affected by a strong repugnance of their own towards circular motion, a repugnance which at a higher level I myself—the man in the control

tower—also share, albeit with less intensity. I feel that I could make my muscles obey orders if I really wanted to do so, that all that is needed is the will—which for some obscure reason is lacking.

June 1976. *Difficulty with buttons.* This developed gradually. I found myself fumbling with buttons and taking longer than usual to unfasten them or do them up. At first it happened only with particular buttons which were awkwardly placed, and I thought little about it. I soon realized, however, that this was another expression of parkinsonian clumsiness. Shirt buttons gave the most trouble, because of their small size, but trouser buttons were almost equally difficult.

September 1979. *Sorting papers.* One of my peculiarities is that I have always enjoyed putting mixed-up papers in order. I have often caught myself, 'accidentally on purpose', getting papers I was working with in a tangle, just for the pleasure of tidying them up. Towards the end of 1979, however, I became aware that I was finding it increasingly difficult to handle papers of every kind, especially if they varied in size. They seemed to stick together and to resist my efforts to separate them. My fingertips appeared to have lost some of their sensitivity and to have become unnaturally smooth and dry; at the same time my fingernails obtruded themselves on my notice, as if they were keen to usurp the functions of the fingertips.

November 1979. *Difficulty in handling money.* This awkward symptom manifested itself whenever I tried to count paper money, or stow it in my wallet, or to sort out my loose change. When I drew a number of new five pound notes from a Cashpoint dispenser I had to accept them on trust, as I should have found it next to impossible to count them. Worn notes were easier to handle, but if crumpled or limp they were difficult to sort neatly for insertion in my wallet. Faced with this problem, I would place the open wallet on the counter and try to slip the notes into place. They would resist like some malevolent living creature, jamming themselves under the flap, sticking together, crumpling up, refusing to budge; then my hand would shake violently, and to cover my confusion I would give up the struggle, close the wallet as best I could and put it in my pocket. Sometimes I was subjected to further embarrassment when the wallet jammed in the top of my inside breast pocket and stuck there defiantly.

When these things happened the same thought always arose in my mind: any thug who saw me fumble and shake would mark me down as an easy victim for mugging.

At about this time I also began to have some trouble in picking out coins carried loose in my jacket side-pocket or from a mixed collection in my hand. I seemed to experience a little difficulty in distinguishing the coins from the other objects in my pocket—small penknife, pair of scissors, pencil stub. I wondered if there might be an element of asteriognosis in this—loss of the ability to identify objects by touch.

From the middle of 1980 onwards the tempo increased, new examples of clumsiness coming to notice almost continually. The more important of these were the following:

June 1989. Difficulty in picking up papers from a hard surface.

September 1980. Difficulty when turning pages in a book or using the index; I had trouble in finding the place in the index and in locating the indicated page. In this month also I first experienced difficulty in turning in bed.

December 1980. Difficulty in putting jackets or coats on coat-hangers; in tying up parcels; in sorting and folding a newspaper.

January 1981. Difficulty in putting on jackets and overcoats.

February 1981. Difficulty in enveloping a letter; and in using a toothbrush.

May 1981. I became nervous and tense when driving a car, and had difficulty in taking left-hand turns. I had to give up driving at the end of November 1981.

June 1981. Clumsiness when buttering toast.

December 1981. Difficulty in taking a match from a matchbox. Difficulty with fingers when putting on gloves.

Table 2 (Development of Clumsiness) shows how this symptom accelerated from September, 1979 onwards. The latent period from mid-1976 to the autumn of 1979 will be noted; the commencement of the anti-parkinsonian drug Madopar in July, 1977 contributed largely to this period of relative freedom from advance. If we turn back to Table 1 it will be seen that the introduction of Madopar was followed by a slowing down of the build up of symptoms generally for nearly two years.

10

It is now ten years since I experienced what I believe to have been the first symptom of parkinsonism; and I have little cause to grumble. On the contrary, I feel I have been lucky—lucky to have been affected too close to retirement to interfere with my professional life, lucky to contract the disease after and not before the introduction of effective symptomatic remedies, luckiest of all in having such a loving, understanding and capable wife.

Being a medical man has advantages in a situation like mine. However troublesome his symptoms may be, he knows they could easily be a great deal worse. He knows, too, that as a major chronic disorder of the nervous system Parkinson's Disease has much to commend it in comparison with others— General Paralysis of the Insane, or tabes, or multiple sclerosis, or Motor Neurone Disease, for example. There is no stigma attached to it and it does not normally involve mental incapacity to any marked degree. Then there is the clinical interest in the condition itself, with its variability and slow course. Finally, he is aware of the limitations of therapy and does not expect too much from his drugs.

My present condition would have been shattering if it had developed suddenly, but the gentle unfolding and snail's pace progress of symptoms have enabled me to adapt to each new phase as it occurred. One must

Table 2. *Development of clumsiness*

1975	Oct	Stirring tea
	Dec	Circular motions when washing up
1976	June	Buttons
1977	(July	Madopar commenced)
1978		
1979	Sept	Sorting papers
	Nov	Notes in wallet; loose change; finding things in pocket
1980	June	Papers on hard surfaces
	Sept	Turning pages; using index in book; turning in bed
	Dec	Coat-hangers; parcels; newspapers
1981	Jan	Jackets and overcoats
	Feb	Envelopes; toothbrush
	May	Car driving
	June	Buttering toast
	Dec	Matchbox; putting fingers into gloves

accept the inevitable; grousing does no good, and would only make acceptance more difficult. The answer is to live from day to day and let the future look after itself. This is easier than might be expected, for two reasons: The first being akin to the feeling of troops in action that 'it isn't going to happen to me'— one does not really believe that one will ever fall victim to the worst effects of the disease; and the second is something which I suggest may be a peculiarity of parkinsonism. There are certain disorders in which the patient tends to take an abnormally cheerful view of his plight—advanced pulmonary tuberculosis and multiple sclerosis are classical examples. I suspect that something similar is a feature of parkinsonism. When I contemplate the reality of the coming end-stages of my disease, it does not daunt me as, logically, it should. A similar attitude comes over strongly in letters from patients quoted in *The Parkinson Newsletter*, which is circulated to members of the Parkinson's Disease Society.

Here is a typical example:

A member in Inverness has the following suggestion for injury-saving knee pads to avoid hurt in falls. He says 'I use a sorbo rubber foam and the pads measure 9 inches by 6 inches and are 1 inch thick. To hold them in position I use Tubegrip size F . . . I wear them all the time but *not* in bed!'

I may be mistaken, but to my mind there speaks a man who has accepted his disability and is more concerned to pass on his discovery to others than to seek sympathy. Instead of complaining about his frequent falls he takes measures to minimize their effects and is happy with his achievement. I can just see him sitting there wearing his knee pads, with a big grin on his face.

My present state must still be regarded as mild. Apart from some tremor upon awakening, and shaking of the hands when any kind of manipulation becomes to the slightest extent difficult, I am not greatly troubled by 'the shakes'. There is little muscular stiffness.

On the other hand all my movements are slow, my speech is very poor, clumsiness has progressed to a point where it affects everything I do, and there is considerable muscular wasting and loss of power. Walking is difficult—I sometimes feel as if I were wading through water thigh deep—and at times I am unsure of my balance. My memory for recent events is disconcertingly poor, and I am forced to recognize that my mental ability is deteriorating.

This decline of mental capacity is reflected in slowness of thought. In addition to the physical factors responsible for my speech difficulties, there is a mental element; words simply fail to form in my mind. This, and not the mechanical problem, often accounts for my failure to respond to a question. There are other subtle changes. There seems to be some distortion of my body image; I realized recently that when I thought of the relationship of the orbit of the eye and the ear, I pictured them as juxtaposed, with nothing in between.

There is without doubt a psychological element in some of my problems. When faced with what (for me) is a difficult task of any kind, I am apt to develop a troublesome pain in the lumbar region. Worry, for example when scanning a letter from the Inland Revenue, often provokes the same pain. The interesting thing about this is that if I swallow a tablet of Brufen (ibuprofen, an analgesic), the pain usually disappears immediately, and before the tablet could possibly have taken effect.

My loss of memory, especially for recent events, is annoying, but not such a handicap as I should have expected. When writing these lines, or a letter, I have to keep looking back to see what I have just written. When reading I tend to lose the thread when I turn the page, and although I still enjoy reading I retain very little of what I read. Any repeat of a television film gives me as much pleasure as the original, as it all seems new to me. My spelling, never a strong point, is affected; I have to keep checking with a dictionary the spelling of ordinary words, and I find that some slip through despite my vigilance, often with odd results—'symple' instead of simple,

for example. Everyday words look unfamiliar, and sometimes their meaning eludes me: then the more attention I focus on the word, the more it puzzles me.

I must acknowledge, however, that like most of life's little problems, this situation has compensations; it frees me of the burden of memory, and failure to recall a word, or a name, no longer upsets me. 'It's my Disipal', I say, and dismiss the matter.

Apart from my speech difficulty, clumsiness is still my most troublesome problem. Nearly everything I do with my hands is done with difficulty, slowly and often painfully, and done badly. Some things tend to cling to my fingers unwanted, while my abnormally smooth fingertips fail to pick up small objects—postage stamps, for example. I find myself trying again and again to carry through some minor manipulation in an obviously futile fashion, before it occurs to me to try a different approach.

I now know one meaning of the epithet 'dirty old man'. I grow more and more careless about clothing and my appearance generally, my neglected footwear is a disgrace, and it is an effort to take a bath. This is partly due to sheer laziness and partly due to the lassitude which goes with the disease.

I am aware that to outsiders I look a lot worse than I really am. Whenever I meet anybody face to face I cannot help feeling conscious of my fixed expression and gormless look, especially when my mouth settles into an inane, unchanging grin. 'Poverty of movement', as it is called, fixes my head, body and limbs in attitudes which add to my embarrassment; all the normal little twitches and changes of the muscles of the face and neck, the conversational gestures of hands and arms, the shifting of the feet, are wanting, and the best I can manage is an occasional change from one frozen stance to another. Together with my speech problem, this makes me unwilling to meet strangers, or even friends. Chess is the ideal pastime, being played in silence, and yet keeping the mind on the stretch.

An interesting point is that so far as appearances go, I am at my worst when I am alone in the house. As I move about my feet shuffle as if I were wearing loose slippers, my arms hang down lifelessly and my head pokes forward with a fixed expression on my face. I walk with a slow, gliding motion. An observer might imagine I was trying to demonstrate what an advanced Parkinson patient looks like. At the same time, although I disapprove of letting myself go in this fashion, I am conscious of a feeling of relief from tension. So it seems that when I am not alone I must expend some energy in trying to keep up appearances.

My reaction to failing muscular power is interesting. The mind projects it outwards; my strength seems undiminished; it is the outside world which has changed, not me. Everything is heavier, stiffer, steeper; a pot of tea weighs more than it used to, bottle tops are screwed on more tightly, hills present steeper gradients. Before I gave up driving there appeared to be something wrong with the accelerator; for a given pressure of the foot, the response was poorer than it should be. One morning recently I jumped to the conclusion that the clutch had jammed when I tried to depress the pedal in the usual manner. (This last example illustrates the suddenness with which symptoms often develop. I drive the car out of the garage almost every day, so the weakness which foxed me must have developed overnight.)

But the most remarkable thing which parkinsonism has taught me is the mischievous perversity of inanimate objects. My observations have convinced me that these so-called inanimate objects sense the presence of a Parkinsonian and immediately put into operation a malevolent plan. It is a conspiracy of awkwardness and intractability. Watch me putting on a dressing gown or overcoat, or even an ordinary jacket. I draw one sleeve up to my armpit, and reach behind me for the opening of the other. It has disappeared! I try again and again to find it, but it keeps dodging. At last I succeed, and insert my hand. Now the rest of that side of the confounded thing joins the fray, clinging to the material behind my back and wrapping itself frantically round my elbow. The battle swings back and forth but slowly and gradually I gain ground, forcing my arm into the sleeves; centimeter by centimeter I overcome the resistance and draw the sleeve into

place. I bring my other hand across to make the rest of the material conform, and between pushing and pulling I finally triumph. But where is the collar? Ah! There it is, folded down underneath, high up where I can hardly reach and grimly determined not to be dragged out. They have their fun, these inanimate objects, and on a good day—for them—they sometimes get me locked so tightly and awkwardly in their unfriendly embrace that I can neither advance nor retreat and have to be rescued by my wife.

It would be tedious to describe any more of the innumerable examples of P.I.O. (Perversity of Inanimate Objects) which spring to mind.

I have not yet experienced one of the best-known symptoms of parkinsonism, in which the patient's foot 'freezes' to the ground and he cannot take a step. This must be frightening and dangerous when it occurs crossing a street—as it often does. I am, however, familiar with other forms of sudden involuntary arrest of movement. I might be putting a letter in an envelope or sandwiches into a plastic bag—this being the kind of situation when it happens most frequently—when suddenly my hand stops dead and refuses to budge. When this happens, it seems to me that the arrest of movement is always a response to an impediment of some kind, generally of a trifling nature. The letter has gone in crooked or the plastic bag has a small fold which has trapped one corner of the sandwiches. I believe the explanation for the stoppage to be a fault in my cerebral computer; it has been programmed to signal 'STOP!' whenever resistance is encountered, however unimportant that resistance may be.

A patient wrote a letter to The Parkinson Newsletter stating that she had found that she could overcome her own problem if she first took a step backwards. I have tried a similar tactic with other forms of arrest, with some success. It is not easy to imagine how a foot 'freezing' to a spot could be responding to some kind of impediment of however trifling a nature unless the surface underfoot was actually sticky, but that seems unlikely. It occurs to me that the problem might be due to auto-suggestion.

It is said to be easy to hypnotize a hen. You

hold its beak down to a pavement and draw a chalk line away from the beak in the direction in which it is facing. Release the hen and it will stay there as if pinned down by its beak, or so I have been told. Never having had a hen, a piece of chalk and a pavement all at my disposal at the same time, I never tried the experiment for myself.

Could the Parkinsonian with his foot glued to the road be responding to a suggestion from a line on the pavement or some other irregularity of the walking surface, prompting his cerebral computer to give the order to stop? I do not know. No doubt I shall sooner or later be able to offer a solution based on personal experience.

(Thompson 1989)

COMMENTARY

Thompson's account is particularly interesting in that it is based on detailed diary accounts that he was accustomed to keep. The first symptom that he, in hindsight, attributed to his Parkinson's disease (PD) was not a motor one, nor a cognitive one, but an over-reaction in his emotions when recounting a story. Thompson was able to pin-point the symptom to a particular time and place, and to retain a vivid recollection of its occurrence, suggesting that his long-term autobiographical memory mechanisms were quite intact at the time. There was a gap of about 18 months from these first symptoms and the realization that he may have PD, and this only after a colleague hinted that it may be the cause of Thompson's difficulties. Thompson had attributed his symptoms to the side-effects of antidepressant medication.

Thompson succinctly summarizes his own peculiar medical perspective to his condition. 'Being a medical man has advantages in a situation like mine. However troublesome his symptoms may be, he knows they could easily be a great deal worse . . . There is no stigma attached to it [Parkinson's disease], and it does not normally involve mental incapacity to any marked degree. Then there is the clinical interest in the condition itself, with its variability and slow course. Finally, he is aware of the limitations of therapy and does not expect too much from his drugs. 'My present condition would have been shattering if it had developed suddenly, but the gentle unfolding and snail's pace progress of symptoms have enabled me to adapt to each new phase as it occurred' (p. 194). As a general rule, it is probably the case that it is easier for patients to cope with slowly progressive neurological conditions rather than acute neurological conditions of similar severity such as stroke or head injury.

In terms of his everyday difficulties, Thompson reported that his clumsiness was the most debilitating and annoying. The occasional frustrations in having to manipulate and interact with items such as clothes leads him to coin the phrase 'perversity of inanimate objects'. Thompson pointed to an oft-forgotten sequel of his motor symptoms, namely their effect on his social interaction. In addition to the negative effects on others of his 'fixed expression and gormless look', he did not have available to him motor accompaniments of communication in social settings, such as gestures or facial movements. He found himself unwilling to meet strangers or even friends, and noted that for him chess was the ideal pastime—it occupied the mind, but required little in the way of communication and related body movements. These observations highlight the effects on social adjustment of motor symptoms that at first sight would appear to have purely physical consequences.

Another fascinating insight, which only a PD patient can report, is that when Thompson found himself alone he appeared to have much more severe Parkinsonian symptoms than when he was with others. It is as if he had to make an effort to make up appearances when in public, and that not having to concentrate in this way when he was alone was somewhat of a relief to him. This observation points to a cognitive component to some forms of automatic motor activity, perhaps related to 'cognitive effort', 'volition', or 'concentration'. It is as if such forms of motor activity normally occur at subconscious (and perhaps subcortical) levels, without direct mediation of mechanisms related to awareness, mechanisms that may normally be cortically mediated.

Parkinson's disease: doctors as patients

Compiled by J. Williams

J. Williams presents accounts written by eleven doctors, and their respective specialities are indicated at the beginning of each article.

Patients with newly-diagnosed Parkinson's Disease are often anxious about the effects of the illness on their lives. Very little has been published on this subject, so, to help remedy this situation, a collection of 43 autobiographies was recently published by the Parkinson's Disease Society under the title 'Parkinson's Disease & Employment'. These essays gave some insight into such topics as early retirement on health grounds, the reactions of employers and colleagues to the patient's problems, the effects of the illness on promotion prospects and the various techniques adopted by patients to help in coping with the illness. A wide range of occupations were represented but, unfortunately, no accounts by doctors were received. What makes the medical profession of special interest is the doctor/patient relationship. The quality of this relationship is one of the most important factors determining the patient's ability to cope with the illness and its treatment, as Ruth Pinder (1991) has recently shown.

As patients we expect our doctors to be sympathetic and knowledgeable about our problems; but can another person ever really know how we feel? Appearances can so easily mislead. Few non-patients can be persuaded that the writhing movements induced by L-DOPA are much less distressing to the patient than is the inability to move freely. The correct interpretation of the facial expressions of a parkinsonian patient is also very difficult. We feel that only if our doctor should happen to suffer from PD could we converse with complete understanding.

The eleven medical autobiographies which follow complement the earlier set by lay-patients. While we must not draw unwarranted conclusions from such a small number of cases some points are worthy of note. An important way in which the patient/doctor can help all patients arises from his or her ability to speak authoritatively about symptoms which a lay-patient would hesitate to mention because of fear of rejection by the doctor, a fear which is often well-founded, in view of Duvoisin's (1990) advice that 'one must always regard the patient's account of symptoms with healthy scepticism'. The late Dr. A. W. S. Thompson FRCP provides an excellent example in his account of "false emotionalism" which he identified as the first symptom of his own developing parkinsonism (Thompson, 1989). [By this term, Thompson denoted a tendency to over-react emotionally to a situation, even to the extent of causing social embarrassment].

A second notable feature of the medical autobiographies is the virtual absence of any mention of psychological aspects of coping with PD. Most lay-patients, by contrast, regard this as an important element in managing the illness. Training methods for the rehabilitation of effective bodily posture and movement (such as Conductive Education and the Alexander Technique) receives little attention in the doctors' accounts. They are, however, at one with non-medical patients on the deleterious effects of stress on the severity of the symptoms of PD and it is clear that, in general, the practice of medicine is not favourable in terms of the continued employment of those afflicted with PD.

REFERENCES

Duvoisin, R. C. (1990). The differential diagnosis of Parkinsonism. In *Parkinson's disease*, p. 431 (ed. Stern). Chapman and Hall, London.

Pinder, R. (1991). *The management of chronic ill-*

ness: *Patient and doctor Perspectives on Parkinson's Disease.* Macmillan Press, London.

Thompson, A. W. S. (1989). *On being a Parkinsonian.* (Obtainable from R. Beren, 55 Merrick St., Rumford, RI 02916, USA).

DR. A. (PSYCHIATRIST)

Some 10 years ago I was sitting in my dentist's chair. He was pressing down on my lower jaw when suddenly the jaw went into clonic spasm, opening and shutting beyond my control. I realised then that I had Parkinson's disease and a visit to a neurologist confirmed my diagnosis. I am 81 years old and, thankfully, the PD has not progressed much these 10 years. I retired officially at 65, but in fact continued as my own locum for 3 years and then worked as locum in another post for a further 5 years. I finally stopped work not because of PD but because of failing eyesight from cataract and glaucoma.

I found that the chief handicap from PD was extreme slowness of writing (printing was easier than trying to write cursive script). My first neurologist put me on Amantadine and Sinemet and this helped for a number of years, though it gradually became of limited value. I have always been interested in teaching and I continued lecturing after leaving hospital work. In the past few years my voice has been severely affected by PD and, regretfully, I had to abandon teaching. I had some sessions with a speech therapist and she displayed my voice on a computer screen, which showed the raised pitch. My dear wife is, like me, partially deaf so communication is difficult.

Altered posture, which is resistant to therapy, is another problem. I have kyphosis and scoliosis (curvature of the spine forwards and sideways, respectively) and the exercises suggested by the physiotherapist did little to remedy this.

I was warned when I started treatment with Sinemet Plus that I would eventually develop ballismus (involuntary throwing movements). I therefore kept to the minimum dose for about 7 years. By the end of this time I was very stiff, so I resolved to try a bigger dose. A geriatrician kindly admitted me to hospital to monitor the response as the dose was increased from $2 \times \frac{1}{2}$ tablets daily to 6 tablets daily. It resulted in a wonderful sense of freedom, but after a honeymoon period the promised ballismus developed in my right shoulder. I compromised by cutting back to 3 tablets a day, taken in the form of $\frac{1}{2}$-tablets when I am busy with handwork. The only side-effect is mild ballismus which is tolerable and in any case disappears at rest. I still take Amantadine, though its beneficial effect is said to wear off. Recently, I inadvertantly ran out of capsules and felt distinctly worse, though this may have been a psychological effect. A short time ago I went to another neurology professor in connection with the brain bank project and he put me on Selegiline in addition to my other medication.

An irritating symptom of my PD is dribbling of saliva, especially when my attention is preoccupied with some task. I cannot take anticholinergics because of my tendency to glaucoma. It is easy to get confused about medication, so I set out my daily doses first thing in the morning and I keep absorbent tissues in my pocket to deal with dribbling. I can walk about a mile, though slowly: I gave up driving 3 years ago so we go out on foot or by minicab, though all too seldom. Apart from glaucoma, cataract and extreme myopia, I also have a 'lazy' left eye. I used unconsciously to suppress the image from that eye, but now I cannot do this and have double vision. This adds to the problem of turning and keeping my balance and I have fallen twice, once upon getting up from the table after sitting in an ordinary dining chair without arms. I now have stable chairs with arms. I really should have the cataract operation but my wife is reluctant to agree.

The occupational therapist at the centre for old people was most helpful. She visited our home and swathed the tops of the corner posts of the bannisters with soft material, fearing that I might fall. In fact I can manage stairs without too much trouble: we have a stair lift, but we seldom use it. Likewise the OT supplied me with a plank and steps for getting into the bath, but since having a bar fixed to the wall at the side of the bath I do not use them. The OT also fitted velcro to one of my shirts, but I can still manage the buttons. However, a built-up spoon for the left hand is particularly valuable to me, and as my left side is still relatively good I can eat soup and other soft food with this spoon.

In 1935, when I was studying for my Diploma in Psychological Medicine, I took the 'chronic clinic' in the neurological department of my teaching hospital. This included a number if PD patients. There was little we could offer them apart from Stramonium and other anti-cholinergic drugs and admission to a long-term hospital. In 1938 I had charge of a number of survivors of the encephalitis lethargica epidemic and they had parkinsonism. Then there were medical colleagues with PD: there was an old man who came out of retirement during the war to release a colleague for more urgent duties. I particularly remember a psychologist colleague who ran a course for M.O.H.s with great gusto from her wheelchair. There was nothing wrong with her voice. We have come a long way during my professional lifetime in the medical and social provision for PD but there is still a long way to go and an urgent need for research.

DR. B. (PHYSICIAN)

I am now aged 75 and retired from Harley St. 2 years ago. We used to live in London but decided to move to the Suffolk countryside when I retired. My wife, who is an ex-nurse, is in good health. Shortly after retirement I began to notice some unsteadiness of gait, difficulty in managing a knife and fork at meal times, illegible handwriting, increased salivation and emotional instability (sentimental rubbish on television makes me cry). I also find it difficult to get out of a chair and particularly out of the bath. These symptoms led us to suspect the diagnosis, but my son, who is also a doctor, insisted that I see a neurologist. So, a week ago I did so. The neurologist examined me with kindness and skill and diagnosed PD. One question he asked particularly rang a bell; 'Do you have difficult turning over in bed?' I certainly do.

As to my attitude to the disease, let me say that I am 75 years old and have a good wife, so I've no cause to grumble and don't. I've always felt Montaigne expressed my own philosophy when he said, 'When my time comes, I hope I'll be in the garden, planting cabbages'. I plan to carry on with my garden as long as I am able, and despite evidence to the contrary, I hope to live for ever.

DR. C. (GENERAL PRACTITIONER)

I am a medical practitioner, now aged 58, who has been taking drugs for Parkinson's Disease for the past 5 years. Without going into great detail, I will explain. I was injured in a road accident in January 1985, suffering a fractured pelvis and severe bruising of the lower back. Later that year I had surgery for spinal cord decompression from which I made a good recovery. However, my walking ability was not good. I started reasonably well but soon had great difficulty in putting one foot in front of the other; my limbs felt stiff and if I attempted to raise my leg there was marked difficulty. As this condition got worse I finally saw a consultant neurologist in December 1986.

The neurologist suggested that I try Valium, which I rejected because of its dependency problems, then another muscle relaxant (Norflex) which I had previously used for stiff neck but had had to stop because it lowered my blood pressure. He would not give me a diagnosis, but said he would write to me after he had thought about it. I was very disheartened when I left him. However, he did write to me some weeks later, suggesting I start taking Madopar in the appropriate introductory way and then go to see him again in a month's time. Of course, I looked up the drug and found, rather to my consternation that it was prescribed for PD. Nevertheless, I started to take it and one evening, when I had reached a dose of 3 tablets a day, I took my dog out as usual and suddenly found I could walk normally, without effort. My joy was immense; I had forgotten how lovely it was to be able to walk normally.

The neurologist asked me to stop the drugs for a trial period of one week, but I reduced this to one day because after that time I felt the stiffness recurring and I really felt I could not face going back to the state I had been in prior to medication. Over the next 6 months I had to increase the dosage of Madopar to achieve the effect, but then heard from a colleague of another drug which could be useful, Selegiline. I now take Madopar 62.5 mg × 4 daily and Selegiline 5mg × 1 daily. I also take Hormone Replacement Therapy, which has greatly improved my energy. It was started to avoid the risk of osteoporosis, which could be a real problem for me since I have a double spinal fusion.

I do sessional work in Community Medicine (on average 2 sessions per week) and I do some home visits. If I am asked to fill in for colleagues, and work for 3–4 sessions in a week I begin to get very tired and achy and increasingly stiff, despite the medication. Nevertheless I can get by without increasing the dose.

As far as most people can see, I am a normal person and I just hope no one sees me when, sometimes quite unexpectedly, I run out of power. It is the unexpectedness of this happening that makes me careful not to accept too many outside invitations as I feel that both I and other people would be embarrassed. So it is usually only my husband and children who see me at my worst. I sleep well but do sometimes have tight thigh muscles and at times find it difficult to turn over in bed (but you can evolve a technique of pulling on your nightie and pulling yourself over). I sometimes have difficulty in starting to pass urine, and also sometimes in stopping but I have no real problems there. I can run a home and cope with the usual family chores, so long as I allow myself a sit-down period several times a day.

A heavy protein-rich meal and alcohol make my symptoms worse, so I do not drink alcohol when I am dining out. It saves me the embarrassment of staggering from the table as though drunk. Several members of my family are vegetarians so we don't eat much meat and vegetarian meals suit me.

I'm not sure whether I am a better doctor for having this complaint, but it certainly makes me appreciate what I have and understand a little of what it is like to be disabled.

DR. D. (INDUSTRIAL MEDICINE)

Many years ago I had to describe PD as part of a course in neurophysiology at a college in India. I startled the students by entering the lecture theatre imitating a patient with advanced disease. I little thought that one day I would experience many of the symptoms for real. After about 10 years of tropical medicine in India and Uganda I was appointed Director of a treatment centre for chest diseases in this country. I retired from this post 12 years ago at the age of 65. I was 71 when I first noticed tremor in my left hand. Dr. X at Queen's Square confirmed the diagnosis as Parkinson's Disease 6 months later and since then I have seen him annually.

At present my main symptoms are: (i) Tremor, which has increased slowly but is still confined to my left hand and it amounts to no more than a minor embarrassment. (ii) Painful cramp in my left forearm when walking and which is relieved by giving the arm a parcel to carry. (iii) Excessive salivation during the last 3 years and this has increased in recent months so that involuntary dribbling occurs fairly often. For 2–3 years I have noticed a constant production of mucus from the pharynx and during the past year I have had a watery nasal discharge. (iv) My gait has been slightly unsteady for about a year. (v) When my bladder is full I have to empty it without delay or risk wetting my clothes.

During the first 5 or 6 years I avoided medication because my PD was no more than a minor nuisance. Also I had heard from several authorities that after a few years the potency of the drugs was often lost, so it seemed wise to postpone treatment as long as possible. During the last 12 months I tried Madopar (125mg × 3 daily) but I obtained no benefit and side-effects (mainly bouts of ataxia) were frequent. So I stopped taking the Madopar. Then I moved into a new flat and this seemed to aggravate my ataxia quite severely. My GP started me on Sinemet Plus

(1 tablet × 3 daily). The ataxia improved quickly and my tremor and bad handwriting were both improved.

DR. E. (GENERAL PRACTITIONER)

Most of my working life has been in general practice; half in family practice, half in student health; and then 4 years part-time in HM Inspectorate of Prisons, until I retired in 1986 at the age of 65. My first symptoms of PD began in 1988, when I noticed that I was getting slower, both mentally and physically. I put this down to reactive depression after the tragic death of our youngest son a few months earlier, but then the start of tremor in my right hand, increasing inability to write (even as badly as usual) and increasing fatigue and loss of mental alertness made me seek advice. I was referred to a consultant neurologist in 1989, by which time the diagnosis was obvious (at least to him). When I was diagnosed I naturally read all I could on the subject and concluded that, even more than most, prognosis in PD was very difficult.

I now take Madopar (62.5mg × 3 daily) and Selegiline (5mg × 2 daily) without side-effects and with great improvements in my condition. I still cannot write, though I can type and I am practising with my left hand. Tremor is variable and generally worse when walking or being driven in the car, or at unguarded moments (especially stressful ones). I can do woodwork but I sometimes have problems with buttons or with small change. The depression has lifted and my mental agility is much improved. Walking is rather an effort (like walking in deep shingle) but I try to walk a mile every suitable day. I swim 2 or 3 times a week and I maintain and alter a large garden. We entertain a lot and travel a good deal. I still umpire for the Amateur Rowing Association. My family are concerned and very supportive and my wife helps me even more than usual while encouraging me to persevere with exercises and writing practice. I seem to be one of the fortunate ones with late onset PD and reasonable control with minimal medication, which enables me to continue most of my activities

and to take great pleasure in life. Since my student days I have generally been on some committee or other, looking ahead and planning for the future. However, when I retired I determined to stop this and to 'live each day as it were my last'. I do not worry about what the future may bring. Perhaps I should add that religion plays no part in my life.

DR. F. (GENERAL PRACTITIONER)

'Dad, why is your thumb going up and down?' my daughter asked as I drove her to school. I was 39 and this was my first symptom of Parkinson's Disease. Over the next few years other symptoms appeared. My writing deteriorated and I developed an intermittent tremor of my left hand which was aggravated by activity of the right hand such as writing or shaving. Tiredness, tension and excitement made things worse. The loss of the natural swing of my arms when walking, a tendency to drag my left foot, loss of my sense of balance, an ataxic gait and spread of the tremor to my left leg and then to the right limbs: all these appeared by the mid-1980s. Other symptoms, such as tiredness, slowness of movement, insomnia and constipation also caused problems. Apart from these symptoms there were also the side-effects of Sinemet, particularly involuntary movements.

The intermittent tremor of my left hand caused me a little concern and it wasn't until 1976 that the diagnosis of PD occurred to me. Three years later I consulted my GP and he confirmed the diagnosis. I had no treatment until 1981, by which time my writing had become a major concern, along with slowness of movement and difficulty in examining patients, especially away from the security of my own consulting room. Getting in and out of my car, going up and down stairs, kneeling down in cramped conditions beside a patient's bed; all these things posed problems. General Practice which I had enjoyed so much was becoming a struggle.

The attitude of patients was mixed. Some were sympathetic, some embarrassed, some were quite critical, a few were hostile and one or two thought I was drunk. Disipal (an anticholinergic drug) afforded no benefit and caused a dry mouth and consequent difficulty in talking, particularly towards the end of a long surgery, and a marked deterioration in my close vision.

I was referred to a neurologist in 1982. He agreed with my GP's diagnosis and they were both most helpful and were prepared to discuss at length any problems I had. This was a remarkably beneficial factor in my treatment. Sinemet (110mg daily) was started and it gave immediate and considerable benefit to my physical symptoms and wellbeing. Gradually the benefits lessened and the dose was increased to 220mg × 4 daily. With such high doses involuntary movements of trunk and limbs developed. The dose was reduced to 165mg every 4 hours and 110mg at night. This reduced the dyskinesia and also my difficulty in turning over in bed. Finally, Bromocriptine (10mg, 4 hourly) was introduced and this is my current regimen. Eldepryl (Selegiline) was tried twice but it resulted in a marked increase in all my symptoms and was therefore discontinued. My worst symptoms are now tremor, dyskinesia, bradykinesia (slowness) and ataxia (staggering gait). They vary enormously from minute to minute and day to day and, paradoxically, I can have simultaneous tremor in my left limbs and dyskinesia in my right.

By late 1985 I knew I would have to consider retirement. The first stage had been to opt out of night duty and employ a deputising service. I discussed my intentions with my 3 partners early in 1986 and it was agreed that I should go on sick leave on the 1st July and retire 6 months later.

I did not enjoy my remaining weeks in general practice. Consultations took longer and I tended to fall behind with my appointments. House calls took much longer and I used to arrive home exhausted. I had the impression that the arrangements had been efficiently but unsympathetically organised by my partners, who felt I must do my 'full Share' until the last minute. When I woke on the 1st July 1986 it was as though a great weight had been lifted from my shoulders.

My wife and I moved house at this time from a large house and garden to a small

house and garden. The Occupational Therapy Dept. fitted a few aids and I have a wheel chair for shopping trips. As a family we all discuss my problems quite openly and I receive generous help and support. We continue to enjoy occasional lunch and dinner parties so long as we know our hosts and guests well. My table manners have deteriorated and I sometimes need help with cutting up meat. Involuntary movements of my legs sometimes cause trauma to those of adjacent guests. I try to avoid cocktail parties: I spill my drinks if standing up and if sitting tend to be treated as an ashtray or a social leper with whom the occasional guest will spend 5 minutes before 'circulating on'.

DR. G. (GENERAL PRACTITIONER)

I was born in 1940 and entered full time General Medical Practice in 1965, retiring because of PD in 1990. I was first aware of the symptoms of PD in 1984; I noticed that my writing had become almost illegible, I was abnormally tired and I had an occasional tremor of my right arm and hand. Routine tasks, both medical and non-medical became much harder to carry out and my movements became progressively slower and slower. I made the diagnosis myself but I did not tell my partners or my wife and family until December 1984 when I had referred myself to a consultant neurologist, who confirmed the diagnosis.

My speech became rapid and slurred during the next couple of years. At first I tried Disipal (an anticholinergic agent) and Amantadine but neither drug helped me. I also tried Imipramine for my depression but it was of no benefit and aggravated my speech problems. I then tried Madopar (62.5mg 4 hourly) and I could scarcely believe the dramatic improvement. After 2–3 years I increased the dose to 125mg, 4 hourly, due to a slow deterioration of my condition. I am still taking this dose. For several years I have also taken Eldepryl (5mg × 2 daily) in the hope of slowing the progress of the disease. For the past 2 months I have been taking part in a trial of a new drug which is said to enhance the effect of L-DOPA. The results are slightly encouraging, but it is early days.

In an effort to improve my writing I attended Occupational Therapy. Despite the therapist's efforts there was no improvement. As this was the problem causing me the greatest concern I tried to find a different way around it. I contacted a Pharmacist in Manchester and he devised a program for me to use on my Amstrad PCW8512 which enables me to have all my prescriptions printed. I also underwent speech therapy, which I find beneficial and I am still receiving it.

Since my increasing disability prevented me from performing my profession properly I seriously considered retirement. During the winter months I stiffen up considerably when walking in cold weather and my speech is also much worse in the cold. The final incident was that one winter's day, following a heavy snowfall and drifting, I became stuck in a snow drift while visiting a patient. I had to rock myself backwards and forwards for some 5 minutes before I could free myself and carry on walking. By the time I arrived at the patient's house I was exhausted and almost incoherent. After working part-time for 3 months I retired in April 1990. I felt it was my duty to inform my patients (a) that I was retiring and (b) the reason. Most of them were very sympathetic and I found great difficulty in coping with this role reversal. Some, however, became aggressive and felt that I had let them down.

After my PD had been diagnosed I became much more aware of the symptoms and signs of PD in my patients and it was very gratifying to see the dramatic improvement when they were prescribed L-DOPA. It was not until I had retired that I had appreciated how much the stress of trying to carry out my duties aggravated my symptoms. Once I had retired my family and friends were very understanding in that they did not treat me as an invalid but were always ready to help me with any physical task I found difficult. Retirement does not mean that I have become a 'couch-potato' since I set myself small tasks every day: short walks, minor DIY jobs and helping more around the house.

To keep my brain active I attempt crossword puzzles and play weekly bridge. Despite my forebodings I am enjoying my retirement more than I dared hope and as I am not yet too severely affected I am fully independent. I am a member of the PDS and look forward to receiving the Newsletter and the Yapper magazine. When reading the medical literature on PD I think that most articles are too pessimistic. I feel confident that the many trials of drugs or operative therapies will soon produce a dramatic breakthrough in the treatment of PD.

DR. H. (GENERAL PRACTITIONER)

I retired from general practice 7 years ago and worked as a medical ophthalmic practitioner (I had been a clinical assistant in ophthalmology for 30 years). Four years ago I began to feel very tired. My writing became smaller and almost illegible and I had an occasional tremor in my right hand. I also had difficulty in putting my right hand into my trouser pocket. While sitting relaxed or reading I developed pain in the muscles of my right hand. The severity of the pain would increase, but was immediately relieved if I moved my fingers. This symptom lasted about 4 months. I could never find anything that would bring it on. About this time my youngest daughter got married and on looking at the wedding photographs I realised that I had a Parkinsonian face. I saw a consultant and he confirmed the diagnosis. He suggested that I take Selegiline 5mg × 2 daily, but I discontinued this after one week because of headache.

I gave up work, as I felt I could not manage and at that time I was not keen to be on medication. I went around slowly but I found that my other interests were suffering. My fly fishing was inaccurate and I had a 'Twitch' at the end of each cast. I used to play snooker once or twice a week and I found that using the cue was becoming more difficult. I used also to sing in a choir and found that my voice was higher and weaker. To combat these difficulties I started small doses of Sinemet Plus (1 tablet) 30 min. before my activities. Eight months ago it was suggested that I should try Selegiline again. This time there was no difficulty and I have maintained this regime ever since. Five years ago I had a prostatectomy which relieved the symptoms of prostatic enlargement without affecting frequency, which was due to a small bladder. It was, however, greatly improved by Selegiline. One of my many symptoms was an intense dislike of heat. This always affected my face and became so severe that I would have to leave a crowded room. It was often accompanied by a feeling of suffocation. Medication has improved this problem but not cured it. I have been told by my consultant that I am under-dosed at present but he suggests that I continue like this while I am taking the Conductive Education course at the Birmingham Institute.

In order to attend the Institute I have to travel 50 miles early in the morning, take the course for 3½ hours and then return home. Obviously I could not do this safely by myself, but members of the local Rotary Club take me twice a week. The course consists of exercises which are designed to assist the patient's main difficulties (in my case writing, postural instability and speech). The atmosphere is friendly and relaxed but patients encourage each other and are competitive. The exercises are not strenuous but they are unremitting and are interspersed with tests to discover one's weaknesses. Thus, one may be asked to sing a solo, act a small play or plait a piece of string. I have learned to cope with most of my difficulties and I feel much better. In 3 month's time a fresh batch of patients will be started and we will be instructed in continuing the course by ourselves. It is still too early to evaluate the results but I am very impressed by the beneficial effects of Conductive Education on me.

DR. I. (GENERAL PRACTITIONER)

In 1960, at the age of 30, I developed numbness of my right hand and transient diplopia (double vision) which was diagnosed as multiple sclerosis. The numbness cleared after a few weeks and since then I have had 7 episodes of sensory MS, the latest in 1980. These episodes left me with only minor sensory loss. Otherwise I was fit, active and very happy as a small-town GP. Then, during the late 1970s my golf swing gradually became erratic and I found I had decreased power in my fore-hand when playing squash. During 1979 I had difficulty writing; after 1–2 lines it became small and illegible. That same year I consulted a neurologist who diagnosed Parkinson's Disease. Tremor developed mainly in my right arm and soon afterwards in my right leg. Muscular spasms in my leg gave me difficulty in driving, although I continued to drive until 1987.

Treatment with L-DOPA was started straight away since I was anxious to keep working as long as possible. I began taking L-DOPA, increasing the dose to 0.5g × 4 daily. Although my response was good I was troubled with nausea and vomiting. So, after about a year I changed to Sinemet 0.5g × 3 daily. After a further 2 years I was advised to reduce the Sinemet to 0.25g × 3 daily and to add Selegiline 10mg daily. In addition I was prescribed hypnotics for my difficulty in sleeping (due to tremor, difficulty in holding a comfortable position and difficulty in moving in bed). Recently I have been advised to reduce my Sinemet still further to 0.625g daily, with the addition of Madopar CR overnight to ease moving in bed. During the early 1980s I became hypertensive. This is well controlled by taking Enalepril.

Physiotherapy is readily available to me, as I was fortunate enough to marry a very dedicated and enthusiastic physiotherapist who has made a study of the subject and manages a fine line between loving and nagging me about my gait or my posture. I have also found the PDS booklet 'Living with Parkinson's Disease' very useful. I run through most of the exercises every night.

Speech problems are one of the most distressing aspects of my disease. There is a useful section on this in the PDS booklet and I occasionally see a speech therapist. One of my main problems is inadequate volume. For this I was lent a voice amplifier which, although effective, was very awkward to manage with its batteries, wires and microphone. I have found some help from pacing my walking with music, especially military marches and I can dance quicksteps and waltzes better than I can walk.

When I was first diagnosed I felt it was important to keep working for as long as possible: so, for the good of the practice, I kept the news to myself for 2–3 years. I worked for 8 years after the diagnosis was made and at first there was little difficulty and patients were unaware of my problems. I began by using a pocket dictaphone and my letters and records were typed. I stopped fitting intra-uterine loops, as this always caused tremor and it was impossible for me to remove foreign bodies from eyes. On the other hand, I was able to suture simple lacerations almost up to the time I retired. Injections and venepuncture gave little difficulty but drawing liquid up into a syringe was often difficult. However, this being a small town it eventually became common knowledge that I had PD. I was treated very sympathetically by my patients. Nevertheless, it became more and more embarrassing to examine patients with my tremor, which hardly inspired confidence. By 1987, being then 58, I realised the time had come to retire since I was also having difficulty with speech, driving and night calls.

Personal relations have been affected by my illness. I am much more dependent on my wife and, to a lesser extent, on my 4 grown-up children for help with everyday tasks such as dressing, getting out of a low seat, being driven and particularly in getting comfortable in bed. Our friends have been understanding over a long period.

There has been one positive aspect to my illness. I was able to forge a special bond with the PD patients in the practice. Most of them came to me. Nevertheless, my experiences as a patient proved to be a double-edged sword; to know that I too was suffering from PD was a help to patients as long as I was coping well. If I appeared to be out of control then a patient might well get a very bleak picture. As a doctor I might want to protect them from this. My policy on giving patients information about their condition was quite flexible. Naturally I told them what the diagnosis

was, and something about drugs and their possible side-effects. But whether I raised wider issues, such as the likely effect of PD on their work or on their families might depend on such factors as age. Generally, I would say more to young patients than to elderly ones, some of whom I felt did not want to know. In some cases I would discuss things in more detail with the family than with the patient. The role of the carer is of very great importance and the outlook is equally bleak for both of them.

I think the GP has many advantages over the hospital specialist, when it comes to the management of chronic illnesses like PD. You need to be aware of the total family set-up. Also, monitoring the effects of the drugs needs to be done over fairly short time intervals.

Finally, here is my collection of symptoms:

(1) Tremor of arms, mainly at rest or if stressed or self-conscious.
(2) Difficulty in walking; at times I can walk for several miles but if I am 'off' I have great difficulty with festinant gait.
(3) Difficulty in initiating movements, especially in bed or in getting up from an armchair.
(4) Difficulty with fine movements such as writing and using a knife and fork.
(5) Problems with bladder sphincter. In the 'off' state there can be overwhelming urgency, so that slowness in getting through one's clothing can lead to occasional accidents.
(6) Anal sphincter: I tend to be constipated but there is also a feeling of urgency and poor control.
(7) Postural giddiness.
(8) Very infrequently I experience dribbling.
(9) Speech problems with poor volume and lack of clarity.
(10) Naturally, all these problems play havoc with one's sex life.

DR. J. (MEDICAL OFFICER)

I was born in Ireland on the 30th August 1922 and qualified MB BCh (NUI) in 1945. I was diagnosed as a PD patient at the age of 56. I was the only Medical Officer working in a Mission Hospital in Zululand S.A. I first noticed a tremor of my thumb and index finger when at rest. Otherwise I felt very well. I thought of PD as a possible cause, but then said, "It cannot be; I am too fit". I was jogging daily and swimming a good deal. I then thought that it might be due to anxiety, alcohol or an over-active thyroid but I could not fit myself into any of these categories. The tremor gradually became worse and surgical procedures, which I could do before, became more difficult (as also did making decisions).

When on holiday in England I was seen by a neurologist who immediately diagnosed PD and put me on Madopar, Bromocriptine and Selegiline. I read in a medical journal that one should put off taking Madopar for as long as possible, because of its diminishing usefulness over a period of time. Also, I had no difficulty in walking and talking, though I was aware of loss of energy and confidence.

I returned to the Hospital and told my colleagues of my trouble. They arranged for a doctor to help me. This was a great help, although it was irregular help and I had long periods when I was alone. I found the work more exhausting and so, at the age of 63, I resigned.

I now have great difficulty with walking, with frequent falls, a fractured patella and severe osteoarthritis. I had a right knee joint replacement 6 months ago: it has not really improved my walking a great deal, but I do not have pain. Friends, neighbours and relatives could not have been more helpful and understanding and I would say the same for our Zulu staff. [This part of Dr. I's account was written on 23rd July 1991. It was resumed on the 18th November 1991] Sorry, I mislaid this letter, I get frequent on/off reactions. Dispersible Madopar and Apomorphine are a big help and I carry them with me at all times. I cannot walk more than a couple of hundred yards. I salivate a lot and at times I have difficulty speaking. I feel best in the mornings and weaken as the day goes by. I sleep badly. I wake early but cannot get out of bed until my Madopar Dispersible acts. I get depressed at times but I suppose that on the whole this is not a problem. My memory is not too bad and, on the credit side, I go trout fishing. Last week I hooked and landed a 5lb trout. I stopped driving a few years ago and this is a big loss. One of my biggest handicaps and fears is in being invited out to tea or any social gathering. I am fine for perhaps 20 minutes, then tremor takes over and I feel lost and miserable. I know I can avoid such gatherings, I don't go very often, but then one becomes a recluse and that is not good either. I am lucky in that my friends and relations assure me that they understand. I know that they do and I appreciate it, but it remains a miserable feeling. Also, when I get violent tremors I fear that I will not recover from it.

MR. K. (OPHTHALMIC SURGEON)

I am an ophthalmologist who has had Parkinson's Disease for 20 years, not knowing it for the first 2 years. During those 20 years my brain has been active analysing various aspects and effects of the situation. Here is one of those analyses, entitled 'When You Stop Being Afraid'.

This was the answer to a question addressed to my chief, after I had assisted him in a series of eye operations at the Oxford Eye Hospital. He was one of the best eye surgeons in the world. My question to him was 'When does one become a good eye surgeon?' At that time I had already fulfilled the requirement for taking the Specialist Certificate in Canada and I was now starting a 2 year appointment at the Oxford Eye Hospital as First Assistant to the Chief. My rank was Senior Registrar, the highest training level in Great Britain. I had performed many eye operations but had not attained the level of confidence I sought. At that time, and since, I performed every operation at least 3 times: once in my mind before the operation, once again during the actual operation and once again afterwards, analysing what I had done.

Shortly after my question I was analysing a difficult operation I had just done when I realised that I had not been afraid. I had become a good eye surgeon. This was the start of my development as a good eye surgeon, I remained a good eye surgeon for 20 years. Then, one day, at the height of my career it happened—a sudden tremor in my right hand lasting only a few seconds. I lost my status as a good eye surgeon. I was devastated, not having the slightest idea why this had happened. I completed my operations for that day but I couldn't bring myself to go back to the operating theatre after that; ever again.

I made feeble excuses to my patients and sent them to other doctors for their operations. Little did I know that I had started on the downward path of Parkinson's disease. It was not diagnosed for 2 years, during which time my confidence for doing even minor office procedures went down and down. My rigidity and jerky movements became worse and affected my whole life. I was embarrassed playing golf with my friends who were puzzled by the degeneration of my game. I played the trombone in a small band and wondered why I couldn't move the slide fast enough. I couldn't eat soup with a spoon. All my activities slowed down and my muscles ached. After 2 years of mental anguish the diagnosis of PD was made. It was a great relief to my wife and me to have an answer to my problems. My health improved dramatically after the beginning of treatment and many people thought I might resume operating, but I never regained normality or recovered self-confidence or overcame the ultimate obstacle—fear.

(Williams 1992)

COMMENTARY

The collection of accounts compiled by Williams brings home a simple point—that in most cases, Parkinson's disease (PD) strikes when the person is nearing retirement or has just retired (although the case of Todes is a notable exception in this respect). While the effects of the disease may not be as devastating as if it occurred much earlier, the other side of the coin is that the symptoms of PD are set on top of other medical symptoms associated with growing old—poor vision, poor hearing, etc. There must come a point where yet one more handicap is seen as the 'straw that breaks the camel's back'. Whereas younger patients may be able to use other intact functions to help compensate for the symptoms that are associated with PD, this privilege may not always be available for the typical PD patient.

Another feature, one that may be unique to PD, is the central role that drugs play in the management of the condition, especially in the early stages, and the variability in motor symptoms that accompanies the effectiveness of the drugs. In other neurological conditions, such as stroke or head injury or Alzheimer's disease, the disability seldom has any ready medication associated with it. One wonders whether the degree of stress and uncertainty that is sometimes associated with drugs and their side-effects adds to the psychological burden that PD patients already have.

GENERAL COMMENTARY

1. Parkinson's disease and dementia

The risk of dementia occurring in Parkinson's disease increases with age, so that by the age of 85 years, the risk of developing dementia with PD is considered to be 65%

(Mayeux 1992). The extent to which dementia is found in a particular study will also depend on the exact neuropsychological test procedures used to test for the presence of cognitive impairment, and the criteria used for interpreting test scores as indicating the existence of dementia. The presence of depression will also tend to exacerbate test deficits in PD patients, especially on memory tasks (Tröster et al. 1995).

Many of the authors of the articles in this chapter reported cognitive symptoms as part of their clinical condition. In none of them, did it appear that a significant degree of dementia was present, although this may have been related to the stage at which the self-reports were written. Perhaps self-reports written at much later stages of the illness would have revealed more widespread or more severe cognitive impairment.

For the **Anonymous** author, it was a memory symptom—forgetting his patients' faces and what he had prescribed for them—rather than motor difficulties, that seemed to trigger his decision to leave general practice and go back to work as a doctor in the navy, though he only survived in that working environment for a couple of months. **Todes** noted that as the disease progressed, 'continuous recall of events is disrupted and thoughts of a conceptual nature become less readily available' (p. 172). In current cognitive parlance, it would seem that he was suffering from both an 'episodic' and a 'semantic' memory difficulty. The former has been well described in some PD patients (Kapur 1988; Yanagahira and Peterson 1991), but semantic memory difficulties have been less well documented and appear to be less frequent. They usually relate to retrieval of factual knowledge, and they are usually related to cortical pathology. It is worth noting that, in his subsequent book, one of **Todes**' letters to NHS managers is interpreted by others as showing his 'inability to grasp issues and to come to conclusions when presented with certain facts' (**Todes 1990, p. 90**). While the major pathology in PD has been considered to be subcortical in nature, affecting the basal ganglia, there is now evidence that cortical damage in the form of Lewy body disease is more prevalent in PD patients than had hitherto been thought (Marsden 1994). It remains possible that this cortical pathology may play an important role in some of the cognitive symptoms associated with PD.

Todes reported that alertness and memory were increasingly affected by the disease, and that recent and 'medium-term' memory became affected. He reported that childhood memories did in fact become *more* accessible! Although some investigators have reported impairment in retrograde memory tests in certain PD patients (e.g. Sagar et al. 1988), this has mainly been on public events tests, with particular impairment in the ability to date public events. In the Sagar et al. (1988) study, there were some deficits in recalling public and personally experienced events from more recent years, with more distant memories relatively spared. In general, deficits in memory for past events was much more evident in those PD patients who had a significant degree of dementia. My own clinical experience with PD patients is that in most cases there is a relative sparing of memories that predate the onset of the illness. **Todes** noted that drug overdosage, leading to dyskinesia, also adversely affected recent and long-term recall, and the role of medication in long-term memory deficits needs to be borne in mind.

On a holiday trip to Europe some months before his diagnosis, '**J. Doe**' experienced disorientation, which seemed to comprise an inability to accommodate to rapid shifts in time and place. Although it is difficult to be certain as to the significance of this symptom, I wonder if this could have been a subtle manifestation of a memory deficit or to a cognitive inflexibility that is sometimes invoked in discussions of PD deficits.

Thompson thought that his memory difficulties were due, in part, to his antiparkinsonian medication. One particular memory symptom (p. 191) is interesting, and it related to difficulties he had in sleeping in a preferred position in bed: 'I could not remember how to dispose my trunk and limbs for ease and comfort when lying on either side'. The type of 'procedural' memory symptom could perhaps be related to the difficulties on motor/perceptual-motor learning tasks that have been found in some studies of PD patients (Heindel *et al.* 1989), although in this case one is talking about recall of an established pattern of motor behaviour rather than the learning of a novel motor sequence.

In addition to the cognitive changes such as slowness of thought and deteriorating memory, **Thompson** notes that at one stage in his illness 'words simply fail to form in my mind', that he found himself having spelling difficulties, and that he was sometimes at a loss to understand the meaning of written words. These symptoms, although appearing to be relatively mild in severity, suggest that in at least some PD patients there may be a subtle form of language disorder, perhaps related to cortical Lewy body disease, and find echoes in some semantic memory symptoms offered by **Todes** (cf. Matison *et al.* 1982).

Although **Thompson** reported that his memory difficulties were more of an annoyance than a handicap, he reports quite a severe symptom, and one that tends to be associated with more severe memory loss—namely, when he sees the repeat of a television film, it gives him as much pleasure as when he first saw it, since it all seems new to him! He also reported a positive side to his memory lapses—'It frees me of the burden of memory, and failure to recall a word, or a name, no longer upsets me. "It's my Disipal", I say, and dismiss the matter' (p. 196).

2. Parkinson's disease and mood state

Mayeux (1992) stated that as many as 40% of PD patients will become depressed during their illness, and that 25% of these patients will experience depression prior to the onset of overt motor manifestations of PD or within a year of their onset. It is interesting how in some cases a period of depression precedes the onset of Parkinson's disease. It remains possible that such depression, or a related change in temperament/mood state, is a marker for some cases of PD. One of the authors of the self-reports, **Todes**, has argued elsewhere (Todes and Lees 1985) that traits related to depression, such as introspection, passivity, and emotional inflexibility, may be present in the years prior to the occurrence of the clinical symptoms of PD and may represent premorbid personality features of PD patients in general. A number of the authors in this compilation brought out rather unusual symptoms, such as a heightened emotional response to what previously was a relatively minor stimulus. In a number of cases, stress or some other emotionally laden event would greatly exacerbate a particular motor symptom that was otherwise very mild or relatively dormant.

'**J. Doe**' had major emotional symptoms for five years prior to the diagnosis of his

Parkinson's disease, these being characterized by a profound sense of emotional instability. Another case for whom emotional symptoms appeared to be a precursor to the disease was that of **Thompson**. The first symptom that **Thompson** attributed to his Parkinson's disease was an over-reaction to his emotions when recounting a story. It is interesting that he also found himself, presumably at a later stage of his illness, being careless about his appearance and his personal hygiene. It is difficult to say if this was secondary to the PD disease process, since frontal lobe dysfunction has often been reported in PD patients, or to some remnants of the depression that **Thompson** suffered prior to his Parkinson's disease. It is worth noting that inferior orbito-frontal hypometabolism has been reported in some PD patients who suffer from depression (Mayberg *et al.* 1990).

3. Parkinson's disease and control mechanisms

Can a general model of disordered inhibition explain motor, cognitive and mood changes in Parkinson's disease? **Thompson** attributed much of his slowness to a dis-inclination/loss of will to do certain things. 'I feel that I could make my muscles obey orders if I really wanted to do so, that all that is needed is the will—which for some obscure reason is lacking' (p. 193). Perhaps this 'loss of will' may have reflected some degree of frontal lobe dysfunction that has occasionally been reported in PD patients (Owen *et al.* 1990). This has sometimes been referred to as 'abulia', to denote apathy, slowness of thought, etc. Excessive inhibition in the case of his motor symptoms could be seen in his account (p. 197), where he noted his 'cerebral computer' appeared to malfunction by freezing on a motor activity when-ever any minor resistance was encountered. One wonders whether **Thompson**'s report of losing control of his threshold of emotional expression, the first and most dramatic symptom of his illness, could also be considered a form of breakdown of inhibition, similar to that which may have governed some of his later parkinsonian motor symptoms. Over-reaction to an external stimulus, not being able to inhibit an exaggerated response to that stimulus, could therefore be a common thread run-ning through a number of his difficulties. It is often quite possible, therefore, that there are common circuits within the basal ganglia, linked to circuits in the frontal lobe and cingulate region, that are concerned with the regulation of movement, thought, and emotion.

The self-report articles also highlight the presence of multiple neural routes for the control of motor activity, either in terms of multiple pathways or multiple sources of innervation of the same pathway. One of the fascinating observations by PD patients is that in certain situations there may be a paradoxical sparing of motor function (e.g. the author of the **Anonymous** contribution reported that it was easier for him to walk backwards than forwards). There is also the oft-quoted anecdotal observation of PD patients being able to move quickly out of situations of extreme danger, such as fire or a car approaching as they walk across the road. It is pre-sumed that some other motor pathways, or some latent sources of innervation, suddenly come into action when such a novel and life-threatening situation occurs. **Thompson** gives a graphic description of his problems in carrying out the simple, once very automatic, task of stirring a cup of tea. 'The essence of the problem was the failure of the automatic control mechanisms to function normally. It is these mechanisms which enable us to carry out simple operations without thinking about them . . . I find myself reacting like a child who has never done such a thing before . . . It surprises me even more to learn, by observing myself in action, how badly one carries out a simple task when one is forced to take thought in performing it. When the automatic mechanisms pack up, efficiency goes with them' (p. 192). Conversely, there is the observation in a number of the articles that when he/she really concentrated, the PD patient could bring about some improvement in motor functioning.

On the basis of such observations, it is possible to speculate that, while most forms of motor activity require the operation of a distributed network of cortical, subcortical, and cerebellar mechanisms, there may be two dissociable neural systems for many forms of habitual motor activity such as walking, reaching out, etc. One is primarily a subcortical striatal system that is damaged in PD patients. The other is primarily a cortical system which is mediated by frontal lobe structures and requires awareness and specific cognitive effort on the part of the PD patient. Both systems would interact with other structures, such as the cerebellum, to produce movement. It could be argued that for certain motor activities basal ganglia systems largely take over control from cortical systems when the movements become more automatic and much less under conscious control. It is practically impossible as an adult to routinely bring over-learned, habitual motor activities into continual conscious awareness, but one may presume that when PD patients talk about 'concentration' they refer to a conscious effort to produce certain movements that are no longer possible through more established, 'automatic' pathways. For further discussion of the role of the basal ganglia in automatic and controlled motor activities, the reader is referred to an excellent review paper by Marsden and Obeso (1994).

REFERENCES

Heindel, W. C., Salmon, D. P., Shults, C. W., Walicke, P. A., and Butters, N. (1989). Neuropsychological evidence for multiple explicit memory systems: A comparison of Alzheimer's, Huntington's, and Parkinson's disease patients. *Journal of Neuroscience*, 9, 582–7.

Kapur, N. (1988). *Memory disorders in clinical practice*. Butterworth, London.

Marsden, C. D. (1994). Parkinson's Disease. *Journal of Neurology, Neurosurgery and Psychiatry*, 57, 672–81.

Marsden, C. D. and Obeso, J. A. (1994). The functions of the basal ganglia and the paradox of stereotaxic surgery in Parkinson's Disease. *Brain*, 117, 877–97.

Matison, R., Mayeux, R., Rosen, J., and Fahn, S. (1982). 'Tip-of-the-tongue' phenomenon in Parkinson's disease. *Neurology*, 32, 567–70.

Mayberg, H. S., Starkstein, S. E., Sadzot, B., Preziosi, T., Andrezejewski, P. L., Dannals, R. F., *et al.* (1990). Selective hypometabolism in the inferior frontal lobe in depressed patients with Parkinson's Disease. *Annals of Neurology*, 28, 57–64.

Mayeux, R. (1992). The mental state of Parkinson's Disease. In *Handbook of Parkinson's disease* (2nd edn) (ed. W. C. Koller), pp. 159–84. Marcel Dekker, New York.

Owen, A. M., Downes, J. J., Sahakian, B. J., Polkey, C. E., and Robbins, T. W. (1990). Planning and spatial working memory following frontal lobe lesions in man. *Neuropsychologia*, 28, 1021–34.

Sagar, H. J., Cohen, N. J., Sullivan, E. V., Corkin, S., and Growdon, J. H. (1988). Remote memory function in Alzheimer's disease and Parkinson's disease. *Brain*, 111, 185–206.

Todes, C. and Lees, A. J. (1985). The premorbid personality of patients with Parkinson's Disease. *Journal of Neurology, Neurosurgery and Psychiatry*, 48, 97–100.

Tröster, A. I., Stalp, L. D., Paolo, A. M., Fields, J. A., and Koller, W. C. (1995). Neuropsychological impairments in Parkinson's Disease with and without depression. *Archives of Neurology*, 52, 1164–9.

Yanagahira, T. and Peterson, R. C. (ed.) (1991). *Memory disorders. Research and clinical practice*. Marcel Dekker, New York.

Brain tumour   5

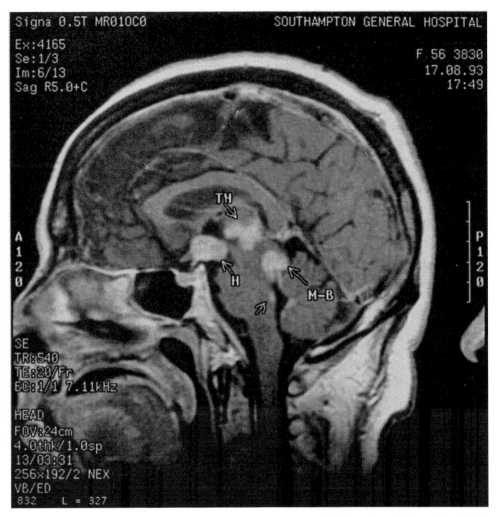

Figure 8. Fifty-six-year-old man with a tumour (primary cerebral lymphoma) that affected the mammillary bodies of the hypothalamus (H), medial parts of the thalamus (T) and midbrain (M–B) portion of the brainstem. He had significant impairments in retaining new information, but his pre-illness memories were relatively intact.

INTRODUCTION

The incidence of brain tumours is considered to be around one new case every year in a population of 20 000. There are various types of brain tumours. Malignant tumours can arise from the glial cells that form the connective tissue of the brain, being classed as 'gliomas', or they may represent off-shoots (metastases) from primary tumours elsewhere in the body. Astrocytomas are a form of glioma, and are graded according to degree of malignancy (grade 1 is the least malignant, grade 4 is the most malignant). A class of more benign tumours (meningiomas) arise from that part of the brain covering called the meninges. The effects of a brain tumour on cognitive functioning will depend on the tumour type—for example, gliomas will have more adverse effects than meningiomas, and tumour location— frontal lobe and temporal lobe tumours will be more likely to have effects on psychological functioning than tumours in other sites. More general factors that are important in determining degree of functional disability include the general brain swelling that results from the growth of the tumour, the specific displacement or distortion by the tumour of particular brain structures or blood vessels, the effects of the tumour on the flow of cerebrospinal fluid, the occurrence of specific clinical conditions, such as epilepsy, that may themselves adversely affect psychological functioning, and specific toxins or other substances that are secreted by the tumour. Therapeutic interventions to treat the brain tumour may in themselves have their own side-effects—surgical removal of the tumour carries a certain risk, and both radiation therapy and chemotherapy have occasionally been associated with particular neuropsychological side-effects.

Three of the brain tumours in the following reports (**Anonymous 1952; McCool 1985, 1987; Arthur 1984**) were astrocytomas, one was a medulloblastoma (**Mainwaring 1990, 1993**), and the remaining case was one of a pituitary cyst, probably a pituitary adenoma (**Anonymous 1977**). The precise grading of the astrocytomas is not reported in the relevant papers, although the one of **Arthur** must have been very malignant, since the patient only survived for nine months after the onset of symptoms. Only two of the tumours (**Arthur; Anonymous 1952**) directly affected the cerebral hemispheres, in the former case—both hemispheres, and in the latter case—only the left hemisphere, and so the papers provide more general clinical observations, rather than specific cognitive insights, into the effects of brain pathology.

FURTHER READING

Lishman, W. A. (1987). *Organic psychiatry* (2nd edn), Chapter 6, pp. 187–206. Blackwell, Oxford.

Cerebral tumour

The doctor in this anonymous article may have been working in laboratory medicine (he refers to using a microscope in his work), but apart from this there are no other firm clues as to his particular speciality.

When I was a boy of 15 or 16 I had an attack of malaise, ushered in by the most severe headaches I have ever had. The local doctor ordered me a mixture which stopped the headaches though the malaise continued for another fortnight. I think it was at this time that I saw bright spots moving about rapidly for an hour or so, with no associated pain or other discomfort.

My progress at school was uneven. I entered for the junior-grade intermediate examination when I was a year under age, and unexpectedly passed. Next year, being the right age, I went up again, and failed. My school reports often said 'Could do better'— but I don't regard this as at all diagnostic! Next year I unexpectedly passed the middle grade. When I entered college I took my place at the tail of the brighter ones, or at any rate in the van of the ruck. However, I did not manage to keep this up for more than a year or so.

For many years after this I had vague symptoms which I did not take very seriously. It is so difficult to know what is the normal. From time to time I would lose my appetite, and I used to sweat a lot, especially on exertion, so that a bunch of keys in my trouser pocket was usually rusty. Occasionally I noticed the little and ring fingers of my left hand twitching, and now and then I had a feeling that some disaster was about to happen. Sometimes I was irritable, and sometimes I made caustic remarks; but many of us do.

When I was abroad, at the age of 35, I had a more severe attack of malaise, accompanied by bradycardia and giddiness, and shortly afterwards I had my first epileptic attack. In the middle of the night I was awakened by a pain in my back so severe that I had to take opium for it. In addition, my tongue was sore and my pillow bloodstained.

There was no enuresis in this attack or in any subsequent one. When consulting my doctor about my back I mentioned the question of epilepsy, but he did not take the suggestion very seriously. Later my back was X-rayed and a deformity was found; I was admitted to hospital, where the final diagnosis was Scheuermann's disease. (This is of the same nature as Schlatter's disease, but in a different site.) While I was in hospital I noticed an occasional sinking feeling in the precordium, followed by a forcible heart-beat, and this symptom continued intermittently up to a few weeks ago.

About nine months after my first fit I had several more at night, and as these were noticed by other people a diagnosis of idiopathic epilepsy was made. The attacks now assumed a pattern: they nearly always occurred at night; I nearly always injured my tongue, but was never incontinent; and my muscles were always stiff afterwards. Sometimes my appreciation of colours and sounds was heightened after the fit.

Up to this time my mind had been pretty clear; but now I began to have a peculiar sensation as though my thoughts were being rapidly revolved. I could almost hear the buzz! This happened many times a day, but it was all over so quickly that it caused me little inconvenience and did not interfere with my usual activities; my train of thought continued its course practically uninterrupted. I also noticed that if I was in a brightly lit room and the light was suddenly put out, there was a subjective image of brightness which flickered about 10 times a second for several seconds. Later I lost the bright image which normally follows pressure on the eyeball— 'seeing stars'. I was on a poor diet, so I went home to Ireland and enjoyed unrationed food for a few months, with excellent results; I put on weight rapidly, my psychological symptoms disappeared, and I soon felt quite well. So, taking the optimistic view, I decided that the whole thing was a matter of malnutrition, and returned to work.

I now had to live in lodgings, and the wartime diet there was very poor. About two months after I had resumed work I had rather an alarming experience. While walking with some friends I suddenly felt as though a flash of lightning had passed through my brain. I did not tell anyone about it—indeed, I had become rather secretive about the whole business. A few weeks later I had a similar attack. About this time I had nocturnal cramps in my calf muscles, and I often found difficulty in emptying my bladder at one go; sometimes it took several attempts, each producing some urine, before the bladder was empty. A few months later I began to have trouble with my eyesight. I had my eyes tested and wore the glasses ordered even when using a microscope: they gave me some relief.

I now had my first epileptic attack when not in bed. I was talking to a colleague when I suddenly had the most awful feeling of terror I have ever experienced. The whole world seemed to be slipping away, leaving me isolated and helpless. When I came to, I found myself on a stretcher on my way to a ward. When I was better I went to a well-known hospital and had the routine investigations for such a case; the diagnosis was as before—idiopathic epilepsy.

Then I began to have more severe psychological symptoms. The moving lights recurred, though they did not last so long as before. Several times I felt an urgent desire to speak to anyone who happened to be close by, whether I knew them or not; I did not know what words I wanted to say, so the result was an intense mental conflict. Occasionally, after I had gone to bed, I had a feeling of acute loneliness, almost amounting to fright. In the daytime I sometimes used to sit at my desk gazing into space for long periods, unable to concentrate on my work. If I suddenly stood up, I had peculiar feelings which I cannot describe, lasting a second or two. Sometimes the same thing would happen just before I yawned. I also noted that when I

took off my hat the rim left a horizontal mark on my brow which remained visible for an hour or more.

For domestic reasons I had to return home, and the day after I got back I went down to the village to make some purchases. I can remember walking out of a shop, but just after that I must have fallen heavily, striking my head such a resounding crack on the pavement that the shopkeeper came running out to see what had happened. I was taken to hospital on the fire-engine, which happened to be there at the time, and apparently I could speak on arrival, as I gave my name and address correctly. I cannot remember that part, but I have a confused recollection of being in a small ward where something amused me very much. That night I lost consciousness for about a week. I was found to have a fractured skull. When I came to, I could read a little but could not speak or even grasp what was said to me. After I had been some days in this state the matron came in on her morning round and said as usual, 'Good morning, Doctor', to which she was delighted to hear me reply, 'Good morning, Matron'.

My senses of smell and of taste were severely affected for about six weeks after this fall; most of the good tasted peculiar and not very appetising. Swede, a one-time favourite of mine, I still cannot eat; even other vegetables cooked in the same pot taste of it, and a most unpleasant taste it is. At first I could not enjoy the taste of whisky, and both beer and stout tasted like water. Luckily I have since fully recovered my taste as far as drinks go.

I went back to my job, but after about three months my epileptic fits were obviously becoming more frequent, so I had to resign. I returned home, hoping that the better food would have the same good effect as before, but I gradually got worse and developed some new symptoms. One was a greatly increased sensitivity to noise, so that the barking of dogs would upset me badly. When their noise was more than I could stand I used to dash out into the street to try and stop them barking. Usually, of course, by the time I got there they would already have stopped. There was also a curious tendency to lacrimate for no particular reason, and without the usual emotion. But I also had become more emotional, and was much more easily moved by sad passages in films or novels. My memory had got very bad. I had to write down any instructions or messages to the most minute detail. Here, for example, are the instructions in my notebook for finding the materials for making tea. 'Teapot in cupboard facing one in kitchen. Milk in frig. 5 teaspoonfuls of tea. Sugar, find.' This loss of memory made my everyday life more difficult. Thus, travelling across London by Underground, I put the ticket in my pocket, but when I had to produce it for the collector I could not find it and had to pay the fare again. I must have looked several times in the wrong pocket, and of course later on I found it easily.

My fits were by no means always complete. They often stopped at a stage when I was making involuntary repetitive noises. Once when out for a walk I went through the pedestrian's wicket gate at a level crossing and noticed that the spring was rather stiff. I said to myself, 'That spring is too stiff' and then my thoughts, so to speak, 'stuck', so I went on thinking 'that spring is too stiff', 'that spring is too stiff', as if my brain was a gramophone and the needle had stuck in the groove.

Another occasional trouble was the failure of my subconscious mind to make the subsidiary decisions—for instance, when writing something down I had to stop and think out all the separate actions, instead of occupying my mind entirely with what I intended to write. There were also curious variations in appetite. Once I had three breakfasts one morning and still had an excellent appetite for lunch. Another symptom is difficult to describe. On going back to revisit a once-familiar scene, some people are conscious of a difference in the atmosphere. Everything is in its familiar place and looks the same as expected, yet there is a different feeling about it all. I used to notice this difference of 'atmosphere' or 'background' nearly every day, sometimes for a week at a time. I even noticed myself how stupid I was becoming.

I was then fortunate enough to visit a neurological surgeon, and after a consultation with one of his physician colleagues I was admitted to a world-famous hospital. Here I had a more detailed and complete examination than ever before, and in a few days my cerebral tumour was found. I was very pleased, for I had never been satisfied with the diagnosis of idiopathic epilepsy. The tumour—an astrocytoma—was successfully removed a few weeks later.

In the seven months which have elapsed since the removal of the tumour my initiative has greatly improved; my intelligence has become keener: and I have had no grand-mal attacks. I am still taking phenobarbitone twice a day. I still have occasional attacks of confusion or failure to find the right word, and sometimes a spell of acute depression lasting a few seconds. These attacks are unquestionably becoming less frequent, and altogether I am much more cheerful than for several years past.

(Anonymous 1952)

COMMENTARY

The self-report by the anonymous doctor does not refer to the site of the tumour, but it looks as if it may have been in the left temporal lobe. Since epilepsy was a major feature of his condition, some of the observations are quite relevant to the symptoms that accompany seizures. For example, there is the feeling of great fear and helplessness that preceded a daytime fit, suggesting the involvement of medial temporal lobe structures such as the hippocampus and the amygdala. More persistent emotional symptoms included a dissociation between the expression and the feeling of emotion, and also a heightened emotionality to sad items in a book or film. The latter symptom is reminiscent of what is known as pseudobulbar affect, where there is a heightened expression of emotions (Benson 1994, p. 110), and suggests the possibility of more widespread pathology in this case. The inability to remember a sequence of actions (e.g. how to make a cup of tea) may have included several separate memory difficulties—remembering where things were located in the kitchen, remembering the components of an action sequence, or remembering the order of these component actions. One suspects the involvement of left fronto-temporal structures in this particular problem, with apraxia being one of the component deficits, though it is difficult to be more precise without any corroborative evidence about the localization of the lesion.

REFERENCE

Benson, D. F. (1994). *The neurology of thinking*. Oxford University Press, New York.

Pituitary cyst

The doctor in this anonymous article appears to have been a general surgeon.

From late adolescence or early manhood I suffered from severe headaches, almost always after playing golf. Over the years the headaches occurred at irregular intervals. In the autumn of 1963, when I was 50, I had a very severe attack with vomiting that lasted for 24 hours. Perhaps there was a sudden enlargement of the cyst with rupture of the roof of the sella turcica.

Soon after I had a motoring and camping holiday in Europe, driving 3000 miles in three weeks. I was continuously exhausted and had to take to my bed. On several occasions previously I brushed the garage doors with my car: I did not then realize that I was losing my peripheral vision.

I was perpetually tired and anorexic and generally ill and was worse after any exertion. I was laid up for 3 or 4 days after mowing the lawn. I had widespread myalgia especially in the extraocular muscles, with pain when moving the eyes, and in the intercostal muscles. I suspected trichiniasis. My joints, especially the interphalangeals, became stiff and there was limitation of rotation and abduction of the shoulders. My sleep was disturbed by restlessness and involuntary movements sufficiently violent to throw off the bed clothes. I had sudden involuntary jerking of the legs suggestive of chorea to a mind groping for a diagnosis. I lost weight and became very pale.

My mental symptoms are difficult to describe in retrospect. I was apathetic and my concentration failed. My thinking became slow and laborious and there was clouding of mental acuity. I lost hair, mainly from the trunk, axillae, pubis and legs and my beard grew less vigorously. My libido disappeared. I became intolerant of cold but suffered from hot flushes suggestive of testicular failure. In the areas of the special senses, I lost auditory acuity and had severe tinnitus. Apart from the garage door incidents there were no optical signs.

Having been labelled a case of virus disease, after about three months rest at home, I took up my duties again in mid-January 1964, still extremely pale and thin, and lacking in stamina. I can remember suffering from excessive perspiration on operating days, a thing to which I had never been accustomed, but more seriously I found that I had lost the visual acuity of picking up small blood vessels and soon my eyes were becoming reddened. I presume now that this was from continual attempts to accommodation trying to achieve a sharp image on the retina. One morning, in early April, on closing one eye as an experiment, I found that I was unable to read newsprint and this sent me to an ophthalmic surgeon for advice. His opinion was that I was suffering from retrobulbar neuritis, and he ordered a further complete rest.

It was at this point that on seeking further medical advice, I was directed along the correct path. It was revealed that X-rays of the skull showed a large pituitary fossa. Fields of vision were measured and gave irrefutable evidence of bitemporal hemianopia, from pituitary compression of the optic nerves, and the diagnosis was established.

Surgical removal of the pituitary cyst by the transfrontal route was undertaken. On recovering from the anaesthetic, I immediately tested my visual acuity for distant vision, and, to my very great joy, found it sharp and clear, where it had been blurred and misty. Visual acuity and fields of vision both recovered completely.

Maintenance therapy has been empirical and it is concluded that there is about half the pituitary function still present. My daily requirement of drugs is as follows:

Cortisone   25 mgm
Thyroxine   0.1 mgm
Fluoxymethisterone   5 mgm

After six years I remain well and able to carry out the normal routine of general surgery. I do get tired at times, but not unduly so. I seem to have regained my former mental acuity, such as it was, hair growth is normal, libido returned and temperature control seems normal, although I believe that the effects of chilling would still be prolonged. My warning signal, should I forget my drugs, is the onset of tinnitus, which I imagine is a cortisone-lack effect.

May I take this opportunity to express my deep gratitude for the most incredible surgical expertise, which had me travelling home on the 10th post-operative day to convalesce and recover. The diagnosis seemed to be the difficulty, and I trust that this account may help to expedite this in other sufferers from the disease, which does not seem to be well described in standard text-books.

(Anonymous 1977)

COMMENTARY

The symptoms from the doctor with a pituitary cyst included a severe headache, with vomiting, that lasted 24 hours, and a loss of peripheral vision that meant he brushed his car against the sides of his garage. A significant degree of fatigue was also a prominent early symptom. His clinical profile suggested that his lesion was a pituitary adenoma. Pituitary lesions are seldom associated with marked cognitive difficulties but this doctor did have symptoms of slow thinking, impaired concentration and a degree of apathy, which are sometimes seen after such pathology (Lishman 1987). Note that his diagnostic label was one of 'virus disease', even after the occurrence of all these symptoms, and also 'hypothalamic' symptoms that included loss of hair, loss of libido, and a change in temperature threshold that included excessive perspiration. Major visual symptoms that the doctor complained of, such as not detecting small blood vessels while carrying out operations, only resulted in his being offered a diagnosis of retrobulbar neuritis!

REFERENCE

Lishman, A. W. (1987). *Organic psychiatry* (2nd edn). Blackwell, Oxford.

An astrocytoma

Leonard Arthur

Leonard Arthur was a consultant physician, specializing in paediatrics.

At the end of March, 1983, I challenged my daughter to squash, and was struck by my inability to serve even a drop shot into the opposite court. My increased right knee jerk ended the fantasy that I had damaged my shoulder; the neurologist diagnosed a small astrocytoma.

A right hemiparesis developed in April, 1983, and an arteriogram demonstrated an inoperable tumour in the left hemisphere. Radiotherapy produced an apparently good resolution, but later a right-sided lesion developed and there was further progression of the left-sided one. For the first two months, while I had my radiotherapy, I continued to work, missing only one clinic. I began to be utterly complacent about my lesion. I had no sensory loss at this stage. It was not until the second or third relapse, which occurred roughly every two months, that I got sensory loss on the right side. I should have realised then that each step was a progressive deterioration; but such is the power of optimism and denial that it was some time before I accepted the truth. This was the perfect summer of 1983. I leap from optimism to pessimism. Each time a plus, is followed by a minus.

I want to write about the signs that people seldom write about, such as the fleeting wisps of headache that sweep across the left side of my brain, which I now believe to be musculo-skeletal symptoms produced by twists to my cervical spine.

I had quite a lot of bruising down both arms, presumably due to steroids. I identified the cause as my plastic wristwatch strap on the left and, more surprising, much bigger bruises on the right which appeared to be caused by my plastic wrist name tape. Finally I took them both off and bought a nurse's watch which I pinned to my left breast. In the midst of this a left pleural effusion, caused by a pulmonary embolism, developed. It caused me severe pain and almost asphyxiated me. The cause of a brown stain that appeared on my finger and toe nails was immediately identified by a staff nurse as high-dose steroids. Nobody else was able to confirm this and it did not reappear when I went back on high-dose steroids.

Steroid myopathy appeared within four days of the start of high-dose steroids in April. It was painless and the neurologist found my muscle weakness difficult to assess. I used to sit down as if pole-axed and it made it more difficult for me to take exercise with my good side. When steroids were first reduced to low levels I felt the improved power, it was very pleasant. However, I had to resume high-dose steroids when epilepsy developed.

Because my appetite has remained normal and I have cause for far less exertion I have put on weight round my middle and now resemble Toad of Toad Hall. Efforts to rein in have not been entirely successful.

At first I thought that I was 'high' on steroids, but I do not seem to have changed very much over the last four months or so. My wife says I was definitely 'high' at the start. The great thing is that I have not become depressed; but then I have always been a fairly optimistic person. Other steroid side-effects have been remarkably absent. I needlessly feared vertebral collapse, diabetes, cataracts, psychotic changes, ulcers, and dyspepsia.

I used to have a serviceable tenor voice. I can no longer sing in tune. I cannot connect this with any neurological sign. I have been on dexamethasone for the last six months. Every time I have reduced my steroids I have had recurrence of symptoms, which means I have not been able to try the effects of minimal or no dosage.

Having neglected and despised my left

hand for 56 years, I have suddenly found myself completely dependent on it. At first I relied on my right hand to supply direction and the left hand (unharmed) simply provided the motive power. But soon I found my left hand taking over all sorts of specialist movements. My biggest problem was reciprocating movement—eg, cleaning teeth and shaving. It was wonderful how my uncomplaining left hand got on with the job. Even writing with my left hand was not too bad, although very laborious. It is said that your left-hand manuscript has many of the char-acteristics of your right-handed script (I speak as a right-handed person). I made a vow that if I ever got my scholarly script back I would never be guilty of hasty or slovenly writing. Alas, I do not think I shall be given the option of the right-hand script, but miracles can happen. I am reminded of this by Christy Brown's classic *My Left Foot*, 1970. This autobiography should be compulsory reading for all paediatricians.

(Arthur 1984)[*]

[*] Dr Arthur died on December 25, 1983.

COMMENTARY

Similar to what we have seen in other accounts, Arthur appeared to have symptoms of denial/excessive optimism in the early stages of his illness. Since his left hemisphere tumour was considered inoperable, this account provides more detail on the role of steroids and their side-effects. The balance that needed to be drawn between too little and too much steroids reminds one of the drug-balance problems that are described in the accounts of Parkinson's disease patients. Arthur's specific problems included putting on weight, being unable to sing in tune, difficulties with motor tasks that required bimanual co-ordination, and a difficulty in writing with any degree of fluency using his left hand. Being unable to sing in tune, or 'amelodia', has been associated with right inferior frontal/right anterior parietal lesions (Benson 1994), and in Arthur's case it is of note that after his initial left hemisphere lesion he developed a further right hemisphere lesion, which may have been the source of his amelodia.

REFERENCE

Benson, D. F. (1994). *The neurology of thinking*. Oxford University Press, New York.

In memory of a brain tumour

J. A. McCool

J. A. McCool was a medical student at the time of his first article, and a junior hospital doctor at the time of the second article.

Everything began with an apparently innocuous headache as I awoke one December morning. It cleared up around 11 am and I thought nothing of it, though virtually my only experience of headaches had been during 'the morning after'. The next morning, however, I again woke with an identical headache—a diffuse, throbbing pain in time with the pulse, brought on by head movement, stopping abruptly after seven to eight beats, then recurring with the next head movement. It, too, abated by midday. And so it went on. Each morning I would awake with the headache, be clear of it by noon, only for it to reappear the following morning. This pattern continued for three months; during this time the headaches had become gradually more severe and were lasting longer throughout the day, sometimes till early evening.

Then, suddenly, things changed. I woke one morning with a catastrophically severe headache, constant and boring, refusing to go away. From then on I also began to feel nauseous and to develop a slight unsteadiness on my feet. When the 'effortless' vomiting started there could be no more delay in presenting myself to the neurologist. At this stage I was only two months from my final examinations. When no physical signs whatever were found on examination, and the skull *x* ray examination and blood tests were normal, the consensus of opinion was that I was suffering from 'tension' headaches. This diagnosis was completely unacceptable to me; I *knew* that these were not 'tension' headaches. Everyone else knew five days later. I had had to wait five days in hospital, without further investigation or treatment, for a computed tomography scan, there being only one scanner in Northern Ireland at that time. The scan confirmed my fears—a tumour. It was Holy Thursday.

The next day all the doctors, apart from the houseman, went off on holiday. Their sudden absence left me feeling somewhat abandoned, and the irony of my hapless position, during Easter, a time of celebration, was not lost on me.

'YOU'RE WITH THE FIRST DIVISION'

I was glad, a week later, when the day of the operation dawned. I felt no apprehension that morning, happy that the waiting was at an end. I had complete confidence in my surgeon, and I just wanted to get the thing over with, so that I could get on with the business of recovery. As I was wheeled out of the ward towards the theatre, it seemed odd to be lying flat on my back, being trundled along corridors that I had trodden many times as one of 'us'—now I was indisputably one of 'them'. The last thing that I remember was admiring the skill of the anaesthetist as he painlessly fed an arterial line into my arm. 'Don't worry', he said, 'You're with the first division'. And then oblivion.

I do not remember being in the recovery room or returning to the ward; I spent the first 24 hours in a shadowy state of consciousness dimly aware of my surroundings, occasionally drifting awake to find myself with an atrocious headache. Fortunately, and to my surprise this was effectively controlled by dihydrocodeine tartrate given intramuscularly. I was out of bed the day after the operation, and, once out, I was eager to attempt a short walk. I expected to be completely ataxic and was a little apprehensive about actually confirming this to myself, but I was delighted to find that, although I was slow, I was fairly steady, and felt no giddiness or dizziness at all. So encouraged was I that I wanted to walk all round the ward and had to be firmly directed back to bed by my supporting nurses.

In other respects, for the first couple of days, I was virtually helpless and completely reliant on the nursing staff. Having the most basic and intimate things done for me was an odd experience, but I felt no sense of embarrassment, only of necessity. During this time, the kindness and sympathy of the nursing staff was overwhelming, and this, together with the highest level of efficiency and competence, made their care unsurpassable.

During my postoperative period many of my friends thought that I had undergone a personality change: I was irritable, tetchy, and sullen. The houseman on the ward told me some months later that, at one stage, I had been suffering from a mild acute confusional state and had even been a little dysarthric at times. This was certainly news to me. I was completely unaware of any of it and had considered myself to have been at all times in a perfectly normal state of mind. I do admit to being somewhat irritable, but surely this was understandable after such an operation, when you are scarcely likely to feel at your best.

CACOPHONY OF TELEVISION NOISE

In fact, the main thing responsible for my irritability was noise and especially television noise. It seemed to come at me from all sides and was as demoralising as it was unrelenting. The patients' sitting room in the neurological ward in which I stayed before my operation was dominated by a large television set. This was left on all day at ear shattering volume. The door to the television room was open, of course, at all times, and the noise reverberated constantly throughout the ward, making any semblance of peace and quiet impossible.

Even in the neurological ward television noise was a persistent torment. Many patients had a portable television by their bedside and often three or four would be blaring away,

each one switched to a different channel and each seemingly trying to outdo the other. The resulting cacophony was intolerable. Surely in any ward, but especially in a neurosurgery ward, where many patients have had a craniotomy, this should not be allowed to go on? Each patient has as much right not to listen to television if he does not want to, as another has to listen. Many patients may be suffering; as I was, from headaches, and they were made a great deal worse by this continual noise. Headphones should be mandatory for those wanting to watch television, so that the thoughtlessness of some is not allowed to disturb the peace and privacy of others.

After the operation I found that I had become more sensitive to noise in general, and that any loud noise, if in any way sustained, was liable to precipitate an immediate headache. I could accept the necessity of the clamour of busy ward activity. It was the unceasing barrage of television noise to which I objected, and which seriously undermined my morale and confidence. This was by far the most dispiriting aspect of my entire hospital stay.

I was discharged home 10 days after the operation. By this time, my weight had fallen to eight and a half stone from a combination of postoperative sickness and no great love for hospital food. I was so thin and had lost so much weight from my legs during my weeks of inactivity that my greater trochanters bulged like a pair of budding horns; they made lying on my side and trying to get to sleep at night most uncomfortable.

RADIOTHERAPY AND ITS AFTER EFFECTS

Anyhow, I managed and the following week I was off to hospital again for radiotherapy. Before the actual treatment began a few days were spent on making a mask. This included the disagreeable business of having my face covered with vaseline and my head encased in plaster of Paris. Yes, they do leave a hole to breathe through.

The treatment itself was painless but

within a few hours of it starting I developed headaches and vomiting almost identical to my original symptoms. It seemed that radiation induced local inflammation and oedema were blocking the cerebrospinal fluid and giving rise to another spell of raised intracranial pressure. Dexamethasone was duly prescribed and it was immediately effective; little did I realise that this was the beginning of a long running steroid saga. For the duration of the treatment the dexamethasone remained necessary to control the headaches and vomiting, and I expected to be able to stop it within around two weeks of the treatment coming to an end. The effects of the radiotherapy, however, persisted well beyond the end of the treatment period, and I found myself still needing the steroid during all this time. The continued intake led to progressive stomach problems, requiring the introduction of cimetidine and an antacid; I felt continually unwell since I was always testing myself against the lowest possible dosage, and I began to despair of ever being able to get off the stuff. In fact, it was four months after the radiotherapy had ended before I succeeded in stopping the drug—four months of convincing demonstration of the problems of steroid usage.

The course of radiotherapy lasted four weeks, and the option of attending as an outpatient was available from the end of the first week. I took it without delay—even though it meant a 60 mile round trip from home to hospital—for one main reason. Each morning in the hospital, despite being in the 'relaxed environment' of the radiotherapy unit, I was abruptly wakened at 6 30 am sharp. I found this extremely discouraging and unnecessary—I did not get my breakfast until at least a full hour later. For some reason I was being deliberately deprived of a valuable hour's sleep. Similarly, in both of my previous wards, I was usually awoken between 6 30 and 7 00 am. Certainly, never once was I allowed to sleep beyond 7 30 am. I had always assumed that a basic premise of hospital treatment was to promote rest, but obviously I had been mistaken. As a hospital patient, weakened and ill, I needed as much rest as possible, yet it was wittingly taken

from me. I fail to comprehend this policy of denying rest to the ill. Why was this practice originally adopted and why, in these 'enlightened' days, does it continue?

As a medical student, I have been repeatedly taught about the importance of confidentiality. I acknowledge that I may be more sensitive to this issue than many of my colleagues, but I admit to being most upset that within hours of my tumour being diagnosed most of the students in my year knew about it. I suppose that they had to talk about it— the shock of seeing one of themselves 'struck down' must have made them suddenly aware of their own mortality and their vulnerability even as healers. And to talk of these things allowed them to reassure each other and to re-establish their sense of security as doctors as opposed to being patients.

IMPORTANCE OF FULL INFORMATION

It is often said that hospital patients feel unhappy that information concerning their condition is deliberately kept from them by the doctors. Having now been a patient myself, I fully understand and endorse other patients' grievances about the lack of information given to them; although no information was withheld from me—being a medical student—I would have found it intolerable had I suspected otherwise. It is the patient's body and the patient's illness and, if he so desires, he must be told the whole truth. It seems to me sheer arrogance for anyone to decide that such and such a person would be better off not knowing, for example, that his illness was terminal. The patient must be given the full details about his diagnosis and prognosis because it is his future, not anyone else's, and it is only he who can make the necessary decisions about it.

Lest the foregoing may suggest otherwise, let me make it clear that I was impressed and happy with most of the care that I received while a patient. This was especially true of the early postoperative stage when the nursing staff were kind and helpful. For when something awful happens it is help and understanding that you need—not pity. I discovered what a useless commodity pity is.

A lot of people these days mourn the passing of the old time doctor, the family friend, always available, and always ready to listen and dispense advice. They decry contemporary 'hi-tech' medicine for its loss of intimacy and warmth, and for its increasing distance between doctor and patient. Yet who would argue that today's medicine is not infinitely preferable to the 'old time medicine', impotent and largely ignorant, for all of its warmth and wealth of reassurance. For in the end, to paraphrase Lewis Thomas, if I develop a brain tumour I want as much comfort and friendship as are available, but mainly I want quick and effective treatment so that I may, if that is possible, survive.

(McCool 1985)

Brain tumour

J. A. McCool

It was the beginning of December 1982, halfway through my final year of medical school when it started. I had just shifted accommodation to commence an obstetrics course. After my first night's sleep at the new hospital, I awoke normally but, on sitting up, quickly developed a peculiar, throbbing headache: six or seven beats, in time with the pulse, each beat progressively more severe, then suddenly disappearing. As I got out of bed, the same thing happened again, and over the next couple of hours it became clear that it was *head movement*, especially standing up from sitting or vice versa, or a sudden glance to the side, that brought on this crescendo of pain. A couple of hours later the headache went away, and I thought no more of it. Till the next morning that was, when the pattern of the previous day's headache repeated itself exactly. And the next morning, and the next, and the next . . .

I wasn't worried at this stage about the headache; I was too busy wondering what was causing it. A friend there had also developed a morning headache, so we thought at first that maybe the rooms were too stuffy. That night we slept with the radiators off and the windows open. But the next morning the headaches were still there—the only difference was that we were now freezing as well! Soon after this my colleague's headache disappeared, but mine persisted, unchanged. I tried changing every variable factor in my room—pyjamas or no pyjamas, foam pillows or feather, position in bed, heating,

ventilation—but none of them made any difference; the headache remained.

After a while I got used to its being there in the morning and largely ignored it. I carried on, ostensibly as normal, over the next three months, but all during this time, the headaches were becoming more severe, often lasting till late afternoon or evening.

There was one occasion, about a month after the headaches had begun, when I seriously considered its implications. I knew that the temporal pattern of my headaches was characteristic of raised intracranial pressure; I knew that the most likely cause of raised intracranial pressure was a brain tumour; I also knew that I could offer no circumstantial explanation for the headache. Logically, then, it seemed that I might actually have a brain tumour. However logical this conclusion may have been, I immediately dismissed it as being impossibly unlikely and dropped my search for the cause of the headache forthwith. I had, now and again, discussed my headaches with a good friend, also a medical student, but in any of these chats, as soon as it seemed that the headaches might be serious, he carefully steered away from the subject.

Then things changed abruptly. I awoke one morning, around the middle of March, to blindingly severe headache—constant, boring, completely confidence-sapping. From that morning, I also developed a more or less permanent nausea with bouts of 'effortless' vomiting and a mild unsteadiness on my feet.

This was, of course, alarming, since I knew there to be no obvious reason for it, and very unpleasant. When, a couple of days later, I put these symptoms together, there was really only one conclusion: that I had raised intracranial pressure—and that meant brain tumour! Naturally, this was not a comforting thought and my mind recoiled from it automatically.

I hadn't been to see a doctor about the headaches. Why not? I don't really know; perhaps I thought they would go away of their own accord, perhaps there was an unconscious inability to admit that something was actually wrong, or perhaps I just didn't want to bother the doctor with a mere headache (not wishing to appear a hypochondriac), or probably a combination of all these reasons and more—but now it was a different story. I was still reluctant, however, and eventually it was my girlfriend who insisted that I see about it.

Being a student, I went to the general practitioner at the Student Health Service. He immediately realised the seriousness of the headache and sent me with a covering letter to a consultant neurologist of the Royal Victoria Hospital (the main teaching hospital in Belfast). I met the consultant the following day, and after listening to my story and examining me, he asked what I thought was wrong. I replied, 'Raised intracranial pressure'. He then explained that he had given me a thorough examination and that he could find no abnormality, and also that he had particularly studied my fundal veins and found them to be pulsating normally. This meant, he said, that I could not have raised intracranial pressure. However, he continued, he considered that I was a calm person, and he believed me that these headaches were not functional. To this end, therefore, he arranged some blood tests and a skull X-ray and told me to return in three days' time, when we could discuss the results of the X-ray and blood tests and see whether three days' 'reassurance' had made any difference.

Unfortunately, his well-meaning words did not cheer me. Okay, he reassured me that I had no raised intracranial pressure (and, therefore, no brain tumour), but I was instinctively dubious about his means of ruling this out; i.e., that my retinal veins were pulsating normally. And, if I did not have raised intracranial pressure, what, then, was causing the headaches? Consider my position: I had no physical signs whatever to corroborate my history, and I was complaining of headaches only two months prior to my final exams. It was understandable that any doctor in the circumstances, asked to make a diagnosis, would probably have said, 'tension headache'. The snag was, I knew that they were not tension headaches; I had never got particularly nervous before exams and had previously done many important ones without getting headaches, and, anyway, I wasn't that type of personality. *I* knew all this, but everyone else remained to be convinced. On one hand, logically and objectively, I could understand those who were saying that these were tension headaches, but on the other, because I *knew* that they were not and because it was happening to *me*, I couldn't.

I went back to the consultant after three days and described to him how I had been no better since I last saw him. He told me that had I been other than a medical student, he would have admitted me to hospital at our first meeting, but that he was now doing so and that he would arrange a computerised tomography (CT) scan immediately. At that time there was only one CT scanner in Northern Ireland, and since the waiting time for an outpatient scan was one month, it was necessary for me to be admitted to hospital so I could qualify for a scan within five days. I received no treatment nor underwent any investigations during that period.

The admitting doctor examined me conscientiously and confidently declared that I had no physical signs and that I could not, therefore, have a brain tumour. I was under stress, he said, and had been suffering from tension headaches, though, he 'generously' added, this could be *muscular* tension. Later, other doctors who examined the central nervous system (CNS) found nothing and, blithely ignoring my history (of vomiting and unsteadiness), dutifully reassured me that all was well: that I was suffering only from 'tension' headaches. My friends from the same year, who visited en masse the night before my CT scan, agreed. They clearly thought that I had lost my nerve, that I was 'chickening out' of finals.

By the morning of the scan, faced as I was with this tide of opinion allied with my natural reluctance to accept that I had a tumour, I had convinced myself that it was going to be normal. The trouble was that since I could not convince myself that I had a tumour, and since deep down, I *knew* that the headaches were not functional, what on earth was causing them and how the hell was I going to get rid of them? If the scan was normal, the only alternative was that the headaches *were* functional—yet I knew, quite categorically, that they were not. Was I going insane?

(Writing now, it seems easy to say that I had, in fact, a tumour, but that obviously my defence mechanisms were denying it and would not let me admit it to myself. But at the time, of course, this was not apparent, and consequently, the above dilemma was very real and worrying.)

Following the scan, I returned to my bed and waited impatiently for my release. I had arranged for my car to be left outside the hospital and was eagerly anticipating a rapid acceleration away. I felt no apprehension at all about the results of the scan; I didn't conceive of being told anything other than that it was normal and that I was free to go. My consultant appeared around two o'clock. When he asked me to accompany him to a private room and even when he told me to have a seat, it still didn't click with me—I was still waiting to hear him say that everything was normal and that I could go. What he said was, 'As I'm sure you expected, a lesion has shown up on the scan. There is a tumour in the cerebellum'.

Thinking about it now, I would like to see the expression on my face at that moment to understand better what I was feeling. I suppose there was disappointment, disbelief, desperation, fear, and many other emotions, but I don't remember too well what went through my mind. The consultant assured me the tumour was virtually certain to be benign and that he was hopeful about the prognosis, then left rather quickly. It's difficult to describe what I felt as I stood there. Perhaps it was nothing—it seemed as if half of my mind was detached from it all and was telling the other half how I should react in such a situation. I suppose that it was similar to the 'numbness' that bereaved persons feel on hearing the news of the death, and that my rational mind was trying to tell the 'numbed' rest of me what I was expected to do. I remember being surprised that I wasn't sobbing with grief.

The consultant returned later that afternoon to see how I was and remarked that I appeared to be a lot calmer. This was true—I had, in the meantime, been transferred to another ward, and once the intolerable red tape was over with and I could get settled into bed without being pestered, my mind seemed to withdraw to another place, and there, oblivious to all that was going on around me, I somehow came to terms with the situation. I seemed to have accepted the fact that I had a brain tumour and that there was nothing I could do about it; the only possible way out of the situation was to put my complete trust in those who were looking after me.

The next day my consultant informed me that he had asked one of his neurosurgical colleagues to see me later that afternoon. I immediately liked the man; to me, he gave off an air of immense confidence in his ability. I felt happy that he was the one to whom I must entrust my life.

My friends also turned up that afternoon, looking pretty sheepish, but also appalled that such a thing had happened. I suppose it made them aware of their own mortality. Nevertheless, they were determined to cheer me up and proceeded with the usual good-natured banter until one of them, a renowned wit, said he had a present for me, and produced a short little book. It was short, he explained, because he didn't think I would have the time to read a long one!

The day of the operation came eventually, to my relief. Though I knew I might die during the operation, I was not at all anxious that morning—more glad to be getting it over with. The surgeon had done his best to scare the hell out of me with tales of maybe ending up with a paralysis or a permanent speech defect or a cough or an abnormal gait, but deep down, I always thought that I would survive the operation in tact.

My memories of the immediate postoperative period are very hazy and incomplete. Apparently, when my girlfriend arrived in early evening, soon after the operation, she took one look at me and promptly fainted! Later she told me that I was so white, she thought I had died and no one had told her— she thought that no one could look so dead and yet be alive. I was astonished to hear this, since in my conscious moments during that early postoperative period, I felt no less vital than ever previously. Similarly, I never felt a moment of great relief that I was still alive; I suppose because I had never expected to be dead. Looking back now, it seems as if it took a long time for me to get over the operation, though at the time I remember thinking that things were going much better than I had expected them to preoperatively. I had very little headache and, even though the tumour was cerebellar, very little ataxia.

From the beginning of my experience of being a patient, I was aware of being treated differently from other patients by my doctors because I was a medical student. No procedures were practised on me by junior staff; I was given a private room, if one was available; but most importantly, I was always satisfied that my consultants were being totally open and honest with me, that I was being kept fully informed at all times. I would have found it intolerable had I suspected otherwise. Having now been a patient, I fully understand and endorse other patients' grievances about the withholding of information from them by the doctors. It is the patient's body, the patient's illness, and the patient's right to be made aware of the full picture.

Naturally, following the operation, I was keen to discover the diagnosis, and each time the surgeon came to see me, I asked him about it. On each occasion, he replied that he didn't know yet, that he was awaiting the pathology report. Of course, he *did* know, since a frozen section done during the opera-

tion had shown the tumour to be an astrocytoma, but I guess he was waiting till he decided that I was ready to hear some bad news. A day or so later, as he was removing the huge bandage at the back of my head, he delivered it. He told me that the tumour had been malignant and that I would shortly have to undergo a course of radiotherapy. I was very disappointed. I felt that I had exhausted my resources in recovering from the surgery and that I just would not be able to take a further four weeks of debilitating treatment. Furthermore, I was becoming increasingly intolerant of the relentless noise surrounding me on the ward. Televisions blared constantly, cleaning women with their whining, clanking machines selfrighteously barged about all day long, typewriters clattered incessantly; I felt sure that another four weeks of it would drive me round the bend.

But the therapeutic process was ineluctable, and after five days' rest at home, I found myself back in hospital, this time in the radiotherapy unit. As I arrived, the staff were at pains to assure me that I would enjoy my stay, in the 'relaxed atmosphere', as they called it, of the unit. However relaxed they may have thought it was, it didn't prevent me being woken at 6:30 sharp every morning. I simply could not fathom the reason for this; it was at least a full hour before my breakfast was brought. Meanwhile, it was made impossible for me to sleep since the awakening nurse had, most deliberately, switched on the light, pulled back the curtains, fully opened the window, and finally, having made sure I was well and truly awake, stomped out, leaving the door wide open. I was surprised she didn't empty a bucket of cold water over me for good measure! I found this deliberate taking away of my very much needed sleep extremely discouraging and unnecessary—and yet it was only one example of the wholly illogical and ridiculous rituals inflicted on hospital patients by the nursing profession.

Luckily, I was obliged to remain an inpatient for only the first week of the four scheduled for my treatment. I seized the opportunity to come as an outpatient as soon as the week had ended, and even though this meant a 60–mile round trip every day, it was, nevertheless, a great deal less demoralising than having to suffer such stupid nursing practices.

The therapy itself was painless, but shortly after it began, I developed a familiar headache and vomiting. The radiation was causing oedema around the cerebellum and blocking the cerebrospinal fluid, giving rise again to raised intracranial pressure. I, therefore, had to go back onto dexamethasone and stay on it for the duration of my treatment. However, the effects of the radiation persisted long after the actual treatment period, and it was a full five months before I could get off the steroids completely. I was furious with this problem since, firstly, no one believed that I could be having any difficulty in stopping the drug, and secondly, I almost ended up with a stomach ulcer. I had been prescribed cimetidine in an attempt to alleviate the constant stomach upset I was having, but when I began to develop nipple tenderness, well—enough was enough!

It is funny that now I don't mind in the least talking or writing about my illness, because I remember being upset about the lack of confidentiality as a patient. The importance of the concept of confidentiality had been repeatedly drummed into us throughout our medical education, but it seemed to me as I lay there in the hospital to be nothing more than a charade; it existed only as a concept, not as an actuality. The experience was good for me, though; I myself am now very much more wary about letting slip any information about any patient I may be involved with.

Two years have now passed since I was told that I had cancer; a prominent milestone on the highway of recovery, one is led to believe—yet the subject refused to die. Two years later, a great many of my daily activities are dominated by the fact that I have had cancer. Nevertheless, the matter does not terrify me; I can, and do, talk about it with equanimity. It fascinates me now to observe patients and relatives break out in a cold sweat when the prospect of the word *cancer* looms, to look pleadingly at the doctor to

speak the word, to accept the responsibility, to spare them the horror of the dread word having to cross their lips. It's as if a curse would befall those incautious enough to breathe 'cancer' in other than awed, whispered voices.

But one-twelfth of the world's population are born in the sign of Cancer—they see the word, even look purposely for it, every day in the newspaper. Obviously, it is not the word itself that terrifies but the disease.

Although myocardial infarction is a much bigger killer, people have no difficulty in saying the words *heart attack*. They just do not provoke the dreadful fear associated with *cancer*. I find this surprising since a heart attack is often more sudden, more unexpected, more dramatic, and surely, for the bereaved, more devastating in its abruptness than any cancer. In addition, many cancers are now completely curable; an episode of myocardial infarction is likely to imply widespread vascular disease and a lifelong vulnerability to sudden death. An enduring horror, it seems, still surrounds the topic of cancer.

So, what have I learned from the experience of cancer?

I've learnt what it is like to be a hospital patient, learnt how vitally important caring nursing staff are to patient morale. For my first 48 hours postop, I was completely helpless and totally dependent on the nursing staff to keep me in one piece. I shall be eternally grateful to those nurses in the neurosurgical ward whose tremendous kindness, sympathy, and professional competence carried me through those first few frightful days.

However excellent were the full-time nursing staff, the part-time night staff who came in for one or two nights a week were another matter entirely. There were undoubtedly exceptions, but in my experience, these women were largely unfeeling and concerned with little more than getting the night over with as painlessly and as comfortably for them as possible. From one of these women, I witnessed extreme callousness and actual physical abuse of a frail old gentleman next to me whose only crime was to call for a bottle in which to pass his water.

It seems to me that the attitude of the

nurses looking after one is really of *vital* importance in determining the speed and extent of recovery from serious surgery, certainly whilst still in hospital, and perhaps even later, when at home convalescing.

I learnt what was for me, a future doctor, an important lesson regarding physical examination of a patient. Being subjected to it was an odd experience—you surrender your body to the doctor for him to poke, prod, press, thump, scratch, as he wishes, and you have no control over any of it; you simply lie there as 'relaxed' as possible and yield up your innocence to the doctor's questing hands. It is a very trusting thing to do. I learnt to respect the extent of this trust in any patient whom I may be required to examine in my future career.

I learnt that to experience cancer is not necessarily to undergo a radical or sudden change of personality. Of course, I am no longer the same person; my attitudes to life *have* changed, but this has been a slowly evolving process over the last two years. The appropriate cliché, possibly, is that I should rejoice with each new dawn, rejoice that I have been lucky enough to have been granted another day of life. I *am* very glad to be alive, but this thought is not uppermost in my mind. I still struggle out of bed each morning with the same fretful reluctance.

It is often said that those who have had a close brush with death are no longer concerned with the petty worries of everyday life, gliding above them serenely. This has not been my experience, perhaps unfortunately; neither have I learnt to accept the unpleasantries of life as being better than nothing, better than being dead.

I have imbued the entire episode of my illness with a personal religious significance. I had spent eight days in the neurological ward waiting for the operation and, to my amazement, I never once felt bitter about what had happened to me, never once thought, 'Why me?' or 'What have I done to deserve this?' If previously someone had told me that I was going to suffer from a brain tumour, I would have imagined that I would have reacted bitterly, but when this actually did happen, there was no trace of bitterness,

no thought at all of 'Why me?' Also, during those eight days I remained in very good spirits and not once became depressed or anxious.

I only realised the above sometime after the operation and there seemed to be only one explanation—that God had sent me His grace to carry me through this immensely stressful period.

Many people in my situation, I imagine, would have reacted angrily to God and would consider that He had betrayed them in letting such a misfortune come their way. I didn't, at the time, really believe in God—the question of His existence was impertinent—and was completely areligious (by this I mean that I wasn't for or against religion; it just had no relevance to my life). But naturally, during this preoperative period, with the prospect of death threatening, I thought about God. And as I reflected on these matters and on God's purpose, all my inner grudges, resentments, hard edges, and nastiness seemed to melt away and I was left with an inner peace and a warmth embracing me. I felt some kind of union with God and knew that if I died, I would not fear to meet Him.

I decided that God had seen how arrogant I had become and had sent me the tumour in retribution and concern, to remind me that He was my creator and that I was subservient to Him and must not set myself up as my own God. He dealt me a bad hand in allowing the tumour, but He did not let me die and He furnished many supports along the way to facilitate my recovery. I don't know if God let me live for a particular reason, for some particular purpose, but I do believe that He never meant me to die, that He saw that I had become my own God and sent me a severe jolt to remind me of His deity and to set me back on the right path.

Secularly, it has taken until very recently for me to appreciate that I must insist (to myself) upon my physical health as my number one priority, that all other goals must become subordinate to this aim. It has taken me till now to appreciate that without your health, you have nothing.

But what of the surgeon, the man who held my life in his hands, who saved my life?

What does it take to accept such responsibility, to live with the knowledge that a less than perfect job may spell the difference between life and death for his patients? What does it take to accept as his workplace the human brain, the 'tabernacle' of our bodies? Is it simply a question of doing the job he was trained for to the best of his abilities, or can he be aware of the awesomeness of invading the essential core of humanity, our 'inner sanctum'? And if he is, what sort of courage does this require?

I find it hard to understand that such a man, whose talent and skill are so prodigious, who spends his working hours saving the lives of others, is still a man like all the rest of us, beset with all the hassles and mundanities of everyday life. His dedication and ability don't seem to exist in the same world as keeping his car filled with gas or paying his electricity bill. Surely, I feel, such a man should be spared such trivialities, such indignities.

And how could I possibly thank him, possibly repay what he has done for me? The only way is to become as well and as healthy as I can, and give him the satisfaction of knowing that he has salvaged a life, that whatever I do or become in the future is due to him, and that his work will never be forgotten.

(McCool 1987)

COMMENTARY

Turning to McCool's account, this too has more in the way of practical, rather than theoretical, implications. McCool bitterly complains of the nursing regime in many British hospitals, whereby patients are woken up as a matter of habit around 6.30 in the morning! Sleep for most patients is a precious commodity that they may lose as part of their condition, and it does seem illogical that one aspect of the nursing regime results in it being partly taken away. McCool also points to the difference between the quality of care given by day nursing staff and by night nursing staff, the latter being much less satisfactory.

Both the account by Mainwaring (pp. 238–41) and that of McCool point to poor or absent memory for the early post-operative period. Although post-traumatic confusional states are the ones that most clinicians recognize, it is important to remember that after most forms of major brain surgery, and even after some non-brain surgical procedures where a major anaesthetic has been given, there may be loss of memory for what is taking place in the early post-operative recovery period. This may be largely due to physical causes, although a state of emotional shock may also be present. It is therefore well to remember that patients in such situations will not remember everything that has been told to them or has happened to them—clinical staff, relatives, and the patient himself/herself need to be aware of this fact.

Life without a cerebellum

Clare Mainwaring

Clare Mainwaring was a veterinary surgeon at the time of writing the two articles.

I am not a doctor, but a veterinary surgeon, the 28 year old daughter of two general practitioners. I have just had a medulloblastoma removed from my cerebellum, and am now coping with the aftermath of the surgery, which has left me with diplopia, dysarthria, and severe ataxia. Didn't James Herriot write that it shouldn't happen to a vet? I think that's rather appropriate in my case. There is nothing wrong with my intellectual capacity nor my sensory input, just my motor capability as you would expect with cerebellar injury. My neurosurgeon has told me that I will continue to improve over a year or so and I have to be patient.

Before my disease was diagnosed I thought it was most likely that I had multiple sclerosis. I certainly didn't imagine that I had a brain tumour, but then most people don't, except perhaps Woody Allen and medical students. The issue was complicated by the fact that in May 1989, three months before my surgery, I came back to England, where I had no job, from America where I had been working hard. So as my symptoms became more prominent and less easy to ignore I had more time to worry. Before surgery I experienced mild ataxia and positional nystagmus progressing slowly for about a year. I consulted my general practitioner who referred me to a neurologist who also thought that I had multiple sclerosis. It wasn't until the magnetic resonance imaging showed no evidence of demyelination but a cystic space occupying lesion in my cerebellum that the truth was known. I had to readjust my mental processes. Instead of having a potentially slowly progressive medical disease I had a surgical one that required dangerous and unpleasant treatment in the short term but wasn't going to hang over me for ever. Which is better? To say neither would be to deny the existence of the disease, which is something I have never done. You can't; it's fact and fact is immutable.

My treatment was surgery followed by radiotherapy, which lasted for seven weeks. I do not think that I was adequately prepared for either. I had been warned by the neurosurgeon that I might be worse after the craniotomy, but I was not prepared for my mild ataxia before the operation being replaced by such a severe form that I was unable to walk afterwards, and I have had diplopia ever since. Surgery was, however, recommended, and as this was the accepted course of action I was prepared to go along with it. I would do so again, though I would know more accurately what state I was likely to be in when I woke up. The surgeon warned me that posterior fossa operations often lead to hydrocephalus. I thought that I was going to get hydrocephalus after the surgery: and I did. This led to severe headaches just after the operation, but I remember little about them. I was in intensive care in the neurological centre for 10 days and I remember little of that either. The hydrocephalus was treated at first with temporary drains. These did not work, so a permanent shunt was placed from my fourth ventricle to my peritoneum. I then moved to an open ward where I stayed for about a month. My ataxia quickly improved and by the time that I left I was able to walk unaided. I had other problems with speaking and swallowing which required supreme muscular coordination. My swallowing is now normal and my speech, although still not normal, is now easily understood.

After surgery I had daily radiotherapy for seven weeks. Again, I don't think that I was adequately prepared for the effects of the irradiation. I was told that I might feel a little sick, but I was not prepared for the extreme nausea, vomiting, and simultaneous shivering and sweating that occurred during the first week of treatment. To counteract the sickness I had been given metoclopramide tablets. But they produced a dystonic reaction, so that for one day I had torticollis and open mouth with protruding tongue. After we realised the metoclopramide was to blame I was given domperidone. This did not stop my nausea and vomiting but at least it didn't produce any side effects.

For the radiotherapy I had to wear a specially made Perspex mask over my face and lie prone while my central nervous system was irradiated for seven weeks. My whole central nervous system was irradiated because it is believed that medulloblastoma could metastasise through the cerebrospinal fluid to other parts of the system. Radiotherapy makes hair fall out in the irradiated area, so my scalp hair has gone. During the radiotherapy I had to keep in mind the benefits of this treatment as it seemed to be full of bad things: the hair loss, the sickness, and the need to lie still every day for seven weeks. After magnetic resonance imaging, three computed tomograms, and seven weeks of radiotherapy I certainly know how to lie still until I am told that I can move. Thankfully, radiotherapy was not combined with chemotherapy as I understand medulloblastomas are not as aggressive in older people as in young children.

The radiotherapy ended over two months ago. At present I am in my parents' house, which I thought I had left for ever nine years ago. I am not working and I am getting more bored and apathetic daily. I suffer frequent frustration and humiliation, which I am learning to live with. I long for the days when I didn't have diplopia and I didn't have to wear an eye patch. Though I can walk unaided, I have problems in the dark, wearing high heels, and moving slowly, particularly in crowds. People who saw me in hospital just after the craniotomy comment on how well I look and how much I have improved. This is nice, but I can't help thinking of healthy friends of the same age.

I need a job to re-establish my sense of self esteem. Unfortunately, my ataxia, which affects my left arm and hand as well as my legs, prevents me doing a lot of jobs. I can perform gross but not fine movements, so as a left hander I now have to learn to write with my right hand. According to the neurosurgeon lots of people have to do this, but I don't find that very comforting.

Such a profound event has changed my attitude towards life. At 27, which I was when the diagnosis was first made, I had most of my career ahead of me and I felt as though I was immortal. Awful things like this happened to other people. I have certainly become more fatalistic. On many occasions I have thought, 'Why me?', but that's rather a futile question in the long run—you just have to answer 'because' and accept facts. I find it ironic that it should be my brain that has gone wrong, as I was quite friendly with it beforehand. It got me several firsts at Cambridge: I used to consider it my greatest attribute. Now I'm not so sure.

Among this plethora of bad events two good things have emerged. Firstly, my illness, vomiting, refusal to eat, and the awful food at the hospital resulted in my losing two stones in weight. As I had been trying unsuccessfully to lose weight for about 14 years this is quite an achievement. Secondly, I have acquired a lovely tortoiseshell cat from a lady I travelled with to the radiotherapy centre every day. As I had to leave a cat in America I very much wanted another one. She has proved to be just what I needed.

I used to think that the cerebellum was not that important, just a rather archaic piece of brain tacked on at the back. Now I know its full use and what an important part of me it is.

(Mainwaring 1990)

Life without a cerebellum: update

Clare Mainwaring

Three years ago I explained that I was a veterinary surgeon who had suffered a cerebellar medulloblastoma in 1989 at the age of 27 (*BMJ* 1990; **301**:447). This was treated with surgery and radiotherapy. Luckily there is no tumour regrowth but I am left with ataxia, diplopia, mild dysarthria, and intermittent severe pain of my neck and back. The first three are showing no inclination to improve, so I must regard my present neurological capabilities as those which I can expect for the rest of my life.

I have had the pain since December 1989, but despite multiple treatments from multiple consultants at multiple hospitals it remains unchanged in frequency and severity. I have now resorted to alternative therapy— osteopathy. It is too soon to say whether this is helping or not. As a veterinary surgeon I have been educated in classical medicine, and the concept of alternative remedies is foreign to me. But the persistence of the pain is distressing and as conventional medicine has failed to help me for over three years I am prepared to try other means.

My physical problems are compounded by psychological ones. I also suffer from depression, which was not caused by my physical problems but has no doubt been exacerbated by them. The disease reared its ugly head when I was suicidally depressed just before my brain tumour was diagnosed. I have suffered from it many times thereafter. I think that my psychological problems, which are still present, would have been reduced by better adjunctive therapy when I first had surgery. I received no psychotherapy, occupational therapy, or speech therapy, and only a little physiotherapy. All of these are important for a patient with a disease whose outcome has such a profound influence on all aspects of life. I do not know why I did not receive better therapy while I was in hospital. Everything was such a blur at the time so I did not realise the deficiency until after I returned home.

My disabilities have had a major effect on my career. At first I did not know whether I was going to be able to return to my profession, but as I improved it seemed that I was. But how was I to go about this to make a living. Fortuitously, I had chosen to specialise in canine and feline internal medicine, which is one of the least physical specialties. But I still needed a lot of help in many aspects of clinical work.

For over a year after my radiotherapy I was jobless. But I could not bear the inertia and wanted to show that I was capable of working. I was offered a year's post as honorary resident in radiology at the University of Liverpool. This fulfilled the criteria but as the job was unpaid I had to rely on social security. After this I moved to London to study for a PhD. This was funded by a grant from the Wellcome Trust, but the project was fraught with difficulties, particularly my physical disabilities, and I quit my studies after 14 months.

I had to look my future squarely in the face. I had spent my time since my craniotomy in non-clinical pursuits, but I longed to return to clinical work. There is a major difference between veterinary medicine and medicine; the latter is more specialised. Most vets in clinical work are in general practice. This was impossible for me as I could not drive, do out of hours work unaided, or perform surgery.

I decided to tailor a job for myself and I set myself up as a self employed consultant in canine and feline internal medicine, a subject in which I am acknowledgeable. Unfortunately, compared with the United States, private referral services are in an embryonic state in Britain. In five months I saw only three cases, so this idea has been a failure. I have to accept that clinical work is a closed book to me. I spend most of my time at home with little money coming in. I am investigating several non-clinical possibilities, both in and outside the veterinary profession. I do not want to leave it but I may be forced to do so.

There does not seem to be a shortage of non-clinical jobs for vets, but there are none at present. Having worked predominantly in clinical veterinary medicine my knowledge of non-clinical possibilities is poor. I started my investigations by writing to the Royal College of Veterinary Surgeons and the British Veterinary Association. They gave me several names, addresses, and telephone numbers to start my job search.

On the other hand, my social life is a success story. I live in a lovely flat with my husband and two Abyssinian cats. The wedding was in the chapel of my Cambridge college. I know that I am lucky and I am looking forward to sharing the rest of my life with a lovely man, but my happiness is tinged with regret that my life will be marred by pain and physical disabilities.

It is hard to imagine all the far reaching consequences of major disease unless you suffer them. My cerebellar ataxia causes me to have a drunken gait, which makes many people stare at me. My poor balance makes walking difficult and I frequently bang into obstacles and sometimes fall over. This results in bruises and grazes. Occasionally, the outcome is more serious. I celebrated my fiancé's proposal in Paris by falling over and breaking my right fifth metatarsal.

I have attempted to show how a relatively small lesion has had an enormous effect on many aspects of my life. Three years ago my tale was largely one of woe. It is little changed but I hope that life will be better in the years to come.

(Mainwaring 1993)

COMMENTARY

Mainwaring's lesion, a cerebellar medulloblastoma, mainly resulted in physical symptoms such as difficulty in walking, motor difficulties in writing, and double vision. In terms of specific diagnostic issues, her case provides an example of the difficulty in distinguishing multiple sclerosis from a cerebellar tumour in a young lady with clinical features that include ataxia and nystagmus. There are also a few general lessons with regard to patient management that arise from her article. She points to the importance of non-medical therapies, such as counselling with regard to the side-effects of treatment, and speech therapy/occupational therapy to help deal with everyday adjustment after leaving hospital. She considers that these may help to reduce the likelihood of significant depression occurring as a result of the various disabilities associated with a major illness. She notes that semi-platitudes—such as 'Lots of people have this difficulty'—do not help! It is interesting that she did not report major cognitive difficulties. Recent functional imaging studies (Posner and Raichle 1994) have pointed to the importance of the cerebellum in a wide range of cognitive tasks, ranging from attention to language. In general, lesion studies have appeared to yield evidence of minimal or rather subtle cognitive deficits (Grafman *et al.* 1992), and there remains a relative anomaly *vis-à-vis* functional imaging data from normal subjects.

REFERENCES

Grafman, J., Litvan, I., Massaquoi, S., Stewart, M., Sirigu, A., and Hallett, M. (1992). Cognitive planning deficit in patients with cerebellar degeneration. *Neurology*, **42**, 1493–6.

Posner, M. and Raichle, M. (1994). *Images of mind*. Freeman, New York.

Stroke 6

INTRODUCTION

The incidence of stroke is estimated to be around two new cases every year per 1000 individuals, and it is estimated that in a community of 1000 people there will, at any one time, be around five individuals who have suffered a stroke. Strokes are usually divided into two types. One type of stroke, which probably accounts for around 85% of stroke cases, is a cerebral infarct. This results from blockage in an artery, with a resultant lack of oxygen to brain tissue supplied by the artery or by its branches—this type of stroke generally affects the older population. In the second type, there is a rupture of the wall of an artery, with resultant haemorrhage and destruction of neighbouring brain tissue—this type of stroke may affect both younger and older people.

Strokes represent a particularly fruitful source of observations from medical minds that have been afflicted with a major, acute insult to the brain—this is partly because, compared to other common neurological conditions, such as head injury, there is a much lower incidence of amnesia for events around the time of the insult (Grotta and Bratina 1995). Thus, stroke patients will tend to retain more vivid recollections of their feelings during the acute stages of their illness. This may be due to the more diffuse pathology, and greater temporal lobe involvement, in head injury compared to stroke.

As in the case of brain tumours, the effects of strokes on psychological functioning will depend on factors such as the age of the individual, the location of the stroke, the size of the area which has been damaged as a result of the stroke; and other factors such as any generalized brain swelling caused by the stroke and the effects of the stroke on the flow of cerebrospinal fluid. In general, cerebral haemorrhage will result in more notable effects on brain function than a cerebral infarct, though other factors such as those mentioned above will also determine the overall level of functional disability that ensues.

Cerebrovascular dysfunction may also be manifest in milder ways, often as transient abnormalities in cerebral blood flow. This may take the form of 'transient ischaemic attacks', where there is a temporary reduction in blood flow in a particular artery, with resultant lack of oxygen to a part of the brain and a temporary neurological deficit. Transient global amnesia (TGA) and migraine are also thought to represent a disturbance of cerebral blood flow, perhaps due to spasm of certain arteries, though the precise nature of this disturbance remains uncertain. Cases of TGA and migraine are presented in Chapters 2 and 3 of this book.

While a number of other articles in the book (e.g. **Moss, Kolb**) are also based on patients who have had a stroke, the papers in this section give greater prominence to the clinical and everyday problems associated with a major cerebrovascular event. Five of the articles relate to strokes that involved the right hemisphere (**Brodal, Kyle, Howell, Smithells,** and **Medawar**), one stroke compromised the left hemisphere (**Buck**), and in the remaining two cases there was involvement of the brainstem (**Goldberg, Coubrough**). It would seem that **Medawar**'s case was the only one of cerebral haemorrhage, and the only one that required surgical intervention, while the others were due to cerebral infarction and were treated by solely medical means.

REFERENCE

Grotta, J. and Bratina, P. (1995). Subjective experiences of 24 patients dramatically recovering from stroke. *Stroke*, **26**, 1285–8.

FURTHER READING

Caplan, L. (1993). *Stroke* (2nd edn). Butterworth–Heinemann, New York.

Skilbeck, C. (1992). Neuropsychological assessment in stroke. In *A handbook of neuropsychological assessment* (ed. J. R. Crawford, D. M. Parker, and W. W. McKinley), pp. 339–61. Lawrence Erlbaum, Hove, UK.

Wade, D. T., Langton-Hewer, R., Skilbeck, C. E., and David, R. M. (1985). *Stroke: A critical approach to diagnosis, treatment and management*. Chapman & Hall, London.

The language disorders

McKenzie Buck, Ph.D.

McKenzie Buck appears to have been working as a psychologist around the time of his stroke.

In light of professional contacts with stricken patients during my post-stroke years, it has become evident that my personal experiences are markedly similar to the majority of those expressed by other patients and their family groups. It is important to stress that patients with similar degrees of recovery are those who were fortunate in having family members demonstrate positive warmth, affection, and acceptance as a result of continuous professional guidance.

Unfortunately far too many immediate families, as well as professional personnel, seem to concentrate on isolated behavioral and physical problems. If we are to provide maximum assistance, the patient must be viewed as a total human being. Sole concentration upon the deviated aspects of the illness is bound to have a negative effect upon well members of the family for they, too, may demonstrate obvious behavioral changes that can be detrimental to the patient's adjustment.

A stroke is actually a family illness and assistance should be readily available for the entire household.

The side effects of brain damage may markedly deter the recovery process. When there is a history of neurological trauma, such as a stroke, epilepsy is apt to develop, This is not a shameful disorder and is a condition that has nothing to do with insanity or heredity. Physicians now know that approximately 8 out of every 10 persons who have seizures can lead relatively normal lives. We in the behavioral areas must do our utmost to recognize symptoms that may reveal one of the many types of seizure patterns and thus assist physicians in their diagnostic procedures.

Epileptic attacks are most assuredly frightening for both the patient and his family. I can speak of this with firsthand information.

Shortly after my first stroke in 1957, I experienced a severe convulsion. It was not until this extreme attack occurred that a *Jacksonian* type of epilepsy was recognized. Since this time, medication has controlled the severity and frequency of such episodes. This kind of attack is similar to the *Grand-Mal* seizure in that there may be a total loss of consciousness. However, immediately after the stroke, I was one of the vast number of stricken patients who did not experience a complete loss of consciousness; consequently, it was extremely difficult to diagnose without an accurate observational report from my own family group.

Without a competent degree of language recovery to assist in my description of sensations, it was impossible for laymen to understand periods of extreme irritability and increased aphasic type disruptions. One of the major psychological avenues of relief and adjustment was highly dependent upon my ventilating feelings of fear and depression that were so easily stimulated by the approach of the epileptic attacks.

Such attacks, far too often, are simply interpreted as patterns of functional obnoxious behavior, and often result in a patient's being dropped from therapeutic programs prior to interprofessional consultations.

As one may readily understand, the lessening or complete removal of such attacks may greatly contribute to emotional and intellectual improvements in such patients. The family must maintain close contact with their attending physician, thus assisting him in the acquisition of information that may be pertinent to thorough medical treatment.

We as professionals are obligated to provide careful family instruction to assist in lessening the fears that may exist in the minds of those within the household. Such a procedure is far more important to patient recovery than any retraining techniques recommended in our literature. As may be well recognised, *your* best learning situations were those in which you experienced the least amount of depressing threats.

It is important to be continually aware of the fact that the patient may have an extreme inability to quickly recall both current and past events. The stricken patient can suffer drastic emotional disturbances all too suddenly when we do not have a thorough understanding of this behavior. If he is subjected to a continuous sequence of unreasonable demands, he has no choice but to voluntarily remain silent and completely withdraw from any social situation. When this occurs, the depressive psychological overlay may stimulate extreme suicidal plans and/or actual attempts.

If we can only recognize our own limitations in trying to follow a highly technical discussion of some topic such as atomic energy, we may gain some insight into the conversational problems being experienced by the stricken patient. For example, in reading the newspaper we 'normals' seek articles that have a personal appeal. These bits of information usually have a vocabulary that is easily understood, resulting in an appropriate interpretation of the content. We tend to ignore articles utilizing a lengthy technical vocabulary.

This type of behavior is actually no different from that of a patient who has even more difficulty with memory spans and language interpretations. We must be extremely cautious, when speaking with stroke patients, to utilize a simple vocabulary combined with a frequent referral to the topic being discussed.

An example of the extreme limitations in memory may be demonstrated by a discussion of my own deviations immediately following the stroke. For a matter of several months, it was not uncommon for me to eat a large breakfast at 8 a.m., then by 9 a.m. be wondering why I had not had breakfast. During this hour my internal body pressure from the food intake had often completely disappeared. Aside from the basic necessities of survival—combined with an attempt to acquire a pleasurable experience—there was little else to occupy my mind.

My insightful wife would calmly discuss the fact that I had eaten breakfast and, for the most part, I would have an immediate recall when I was *quietly* reminded of the event.

However, behavior of this type is not as readily understood by personnel outside of the family; we, as professional persons, must keep in mind that the patient usually has an immediate recall of events if they are noted in a kind and easy manner by those within the situation. This kind of behavior is usually not pursued merely to attract attention, for it is most often a result of an extremely short memory span and self-disgust.

When the patient begins to initiate obvious symptoms of insight, it is necessary that we remember he is bound to have some internal disgust concerning his failure in recalling current activities. He is condemning himself enough without suffering an increase of frustration resulting from negative comments by family and clinical personnel. You may assuredly contribute to the alleviation of deep and morbid depression through the quiet acceptance of repeated behavior for, as time progresses, the patient will likely acquire further insight to assist himself in maintaining improved emotional stability.

At this point, it must be strongly emphasized that there is an unfortunate degree of professional failure concerning careful intellectual evaluations. Intelligence tests frequently reveal variations in different types of thought processes. For the most part, the normal individual will acquire scores that are relatively equal in the various portions of the test such as problem solving, vocabulary, arithmetic, etc. This is not necessarily true of the brain damaged patient, however, for he may reveal a high problem solving score in contrast to a very low vocabulary score. In other words, there is not an over-all reduction of scores on all types of tests in the intellectual evaluation.

Prior to any clinical retraining, every attempt should be made to at least estimate the patient's current intellectual ability. If, for example, he has a score in the 60's—such as I experienced initially—extreme care must be taken to avoid an unrealistically high degree of professional expectation. Far too often, this particular means of evaluation is overlooked and retesting is completely absent.

The patient should have repeated intellectual evaluations at least every four to six weeks. In this manner, our clinical procedures may be far more realistic, both in terms of family insights and patient abilities. Forced retraining may destroy even reasonable expectations when the patient is continually confronted with demoralizing results which, in turn, amplify stronger desires for complete withdrawal from society. Again it must be stressed that we are obligated to maintain consistent and lengthy family contact to assist us in the maintenance of appropriate training procedures.

Family and professional personnel must keep in mind that the patient is basically starting over again and it is absolutely essential that we demonstrate as much insight and kindness in this instance as we do with the very young child who is acquiring initial language and social development.

We rarely push, over-pressure, or over-anticipate rapid vocabulary development within the child. A youngster acquires his language through kind, patient, and non-direct stimulation over a period of several years. Perhaps with this in mind, we should re-examine our professional approach to the language problem of the stricken patient.

From a personal standpoint, I found no assistance from direct vocabulary and language drills. The majority of my successes were almost wholly dependent upon my psychological security and the deletion of unrealistic pressures concerning word by word expression in conversations. It was not until the word and language drills were withdrawn entirely that I began to experience a significant degree of reasonable expression. Professionally, we need to examine our own language behavior in order that we may understand the problems involved with the aphasic disorder.

Some persons reading this article may have had very disturbing experiences in classes dealing with public address. Initially at least the greatest difficulties in formulating speeches were concerned with an over-attention to language formation and expression. This resulted in grossly uninteresting presentations combined with emotional traumas that disturbed reasonable communication, leaving the student in a complete state of exhaustion upon the completion of the exercise.

As time progresses, however, such persons may acquire an ability to pay less attention to the sequence of verbal expression, thus returning to a more normal conversational manner. Consequently, a predominance of the efforts can be concentrated upon thought processes of interest to the speaker and contagious to those within the audience. Unfortunately, certain individuals are unable to eventually delete their attention to verbal expressions and, as a result, the message continues to be lost to both the speaker and his listener.

If this occurs among those who have no apparent neurological damage, does it not seem reasonable that a stricken patient should also have markedly similar anxieties? It is important to stress that such a patient is already over-concerned without having negative reactions from those within the immediate environment and clinical settings.

It was not until I found it possible to ignore the 'big ears' of those about me that I began to demonstrate progress in free expression. Language exercises were useless despite the word drills in booklets, pictures, etc. The recovery process was really no different than the initial vocabulary enlargement experiences as a youngster. The less I concentrated upon individual words, the more meaningful my expression became, resulting in fewer fears and thus lessening feelings of inadequacy.

I still have unpredictable periods of difficulty concerning the recall of proper names. Fatigue appears to have no bearing upon the disorder and, quite frankly, I have no explanation for the causation of the apparent neurological short circuits. It is quite evident that I shall be unsuccessful, for the most part, in attempting to explain the problem. My emotional adjustments are far more secure if I simply skip any explanation and proceed as though I feel as normal as those about me. This, as you may well understand, was not an easy attitude to develop and it requires an abundance of self-discipline.

Other patients, with a similar history, have expressed identical reactions to their experiences with word drills, picture games, and over-stimulation. Also, the families of other patients who progressed satisfactorily simply accepted each individual as a *person* who may respond appropriately with extensive patience, courtesy, and time. In view of the preceding, it seems apparent that we need to carefully re-examine our clinical procedures.

In summary, the major considerations in personal and language adjustment of the stricken patient involve far more than language drills in isolation. First of all, careful medical care must be established. Unless the family members have enough information to assist in motivating them to be extremely conscientious, the medical follow-up may be deterred due to their lack of careful cooperation.

As far as any language retraining is concerned, some will be of little value until the overlying psychological disruptions are well-controlled. Undue pressures in solving unrealistic language drills may markedly interfere with both psychological and physical adjustments.

This point is stressed to emphasize the fact that most brain damaged patients have unpredictable periods of extreme neurological and physical fatigue. With fatigue comes discouragement, and any learning process of abstract materials may well lead to chronic states of depressive withdrawal.

Careful family guidance should continually be available, for it is the family who can do most to assist in language retraining. Unless they have a thorough understanding of the total picture, they, too, may join the patient in attempting to escape from the situation.

(Buck 1963)

COMMENTARY

Although Buck's paper is entitled 'The language disorders', it offers more general observations relating to the understanding of patients' needs, emotions and behaviour after a stroke. Buck highlights the importance of dealing adequately with the emotional side of adjustment in the overall management of the patient. He points out that epileptic seizures may be manifest as behavioural and emotional difficulties which result from a need to ventilate feelings of fear and depression that in turn are precipitated by an impending fit.

Buck remarks, 'It is important to be continually aware of the fact that the patient may have an extreme inability to quickly recall both current and past events' (p. 247). His observation suggests that a generalized retrieval failure for both episodic and semantic memories may accompany some forms of dysphasia, although it is not possible to say if one retrieval mechanism serves both types of information. Buck emphasizes the use of simple vocabulary when talking to patients with language disorder. He reports an interesting experience of having lost bodily sensory memories of having eaten breakfast one hour earlier—there must also have been an autobiographical memory loss for the event itself, which suggests the presence of significant memory impairment. He indicates that such memory would return if he was reminded in a quiet and tactful manner. He mentions that memory loss may result in frustration, a feeling of disgust with oneself, and that this may then result in emotional difficulties. Inability to cope with these or similar cognitive demands may lead to a withdrawal from any social situation.

In contrast to the views of Rose reported in Chapter 2 on language disorders, Buck speaks out against forced retraining, and against direct vocabulary learning and language drills/exercises—he points out that these may in fact be demoralizing if they result in failure on the practice tasks. He reports that 'most brain damaged patients have unpredictable periods of extreme neurological and physical fatigue' (p. 249), and this also needs to be borne in mind by therapists and relatives alike.

Self-observations and neuro-anatomical considerations after a stroke

A. Brodal

A. Brodal was a renowned professor of anatomy, who specialized in neuroanatomy.

The present report is based on certain observations which the author made on himself following an acute left-sided hemiparesis. They are certainly not unique, but they may be better described by one with knowledge of the brain than by a layman. Some questions may be raised on the basis of these observations, and they may be of interest in directing my colleagues' attention to certain problems. As a basis for an evaluation of the observations, in part purely subjective, it will be appropriate to give a short report of the case and to discuss the probable site of the cerebral lesion.

CASE REPORT

The patient is a 62–year-old professor of anatomy who was suddenly taken ill during a lecture-trip abroad. He had had no serious ailments. About a year before, one evening in the course of a few minutes he suddenly had paræsthesiæ around the left corner of the mouth, in the radial side of the left hand and in the left great toe. There was dizziness on vertical movements of the head. The paræsthesiæ and the dizziness persisted, although in diminishing intensity, for nine months. An examination (Professor K. Kristiansen) as well as X-ray examination of the skull and an EEG two weeks after the onset showed no changes.

The present illness started suddenly when the patient woke up and turned in his bed on the morning of April 12, 1972. In the course of a few minutes an initial heavy, but uncharacteristic, dizziness was followed by dysarthria, double vision and a marked paresis of the left arm and leg. There was no loss of consciousness, no headache or vomiting and no stiffness of the neck. In the very beginning there were paræsthesiæ of the left side of the head, especially the scalp. The patient was immediately brought to the Clinica de Santa Teresa in Coimbra under the supervision of Professor N. Vicente. On the fourth day he was transported to

Oslo by plane and transferred to the Neurosurgical Department at Ulleval Hospital (Professor K. Kristiansen).

The findings in Oslo were like those in Coimbra, except for some signs which had disappeared or become less marked in the first days. Thus the double vision, due to gaze paralysis to the left, receded gradually and disappeared on the third day; the paræsthesiæ on the left side disappeared on the second. The initial nystagmus on looking to the left was less. Otherwise there was a left central facial paresis, slight hypoæsthesia of the left cornea (left corneal reflex the weaker), but no deviation of the palate or tongue, no visual disorder, and only slight nystagmus on extreme left gaze. Sensation was normal. Coordination was impaired corresponding to the paresis. The tendon reflexes in the left leg were brisker than in the right, the left plantar reflex was extensor.

The left-sided paresis was almost a complete paralysis on the first day. It gradually improved, so that on the fifth day some slight movement of the finger flexors and the flexors of the elbow were possible. Strength at the shoulder was better than at the elbow. Extension of fingers, especially the thumb, was impossible. Dorsiflexion of the toes and dorsiflexion and pronation of the left foot were completely abolished, flexion at the knee and hip was weak while extension at the hip and knee as well as plantar flexion of the foot was fairly good.

Investigations of heart (including electrocardiography), blood and urine were normal as were blood pressure and blood cholesterol. Electroencephalography suggested a deeply seated right-sided lesion. Electronystagmography (April 22) did not localize the site of the lesion, except that the peripheral vestibular and acoustic apparatus (pure tone audiometry) were normal. Bilateral carotid and vertebral angiography showed normal intracranial vessels and good communication between the two carotid arteries and between these and the vertebral arteries. A right-sided carotid stenosis was found in the neck, probably caused by an atherosclerotic plaque extending from the right common carotid into the carotid sinus and obliterating half the lumen of the internal carotid artery. Since it was assumed that the hemiparesis was caused by loosening of an embolus from this atherosclerotic plaque it was decided to remove this surgically. This was done on April 27. The post-operative course was uneventful. The patient was discharged from hospital on May 13, one month after the stroke.

During the entire period in hospital and later, the patient regularly received physiotherapy, the first days only passive movements on the left side, later increasingly demanding active exercises. As is usual there was in the beginning a fairly rapid and extensive recovery. Two months after the stroke the patient was, for example, able to button and unbutton his clothes and to handle a fork when eating, although clumsily and with reduced power, and both needed much more attention and energy than normally. Later, a slow but steady improvement took place. After some six months the patient could walk fairly well, and could use his left arm and hand (although not satisfactorily) for most things, and there was a gradual improvement of the initially marked dysarthria and dizziness and mental capacity.

The lesion

The symptoms at the onset and during the further course of the disease make it almost certain that there had been an embolism to the right hemisphere. Although some of the symptoms, such as dizziness and the disturbances of gaze, might be explained by a brain-stem lesion, it is more likely that there was an occlusion of a branch of the right middle cerebral artery causing an infarction of part of the right internal capsule and its surroundings. The obstruction presumably involved dorsal parts of the capsule. The clinical picture corresponded to what Fisher and Curry (1965) have termed 'pure motor hemiplegia,' that is a hemiplegia without somatosensory impairment, visual field defects, dysphasia or apractagnosia. In 6 out of 9 cases of this type which came to autopsy, there was damage of the posterior part of the internal capsule, where the corticospinal fibres are assumed to be located (see Smith, 1967). In these cases the hemiplegias were probably due to thrombosis. The intact visual fields in the present case as in those described by Fisher and Curry (1965) indicate that the optic radiation is undamaged, and that the lesion is consequently relatively high in the posterior part of the capsule. The marked dizziness and the slight spontaneous nystagmus at the beginning as well as the asymmetrical electronystagmographic recordings might be due to interruption of some as yet little known connexions between the cerebral cortex and the vestibular nuclei, as assumed, for example, by Carmichael, Dix and Hallpike (1954). Although the anatomical connexions concerned are not yet known, it is of interest to note that recent research (see Fredrickson, Figge, Scheid and Kornhuber, 1966) indicates the presence in the monkey of a vestibular cortical area in the posterior part of the postcentral gyrus, in what appears to be, cytoarchitectonically, area 2 (see also Boisacq-Schepens and Hanus, 1972), and that recently Gildenberg and Hassler (1971) have recorded potentials in the vestibular nuclei in the cat following stimulation of what they refer to as cortical areas 2 pri and 6a. Furthermore, it is of relevance that occasionally patients have dizziness after stereotactic operations for parkinsonism, when the electrode has presumably entered the internal capsule, but where the brain-stem has not been touched. The problem of the cerebral corticovestibular relations will not be pursued further here (for reference see Markham, 1972). An alternative explanation would be that the dizziness was caused by interruption of cortical fibres acting on the extrinsic eye muscles (see Wagman and Mehler, 1973). In either case it appears that the clinical picture in the present case is compatible with a lesion involving the posterior part of the right internal capsule. A lesion situated in the brain-stem, for example the pons-mesencephalon, could give a rather similar clinical picture as seen in the patient (especially, it could be responsible for the vestibular and gaze disturbances), but a lesion of this location would probably result in damage to the right cranial nerves. It may be noted that in an extensive autopsy material of thrombo-embolic cerebral lesions Jörgensen and Torvik (1969) found that embolic brain lesions are far more common in the region of the middle cerebral artery than in the territory of the vertebral artery (83 against 19, and of the latter only 8 were infratentorial). An embolus responsible for a lesion of the brain-stem would most likely have had to enter through the right vertebral artery.

Although in this case, as usual, one is left in some uncertainly when trying to determine the site of a lesion on the basis of clinical findings, it will be assumed below that there has been an embolism in a branch of the middle cerebral artery supplying the posterior, upper part of the right internal capsule and adjacent territories and, furthermore, that there has been no damage to the left half of the brain.

SOME OBSERVATIONS ON VOLUNTARY MOVEMENTS OF MUSCLES AFFECTED BY A 'CENTRAL PARESIS'

Only some aspects of this extensive problem complex will be considered here. Attention will be drawn to some subjective experiences which are apparently only rarely considered in discussions of hemipareses.

Force of innervation. It was a striking and repeatedly made observation that the force needed to make a severely paretic muscle contract is considerable. The expression force in this connexion refers to what one, for lack of a better expression, might call force of innervation. Subjectively this is experienced as a kind of mental force, a power of will. In the case of a muscle just capable of being actively moved the mental effort needed was very great. Subjectively it felt as if the muscle was unwilling to contract, and as if there was a resistance which could be overcome by very strong voluntary innervation. The greater the degree of paresis of such a muscle, the greater was the mental effort needed to make it contract and to oppose voluntarily even a very weak counterforce. On the other hand only a slight mental effort was needed to bring about a fairly good contraction of a muscle able to work with about half or a little less of its full force.

This force of innervation is obviously some kind of *mental* energy which cannot be quantified or defined more closely, but the result of which is seen as a contraction of the muscle(s) in question. The expenditure of this mental energy is very exhausting, a fact of some importance in physiotherapeutic treatment. To a lesser degree it is felt in all innervations of paretic muscles when they get tired, for example in walking, when one has to concentrate on the process of moving the leg properly, in contrast to that for a normal leg. One can only speculate upon how this mental energy is ultimately transferred to mechanical energy, a question related to the apparently insoluble mind-body problem.

The value of passive movements in training. It is generally agreed that in the physio-therapeutic treatment of pareses, passive movements may be desirable, and often even necessary, to prevent shrinking of joint capsules, ligaments and muscles. There is less unanimity about other reasons for using passive movements, for instance in order to facilitate subsequent active contraction of the relevant muscles. In the patient's experience this undoubtedly occurs, particularly when a muscle is just resuming the capacity to respond to a voluntary impulse. At the beginning it often happened that the patient, even with his strongest effort, was unable to make a voluntary movement of a particular joint, for example, pronation of the foot (the peroneal muscles), but when the proper movement had been made passively by the physiotherapist a couple of times, the patient was able to perform the movement, although with minimal force. Subjectively it was clearly felt as if the sensory information produced by the passive movement helped the patient to 'direct' the 'force of innervation' through the proper channels. The effect was not due to the removal of passive resistance caused by shrinking of structures, since the relevant joints in the cases when the phenomenon could be tested had normal range of passive movements. It may well be that there are subtle neurophysiological mechanisms involved in this 'facilitation' of movements. From introspection it appears, however, that the subjective information about the movement to be executed, its range and goal, is an essential factor. The phenomenon is probably parallel to the learning of all motor skills. Among an original multitude of more or less haphazard movements the correct ones are recognized as such by means of the sensory information they feed back to the central nervous system, and this information is later used in selecting the correct movements in the further training.

Muscle sense. It has been debated whether sensations from muscles (apart from pain) are consciously perceived, and whether they contribute to give subjectively recognized information about movements and positions of joints (for a historical review, *see* Goodwin *et al.*, 1972). A particular question has been whether afferent impulses from the muscle spindles are involved. While some earlier observations in man were interpreted as giving a negative answer to both questions, there is now fairly good evidence to the contrary. It has been demonstrated experimentally in the cat (*see*, for example, Landgren, Silfvenius and Wolsk, 1967; Landgren and Silfvenius, 1969) as well as in the monkey (Albe-Fessard and Liebeskind, 1966; Phillips, Powell and Wiesendanger, 1971) that impulses arising in primary sensory afferents from muscle spindles evoke potentials in the sensorimotor cortex. While it is doubtful whether these impulses are consciously perceived in the cat and monkey, the fact that they reach the cerebral cortex strongly suggests that they are at least involved in motor control. In man, the recent experiments of Goodwin, McCloskey and Matthews (1972) and Eklund (1972) seem to leave little doubt that sensory information from the muscles contributes appreciably to the conscious evaluation of the position of the limbs, and it appears that the muscle spindles are important as receptors for kinæsthetic sensations.

Some observations made by the author are in agreement with the view that information from the muscles reaches consciousness.

In the first weeks following the stroke, very little active movements of the fingers were possible. When the fingers had not been moved for some time, the patient, as is usual, had no feeling of his muscles in the hand and forearm and of the position of the finger-joints, but when making the first movements with the fingers, even very slowly, a feeling of resistance was obvious to him, giving the subjective impression of what could best be described as 'stiffness.' On repeating the movement this feeling increased as did the objectively observed spasticity. This feeling, not being known to the patient before, was at first assumed to be derived from the joints or to be caused by slight œdema of the hand, and was not recognized as coming from the muscles. This became clear to the patient only later when he had some control of his finger movements. It should be noted that the joints were all freely movable, and the subjective feeling could be localized to particular muscles, for example particular interossei. The subjective feeling apparently occurs parallel to the objectively recognizable spasticity. Probably the increased

activity of the spindles (which are numerous in the small finger muscles) facilitates the subjective awareness of the tension of the muscle. Even if these observations, like some earlier observations by Chambers and Gilliat (1954) are made in a pathological condition, they are in agreement with the recent experimental findings, and show that sensations of tension of muscles can indeed be consciously perceived. For a discussion of the possible role of such afferent impulses in the appreciation of movement *see* Granit (1972) and Goodwin *et al.* (1972).

Skilled movements.   For some forty years the patient has used a bow tie almost daily and has tied it every morning. When he had to do this for the first time again after the stroke (some two months later) it was, as expected, very difficult and he had to make seven to ten attempts before he finally succeeded. The appropriate finger movements were difficult to perform with sufficient strength, speed and co-ordination, but it was quite obvious to the patient that the main reason for the failure was something else.

Under normal conditions the necessary numerous small delicate movements had followed each other in the proper sequence almost automatically, and the act of tying when first started had proceeded without much conscious attention. Subjectively the patient felt as if he had to stop because 'his fingers did not know the next move.' He had the same feeling as when one recites a poem or sings a song and gets lost. The only way is to start from the beginning. It was felt as if the delay in the succession of movements (due to pareses and spasticity) interrupted a chain of more or less automatic movements. Consciously directing attention to the finger movements did not improve the performance; on the contrary it made it quite impossible.

The tying of a tie is a particularly good example of what one could call an automatized manual skill, and one which can be broken down into a long series of particular co-ordinated finger movements. Even if we are here dealing with a relatively complicated motor skill which is acquired only by learning, it appears in many ways to be similar to other movements where learning is presumably superimposed upon some inborn capacity, as for example walking. From an analysis of the act of stepping it appears that the basic mechanism of the alternating activation of extensors and flexors in stepping is centrally programmed in the spinal cord, and does not occur exclusively by way of reflexes (Lundberg, 1969, p. 11). Presumably the basic programme is in part modified by learning.

It is relevant in this connexion to recall an important fact which Granit (1972, p. 649) phrases as follows: 'Even those movements which we regard as voluntary are largely automatic. Most of them intrude upon consciousness only at the moment when they are triggered off into action'. What is apparently defective in the patient's tying is not the triggering off of the act. There appears to be a lacking of capacity to let the movements proceed automatically when the pattern is triggered because they cannot be performed with the usual speed.

We can so far only speculate upon where in the nervous system the neurons are situated which form the morphological basis of the neural programme which secures proper sequential innervation of the particular α and γ motoneurons concerned. There is no convincing evidence that the cerebral cortex is the main region. Nothing resembling skilled movements is seen in response to electrical stimulation of the cerebral cortex (Penfield and Jasper, 1954). There appear to be more data in favour of the assumption (see Bates, 1957) that the fundamental patterns of discrete movements are largely organized at the spinal level.

SOME OBSERVATIONS ON COMPLEX FUNCTIONS

Among functions affected by hemispheric lesions those related to speech and mental activities have attracted much interest. Below, some of the patients' observations on writing and speech will be described and briefly discussed.

Writing. Thinking, as most neurologists probably do, that in right-handed persons writing is governed solely by the left hemisphere, it came as a surprise to the patient that there were clear-cut changes in his handwriting after the stroke. Such changes may probably be easily overlooked in cases of right-sided brain damage, as patients do not write soon after a stroke and so are not likely to notice more subtle changes in their handwriting. Even if the situation has changed since 1954, it is appropriate to recall Critchley's words (1954, p. 5) when he says, speak-

ing of the neurologist's habits in examining cases of unilateral brain damage: 'We are apt to ignore those faculties other than speech which may be impaired by unilateral brain disease.'

The patient is right-handed and has always used his right hand for writing and drawing, although to some extent he could use his left hand for simpler procedures such as to hit a nail with a hammer, to stroke a brush of wet paint on a wall, to saw, etc. Fig. 1 shows examples of his handwriting before and after the stroke. It may be argued that the specimens are not representative, and that factors such as tiredness, a more or less awkward position of the right arm and hand when writing etc., may explain the differences, but the changes were observed constantly, and were present even under the most favourable conditions for writing. The main changes were as follows:

There was a tendency for the lines of writing to be uneven or oblique, not horizontal, and the distance between the lines were often uneven. The shape of the individual letters tended to be more irregular than previously, they were less smooth, and the last stroke in the writing (up or down) was sometimes missed or it was incomplete or exaggerated. Furthermore, there was often dropping out of one or two letters or of a word, or a letter which should be doubled was repeated three times (letttter instead of letter). More often than before figures were interchanged, for example he wrote 46 instead of 64. These changes in his writing gradually became less marked, but they could still be noticed more than nine months after the stroke.

While the former phenomena clearly indicate a defective control of the motor functions of the right hand, the skipping or doubling of letters, etc., is scarcely a pure motor phenomenon, but suggests some kind of apractic disturbance related to language functions (see below). It should be noted that there were no signs of aphasia according to the patient's own judgement as well as to the observations of his colleagues and his family.

Provided that the cerebral lesion is unilateral as assumed, the question arises, how are the motor changes in handwriting to be explained? Before attempting to answer this question, it will be appropriate to recall briefly a few data concerning the innervation of muscle (for recent complete reviews, see Evarts and Thach, 1969; Granit, 1970; Brooks and Stoney, 1971).

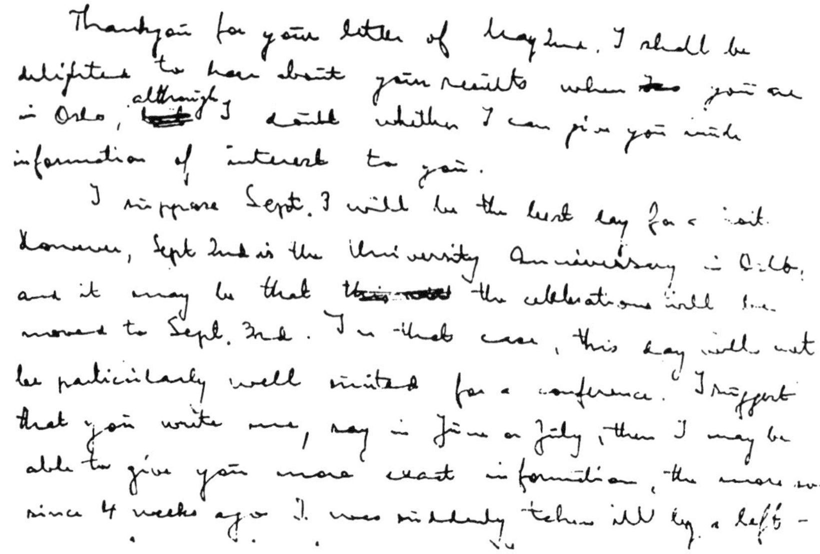
Thank you for your letter of May 2nd. I shall be delighted to hear about your results when you are in Oslo, although I doubt whether I can give you much information of interest to you.
I suppose Sept. 3 will be the best day for a visit. However, Sept 2nd is the University Anniversary in Oslo, and it may be that the celebrations will be moved to Sept. 3rd. In that case, this day will not be particularly well suited for a conference. I suggest that you write me, say in June or July, then I may be able to give you more exact information, the more so since 4 weeks ago I was suddenly taken ill by a left-

A

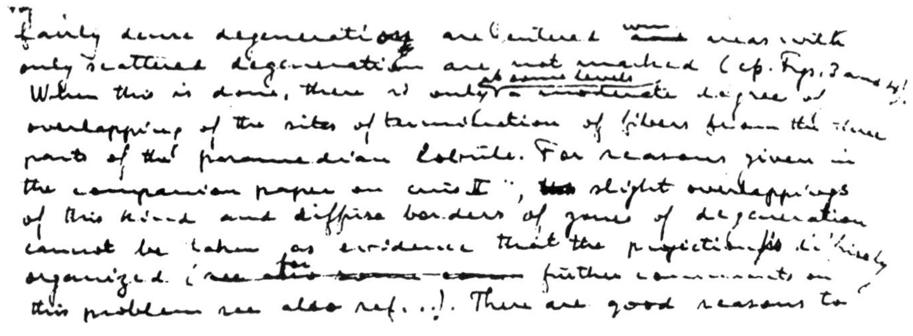
fairly dense degeneration are combined with areas with only scattered degeneration are not marked (cf. Figs. 3 and 4). When this is done, there is only a moderate degree of overlapping of the sites of termination of fibers from the three parts of the paramedian lobule. For reasons given in the companion paper on crus II, slight overlappings of this kind and diffuse borders of zones of degeneration cannot be taken as evidence that the projection is diffusely organized. (further comments on this problem see also ref...). There are good reasons to

B

Figure 1. A, Part of a letter written a month after the stroke on lined paper. B, Part of the first draft of a paper six months before, on plain paper. Note the irregularities of letters, lines and intervals in A.

The classical notion that the corticospinal (pyramidal) tract is of particular importance for skilled and delicate voluntary hand and finger movements appears to be in essence correct, even if it is obvious that a number of other—indirect—routes for corticospinal impulses (through the brain-stem nuclei, the reticular formation and the cerebellum) are involved in addition, and that one has to consider the role of γ- as well as α-motoneuron innervation. It appears that the pyramidal innervation may superimpose speed and agility on the mechanisms subserved by other descending pathways (*see* Lawrence and Kuypurs, 1968). The pyramidal tract units with relatively large and rapidly conducting axons are especially important for the control of rapid, discrete movements (Evarts, 1965, 1966). These fibres to a certain extent act monosynaptically on the motoneurons, at least in the monkey (Bernhard, Bohm and Petersen, 1953; Preston and Whitlock, 1961; Landgren, Phillips and Porter, 1962, and others), and they tend to activate distal limb muscles more than proximal ones. Thus the motoneurons of certain finger muscles, for example, receive larger quantities of monosynaptic corticospinal excitation than do those innervating other forearm muscles (Clough, Kernell and Phillips, 1968). Finally, it is of interest that according to the recent studies in man by Vallbo (1971), in voluntary movements the α-motoneurons (producing skeletomotor contractions) are activated before there is evidence of activity in the muscle spindles as measured by acceleration of their afferent impulses. Thus, fusimotor activity does not seem to be essential for the initiation of voluntary contractions, even if it is necessary in the further process of movement, particularly tracking movements.

The question of particular relevance for the problem concerning us here, is to what extent the cortical control of the motor units of the hand is strictly unilateral. As regards the pyramidal tract fibres, it appears from anatomical studies that the proportions of non-crossing fibres in man show great individual variations (see Nyberg-Hansen and Rinvik, 1963). It appears, however, that the corticospinal (pyramidal)—to a large extent monosynaptic—supply of motoneurons for the hand muscles is almost all contralateral, at least in the monkey (Kuypers and Brinkman, 1970) and presumably in man. Physiologically it appears that most pyramidal tract neurons are related primarily to movements of the contralateral arm (Evarts, 1966). Although movements elicited on cortical stimulation of the motor cortex cannot be taken as mediated only through pyramidal tract fibres, it is worth noticing that ipsilateral finger movements are rarely, if ever, obtained on cortical stimulation in man (see, for example, Penfield and Jasper, 1954).

There are thus good reasons to think that the motor units of the small muscles of the hand, used in writing, are those most exquisitely governed by the contralateral cerebral cortex, and that the corticospinal (pyramidal) fibres are particularly important in the performance of delicate finger movements. It might be assumed, therefore, that an interruption of one corticospinal tract should not interfere with the function of the small hand muscles on the side of a cerebral lesion. To explain disturbances in handwriting in such cases other reasons must be sought.

One might imagine that damage to commissural connexions from the hand region of the right hemisphere to the left may be of importance so that a normally occurring co-operation of the two hemispheres is disturbed. These connexions are quite likely to be affected by an infarct extending from the region of the internal capsule towards the cerebral surface, but recent experimental studies have shown that in the monkey (Ebner and Myers, 1965; Jones and Powell, 1969; Pandya and Vignolo, 1969) as well as in the cat (Jones and Powell, 1968) and the racoon (Ebner and Myers, 1965) commissural connexions between the sensory (especially SI) hand areas are lacking, while they exist between cortical areas 'representing' more proximal parts of the limb. The situation appears to be similar for the precentral region in the monkey (Pandya and Vignolo, 1971; Karol and Pandya, 1971). An affection of commissural fibres is, therefore, not likely to explain the changes in handwriting. If commissural fibres are involved one would, furthermore, expect that patients having had transections of the corpus callosum would show disturbances of writing. Little appears to be found about this in the literature. Gazzaniga, Bogen and Sperry (1965), who studied two cases, briefly state (loc. cit., p. 233): 'Activities that involved speech and writing were well preserved but only in so far as they could be governed from the left hemisphere'. In another study of three cases Gazzaniga and Sperry (1967) found (loc. cit., p. 135) that: 'The right hand . . . was always capable of writing correctly the names and descriptions of visual or tactile stimuli presented to the left hemisphere with no special difficulty evident'. The authors, however, apparently did not examine the patients' handwriting more particularly (see also Gazzaniga, 1970).

It thus appears that one has to look for explanations for the disturbances in handwriting other than damage of commissural connexions. It is now general knowledge that a lesion of the internal capsule and of regions between this and the cortex will interrupt not only corticospinal (pyramidal) fibres, but many others as well, among them afferent fibre systems to the thalamus and cortex and efferent cortical fibres passing to the red nucleus, the pontine nuclei, the inferior olive and several nuclei of the reticular formation. To what extent these various connexions are engaged in the performance of voluntary movements is not known, but it must be considered fairly certain that many of the afferent as well as the efferent cortical projections co-operate intimately with the corticospinal fibres in this process. If some of these efferent fibre tracts act bilaterally on the motoneurons for the hand in the cervical cord, their interruption may be imagined to cause changes in the function of the motoneurons for both hands. While the corticospinal pathway through the red nucleus appears to be, at least mainly, a contralateral route (*see* Brodal, 1969), the corticoreticular fibres, judging from animal experiments in the cat (Rossi and Brodal, 1956; Kuypers, 1958*a*) and the monkey (Kuypers, 1958*b*; Kuypers and Lawrence, 1967), and presumably also in man (Kanki and Ban, 1952; Kuypers, 1958*c*), are to a great extent bilaterally distributed and may play a role. The cerebellum is presumably more directly involved than either of these connexions in the performance of precise voluntary movements, especially in their speed and control. It is of interest, therefore, that the cerebrocerebellar connexions (for a recent review, *see* Brodal, 1972*a*) are to a greater extent bilateral than is generally assumed (it is often alleged that the right cerebral hemisphere is linked to the left half of the cerebellum and vice versa).

There is experimental evidence that the corticopontine projection from the sensorimotor regions is almost entirely ipsilateral in the cat (P. Brodal, 1068*a*, 1968*b*) as well as in the monkey (Nyby and Jansen, 1951). The same appears to be the case in man (Kuypers, 1958*c*; Kanki and Ban, 1952; Martinez, 1955). The next link, the pontocerebellar projection, is in part uncrossed in the cat (Brodal and Jansen, 1946) as well as in man (*see* Jansen and Brodal, 1958). Regarding the inferior olive, the olivocerebellar projection is crossed in the cat (Brodal, 1940), and the same appears to be the case in man (Holmes and Stewart, 1908; Jakob, 1955; Jansen and Brodal, 1958) but the (relatively modest) cortico-olivary projection is bilateral (Walberg, 1956; Sousa-Pinto and Brodal, 1969), at least in the cat, the only animal where it has apparently been studied in some detail. It may well be more developed in man. Clearly, the right cerebral half acts not only on the left but also on the right cerebellar half through the pons and the inferior olive. A more detailed analysis of the cerebellar afferent and efferent connexions supports these data, and makes it clear that the common assumption of a cerebellar half controlling only the ipsilateral half of the body is an over-simplification.

Accordingly, it is considered rather likely that the changes in handwriting in the present case are consequences of an affection of descending pathways from the cerebral cortex other than the pyramidal tract, acting on motoneurons of both sides, directly or indirectly. The hypothesis is ventured that among these pathways the cerebrocerebellar ones may be particularly important. It is of some relevance in this connexion that the number of corticopontine fibres in man is some nineteen millions (Tomasch, 1969), while the pyramidal tract has only about one million (Lassek and Rasmussen, 1939; DeMyer, 1959).

While it is not possible to reach definite conclusions as to the correctness of these views, the observations made might stimulate systematic search for possible changes in handwriting after lesions of the right hemisphere in right-handed patients. We might need to work out far more elaborate tests to study these very delicate movements than those at present used to study co-ordination in clinical practice. It is likely that these defects will also become evident in other motor tasks needing delicate and precise movements, for example piano playing. Is playing with the right hand affected in a skilled pianist who has right cerebral damage?

Speech. As usual after a recent hemiparesis, the patient had marked dysarthria at first. The speech was slurred, in part explosive, and there was a tendency to 'swallow' the last words in a sentence. This dysarthria eventually receded, but even after six months, the dysarthria became obvious with fatigue.

Speech, as is well known, is a very composite process involving a multitude of muscles. Most of the cranial nerve nuclei supplying these muscles have a bilateral central innervation as anatomically verified in man (*see* Kuypers, 1958*c*). At the clinical examination, even immediately after the stroke, there was no deviation of the tongue or of the palatine raphe suggesting, according to general clinical criteria, that the central innervation of the hypoglossal and the ambiguous nuclei (n. XII and X) from one cerebral hemisphere is sufficient to secure balanced function; nor was there any clear evidence of asymmetrical innervation of the respiratory muscles, but there was, as usual, a typical 'central' facial paresis on the left side. One may raise the question: why is there dysarthria in such cases?

Obviously, in the present case as in many others, the marked dysarthria could not be due to the left-sided facial paresis alone. There must be a defect in the finely integrated and co-ordinated activity which is not evident in the performance of simple tasks such as pushing the tongue forwards (m. genioglossus) or lifting the velum palatinum (m. levator veli palatini).

It appears that articulation is not governed from one hemisphere only. Thus dysarthria occurs after left as well as right hemisphere lesions. The peripheral motor neuron groups concerned in speech are supplied bilaterally by direct corticofugal fibres. Vocalization and arrest of speech can be elicited on electrical stimulation of either hemisphere (Penfield, 1954; Penfield and Jasper, 1954).

The fact that dysarthria follows unilateral brain lesions must be taken as evidence that normally there exists a very close co-operation between both sides of the brain in articulation. The ample commissural connexions between the sensory and motor regions of the face (*see* references above on commissural connexions) may be taken as morphological evidence in support of this view. A destruction of the corticofugal supply from one hemisphere of the relevant motoneurons may be assumed to cause a disturbance of the necessary delicate co-ordinated innervation of the peripheral motor neuron groups of the two sides, resulting in disordered movements of the muscles concerned. In addition, it is extremely likely that the interruption of pathways other than the direct corticobulbar pathways is of importance. Considering the delicacy and precision of the movements of larynx, pharynx, tongue, lips and respiratory muscles necessary for perfect articulation, the cerebrocerebellar pathways are presumably important and involved in achieving smooth movements. Dysarthria after cerebellar lesions is well known. The fact that proper articulation needs adequate co-operation of the muscles of respiration became painfully clear to the patient when some two months after the stroke he attempted to shout. The result was very poor, and it was clearly felt that the main reason was a defect in the proper innervation of the muscles of respiration.

Deglutition. During the first two weeks or so there were some slight defects in deglutition, swallowed food and especially drink being more apt than before to enter the air passages. Corresponding considerations may be made concerning this phenomenon as about speech.

Higher mental functions. This heading is here used in a very loose and unspecified sense and without any definition, as a common denominator for some functions which are not covered under the other headings but which were changed in the present patient after the stroke. As might be expected, these changes were present from the beginning, but then became less marked. Even ten months after the stroke they could still be detected.

No attempt will be made here to consider in detail changes in all those functions which, according to contemporary views, are dependent on the right ('non-dominant') hemisphere. Some subjective observations of relevance to the problem of the relative role attributed to either hemisphere in some functions, particularly verbal ones, will be mentioned.

Subjectively the patient noted that he became much more easily tired than previously from mental work, even from ordinary conversation and reading newspapers. There was a marked reduction in the powers of concentration which made mental tasks far more demanding than before. Reading novels did not cause great problems, but it was often quite difficult and needed much concentration to follow the arguments, for example in a scientific paper. In part this seemed to be due to a reduced capacity to retain the sense of a sentence long enough to combine it with the meaning of the next sentence. It appeared subjectively as a reduction of short-term memory for abstract symbols. This is supported by the following observation: when trying to remember a series of figures, for example looking reference numbers up in a list, the limits of achievement even with maximal concentration were reduced, compared with previous capacity. These few observations, along with some others of a similar type, suggest that there is some impairment of certain mental functions.

About two and a half months after the stroke the patient was subjected to psychological tests (H. Bjørnœs), including the Halstead neuropsychological battery test and the Wechsler adult intelligence scale (WAIS). In the latter the verbal IQ was estimated to be 142, the performance IQ 122. The powers to solve spatial problems on the basis of tactile and kinæsthetic clues showed some reduction and there was some finger agnosia on the left. The relatively great difference between the verbal and performance IQ may possibly reflect some reduction of those intellectual functions which are particularly dependent upon an intact right hemisphere. The results of the Halstead battery tests appear to point in the same direction. More marked evidence of right parietal lobe damage was not found.

Mention was made, when describing writing, that there were changes not to be explained by faulty innervation of the hand and finger muscles, but pointing to more subtle aspects of the control of writing: the frequent skipping of letters, syllables or words, or the incorrect doubling or trebling of a letter or syllable, and the interchanges of figures when writing numbers. Such errors also occur, of course, in normal people, and they were known to the patient to happen before he had his stroke, but they were far more frequent and more marked, and although they became less frequent as time passed, they were clearly present ten months after the stroke. Parallel with these were similar tendencies in speech, sometimes a word was skipped, or a syllable, especially at the end of a sentence, or two small words were incorrectly fused.

Changes in writing and speaking like these may perhaps be classified as signs of dysgraphia and dysphasia. The author does not venture to go into the complex field of categorization of disturbances of speech, but it appears that according to current views disturbances as those described are assumed to be caused by affections of the 'dominant' hemisphere. Although only an autopsy would prove that the left hemisphere of the patient is intact, there is no reason to assume that it is not.

The changes in the patient's powers to express himself without defects in writing and speech must therefore be due to the changes in his right hemisphere, and may be taken to indicate that this is not without influence on the expression by verbal symbols, written or spoken.

A scrutiny of only a small part of the vast literature relevant to this question has given some interesting results. Eisenson (1962) compared some patients with damage of the right cerebral hemisphere (the number is not given) with a control group of normal persons with regard to their performance in a series of widely varying verbal tests. It was found that the patients performed less proficiently than did those of the control group with regard to linguistic and intellectual functions, particularly when abstract concepts were involved. It is concluded that in general the results support the view that right cerebral damage is associated with changes in linguistic and intellectual functions. The results of the tests confirmed Eisenson's (1962) impression that in such patients there is an 'increase in the number of words the individual needed to express his ideas, and a looseness of verbalization'. Further: 'There seemed to be more circumlocution, more hunting for the right word in the patients than in adults free of brain damage'. As far as it is possible to evaluate oneself, the present author feels that the above quotation gives a fair description of how he felt the condition in himself.

The findings of Eisenson and others, and the observations made by the present author, suggest that the right ('non-dominant') hemisphere is not without influence on verbal functions, even if overt aphasic disturbances are usually seen only following lesions of the left hemisphere. Penfield and Roberts (1959, p. 249) suggest that homologous areas of the two hemispheres may be necessary for certain intellectual functions. Eisenson (1962) supports a view expressed by Critchley (1961), that while damage of the left hemisphere gives rise to disturbances in ordinary language functions, the right hemisphere might have some higher than ordinary language potential. Eisenson suggests that the right hemisphere may be involved with super- or extra-ordinary language functions, i.e. for high-level language functioning. The present case, where there was no overt aphasia, may be taken to support this view.

DISCUSSION

The observations described concern different aspects of central nervous function. A fully satisfactory discussion of them needs a thorough insight in experimental neurophysiology and clinical neurology as well as neuro-anatomy. Even if the author does not possess such qualifications, it is hoped that his considerations may be of interest to colleagues in the neurological sciences.

The tenability of several of the considerations made concerning speech and writing depends upon the fact that the patient's cerebral lesion is purely unilateral (right-sided). As discussed above, there is no convincing evidence to the contrary.

During a lifelong occupation with the anatomy of the central nervous system, especially its fibre connexions, the author has been increasingly struck by the tremendous complexity in the organization of the brain. Two aspects—apparently contradictory— are particularly conspicuous. There is an extremely high degree of specificity and at the same time a far-going diffuseness in the patterns of organization.

The *specificity of the morphological organization of the nervous system* is amazing. The more we know about the structure of the brain, the more we realize how this specificity can be traced to the minutest levels. It is the rule, rather than the exception, that even a small nucleus can be subdivided into parts or territories which differ with regard to cytoarchitecture, glial architecture, vasoarchitecture, fibre connexions, synaptic arrangements and by its chemistry. This, of course, is the morphological counterpart to the localization of function in the central nervous system. Very small and neighbouring regions may show differences in their function (as in their structure), for example the visual areas 17, 18 and 19, the various laminæ in the cerebral cortex and in the spinal cord. From this point of view the entire nervous system may be considered to be composed of a multitude of minor units, each with its particular morphological organization and its specific task. This view is compatible with much current thinking in clinical

neurology: a lesion of a certain part of the brain, for example the dorsal columns, or the subthalamic nucleus, results in specific symptoms.

If one focuses attention on the fibre connexions of the central nervous system one is struck by another feature in its organization: The *multiplicity of connexions*. As a rule each small region receives fibres from a number of others and likewise emits fibres which pass to many other regions. A particularly well-studied part of the brain where this has been shown to be the case is the vestibular nuclear complex (Brodal, 1972b). There may, of course, be great quantitative differences among the various contingents of afferent and efferent fibres of a nucleus. Nevertheless, a scrutiny of the fibre connexions of the central nervous system as a whole leaves one with the conviction that there are morphological possibilities for an impulse from a certain part of the brain to be transmitted along circumvential routes of varying complexity to virtually every other part of the central nervous system! These multifarious interconnexions between structures presumably provide possibilities for co-operation and integration of function between them and make it increasingly difficult and unjustified to describe a certain part of the brain as simply 'motor,' 'visual,' etc. To take one example: the superior colliculus. This receives not only a major supply of optic fibres and impulses, but is played upon by the acoustic, the motor, the somatosensory and 'association' cortex, the spinal cord, the reticular formation and other sources. On one hand a multitude of small units in the central nervous system can be identified which all have their particular structure and function, on the other hand they are all more or less amply interconnected and dependent on each other.

These views lead to the conclusion that destruction of even a localized part of the brain will cause consequences for several functions in addition to those which are more specifically dependent on the region damaged. In other words, for optimal, perfect function, we need the whole brain. It appears that with our present knowledge of the brain the views of the pure 'localizationists' and those stressing a holistic function of the brain can be reconciled.

When applied to clinical neurology, the point of view outlined above has two consequences. First, in any brain damage one may expect to. find disturbances in function which—according to current views—are not primarily served by the damaged part. Secondly, such 'secondary' or 'indirect' functional changes may often be small and may escape recognition in routine examination, but it may be assumed that systematic studies with adequate methods of such changes may give valuable information on the way the central nervous system functions and supplement conceptions gained from animal experiences.

The symptomatology in cases like the present one may be taken to be compatible with the views presented above. The predominant symptom is the hemiparesis, but there are many other signs of disturbed function. The most striking are perhaps the changes in writing. As has been discussed, it is considered likely that the changes in handwriting are a consequence largely of damage to certain descending fibre connexions which act bilaterally and whose impairment will influence the function of hands and fingers on either side. The intactness of the direct route for impulses from the left cortex to the motoneurons of the right hand and fingers is not sufficient for perfect handwriting. In a corresponding way, even if the motoneurons for the muscles of articulation are bilaterally supplied from the cortex, if the supply from one side is damaged there is obvious reduction of function: dysarthria. Those changes in writing which are perhaps related to agraphia are other examples of disturbances not to be expected with lesion of the right (non-dominant) hemisphere, although the classification of the changes described is uncertain. By some they would perhaps be attributed to lesion of the right parietal cortex only.

In addition to the changes mentioned which can be objectively studied, the patient has found that destruction of even a minor part of the brain causes changes in a number of functions which are difficult to study objectively. They are, however, very obvious to him. They are what one might call general defects in the functions of the brain: loss of powers of concentration, reduced short-term memory, increased fatigue, reduced initiative, incontinence of movements of emotional expression and other phenomena. It may be argued that several of these changes are due to the psychologically depressing effect of having suffered a stroke. (In general depressive reactions appear to be more common in lesions of the left hemisphere than of the right, see Gainotti, 1972.) While this obviously may play a part, close observations of himself has led the patient to the conviction that much of the reduced mental capacities have an organic basis. It has also been astonishing to note how long it takes for these symptoms to improve visibly. Even after ten months if the patient seems to be as he was, apart from his slight remaining pareses, he is painfully aware himself that this is not so.

It may be argued contrary to the view presented here, that in common clinical experience, some consequences of a brain lesion tend to disappear after some time, and there is often what appears to be a complete recovery. One may, however, doubt whether this is ever really true. It indeed seems likely that sufficiently delicate tests might show that even after slight brain damage there are some sequels. Nevertheless, it is often amazing to see to what degree restitution may take place. It is usually explained as being due to a process called 'compensation,' but we know little about what actually takes place in the nervous system during this recovery. While the early restitution occurring, in say, the first two months, may be due to disappearance of œdema, resorption of blood and debris, the restitution occurring later cannot be explained in this way. Since regeneration of transected central axons has never been convincingly demonstrated in higher mammals, it seems in most instances that one must resort to the assumption that intact fibres 'take over' for the damaged ones.

Based on the concept of the brain's great 'reserve capacity' it is sometimes held that some nerve cells (with their axons and synapses) which previously have not been functioning, become active after a brain lesion. This hypothesis can scarcely be tested. One may ask, however, if such 'dormant' cells—if they exist in the fully developed brain—can escape disuse atrophy. It appears more likely that the 'taking over' for the damaged fibres must imply that remaining intact and functioning fibres establish new synapses where the destroyed fibres were previously acting. The physiological study of Wall and Egger (1971) supports this assumption, and there is some recent morphological evidence that this is what may actually occur. Thus Raisman (1969, and Raisman and Field, 1973) in an electron microscopic study of the effects of interruption of two contingents of afferents to the septal nuclei in the rat, has produced evidence that if one tract is interrupted the fibres of the other will extend to supply the denuded synaptic sites belonging originally to the transected fibres. While a reinnervation will occur by this process, it is clear that there will be considerable loss in specificity of neuronal connexions. In the rat the establishment of new connexions appears to be completed after a few weeks (Wall and Egger, 1971; Raisman and Field, 1973). In man it may well be assumed to extend over a longer period.

These views on regeneration seem applicable to the improvement of hemiparesis following a stroke, especially at later stages when an initial temporary functional block of some damaged corticofugal fibres by œdema and so on has disappeared. (In the present case improvement was still noted after ten months.) With the use of the paretic muscles, physiotherapeutic exercises and training one may imagine that two components are active. It is likely that there will be some hypertrophy of muscle fibres belonging to motor units whose motoneurons have retained their central innervation more or less completely and so can be activated. Greater demands are now made on these units than before. Secondly, in view of Raisman's (1969) findings it appears extremely likely that part of the recovery is due to the fact that the terminal endings of preserved

corticospinal, and probably other central fibres, form new terminals which occupy denuded synaptic sites on the motoneurons. Gradually more of the motoneurons originally devoid of cortical innervation will regain it. A corresponding process may presumably take place where other, in part interrupted, cortical efferents, such as cortico-rubral, -reticular, -pontine end. But considerable loss of specificity may be expected to occur, for example a reticulospinal fibre may establish a new synapse on a motoneuron where there was previously one belonging to a corticospinal fibre. Functionally there will presumably be confusion by establishing new patterns of neuronal connexions. Even if such a mechanism were acting optimally, one could never expect complete re-establishment of the neuronal patterns which were present before, and scarcely, therefore, a complete functional recovery of the motor functions.

It seems quite likely that the mechanism which has been discussed is an important factor in recovery after damage to central neurons, and that it has a general application, and is thus also valid for the thalamus, cortex and other regions. We do not know anything, so far, of the factors which stimulate the process, and how training (use) appears to have a beneficial effect. It appears likely that the results of the mechanism described will be less satisfactory the more complex is the organization of the part of the brain concerned.

SUMMARY

The author describes and comments upon some observations he made on himself following a left-sided hemiparesis without hemianopsia and overt sensory disturbances. The hemiparesis was diagnosed as being due to an embolic lesion of the posterior part of the right internal capsule and neighbouring regions. There was no evidence of damage to the left hemisphere.

Some observations of muscular function are interpreted as showing that sensory impulses from muscle spindles are consciously perceived, other observations are compatible with the view that the patterns of automatized skilled movements are to a great extent organized at the spinal level.

Changes in the patient's handwriting (he is right-handed) are discussed at some length. On the basis of present neuro-anatomical and neurophysiological knowledge it is concluded that the motor disturbances in handwriting are most likely due to the interruption of some corticofugal fibre systems which act on the motoneurons of both sides. Pathways through the cerebellum may be particularly important. Disturbances in delicate motor functions, as for example writing, may be more common in pure right hemisphere lesions than generally assumed, but may only be recognized in more refined tests than those generally employed in routine clinical examination.

From what is known of the descending influences on the peripheral motoneurons involved in speech, an attempt is made to explain the fact that dysarthria is commonly seen following lesions of either hemisphere.

Some disturbances of mental functions were subjectively clearly noticed by the patient, and certain changes in his verbal expression, especially writing, were of long standing. The latter phenomena seem to indicate that the right hemisphere is not without influence on language functions.

The observations made by the patient fit in with a view of the organization of the central nervous system which emanates from a life-long occupation with its anatomy: the central nervous system consists of a multitude of minute units, each with its particular structure and specific function. These units are abundantly interconnected in a very complex pattern. Destruction of one part will, therefore, inevitably have consequences for the functions of several others, although these changes may be subtle and need specially designed tests for recognition. The observations which the patient has made on himself are in agreement with this view.

Finally, the improvement which follows a brain lesion is commented upon, with particular reference to the clinical relevance of the recent experimental anatomical study of Raisman (1969). It seems that some of the recovery after a brain lesion may be explained by reinnervation from remaining fibres of synaptic sites which have been denuded as a consequence of the interruption and degeneration of afferent fibres.

REFERENCES

Albe-Fessard, D. and Liebeskind, J. (1966). Origine des messages somato-sensitifs activant less cellules du cortex moteur chez le singe. *Expl Brain Res.*, **1**, 127–46.

Bates, J. A. V. (1957). Observations on the excitable cortex in man. *Lect. scient. Basis Med.*, **5**, 333–47.

Bernhard, C. H., Bohm, E., and Petersen, I. (1953). Investigations on the organization of the corticospinal system in monkeys (*Macaca mulatta*). *Acta physiol. scand.*, **29**, Suppl. **106**, 79–105.

Boisacq-Schepens, N., and Hanus, M. (1972). Motor cortex vestibular responses in the chloralosed cat. *Expl Brain Res.*, **14**, 539–49.

Brodal, A. (1940). Experimentelle Untersuchungen über die olivo-cerebellare Lokalisation. *Z. ges. Neurol. Psychiat.*, **169**, 1–153.

Brodal, A. (1969). *Neurological anatomy in relation to clinical medicine* (2nd edn). Oxford University Press, New York.

Brodal, A. (1972a). Cerebrocerebellar pathways. Anatomical data and some functional implications. *Acta neurol. scand.*, Suppl. **51**, 153–95.

Brodal, A. (1972b). Some features in the anatomical organization of the vestibular nuclear complex in the cat. *Prog. Brain Res.*, **37**, 31–53.

Brodal, A. and Jansen, J. (1946). The ponto-cerebellar projection in the rabbit and cat. *J. comp. Neurol.*, **84**, 31–118.

Brodal, P. (1968a). The corticopontine projection in the cat. I. Demonstration of a somatotopically organized projection from the primary sensorimotor cortex. *Expl Brain Res.*, **5**, 210–34.

Brodal, P. (1968*b*). The corticopontine projection in the cat. II. Demonstration of a somatotopically organized projection from the second somatosensory cortex. *Archs ital. Biol.*, **106**, 310–32.

Brooks, V. B., and Stoney, S. D., Jr. (1971). Motor mechanisms: The role of the pyramidal system in motor control. *A. Rev. Physiol.*, **33**, 337–92.

Carmichael, E. A., Dix, M. R., and Hallpike, C. S. (1954). Lesions of the cerebral hemispheres and their effect upon optokinetic and caloric nystagmus. *Brain*, **77**, 345–72.

Chambers, R. A., and Gilliat, R. W. (1954). The clinical assessment of postural sensation in the fingers. *J. Physiol., Lond.*, **123**, 42P.

Clough, J. F. M., Kernell, D., and Phillips, C. G. (1968). The distribution of monosynaptic excitation from the pyramidal tract and from primary spindle afferents to motoneurones of the baboon's hand and forearm. *J. Physiol., Lond.*, **198**, 145–66.

Critchley, M. (1954). Parietal syndromes in ambidextrous and left-handed subjects. *Zentbl. Neurochir.*, **14**, 4–16.

Critchely, M. (1961). Cited by Eisenson (1962).

DeMyer, W. (1959). Number of axons and myelin sheaths in adult human medullary pyramids. *Neurology, Minneap.*, **9**, 42–7.

Ebner, F. F. and Myers, R. E. (1965). Distribution of corpus callosum and anterior commissure in cat and raccoon. *J. comp. Neurol.*, **124**, 353–65.

Eisenson, J. (1962). Language and intellectual modifications associated with right cerebral damage. *Language Speech*, **5**, 49–53.

Eklund, G. (1972). Position sense and state of contraction; the effects of vibration. *J. Neurol. Neurosurg. Psychiat.*, **35**, 606–11.

Evarts, E. V. (1965). Relation of discharge frequency to conduction velocity in pyramidal tract neurons. *J. Neurophysiol*, **28**, 216–28.

Evarts, E. V. (1966). Pyramidal tract activity associated with a conditioned hand movement in the monkey. *J. Neurophysiol.*, **29**, 1011–27.

Evarts, E. V. and Thach, W. T. (1969). Motor mechanisms of the CNS: Cerebrocerebellar interrelations. *A. Rev. Physiol.*, **31**, 458–98.

Fisher, C. M. and Curry, H. B. (1965). Pure motor hemiplegia of vascular origin. *Archs Neurol., Chicago*, **13**, 30–44.

Fredrickson, J. M., Figge, U., Scheid, P., and Kornhuber, H. H. (1966). Vestibular nerve projection to the cerebral cortex of the Rhesus monkey. *Expl Brain Res.*, **2**, 318–27.

Gainotti, G. (1972). Emotional behavior and hemispheric side of the lesion. *Cortex*, **8**, 41–55.

Gazzaniga, M. S. (1970). *The bisected brain*. Appleton, New York.

Gazziniga, M. S., Bogen, J. E., and Sperry, R. W. (1965). Observations on visual perception after disconnexion of the cerebral hemispheres in man. *Brain*, **88**, 221–36.

Gazziniga, M. S. and Sperry, R. W. (1967). Language after section of the cerebral commissures,. *Brain*, **90**, 131–48.

Gildenberg, P. L., and Hassler, R. (1971). Influence of stimulation of the cerebral cortex on vestibular nuclei units in the cat. *Expl Brain Res.*, **14**, 77–94.

Goodwin, G. M., McCloskey, D. I., and Matthews, P. B. C. (1972). The contribution of muscle afferents to kinæsthesia shown by vibration induced illusions of movement and by the effects of paralysing joint afferents. *Brain*, **95**, 705–48.

Franit, R. (1970). *The Basis of Motor Control*. Academic Press, New York.

Granit, R. (1972). Constant errors in the execution and appreciation of movement. *Brain*, **95**, 649–60.

Holmes, G. and Stewart, T. G. (1908). On the connection of the inferior olives with the cerebellum in man. *Brain*, **31**, 125–37.

Jakob, H. (1955). Zur Analyse konsekutiver Olivenschäden vei vasculär bedingten Kleinhirndefekten. *Arch. Psychiat. NervKrankh.*, **193**, 583–600.

Jansen, J. and Brodal, A. (1958). Das Kleinhirn. *In Handbuch der mikroskopischen Anatomie des Menchen* (Vol. 4, pt. 8), (ed. W. v. Möllendorff). Springer, Berlin.

Jones, E. G. and Powell, T. P. S. (1968). The commissural connexions of the somatic sensory cortex in the cat. *J. Anat.*, **103**, 433–55.

Jones, E. G. and Powell, T. P. S. (1969). Connexions of the somatic sensory cortex of the rhesus monkey. II. Contralateral cortical connexions. *Brain*, **92**, 717–30.

Jörgensen, L. and Torvik, A. (1969). Ischæmic cerebrovascular diseases in an autopsy series. 2. Prevalence, location, pathogenesis, and clinical course of cerebral infarcts. *J. neurol., Sci.*, **9**, 285–320.

Kanki, S. and Ban, T. (1952). Cortico-fugal connections of frontal lobe in man. *Med. J. Osaka Univ.*, **3**, 201–22.

Karol, E. A. and Pandya, D. N. (1971). The distribution of the corpus callosum in the rhesus monkey. *Brain*, **94**, 471–86.

Kuypers, H. G. J. M. (1958a). An anatomical analysis of cortico-bulbar connexions to the pons and lower brain stem in the cat. *J. Anat.*, **92**, 198–218.

Kuypers, H. G. J. M. (1958b). Some projections from the peri-central cortex to the pons and lower brain stem in monkey and chimpanzee. *J. comp. Neurol.*, **110**, 221–55.

Kuypers, H. G. J. M. (1958c). Corticobulbar connexions to the pons and lower brain stem in man. *Brain*, **81**, 364–88.

Kuypers, H. G. J. M. and Brinkman, J. (1970). Precentral projection to different parts of the spinal intermediate zone in the rhesus monkey. *Brain Res.*, **24**, 29–48.

Kuypers, H. G. J. M. and Lawrence, D. G. (1967). Cortical projections to the red nucleus and the brain stem in the Rhesus monkey. *Brain Res.*, **4**, 151–88.

Landgren, S., Phillips, C. G., and Porter, R. (1962). Cortical fields of origin of the monosynaptic pyramidal pathways in some alpha motoneurones of the baboon's hand and forearm. *J. Physiol., Lond.*, **161**, 112–25.

Landgren, S. and Silfvenius, H. (1969). Projection to cerebral cortex of group I muscle afferents from the cat's hind limb. *J. Physiol., Lond.*, **200**, 353–72.

Landgren, S., Silfvenius, and Wolsk, D. (1967). Somato-sensory paths to the second cortical projection area of the group I muscle afferents. *J. Physiol., Lond.*, **191**, 543–59.

Lassek, A. M. and Rasmussen, G. L. (1939). The human pyramidal tract. *Archs Neurol., Psychiat., Chicago*, **42**, 872–76.

Lawrence, D. G. and Kuypers, H. G. J. M. (1968). The functional organization of the motor system in the monkey. I. The effects of bilateral pyramidal lesions. *Brain*, **91**, 1–14.

Lundberg, A. (1969). Reflex control of stepping. *The Nansen Memorial Lecture.* 10 October 1968. Universitetsforlaget, Oslo.

Markham, C. H. (1972). Descending control of the vestibular nuclei: physiology. *Prog. Brain Res.*, **37**, 589–600.

Martinez, A. (1955). Some efferent connexions of the human frontal lobe. *J. Neurosurg.*, **12**, 18–25.

Nyberg-Hansen, R. and Rinvik, E. (1963). Some comments on the pyramidal tract, with special reference to its individual variations in man. *Acta neurol. scand.*, **39**, 1–30.

Nyby, O. and Jansen, J. (1951). An experimental investigation of the cortico-pontine projection in macaca mulatta. *Norske Vid. Akad. Avh. I, Math.-Nat. Kl.*, **3**, 1–47.

Pandya, D. N. and Vignolo, L. A. (1969). Interhemispheric projections of the parietal lobe in the rhesus monkey. *Brain Res.*, **15**, 49–65.

Pandya, D. N. and Vignolo, L. A. (1971). Intra- and interhemispheric projections of the precentral, premotor and arcuate areas in the rhesus monkey. *Brain Res.*, **26**, 217–33.

Penfield, W. (1954). Mechanisms of voluntary movement. *Brain*, **77**, 1–17.

Penfield, W. and Jasper, H. (1954). *Epilepsy and the functional anatomy of the human brain.* Little, Brown, Boston.

Penfield, W. and Roberts, L. (1959). *Speech and brain mechanisms.* Princeton University Press, Princeton, NJ.

Phillips, C. G., Powell, T. P. S., and Wiesendanger, M. (1971). Projection from low-threshold muscle afferents of hand and forearm to area 3a of baboon's cortex. *J. Physiol., Lond.*, **217**, 419–46.

Preston, J. B. and Whitlock, D. G. (1961). Intracellular potentials recorded from motoneurons following precentral gyrus stimulation in primate. *J. Neurophysiol.*, **24**, 91–100.

Raisman, G. (1969). Neuronal plasticity in the septal nuclei of the adult rat. *Brai Res.*, **14**, 25–48.

Raisman, G. and Field, P. M. (1973). A quantitative investigation of the development of collateral reinnervation after partial deafferentation of the septal nuclei. *Brain Res.*, **50**, 241–64.

Rossi, G. F. and Brodal, A. (1956). Corticofugal fibres to the brain-stem reticular formation. An experimental study in the cat. *J. Anat.*, **90**, 42–62.

Smith, M. C. (1967). Stereotactic operations for Parkinson's disease—Anatomical observations. *In Modern trends in neurology* (Vol. 4), (ed. D. Williams), pp. 21–52. Butterworth, London.

Sousa-Pinto, A. and Brodal, A. (1969). Demonstration of a somatotopical patterns in the cortico-olivary projection in the cat. An experimental-anatomical study. *Expl Brain Res.*, **8**, 364–86.

Tomasch, J. (1969). The numerical capacity of the human cortico-pontocerebellar system. *Brain Res.*, **13**, 476–84.

Vallbo, Å. B. (1971). Muscle spindle response at the onset of isometric voluntary contraction in man. Time difference between fusimotor and skeletomotor effects. *J. Physiol., Lond.*, **218**, 405–31.

Wagman, I. H. and Mehler, W. R. (1973). Physiology and anatomy of the cortico-oculomotor mechanism. *Prog. Brain Res.*, **37**, 619–35.

Walberg, F. (1956). Descending connections to the inferior olive. *J. comp. Neurol.*, **104**, 77–173.

Wall, P. D. and Egger, M. D. (1971). Formation of new connexions in adult rat brains after partial deafferentation. *Nature, Lond.*, **232**, 542–5.

(Brodal 1973)

COMMENTARY

In addition to the left-sided hemiparesis brought about by his right hemisphere stroke, Brodal suffered changes in handwriting and other skilled activities using the right hand, changes that were both significant and surprising to him. It remains possible that his right hemisphere lesion affected 'uncrossed' pathways from the right hemisphere to the upper limbs on the right side of his body. Subtle, ipsilateral motor deficits following a unilateral stroke have been documented in subsequent research studies (Jones *et al.* 1989). The converse may also have held in Brodal's case—recovery of function on his paralysed left side may have been due in part to 'uncrossed' pathways from his intact left hemisphere to the left side of his body. The possibility of such a mechanism underlying recovery of function after stroke is highlighted by reports of patients who suffer two separate strokes in each hemisphere, with some time lapsing between each stroke. The second stroke has been shown to result in reappearance of ipsilateral motor deficits, deficits that had initially largely recovered after the first stroke in the contralateral hemisphere (Fisher 1992; Lee and Van Donkelaar 1995).

Brodal was also acutely aware of impairments in neuropsychological functions that are less tangible than motor or writing impairments: 'loss of powers of concentration, reduced short-term memory, increased fatigue, reduced initiative, incontinence of movements or emotional expression . . .' (p. 262). Brodal did not regard these as resulting from secondary psychological changes following his stroke, but as primary deficits of neurological origin. Similar to Kolb, Brodal refers to emotional changes after his stroke. Kolb reported emotional lability and panic attacks after his right hemisphere stroke, whereas Brodal refers to the 'depressing effect' of his stroke. While Kolb interprets the literature (p. 142) as indicating that right posterior lesions are associated with depression, Brodal (p. 262) concludes that left hemisphere lesions are more closely associated with depression. Although right hemisphere lesions may impair the expression and interpretation of emotional behaviour, such as facial affect, and thus indirectly lead to changes that mimic depression, it is probably the case that where there is hemispheric asymmetry for emotional changes, it is in the direction of more significant depression with left hemisphere damage and euphoria/indifference associated with right hemisphere lesions (Heilman *et al.* 1993). However, this dichotomy is by no means an absolute one, and the role of lesion location may be affected by the stage of recovery from the stroke (Iacoboni *et al.* 1995).

Brodal also points out that some ten months after the stroke he appeared clinically to have recovered well, but that he himself was 'painfully aware' that this was not so. Brodal notes: 'It indeed seems likely that sufficiently delicate tests might show that even after slight brain damage there are some sequels' (p. 262). Some of the symptoms mentioned by Brodal such as fatigue, spontaneous lapses in concentration, loss of initiative, etc. are particularly difficult to assess in laboratory/clinic settings, especially where symptoms cover time frames such as several hours or more. In the case of Brodal's particular comment relating to 'delicate tests' showing up 'slight brain damage', there is now an extensive literature on mild head injury (Hoff *et al.* 1989; Levin *et al.* 1989), much of it claiming to show that even patients with mild concussional head injury may show significant cognitive deficits. As far as I am aware, there is not as yet a parallel literature on mild cerebrovascular disease. Even if such a literature were present, I suspect that it might generate an equivalent degree of conflicting findings and controversy as is the case in head injury, since mild psychological deficits are by their very nature difficult to delineate with certainty!

Brodal distinguishes between short-term recovery mechanisms and long-term recovery mechanisms. He relates the former to reduction in cerebral oedema, resorbtion of blood and debris, etc. and the latter to more speculative mechanisms, such as the establishment of new synapses by fibres that remained intact. Other researchers have also outlined two broad stages of recovery of function at the physiological level (Kertesz 1993), although the precise neural delineation of these stages remains to be mapped in detail.

Brodal found that his impairment of 'higher mental functions' was of three broad types:

1. It included a mental fatigue, which limited his capacity to concentrate for an extended period of time in areas such as reading.

2. There was a limitation in short-term memory, whereby it was more difficult for him to retain abstractions such as meanings of sentences, and to connect these with other similar items that were encountered later.

3. It encompassed modest although significant language disturbance. This included impairments in writing, such that he would skip letters, syllables, or words, or such that he would incorrectly double or treble a letter or syllable. In his speech, he might skip a word or syllable, or incorrectly fuse together two small words. Brodal thought that these language difficulties were present to some extent prior to his stroke, but that they were significantly exaggerated after his stroke.

Brodal discusses the possibilities that either the right hemisphere has some role to play in language processing, or that homologous areas in the left hemisphere were in some way compromised, thus contributing to his writing and speech difficulties.

Since the publication of Brodal's paper, there is now evidence that favours the first of the two explanations. Subtle speech comprehension deficits have been noted in some patients with right hemisphere lesions (Brownwell *et al.* 1984; Chiarello 1988; Gardner 1994), and functional imaging studies have also highlighted a role for right hemisphere structures in some aspects of verbal reasoning (Demonet *et al.* 1993). Some of Brodal's writing errors (uneven lines, shapes of letters sometimes incorrect, repeating or dropping out a letter, etc.) have been associated with right parietal lesions, and may in part reflect a 'spatial agraphia' (Roeltgen 1993).

REFERENCES

Brownwell, H. H., Potter, H. H., and Michelow, D. (1984). Sensitivity to lexical denotation and connotation in brain-damaged patients: A double dissociation? *Brain and Language*, **22**, 253–65.

Chiarello, C. (ed.) (1988). *Right hemisphere contributions to lexical semantics*. Springer, New York.

Demonet, J. F., Wise, R., and Frackowiak, R. S. J. (1993). Language functions explored in normal subjects by positron emission tomography: A critical review. *Human Brain Mapping*, **1**, 39–47.

Fisher, C. M. (1992). Concerning the mechanism of recovery in stroke hemiplegia. *Canadian Journal of Neurological Sciences*, **19**, 57–63.

Gardner, H. (1994). The stories of the right hemisphere. In *Integrative views of motivation, cognition and emotion* (ed. W. D. Spaulding), pp. 57–70. University of Nebraska Press, Lincoln.

Heilman, K. M., Bowers, D., and Valenstein, E. (1993). Emotional disorders associated with neurological disease. In *Clinical Neuropsychology* (3rd edn) (ed. K. Heilman and E. Valenstein), pp. 461–497. Oxford University Press, New York.

Hoff, J., Anderson, T. E., and Cole, T. (ed.) (1989). *Mild to moderate head injury*. Blackwell, Oxford.

Iacoboni, M., Padovani, A., Di Piero, V., and Lenzi, G. L. (1995). Post-stroke depression: relationships with morphological damage and cognition over time. *Italian Journal of Neurological Sciences*, **16**, 209–16.

Jones, R. D., Donaldson, I. M., and Parkin, P. J. (1989). Impairment and recovery of ipsilateral sensory-motor function following unilateral cerebral infarction. *Brain*, **112**, 1113–32.

Kertesz, A. (1993). Recovery and treatment. In *Clinical neuropsychology* (3rd edn) (ed. K. Heilman and E. Valenstein), pp. 647–674. Oxford University Press, New York.

Lee R. G. and Van Donkelaar, P. (1995). Mechanisms underlying functional recovery following stroke. *Canadian Journal of Neurological Sciences*, **22**, 257–63.

Levin, H. S., Eisenberg, H. M., and Benton, A. L. (ed.) (1989). *Mild head injury*. Oxford University Press, New York.

Roeltgen, D. P. (1993). Agraphia. In *Clinical neuropsychology* (3rd edn) (ed. K. Heilman and E. Valenstein), pp. 63–90. Oxford University Press, New York.

Personal view

David Kyle

David Kyle was a general practitioner at the time of his stroke.

Two and a half years ago I was the senior partner in a group of six general practitioners in a large rural practice extending over 80 square miles. In addition I was extremely busy reorganising a garden of an acre attached to a bungalow built for my retirement at the top of our previously far too large garden. I had already decided to retire at the end of September 1973 after 38 years in a busy practice and I was looking forward to having some time to myself. I realised that I was going to miss my busy life and my daily contact with so many people. But in August 1973 I was honoured to be appointed chairman of the area health authority to the new county of Powys—a job which would take up to two to three days a week so that at that time all seemed set fair for a happy and useful retirement.

Looking back now it all seems too good to be true but the Fates had their baleful eye on me, and at the end of August 1973 Nemesis overtook me. One morning I felt sick and giddy. Rather than risk falling and hurting myself I knelt and found to my horror that I could not get up again and, though my brain was quite clear, my limbs refused to do what I asked them to do. After a few days in my local hospital to recover from the immediate physical and mental shock, which was considerable, I was moved for a full neurological investigation to the University Hospital of Wales in Cardiff. I had an EEG and a radioactive brain scan, which confirmed the clinical diagnosis but showed nothing adverse and suggested that my condition was due merely to the accumulated wear and tear of 40 busy years as a doctor. I would not have been surprised to have had a coronary, which has always been known as a 'doctor's disease', but the thought of a CVA would never have entered my mind.

And so 'at a stroke' all my bright prospects for a contented retirement were suddenly extinguished. I had to resign the chairmanship of the AHA, I could never again go on country expeditions with my butterfly net, would never be able to plunge about in bogs and marshes studying my favourite dragonflies, I could not dig my garden, or cultivate my vegetables. My vision of a happy future for at least 15 years (my father lived to 90, my paternal grandmother to 98, and my mother is 94) changed to a gloomy and depressing prospect of about 15 years of boredom, dissatisfaction, and inactivity. After two weeks in Cardiff I returned to Brecon Hospital where I was to stay until concentrated physiotherapy made me active enough to go home. After a further six weeks I was able to stagger along the hospital corridors with a walking aid.

So home I came to my poor wife who now had to add to her domestic duties the care of a husband still considerably disabled, my left hand still completely useless. The first thing was to equip the bathroom and lavatory with strong rails and hand supports so that I could help myself by the use of my right hand, which was now almost normal in strength. As a result of much contriving and many adaptations I can visit the lavatory on my own, a great advantage to all concerned. But what I could not do and still cannot do is to fasten the clips which support my trousers. This difficulty has proved one of the most annoying complications of having only one effective hand. There must be some fairly easy method of overcoming this problem but I have not yet thought of it.

And so in the course of time I have gradually become more self sufficient and independent, but I am still unable to dress or undress myself properly, or put myself to bed. I have learnt to put on a tie by fastening the free end to my shirt by means of a clothes peg, but it is easier to use a ready made-up clip-on tie which probably looks a lot tidier than my make-shift efforts. I can also do up my shirt buttons provided I do not start by putting the first button into the wrong hole, a fact which I do not discover until I have fastened them all. The answer to this is to stand in front of a mirror, which always reminds me of the legend of Robert the Bruce and the spider which had to make several attempts to attach its web but did it in the end. I am encouraged by this story (as I am no doubt supposed to be).

I can now look back over almost two years of illness and accept what it has meant to me and what I have learnt from it. Looking right back to the first weeks or so I remember little in the way of pain except for occasional muscle cramps and especially in the legs. But this has responded well to mild analgesic preparations.

I still suffer from days of depression, and sometimes feel that life holds very little for me. At times I am irrationally, but I hope understandably, jealous of the people who are able to move around briskly digging their gardens and doing all the things I want to do. I sometimes dream of being out for a country walk, and it is only then that I feel the joy of a spring in my step and the pleasure of physical activity, when it would be a joy to jump over a ditch or leap timidly from crag to crag. I can still enjoy the caress of sunshine on my body when I sit out in the garden with my shirt off, but the fair weather only aggravates my feelings of frustration that I cannot get on with any work in the garden and the lawn

shines white with daisies. I never thought that I would miss so much the simple pleasures of physical activity such as digging or even lawn mowing, tasks which were at one time a nuisance and a bore but now that all these simple activities of life have gone how important they are and how much their deprivation means to me.

As an ex classical scholar at Cambridge, I still find some solace in the classics and for some time I have been chasing about in long disused corridors of my memory searching for a couplet from my beloved Horace. Eventually I found it, dredged up from deep dark pools of memory whose waters have been undisturbed these 40 years or more.

Si fractus illabatur orbis,
Impavidum ferient ruinae.

The translation in my own rather pedestrian verse is as follows:

If his world should break in pieces
and be all around him laid,
You would find him in the ruins
standing firm and undismayed.

A somewhat Kiplingesque philosophy I will do my best to achieve, but to which I have not yet attained. My world has equally collapsed around me, but I cannot yet claim to be undismayed, though I hope to acquire virtue as time passes.

(Kyle 1976)

How my teaching about the management of stroke would change after my own

Trevor H. Howell

Trevor Howell was a research fellow in geriatric medicine. He died in 1988.

On 28 April 1983 I had a cerebrovascular accident. My left arm became useless; the left side of my mouth felt strange and so did my tongue; swallowing was difficult and I tended to choke when I drank. For some time my arm felt a vibration, as if I had been lying on it for a long time. Fortunately my leg remained quite unaffected and I had no sensory abnormalities.

For the first three days I had to live on semisolids. Solid food tended to accumulate in the corners of my mouth and under my tongue. After this the lips and tongue returned to normal, so that I could eat more normally in comfort. At the same time the movement came back to my shoulder. One odd clinical finding was that when I yawned the fingers of my left hand would move.

After this, shoulder movements became fuller, elbow movements started to come back, and eventually, wrist flexion and extension made their appearance. After two months, the fingers began to flex and extend, but the thumb and index finger recovered less then the others. For several weeks there was considerable oedema of the left hand, including the proximal part of the fingers. This was to produce some difficulties later.

The clinical sequence of events described above produced a number of problems in daily living which had to be solved. Given that I had taught students about these for many years I began to think how my own experience would affect what I taught them. What follows is what I would now say.

THE DOCTOR'S ROLE

When a doctor is called to see a patient with a stroke he usually finds both the sick person and his family in a state of shock and despondency. After examining the patient and assessing his condition his first duty is to encourage them. He must not commiserate that the patient has suffered a serious loss of function, but congratulate them that so much ability still remains. Then he should advise that the affected limbs should be put through their full range of movements several times a day, either by a physiotherapist or by the family themselves, as Celsus advised in the first century AD.

As the patient starts to recover several problems will arise from his residual disabilities. The family should be warned about these and given guidance as to how to deal with them. One of the first will be the question of bathing. If the patient gets into a bath the weakness of his hemiplegic limbs will make it very difficult to get out, even with help. A bath seat, or a plank placed across the bath, will enable him to sit up and use his good arm and hand to help in washing himself. Self help must be encouraged and dependence on others discouraged. When he becomes stronger and can get into the bath unaided, there is a set of movements which will enable the patient to get out of it without help. First, he should sit upright. He then clenches his good fist and presses it on the bottom of the bath. Next he rotates his body to the strong side, flexing his legs as he does so, with his feet on the bottom of the bath. Extension of the legs will allow him to stand up, ready to get out of the bath.

After this, the patient should try to dry himself. He may find that a large bath towel is unsatisfactory, since it tends to fall into folds, which get in the way of his rubbing movements. A small towel is simpler to control, and will make it easier to dry his unaffected limbs and the inner aspect of his hemiplegic arm and leg. Nevertheless, he will have to twist his trunk if he is to rub the outer side of his weak limbs. This may cause a strain in his lower intercostal muscles of the hemiplegic side, which may be painful. It may prove rather hard to dry the upper part of the good arm, and particularly the axilla, if the hemiplegic wrist and hand have recovered only incompletely.

DRESSING

After drying, the next problem is to get dressed. Each garment has its own difficulties. For example, it is not too hard to put on pants with one hand, grasping first one side and then the other alternately, pulling upward. To get trousers in position, however, needs similar movements repeated six or eight times. Even so, the garment tends to droop towards the floor when the grip is released. This is most obvious towards the end of the operation, when it becomes necessary to fix the top of the trousers, either by a button or a clip. At this moment gravity comes into play and the whole garment falls to the floor unless caught in time. In fact, putting on trousers may be fatiguing and exasperating. Nevertheless, the garment can be secured by leaning against a wall while doing up the buttons or zip. If the garment has braces attached these can be looped over an arm to prevent the trousers from descending. It is so easy to put on the garment with two hands and relatively difficult with only one.

Putting on socks may create similar problems. These may be overcome by invaginating the part covering the foot, folding the ankle portion over it. This allows the toes to be easily introduced. Then a one handed pull will bring the sock up into position and the ankle portion can be folded back. Vests, shirts, and coats have their own peculiarities. Getting the weak arm into its sleeve first is not too difficult. But there is then a tendency for the garment to get on top of the head when the other arm is introduced. This may necessitate a series of awkward rotatory movements to grasp the lower part of the shirt or vest or coat to pull it downwards into position. Pyjama tops have a similar problem.

I have already mentioned the need for compensatory movements while dressing. Such movements also become necessary in everyday life. Any object on the weak side of the body may be difficult to reach with the affected hand. Hence the trunk is rotated to allow the good hand to grasp it. This may be quite forcible at times, twisting the intercostal muscles, which become quite painful as a result. This brings us to the problem of sleeping. Patients are always advised to sleep on the sound side. But if they attempt to turn over in bed, the strained intercostal muscles, which are tender, wake them up and they have a broken night's sleep. To one who had previously been a good sleeper that proved more than a nuisance and I had to choose an analgesic carefully to stop the whole sequence.

Re-education in walking is best undertaken by a physiotherapist. When the patient has to put on shoes, however, he may find it difficult or impossible to tie his laces in a bow. In these circumstances, the use of elastic laces which remain permanently tied but allow the feet to enter the shoes without difficulty since they stretch to accommodate them is a great advantage.

There is a definite technique in getting into bed. The patient must approach it closely so that his calves touch the bedclothes. He then sits down and loops the strong ankle underneath the weak one. Rotating the trunk and flexing the knees at the same time will allow him to get on top of the bed. He can now move into a suitable position by leaning on his elbow and ankles, which can be used to let him wriggle into place. Such a manoeuvre is best performed with the strong side towards the head of the bedstead.

I cannot emphasise too strongly that one of my greatest enemies was the frustration which resulted from fruitless struggling to perform tasks which would have normally been simple to carry out unaided. It could cause one to become morose and miserable —distressing both me and all those around me.

TOILET PROBLEMS

An unexpected difficulty arises when a hemiplegic patient goes to the lavatory and wants to use toilet paper. A pull on the roll with the unaffected hand merely unravels the entire roll leaving a yard lying loose on the floor. One has to find some way of anchoring the roll while using the good hand to detach one piece at a time. At first it may be necessary to place the head firmly on top of the toilet roll before trying to detach a section with the stronger hand. Alternatively, several pieces of loose paper may be placed on a shelf or small table within reach.

FATIGUE

An unexpected complication of my stroke was a definite loss of exercise tolerance. This seemed due to several factors. Firstly, there was an element of cerebral shock. Secondly, and more important, was the frequent need to undertake compensatory movements with my right hand. These tended to strain my lower left intercostal muscles, causing pain. Broken sleep would make for a poor night's rest and give a feeling of tiredness next day. Finally, the need for repeated compensatory movements was much more tiring than normal activities of the left hand would have been.

OEDEMA OF THE HAND

Oedema of the hand has been known for almost a century. The best modern account was given by Exton-Smith and Crockett, who found it in 16% of their series of hemiplegic patients.[1] The oedema fluid has a high protein content and it seems to originate in inefficient drainage from the lymphatics resulting from poor and infrequent movement of the muscles. Usually occupying the dorsum of the affected hand, sometimes, however, the oedema may lie on the palmar aspect of the fingers. Here (since fingers recover last and least) it may become organised and make flexion of the affected digits difficult. Hence effective treatment of the

oedematous parts is important. Passive movements will do something towards draining the fluid away. If these are not wholly successful other methods may have to be tried. The use of sinusoidal electrical current is sometimes beneficial in encouraging drainage by making movements in the small muscles of the hand. Where there is an element of spasticity present faradism is contraindicated. When that is absent, however, such a current can cause more forcible movements with benefit to the patient. The use of plasticine or 'putty' has only limited value in restoring movement in hemiplegic hands, as opposed to its effectiveness in arthritic fingers.

In my own case the residual organised protein failed to disappear even on voluntary movement. Hence I went back to my own physiotherapists at Queen's Hospital, Croydon, and asked them to help me with a research project. Our first move was to use the flow pulse intermittent pressure apparatus to squeeze the tissues of my left arm, hoping in this way to remove the inspissated protein residue, which limited my ability to flex the fingers. This might have been much more effective if it had been used earlier, but, though there was some improvement, little pads still remained in the palmar aspect of my proximal phalanges showing pitting on pressure. These diminished immediately after treatment.

Since my own experience had shown that ultrasonics could soften fibrous tissue I asked my physiotherapists to use this. Stiffness in the shoulder was greatly relieved, but the effect on the fingers was only slight at first, but showed improvement later.

It is a common observation that hemiplegic patients disregard their affected limbs. There may be two aspects to this. One, the inattention is due to neurogenic damage. Another, I found, was that having evolved compensatory movements in the good hand, I employed these instead of using the weak limb.

THE HEMIPLEGIC STIFF SHOULDER

A stiff, painful shoulder after a stroke is not unusual. If neglected this can cause considerable discomfort and disability. It must not be allowed to go untreated for long. The most effective form of therapy seems to be intra-articular injection of a mixture of 1 ml hydrocortisone solution in 4 ml local anaesthetic. This should be immediately followed by putting the joint through its full range of movements. Treatment by ultrasonics will help to maintain the increased range of joint activity.

MORALE

I have commented how a hemiplegic patient may easily become morose and depressed. Special efforts should be made to give him every encouragement. He and his family should be told that the leg usually recovers more quickly than the arm. They should also learn that improvement may continue for at least 18 months after the stroke. The more the patient tries to do for himself, the better will be his chance of recovery. But it must also be remembered that a number of 'gadgets' can help him to compensate for his disability: things such as a Nelson knife, may make all the difference to his eating habits, for instance. In fact, it is almost true to say that there is now a special tool or adaptation for every common lesion. Hence the help of an occupational therapist is of great value.

CONTRACTURES

In certain hemiplegic patients the tone in the flexor and adductor muscles is too great for the extensors and abductors. This may sometimes result in joint contracture. Hence every attempt must be made to promote extension and abduction of the affected limbs. Drug treatment is of limited use in these cases, though dantrolene may be used in doses increasing from 25 mg to 100 mg five times a day. In any case, great care must be taken to avoid injury or abrasion to the affected parts, since healing is always poor and chronic ulceration not uncommon. A contracted limb is a great handicap.

CONCLUSION

A stroke is always a great shock, both physical and psychological, to anyone. There is little place for drugs in treatment. Most of the improvement possible must come from the efforts of the patient himself. He should be given every available help and encouragement to guide and help his progress. To discard such a case too early is culpable negligence.

REFERENCE

1. Exton-Smith A. N. and Crockett, D. J. (1957). Nature of oedema in paralysed limbs of hemiplegic patients. *British Medical Journal*, **ii**, 1280–3.

(Howell 1984)

My experience had a famous name

David Goldberg

David Goldberg was, at the time of writing his article, a physician specializing in child and adolescent psychiatry.

I had a stroke. Not that I knew it at the time. I did know that if I moved even slightly the world would spin for the next few minutes. I knew that if I opened my eyes I was entering a world in which I was unable to think. Like a late night B movie I saw two views at once, both circling each other and more, much more. I could not put words to this and my other symptoms—my body was changing, I felt in flux. It was simplest to shut my eyes and lie still rehearsing the presentation which I was due to give the next day.

My wife asked what was wrong. She ran up and down stairs with the vomit bucket and became increasingly concerned as I was only able to repeat that I felt unwell. Despite years as a doctor, some as a neurologist in training, I had inadequate vocabulary to explain what I was experiencing. If I began my explanation sounded vague, full of similies and metaphors. After relaying my cursory description to a friend, a consultant neurologist, my wife returned from the telephone to say that my symptoms did warrant calling out the general practitioner. I knew that I was ill and stopped preparing for the presentation. I began making calculations as to when I would recover from the surgical removal of a posterior fossa tumour and where I would go on my first holiday.

The locum general practitioner asked about my symptoms. I replied as briefly as possible, not wanting to be considered histrionic. Luckily he did not ask me to elaborate as I would have been comprehensible only to myself. As he performed a careful neurological examination, I noted my physical signs. He stopped before finishing, saying that the problem was definitely neurological and too complicated for him. I felt strangely reassured by his puzzlement and that he spent time working out how I could get downstairs to the ambulance.

My body continued to feel as if it was changing, gaining and losing properties, not all unpleasant. I would recite to myself descriptions of my visual and other symptoms. During my first day in hospital I gave my story four or five times when I was examined. I began to find discrete words and phrases to describe my symptoms, adapting and clarifying them in response to the examining doctors' questions. By the end of the day I could summarise my history quite quickly; it was not a description of my experience but did answer the doctors' questions as accurately as possible. The last doctor declared that my story fitted lateral medullary or Wallenburg's syndrome and that the nuclear magnetic resonance scanning would show this. It did.

The scan changed everything. I was no longer asked for detailed descriptions of my symptoms; the puzzle was over. I was happy. My fear of multiple sclerosis, which had been referred to as inflammation, disappeared. It was replaced by the thought that I had a diseased bit of body and the rest was all right. The stroke became an 'it' which troubled the rest of my body. I was no longer preoccupied by the feeling that my whole body was changing and diseased. Diagnosis worked like magic: the whole of me was no longer strange; just a tiny, though important, bit of me. Furthermore, my experience had a name and a famous one, a hero who had saved many Jews at the expense of his own life.

A succession of doctors—physicians, surgeons, radiologists, and researchers—followed as I was investigated to find a cause of the stroke. Most asked me to tell my story. Some inquired more, puzzled, and continued inquiring. They asked about my sensations while they examined me and finally discussed which symptoms they could explain and those they did not understand. I felt reassured by their statements of what they knew and what they could not make sense of. Somehow their acceptance of uncertainty was helpful. Other doctors asked for limited information and tended to make more definitive statements. I thought I was questioning their authority when I answered questions expansively. It was as if expression of ignorance or uncertainty challenged their skill while other doctors saw this as part of their skill.

Most of the time I did not think of my symptoms as they changed. In conversation it was easier to use approximations or technical words. For instance I used the words pain or spinothalamic to refer to what was not like any pain I had ever experienced. It is more a bizarre perception, an afterthought to some sensation of being squeezed and released. When people empathised or referred to pains that they had had I was left bemused. How could they remember it when I could not from minute to minute?

I was pleased when the doctors explained the medical details. But it was hard to think that they were talking about me as only the sensations were real while the lateral medullary stroke was a dark area on the nuclear magnetic resonance scan or a squiggly line on the angiogram. When statistics were mentioned in discussion of a possible operation I was left muddled. Did I want to make a bet on my life? I have always been hopeless at gambling. 'What questions would you ask in similar circumstances?' I asked the neurosurgeon. His manner changed and he told me a story of how, after the discovery of his son's brain tumour, he had had to forget all his neurosurgery. This story helped me in a way I can only guess at.

Other stories told by my doctors were also of more use to me than medical explanations. Even the medical explanations felt like stories which may or may not be true. The personal experiences of the doctors assured me that they and others had difficulty making sense of their symptoms. Even now, two months after the stroke, I still feel a need for my symptoms to be legitimised. Although the textbooks do not describe the return of symptoms when tired, I rediscover them afresh each day. Once I was told that others had described this I feel less frustrated. I was given an explanation that the brain suppresses symptoms until it is time to rest. Symptoms are a message to take it slowly. This is a comforting image which may not be physiologically accurate.

I still do not know what sense, if any, to make of having a stroke at the age of 40. Neither could the doctors who asked my wife if I was a secret smoker. 'It is just one of those things—a one off', I was told. At first I wondered about an explanation but did not come up with one. Some of my friends attributed it to some aspect of my personality and wondered what I should change about my lifestyle. Nevertheless, it did give me an idea that if I wanted to change my life I could use the fact that I had had a stroke as justification. What story did I want to make about the importance of having the stroke? Did I want to leave London and live in the country? I would like to remember the experience of having a stroke but since it is so hard to find the words I do not know how to. What I do remember are the stories of my fellow patients as they also made sense of being ill.

(Goldberg 1993)

COMMENTARY (Kyle, Howell, Goldberg)

Kyle, who appears to have suffered a right hemisphere stroke, notes the tricks, aids and adaptations that he had to use in his everyday adjustment, and the frustration/depression that accompanies the thoughts of not being able to enjoy life to the full. His article brings home the point that every patient with a significant neurological disability should be visited at home by an experienced occupational therapist, physiotherapist or community nurse. Clinical neuropsychology probably has a role to play in design of compensatory aids to help in the rehabilitation of the neurological patient in the community—an excellent starting point for clinical neuropsychologists to start thinking in this direction is the book by Norman (1988).

Howell points to the importance of encouraging the patient and his/her family after a stroke and actively promoting recovery and compensatory strategies, and not just leaving the patient with a rather hopeless prognosis. Like Kyle, he also gives detailed advice on a range of everyday self-care and other tasks. He notes how difficult it is to put on a pair of trousers with only one hand—perhaps every medical student should have this exercise to do as an essential part of their medical training! Howell's stroke affected his right hemisphere. He notes that the disregard of the affected limbs that is often reported in such patients may be due not only to inattention factors, but also to compensatory movements having evolved in the good limb, with a consequent reduction in use/absence of use of the weak limb. Howell notes that improvement may continue for at least 18 months after a stroke. This is important to remember—although the general dictum of the first 3–6 months seeing the most recovery may be correct, it is worth bearing in mind that the slight improvements that occur in the subsequent 1–2 years may result in a particular everyday self-care task being executed without a lot of frustration; this in itself will significantly help the morale and well-being of the patient and his family. It is also worth bearing in mind that some stroke patients may not be as aware as Howell about their recovery of function. Grotta and Bratina (1995) found that only half of the patients in their sample were retrospectively aware of the severity of the neurological deficits in the first 24 hours after the onset of the stroke, and, when recovery occurred, many of these appeared to be unaware of the extent of recovery that had taken place.

The main points of interest in Goldberg's account are: the initial symptoms of 'confusion' and word-finding difficulty, even though the stroke was not in the cerebral hemispheres but in the brainstem; the return of some of his symptoms when he became tired; and the ill-defined symptoms of 'pain' that he suffered.

REFERENCES

Grotta, J. and Bratina, P. (1995). Subjective experiences of 24 patients dramatically recovering from stroke. *Stroke*, **26**, 1285–88.

Norman, D. A. (1988). *The psychology of everyday things*. Basic Books, New York.

A personal account by a sufferer from a stroke

P. Smithells

P. Smithells was a professor of physical education, within a department of physiology.

1

I would venture the opinion after 42 years of professional work, that the majority of people who enter the physical education profession do so because of their motor skills and high ability in learning new skills. I came into physical education from intellectual conviction and not because I had any soupcon of physical perfection. I remained in the field because it provided a continuing intellectual and spiritual challenge.

Learning motor skills never came easily to me. As a small child I had difficulty with my shoe laces, and at kindergarten prevailed on an older girl to attend to my shoes. Later on though I learned to tie a bow with a secret knot and mastered the art of knotting and lashing so useful in camping and outdoor life. I became a person who used his hands a lot, in speech, in acting, in play, as well as in conjuring.

2

In July 1975, shortly after retiring, I found it difficult to hold a chisel, could not tie my shoe laces and became a little confused about left and right, and in fact found my body very disobedient when doing practical tasks. This was in a sense like returning to my over-grown adolescence and its awkward body. In August 1975 I fell off a ladder breaking six adjacent ribs on my left side, a singularly painful experience. I realised that long-established neuro-muscular patterns were not working or were at least impaired.

I went then to an ophthalmologist who was testing my optical fields routinely and he immediately rang the neurologists at the hospital who agreed to see me the following day. After a few tests it seemed possible that I had had a parietal lobe stroke, which explained to me the lack of feedback from the muscles and joints on my left leg and arm. When I was admitted to hospital the neurologists recommended that I have an arteriogram, a procedure which I did not relish, but which was very skilfully carried out. The findings were inconclusive with no impairment of carotid blood supply. Difficulties with my left hand and leg became gradually worse with little remission of symptoms until September 1975 when physiotherapy was started and proved immediately helpful. I continued to walk whenever I could but there was speech impairment and ptosis of the left eye and weakness of the cheek and mouth. All function of my left hand disappeared but I could still walk with a dragging action for I had not kinaesthetic sense, the bio-feed-back mechanisms having been knocked out.

3

I continued to write, but my handwriting always difficult, became even more undisciplined losing both horizontal and vertical accuracy, even though carried out by my unimpaired dominant hand. The worst blow was the loss of will-power. I had often pondered on where the seat of the will could be neurophysiologically speaking, and now conclude that it must be in the intact upper motoneurone. It is a blow to the ego not being able to move a limb when you want to. It also is a very strange experience and as such disorientating. This led to a lot of sartorial confusion buttoning shirts and cardigans wrongly and putting on ties inaccurately. One has the feeling of shabbiness. Eating is a messy performance at first but then one learns to use a combined fork and knife with the one hand and not to eat soups that require full control of mouth and throat. Cutaneous sensations being diminished, one is unaware about what is on the face on the affected side where the menu is there for all to see. One's total postural reflexes alter and in walking one's pendant useless arm is apt to become very cold and somewhat oedematous, producing a general spinal twist, of a scoliotic kind. I was apt to scuff the sole and inner edge of my weakened left shoe though later walking with a stick helped to diminish this unwanted abrasion. My head poked forward in walking producing a long kyphosis and a wobbly cervical spine, which led to some restriction in chest movement and breathing. One general reaction was my perpetual state of drowsiness and ennui, so that if I took my usual post-prandial sleep, it was apt to go on far too long. I used a timer with an alarm to control this tendency. After a sleep I was very slow to pick up in vitality of perception and action and would stumble around in an unco-ordinated fashion, blundering hither and thither.

One of the curious effects of the stroke and what an appropriate term, was a loss of timbre in my voice which had always been deep and resonant, and I became slightly enunuchoid. I used to read poetry in public and broadcast and my voice became to me an instrument which I could no longer play properly. I do not know who coined the word 'stroke', but it is such a one-fell-swoop experience that I think stroke is a singularly appropriate term for the sudden cutting-off of competence. I had always been in previous illnesses a quick healer, so living with the slow recovery of a stroke has been a salutary

lesson in accepting the inevitability of age and the inevitable decrepitude of old-age.

Remarkably the one mechanism that has never wavered has been my appetite for food, and for learning, and for delving into the past. I am blessed with almost total recall in terms of memory so that I can remember the absolute detail of what happened 20 and 30 years ago, including topics of conversation on the last occasion of meeting. I have no difficulty with names and faces, and although I have now moved far away from where I did my 30 years of University teaching, visits from old graduates passing through bring instant recall and much pleasure through being able to reminisce about the past. I hope I have not become a bore, the most unforgiveable of senile traits. I have had a very happy and exceedingly busy life with interesting people and challenges all the way.

4

On 14 November 1976 I suffered a second stroke and am now totally paralysed on the left side except in my speech and some aspects of recall, so that this account is not written with the clarity of my former self. I am rather tired and unable to sustain consecutive thoughts unless reminded by my wife. I do hope that this scrappy account may give a grain of insight into the stroke condition or alternatively warn people to restructure their lives if their jobs are their lives.

Professor Smithells died in January 1977 after a third stroke.

(Smithells 1978)

COMMENTARY

Smithells' account is from one who was not medically trained, but—because of his professional background in physical education—Smithells had unique insights into the loss of motor skill that accompanied his stroke. It is interesting that the onset of his difficulties appeared to be gradual rather than sudden, with the initial occurrence of difficulties in tying his shoe-laces, minor left-right confusion, and a general awkwardness/loss of control of his body movements. He probably had some subtle spatial deficits, since his writing with his intact, right hand suffered from loss of vertical and horizontal accuracy. The loss of will-power for things that were previously 'willed' automatically led to frustration and difficulties in many everyday motor tasks, such as putting on clothes, eating, etc. Smithells reported that his power of recall, particularly for longer-term past events, remained clear—even putting names to faces, a notorious memory symptom in many forms of brain disease, was not affected. This relative preservation of memory function is often present in cerebrovascular disease, where there may be focal cortical involvement with sparing of critical temporal lobe and limbic-diencephalic structures. It is also worth noting that he found it therapeutic to reminisce about the past with friends and former students. This highlights the dictum that a key part of the everyday activities after a major neurological event, such as a stroke, should include the patient taking part in those activities that are both enjoyable and are subsumed by spared neuropsychological functions. Memories and skills that are well-established/over-learned are rarely affected in brain disease, and they should be used as a platform on which to build either therapeutic interventions or activities simply to pass the time of day.

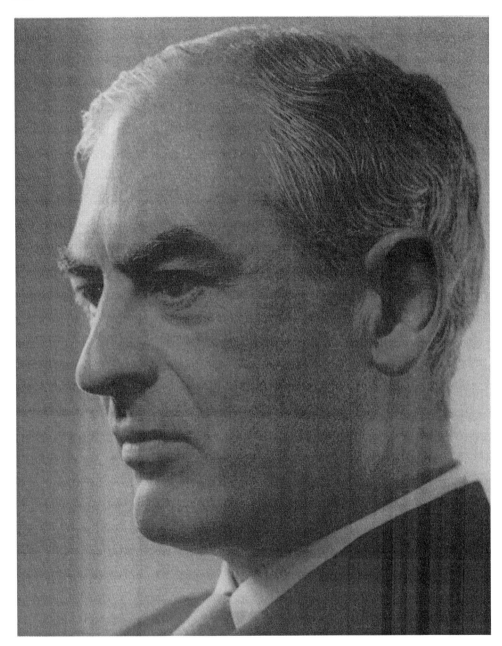

Figure 10. Sir Peter Medawar.

Memoir of a thinking radish

Peter Medawar

Sir Peter Medawar (1915–87) was an immunologist who shared, with Macfarlane Burnet, the 1960 Nobel Prize for Physiology or Medicine. He was a zoologist by training, being Professor of Zoology at the University of Birmingham (1947–51) and then at University College, London (1951–62). He subsequently became director of the National Institute of Medical Research, London from 1962 to 1971, and after this he was head of the Transplantation Biology Section of the Clinical Research Centre, London.

ILLNESS

While I read the Lesson I became aware that something was going wrong: my speech became slow and rather slurred and I felt as if I was somehow being dragged down on my left side. I completed the Lesson, however, and was supported by a verger back to my place, hoping to look as if nothing was happening. Jean realized that I was having a stroke. She said to the Cathedral dignitary sitting next to her, 'My husband is having a stroke. I must go to him.' He tried to reassure her, 'Don't be concerned, dear lady, it's probably the acoustics.' She boldly came to my seat and I was helped down the aisle and transported as quickly as possible to the Royal Infirmary, where I came under the care of Mr John Simpson FRCS. It was all monstrous bad luck, because at this time Dr Jim Whyte Black had not yet devised beta blockers, which slow the heart-beat and could have preserved my health and my career. As it was, it soon became clear that I had had a massive bleed in my right cerebral hemisphere. As soon as he heard of this disaster, the Professor of Medicine in University College London, Sir Max Rosenheim, who had been advising me, came straight to Exeter. A doctor, Jean, and a nurse took me up to London by train and in accordance with Max Rosenheim's instructions I was transported directly to McAlpine Ward in the Middlesex Hospital, in order to come under the care of Michael Kremer, whom Max rated the foremost neurologist in England. McAlpine was an eight-bedded ward in the

charge of Shirley Kean, known throughout the hospital for her expertise as a nurse and, I may add from my own knowledge, her psychological insight and her belief in the efficacy of the form of therapy known as TLC (tender loving care).

A right-sided cerebral haemorrhage impairs the use of the left arm and the left leg, and the left half of each eye. There was also some anxiety about the possibility of mental impairment. Two circumstances put Jean's and my physicians' minds at rest on the subject of my higher faculties. The first was that I had said shortly after my stroke, with reference to my having read the lesson, 'Human beings simply don't realize the risks they run when they meddle in the supernatural.' I learned later that this remark had come to the ears of the Bishop, Dr Mortimer, who was said to have thought it—as I did myself—rather funny. The second piece of evidence was proffered my first night in the Middlesex Hospital after the operation to remove the blood clot from my brain. Jean stayed with me all night because my fate was uncertain. I myself, habitually sanguine, had considered and dismissed the possibility of dying. I was so deeply unconscious after the operation for the removal of the clot that Dr Kremer encouraged Jean to get me to wake up and take notice. She accordingly leaned over, bringing her pretty face close to mine and whispering words to bring me to my senses and say something to her. My first words were 'Entire visual field is agreeably occupied'. I thought this remark apposite and well turned and it repudiated the case that my mind had deteriorated beyond hope of recovery.

Getting better after a stroke is a weary and lengthy business. It is a matter of time more than anything else and of course of the skill of the physiotherapists. In this latter respect I was very well served and marvelled at their patience and willingness to crawl on the floor to pull my left leg for me in my first lessons in walking. I had one frightening setback, though—more than two months after my original operation I developed a violent headache that was judged to be due to a substantial brain abscess caused, it turned out, by bacteria which presumably entered the original wound through the drainage tube necessarily inserted into it. This called for another, very urgent operation, which, not unexpectedly, caused further scarring and neurological damage. My mind wandered a bit after this second operation and I can remember some confused and unreasonable thoughts: I complained urgently to Jean that lying under my bed was an enormous radioactive skate which could not but be a danger to other patients. It was also discovered that I had lost the left half of my field of vision in both eyes. Even this disability made its contribution to the human comedy by making it possible for the more audacious nurses to creep up on the left-hand side of my bed, reach over, and help themselves to chocolate truffles or any of the other delicacies my friends had brought me. My visual defect incidentally, was identified using the simplest possible apparatus—passing a bunch of jingling keys past my visual field from left to right while I looked straight ahead. My condition was discerned by Dr Graham Bull, a very intelligent and accomplished physician who later became Head of the MRC's Clinical Research Centre and thus in a year or two my boss.

Life in the ward during convalescence was not without its distractions. Jean came for about half of every day, in spite of being preoccupied and harassed by administrative problems in the Family Planning Association of which she was the chairman, bringing nourishing home-made soup ('nerve soup', I called it) and news of the outside world. With

Sister Kean's connivance we also kept at bay a number of people who, though I had no wish to see them, wanted to see me, more out of curiosity than compassion. But my true friends and my children—and sometimes theirs—were a joy and they also gave much pleasure to the nurses and other inmates of the ward. With characteristic wisdom Dr Kremer allowed me a modest ration of B and B (Benedictine and Brandy) to recruit my spirits from time to time, and I, having been educated at an English public school, thought hospital food tasty and agreeable and always looked forward to my 'wittles'. Physiotherapy proceeded daily and I enjoyed it when not hopelessly slugged by the injudicious practice of administering sleeping tablets at night.

After four or five months I was judged fit enough to go to a rehabilitation centre that turned out to be the worst medical institution of any kind I have ever known—a tragic example of how what might otherwise have been a good place was morally undermined by a self-important and in my opinion incompetent director. I was taken to this little man for a first appraisal by Jean and a close friend, Dr David Pyke, who was also Registrar of the Royal College of Physicians. I did not look for or expect anything but civility and a sound medical judgement, but this was not to be my lot. The director was evidently much put out by my being a Knight and a Nobel-Prize winner. He'd show me, he must have thought, when he bustled into his office past the three of us, waiting at the appointed time. Instead of saying, as a normal human being would, 'I'll be with you in just a second', he disregarded us completely and stalked into his office. When I entered, the clinical appraisal began. Of my left arm, after a perfunctory examination he said, 'Your arm will never get better: it's not worth my while to prescribe any treatment for it'. The treatment he did prescribe was not, as I had hoped, that I should be given lessons in walking, but that I should have lessons in how to propel a wheelchair using only one arm and one leg. He also arranged for me a psychological appraisal, the design of which was so disgracefully bad it deserves to be recounted in detail. I was sat before an apparatus rather like a typewriter with one row of perhaps fifteen numbered keys alternating in colour. The depression of one of these keys either lit up a cheerful little light-bulb or made the electronic equivalent of a refined fart. The exercise was to traverse the keyboard from left to right depressing as I went along only those keys that would cause the light to come on, eschewing farts. 'Take your time', said the psychologists, 'and have as many goes as you like'. I tried again and again, starting off all right by recognizing a pattern in the colours of the keys but always ending with farts. I became increasingly exasperated and eventually—for this is one of the most disagreeable sequelae of a stroke—rather tearful. The psychologists decided I was mentally impaired and told Jean so—a judgement with which she did not agree, though she might easily have been upset. The truth is that these psychologists did not suspect or look for evidence of the eye defect which should have been as obvious to them as it had been to Graham Bull when he had asked me to draw a man for him—in a matchstick form, if I couldn't do better. I had drawn a matchstick man, gave him a fine head of hair but no right arm or right leg, these being outside my field of vision. Although he had a much better clue than Graham Bull had, the director was not attentive enough to discern that anything was amiss.

The exercises at working a wheelchair with one arm and one leg were in full swing when I had a surprise visit one afternoon from Sister Kean and the head of the Physiotherapy Department at the Middlesex Hospital —a friendly call to see how I was getting on. They were scandalized that I was not walking and that no attempt had been made to teach me to do so. I had indeed deteriorated seriously, having received no treatment whatsoever, though my room-mate—a doctor of science—had been gravely instructed by the occupational therapists in how to toast bread by holding a pre-cut bread slice between forefinger and thumb, dropping it into an electric toaster, and switching on the electric current. It was the kind of toaster, I suspect, that would announce the completion of the operation by playing the 'Star-Spangled Banner' as the toast leapt out of the instrument on to one's plate. The occupational therapists tried to teach me to tie a shoe-lace with one hand but, whether through my stupidity or their inability to teach, it was a knack I never mastered. Living in this remedial centre was a real pain. The male nurses I came across were homosexual to the extent that I dreaded being bathed or conducted to the lavatory by them; I was also dismayed to find when I returned from a weekend at home that the attractive picture of Jean I kept in my bedside drawer to spirit me up from time to time had been neatly torn across, leaving a pile of fragments that could not be reassembled.

Another of the trials of the stroke or MS victim is to hear the views of amateur theologians who see misfortune as a manifestation of divine benevolence. Thus a speaker on BBC Radio 4's popular morning 'God-spot' said that one of the lesser benefactions of a disabling illness was the opportunity it created for others to display magnanimity and helpfulness that would make them feel good. I was not impressed by this argument.

Another indignity I had to submit to was a drawing class where I was required to execute a still life consisting of a bottle of gin (empty) and a glass (the art teacher told Jean 'I always think it does "them" good to do something different'). It didn't do me a bit of good because of my loss of vision and because I am in any case a wholly verbal type with not much visual sense. This episode resolved me to quit the premises, beginning with long weekends at home. My action was strongly opposed by one or two of the psychiatrists with their overall pockets full of anti-depressants. They warned Jean that if I went home even for a weekend I would probably refuse to come back at all. All this determined us to cut short the proposed stay of several months. When Jean informed the director of this, he said grimly, 'On your own head be it'.

My stay at this supposedly remedial centre had been a complete waste of time. The lack of treatment had made me worse and pop music, piped from morning till night, had left me no peace or opportunity for real rest. I was very low indeed after my stay in this ghastly place, having lost my habitual *joie de vivre* and also to a large extent quickness of mind and verbal fluency.

The tearfulness I have referred to is the most embarrassing long-term effect of the stroke, as many other stroke victims have observed. This readiness to dissolve into sobbing is *not* a sign of misery or depression, though goodness knows there is reason enough for it to be so: it is physiological in origin and is not uncommon after extensive injuries to the brain. It is true that sad situations in plays or, characteristically, at the end of operas would provoke weeping—but then, happy endings did also. A moment of glory is a more dangerous trigger than the denouement of a tragedy such as the ending of *Othello*, whether opera or play. As everyone knows, it is an invariable characteristic of tragedy that one feels that all the mischiefs and misunderstandings could be circumvented if only one could join the cast and say a few reassuring words to the principal characters—'Watch out for that Iago,' you whisper urgently, 'he's up to mischief; and by the way don't read any significance into that handkerchief'.

Tragedy is bad enough, God knows, but moments of glory are even worse: in Beethoven's *Fidelio* my undoing is not the miserable plight of the unjustly imprisoned Florestan, but the moment when his faithful wife (alias Fidelio) draws a pistol on the wicked prison governor and distant trumpets from the prison tower announce the arrival of the sheriff's posse—of justice, therefore, and freedom. Fidelio usually gets an ovation at the end of the opera, but my tribute is more often tears—especially if Fidelio is Gwyneth Jones. All this is much more moving then an ostensibly more tragic situation, such as the end of *La Bohème*. The heroine Mimì, surrounded by loving friends, sinks into the last minutes of her life. The extremities are cold, the pulse barely perceptible, and the breathing very light and shallow. Her friends pool and sell their trinkets—one, his overcoat—and propose the preposterous remedy: 'send for some medicine!' This ludicrous suggestion provokes, for a medical

scientist, laughter rather than tears. I am pretty sure that Sir William Osler must have heard this Edwardian favourite and I wonder if it gave him cause to question the wisdom of his famous teaching that medicine in his time was totally inefficacious. A cognate situation, as I told the Royal College of Physicians in a brief address on disability, occurs in *La Traviata*, in which the proposed remedy is even more absurd: 'send for a doctor, send for a doctor!' The College seemed to share my delighted amusement and its President proposed a light dose of Mozart.

I went back to full-time work as soon as I reasonably could, and with the support of my staff I went through the motions of being Director. But I felt as if my life had been transposed to a lower key, especially as the loss of the use of my left hand denied me what had until then been the deep pleasure and intellectual stimulus of working at the bench. The great enemy of which I became acutely aware was *tiredness*, and I spent the working day longing for the evening to come and the working week longing for the weekend—this in spite of having lunch in my room and an after-lunch rest, all arranged for me by my secretary Pauline Townend, whose attentiveness and considerateness helped to keep me afloat at this difficult time. Because we were embarking upon a new project in which I specially wanted to play a practical part, I did begin by sitting beside Mrs Ruth Hunt, using my right hand for various delicate technical procedures while she supplied the office of the left hand. This procedure continued, until with great tact and very good sense Ruth delicately intimated to me that we should get on much better and more quickly if she were to do the whole job herself. I gladly accepted her advice and henceforward she became my right hand as well as my left, with the advantages she had foreseen. Although Ruth was classified as a technician in terms of administrative nomenclature, her skill and intelligence had for some time past effectively made her my research assistant. We collaborated well and in 1985 she also qualified for an M.Sc. degree.

Just now the MRC was going through a difficult period. Thanks mainly to the—in my opinion—injudicious advocacy of Lord Rothschild, the government was engaged in reorganizing the funding of the Research Councils on the basis of the retail trade: customer–contractor was to be the principle, in which the scientist was to put up a research proposal to the government and if the government approved, the scientist would be given a contract to undertake it and bring about the desired result. This was a very bold innovation and had not been the basis on which research had hitherto been conducted. Nor was it the proceeding that had given us penicillin, insulin, the discovery of the blood groups, the elucidation of the causes of myasthenia gravis, the transplantation of tissues, or the discovery of the genetic code. Scientific discovery cannot be premeditated.*

With these difficulties impending, the Council not unnaturally thought it would be well for all parties if their oldest and largest research unit were henceforward to be administered by a younger man, physically fit. When I had been recruiting staff in the past, I always made the point of telling them that the Council was a good employer and that if they did well they would be properly looked after. In my case the Council now had a chance to earn the opinion I had formed of them and they rose to the occasion: it was decided to transplant me and those of my immediate colleagues who would accompany me to the Clinical Research Centre, newly built on the site that also housed the big and very well-equipped regional hospi-tal—Northwick Park Hospital, a mile or so from Harrow-on-the-Hill.

This judgement was of course a blow to me but I could see there was a lot of sense in it. I am essentially a managing-director type and newly appointed managing directors usually do any good they are going to do within five years of their appointment, though the fulfilment of their plans is likely to take somewhat longer than that. I had been Director of the National Institute for nine years, during which the talents of its scientific staff had included immunologists of international reputation such as John Humphrey, Ite Askonas, Leslie Brent, Avrion Mitchison, Martin Raff, Elizabeth Simpson, and David Dresser; not to mention a number of scientific guests including Sol Berson, co-discoverer of immuno-electrophoresis, who set us an awe-inspiring example of total commitment to scientific research; Eugene Lance, the orthopaedic surgeon, and my old friend H. Sherwood (Jerry) Lawrence whose endeavour to demonstrate that a cell-free extract might be a vector of cell-mediated immunity I had followed through all its excitements and setbacks for some twenty years, since we had worked together in University College. With this galaxy of talent it is not surprising that the NIMR came to rank as the principal centre of immunological research in the world. I had done what I could, therefore, and was in a mood to start on a new life in which, being now relieved of administrative chores which I admit I had found increasingly tiresome, I would be able to devote myself uninterruptedly to research and writing.

(Medawar 1986)

* See my book *The limits of science* (New York, 1984; Oxford, 1985).

COMMENTARY

The fear that a patient with an illness or injury to the brain may have 'lost his senses' is an understandable one. Rollings (1989) refers to the feeling of fright and the need for simple reassurance during the acute stages of admission after a stroke. Webb (1994) also refers to feelings of fear as a persistent symptom—fear of major disability, of a further stroke, etc. Indeed, throughout many of the articles in this book it has emerged that the clinicians who found themselves as patients had one of two main concerns—was the illness a life-threatening one, such as cancer, and were they 'losing their mind'. Medawar offers a simple diagnostic test for ensuring that one's mental faculties are well preserved—can the patient, as Medawar could in the early stages of his own right hemisphere stroke, show by his verbal utterances a wit and a sense of humour that conveys the remnants of intellectual vigour? [One could also argue that this applies equally well to non-verbal behaviour after a left hemisphere lesion—witness the case of Moss, who in the early stages of recovery from his stroke, when his condition appeared rather despairing, fondled his wife with a 'familiar twinkle in his eye' (1972, p. 26), thus reassuring her that in some respects his mind was still as sharp as ever].

In his account, Medawar recalls being rather confused after one of his operations—he remembers thinking that there was an enormous radioactive skate under his bed. Many patients in the post-traumatic or post-operative 'confusional state' may have amnesia for what they have said or for events in general that they have experienced. The presumably accurate recollection by Medawar of his confusional state is an example of the exceptions that can occur, and suggests that whatever neural mechanisms may be responsible for such 'confusion' are distinct from those that are responsible for laying down traces into long-term memory. This could, therefore, be seen as an example of confusion without amnesia, since the patient subsequently appeared to have a good recollection of events that occurred during the time of the confusion.

Several interesting points emerge from Medawar's description of his time in the rehabilitation centre. He appears to have been treated in a rather perfunctory manner; he encountered a variable quality of nursing care; he was from the start encouraged to use aids rather than given mobilization to improve his existing abilities; and the psychologist appears to have totally missed out Medawar's visual field defect when conducting a visual attention task that comprised an horizontal array of stimuli. It is uncertain if Medawar, when he points to missing out the right-hand side of the match-stick man that he constructed (p. 285), is referring to the right-side of the man itself, or whether he is referring to the right half of his own visual field. If the latter is the case, this may either be an error on Medawar's part, or it may be an example of right-sided neglect after right cerebral lesions—a rare phenomenon, but one that has occasionally been reported (Weintraub and Mesulam 1987). It is regrettable that the psychologist seems to have made the bland statement that Medawar was 'mentally impaired'. To a patient and to his carer, this may have various connotations that are out of step with those intended by the psychologist.

Medawar gives a graphic description of the tearfulness which he suffered, often brought on by a happy rather than a sad event, such as part of a play that he was watching. He insists that this was physiological rather than psychological in origin. Pathological crying has in fact tended to occur with left rather than right hemisphere lesions (Sackeim et al. 1982). However, it is of note that 'ictal crying' as an epileptic phenomenon has been more often associated with right hemisphere than left hemisphere foci (Offen et al. 1976), and it remains possible that Medawar's episodes were in fact epileptic in nature. Medawar also points to tiredness as a sequel to his stroke, something that appears to run through most of the accounts of this book. Later in the same chapter, Medawar offers 13 aphorisms about how to survive in a British hospital after suffering a disabling neurological illness. (These are reproduced in the Overview chapter at the end of this book (pp. 404–5)). They are probably worth printing and putting up in every ward that cares for neurological patients!

REFERENCES

Moss, C. S. (1972). *Recovery with aphasia.* University of Illinois Press, Urbana.

Offen, M. L., Davidoff, R. A., Troost, B. T., and Richey, E. T. (1976). Dacrystic epilepsy. *Journal of Neurology, Neurosurgery and Psychiatry*, **39**, 829–34.

Rollings, D. (1989). On the receiving end. *Nursing Times*, **85**, 57.

Sackeim H. A., Greenberg M. S., Weiman A. L., Gur R. C., Humger-buhler J.P., and Geschwind, N. (1982). Hemispheric asymmetry in the expression of positive and negative emotions: neurologic evidence. *Archives of Neurology*, **39**, 210–18.

Webb, M. F. (1994). My stroke—'mens sana in corpore non sano'. *Journal of the Royal College of Physicians*, **28**, 474–5.

Weintraub, S. and Mesulam, M. (1987). Right cerebral dominance in spatial attention: further evidence based on ipsilateral neglect. *Archives of Neurology*, **44**, 621–5.

On the receiving end

Fiona Coubrough

Fiona Coubrough worked as a nurse in an intensive care unit.

I was at home on my night off and was due to drive back to work the next morning for a late shift. However, I had had a headache for a few days. It was worse than a simple headache, but not severe enough to worry me. What's more, it did not really fit any of the symptoms I had learnt about during my neurology course.

I was on the telephone to my mother to say I had not gone to work because of this nagging headache, when all of a sudden the room started spinning round. I was sick, then I fell to the floor, dropping the telephone beside me. My mother alerted my father, who called for an ambulance.

A fit and healthy nurse cannot have a stroke at the age of 31, can she? Yet one day I was an active person arranging my next game of squash—the next I was paralysed.

I remember lying on a trolley in casualty being stimulated with a piece of cotton wool and being pricked with a sharp pin. But I could not move my body or nod or shake my head in response. This, I have since learnt, was either owing to oedema during the acute stage or to neuropraxia—a temporary disruption along the nerve fibres. I heard a doctor say to the nurse: 'I don't think there's anyone in there'. At that stage I could not answer, although a voice in my head was screaming: 'But there is and I can hear and feel everything'.

No one who works in an intensive care unit expects to be a patient in one. But that is where I was whisked off to. So many times I had drawn up paralysing and sedating drugs ready for intubation; now it was my turn to receive them. An endotracheal tube was necessary for my airway management. The drugs work well—I can vouch for that! I also dreaded being suctioned. It was so painful. It made me cough violently and took my breath away.

Having a nasogastric tube was another awful experience and I would hate to go through it again. It was so irritating and I desperately wanted to remove it with my recovered good arm. But what was the point? As a nurse I knew it would only be replaced by another. I swear I could feel the liquid feed going down my oesophagus. 'That's impossible', I was reminded, but I am sure I could.

I am sure, too, that I could feel the blood being gently drawn out from my arterial line. If my intravenous antibiotics were given to me well diluted with water, they stung less. It also hurt less when they were given slowly.

At the other end, as it were, I had to have a urinary catheter passed. Even though I know the significance of having to have hourly urine measurements in ICU, I still resisted the catheter as much as I could. The nurses, of course, won.

I hated being alone in my room. I wanted to be watched constantly. What was happening to me? Had anyone told me? I suppose a doctor must have, but when? And what had been said? I knew I had developed a right-sided weakness, but what had caused it? Was I going to be all right? I needed to be reminded of my diagnosis several times a day at first, to make it sink in and to make me realise it was all for real. I was so frightened. Having my hand held and being talked to reassuringly really helped a lot.

In the ward, 10 days later, I had my second stroke—an extension of the first. This left me unable to speak. My mind was in a state of confusion. I refused to believe this could be happening to me. I used a spellboard to spell out 'I don't want to speak to anyone'. The truth was I couldn't speak to anyone. I used to try and talk to myself—to prove I could—while I was alone in the sideroom, with the door closed. But not a sound would pass my vocal cords. It was all so frightening.

Soon, it was time to have the catheter removed, although I was warned that if I was incontinent I would have to have it back in again for a while longer. No sooner had it been removed than I was wet. I felt terribly embarrassed, but was told not to worry about it. But I did. My muscle tone gradually returned, helped by pelvic floor exercises.

As I became more mobile, I was brought the commode—occasionally excreta-stained. Why could the time not have been taken to give it a good clean? I was also frustrated by the number of times I was left on a commode without a call bell in reach, hoping and listening out for a passing nurse to rescue me. Had I ever done this to patients—promising to return a few minutes later, then inevitably getting caught up in something else?

For quite a few weeks after my strokes, I had no tone in my trunk. When I was propped up on the edge of the bed by the occupational therapist for dressing practice, I would fall over backwards, just like a floppy doll.

The next setback was that the nasogastric tube had to be passed again as I failed the swallow assessment. My throat was often sore, relieved only when my mother brought in an ice lolly for me to suck. I found that it was better when my nasogastric tube was removed very quickly as it minimised the gagging; this was different from the way I had always removed them—gently and slowly. 'It's better for patient comfort', we had been taught.

A speech therapist taught me how to turn my head to the right when I swallowed to prevent any fluid from trickling into my airway, because of my impaired swallow reflex. For this reason I was allowed only soup, ice-cream and yoghurts. Consequently I was always starving.

I also had a troublesome time coping with my seasonal hayfever. I did not have the strength in my chest to take a deep breath before blowing my nose, and I was reluctant to take any anti-histamines in case they made me sleepy and marred my physiotherapy sessions. So I could only wipe my nose as it ran, which was frequently. I got through numerous boxes of tissues until I was eventually persuaded to take hayfever tablets guaranteed not to cause drowsiness.

The first time I made an attempt at applying my make-up with my left hand, I attracted lots of wolf-whistles from the nursing staff, which made me feel quite embarrassed. What was the big deal about applying make-up? I suppose they thought 'all dressed up and nowhere to go'! But I have worn make-up every day since I was 17, and I don't feel properly dressed without it.

Before my strokes my first cup of coffee in the morning was vital to me. So I really missed it when I had to go for a bath instead, fitting in with the ward's busy bath schedule. I was frustrated when I was taken for a bath, with the clothes I was to wear that day rolled up in a convenient accompanying ball, as I had always taken pride in my appearance, and would not have countenanced wearing badly creased clothes under normal circumstances. Was I just being too fussy? It was in the bath, in fact, that I cried most, as I realised how dependent I had become.

The disadvantage of being 'neuro-trained' is that I fully understood what had happened. A magnetic resonance imager (MRI) scan confirmed that I had had a pontine infarct. I know that the pons is part of the main motor-fibre pathway, and that I can only hope that the fibres can refind their pathway, or find that an 'alternative pathway' as quickly as possible.

The days in hospital were very long and quite boring. Every day was the same. It was hard to keep track. I would be sweltering in the summer heat wearing my recommended anti-embolism support stockings and my thick plastic ankle support splint. In the past, during the summer months I walked barefoot or in flip-flops. Now I had to wear well-supporting trainers as I could not keep anything else on my foot. It is surprising how much you take for granted the small muscles in your feet which help you hold sandals in place.

I was glad when evening came, because my boyfriend would come and visit me. We often took a walk with my wheelchair down to the local pub. It was so nice to get out for a while and get some fresh air. I could not drink anything alcoholic as my tastebuds had altered and become hypersensitive. Any strong, spicy, or hot foods were out. Even eating an orange made me grimace, and I had to let all my 'hot' drinks become lukewarm before I could bear to drink them.

My recovery continues with lots of physiotherapy, speech therapy and occupational therapy for which I am grateful. I never knew walking was so difficult, involving so much work at hip and pelvis level. I try to help improve my walking by placing the wheelchair a bit further away from the bed each day. It takes a lot of confidence and retraining.

I am making good progress, so I am told. Four months is a very short time in which to recover from such an episode—I have told many patients this in the past. But I didn't quite appreciate what a frustrating and tearful uphill struggle it is. Tasks that used to take a few minutes now take such a lot of time and effort, and I have to learn to do everything one-handed. I am also having to learn to write left-handed. I do lots of crosswords, which are a good incentive to improve my handwriting. I have also learnt the knack of washing and drying my hair one-handed.

I refuse all offers of help because, after all, I have got to learn. I am so grateful to my boyfriend for giving me so much motivation and encouragement and for sticking by me. I don't know what I would have done without him. I think I would have given up this fight long ago.

This experience is bound to change my nursing practice, providing I make a full recovery and am able to return to work. It has made me understand what nursing is really about, and I have had to learn to be the recipient of care, and not the giver.

(Coubrough 1992)

COMMENTARY

Coubrough gives a graphic account of the comforts and discomforts of aspects of her nursing care during the early stages of recovery from her pontine stroke. From the neuropsychological point of view, her comments when she was 'mute' but had full language skills are of particular interest. She had use of a spell-board, which appeared to be of limited benefit. Although more sophisticated communication devices do exist, there must be scope for research by neuropsychologists and language therapists which would enable rapid and successful communication to be possible in such settings. Brainstem strokes, such as the one that Coubrough suffered, are thankfully quite rare, but they highlight the frustrations and psychological difficulties that accompany having to cope with basic self-care needs and being dependent on the understanding and co-operation of others. Although it is unlikely that she suffered persistent memory impairment as such, she did indicate that she needed at first to be reminded of the diagnosis several times a day. It remains possible that there was a transient subtle memory deficit directly due to her lesion (cf. Howard et al. 1992).

There are a number of key practical points on the everyday management of neurological patients that emerge from Coubrough's article, and it is worth outlining them:

1. Don't assume that, because a patient cannot speak, the patient cannot feel and understand everything that is going on around him/her.

2. Being suctioned and having a nasogastric tube is painful. The nasogastric tube gives less pain when it is removed very quickly rather than gently and slowly.

3. Give intravenous antibiotics slowly, and if possible diluted—they hurt less that way.

4. Repeat information to a patient many times—for various reasons, it may not sink in the first time.

5. Self-image is important for patients—they care how they look to others, even when they are in a hospital ward.

6. Find out patients' feelings, and why they feel the way they do.

7. Patients may be bored and need stimulation during their hospital stay. Try to make each day different, but with regular events happening on particular days. This will help to maintain patients' sense of time.

REFERENCE

Howard, R. S., Festenststein, R., Mellers, J., Kartsounis, L. D., and Ron, M. (1992). Transient amnesia heralding brain stem infarction. *Journal of Neurology, Neurosurgery and Psychiatry*, **55**, 977.

INTRODUCTION

Head injury is one of the most common types of damage to the brain, especially in younger age groups. In Great Britain, with a population of around 60 million, 23 000 people suffer a moderate or severe head injury every year.

Head injury can be classified into two types—blunt or closed head injury, where the covering of the brain, known as the dura mater, is not torn; and open head injury, where there is a fracture of the skull and a tearing of the dura mater. In closed head injury of any significant severity, there is loss of consciousness or 'concussion'. The severity of concussion can be gauged by instruments such as the Glasgow Coma Scale, which assesses functions such as motor responsiveness, verbal responsiveness, and eye opening. A further index of the severity of a head injury is the degree of memory loss for events which occurred after the head injury patient has recovered from a period of unconsciousness (i.e. duration of post-traumatic amnesia).

The cortex of the frontal and temporal lobes are particularly susceptible to bruising in patients with closed head injury, and this probably explains the predominance of changes in memory and temperament that are the hallmark of the long-term deficits associated with closed head injury. In addition to focal damage that results from such bruising, or from blood clots that may form as a result of the head injury, there is invariably some degree of diffuse pathology that involves white matter beneath cortical areas. More diffuse pathology may also result from generalized brain swelling, disruption of the flow of cerebrospinal fluid in the brain, and from lack of oxygen to the brain, which arises from factors such as reduction in cerebral blood flow.

In some patients with open head injury, there may be no loss of consciousness yet the patient will still be left with significant neuropsychological deficits. The pattern of deficits will depend on the particular site where the focal brain injury was sustained.

The articles in this section provide a relatively good cross-section of the types of head injury that one meets in clinical practice. All of the patients recovered well enough to be able to recount their experience—to this extent, there is the absence of any case with severe residual cognitive impairments. The **Marshall and Ruff** paper refers to a case of mild head injury, an area that has, until recently, been rather neglected in head injury research. The cases of **Freedman, Linge**, and **LaBaw** represent more severe head injuries, and give a good indication of the types of difficulties encountered by patients and their families after a severe head injury. The reports by **Ostrum** are a little more atypical of what one sees in neuropsychological practice, with the relative absence of direct cortical pathology. However, they do highlight some of the more general psychological sequealae of a severe head injury that results in major disability.

All of the cases in this section would be classified as 'blunt' or 'closed' head injury. Cases of open head injury, such as penetrating missile wounds, are a quite distinct type of injury with a different clinical and neuropsychological profile (Grafman and Salazar 1987). I have yet to encounter an equivalent self-report of such a head injury.

REFERENCE

Grafman, J. and Salazar, S. (1987). Methodological considerations relevant to the comparison of recovery from penetrating and closed head injuries. In *Neurobehavioural recovery from head injury* (ed. H. S. Levin, J. Grafman, and H. M. Eisenberg). Oxford University Press, New York.

FURTHER READING

Lezak, M. (ed.) (1989). *Assessment of the behavioural consequences of head trauma.* Alan Liss, New York.
Richardson, J. T. E. (1990). *Clinical and neuropsychological aspects of closed head injury.* Taylor & Francis, London.
Rosenthal, M., Griffith, E. R., Bond, M. R., and Miller, J. D. (ed.) (1990). *Rehabilitation of the adult and child with traumatic brain injury.* F. A. Davis, Philadelphia.

Thirty-five months of recovery from trauma, a subjective report. Closed brain injury

Wallace L. LaBaw

Wallace LaBaw was a physician at the time of his injury.

'In 1965, 52 million accidental injuries killed 107 000, temporarily disabled over 10 million and permanently impaired 400 000 American citizens at a cost of approximately $18 billion. This neglected epidemic of modern society is the nation's most important environmental health problem. It is the leading cause of death in the first half of life's span . . . 49 000 deaths in 1965 were due to motor-vehicle accidents . . .' So speaks the National Research Council.[1] The Medical School at George Washington University is among the first to formally recognize the magnitude of this health hazard. The school is sponsoring traumatology as a new medical specialty, this announcement being a recent feature of the annual meeting of the American Association for the Advancement of Science in Washington, D.C. Specialized centers for clinical research in shock and trauma manned by basic and clinical scientists have been installed in highly sophisticated laboratories in a limited number of medical centers. Such units for research on head and neck injuries are vitally needed.[2] Robert L. McLaurin, MD, head of the Division of Neurosurgery, who has documented metabolic changes accompanying head injury,[3] is moving to 'establish a clinical research center on head injuries which would pursue the systemic metabolic, the intracranial pathophysiologic, and the cerebral metabolic aberrations simultaneously' (Personal communication) at the University of Cincinnati, one of several other centers also joining the attack. Such efforts will eventually reveal a wealth of new objective information concerning head injuries. But subjective data need be known, as well, how the patient sees his own accommodation.

As the result of the work of the Cornell Research Group and the Trauma Committee of the American College of Surgeons, great strides have been taken in automobile design already, with more to follow. But many spokesmen admonish us that we are not knowledgeable enough about the medical management of trauma, much of which is promulgated by the automobile. We are obligated to foster our own efficiency regarding this, and both the subjective and objective views of the trauma victim are needed to augment and catalyze the process.

I sustained a closed brain injury on October 3, 1964. I consider the residual deficits minimal. The chronology of recovery from such which is concomitant with neurologic tissue repair is not thoroughly documented in the medical literature, particularly from a subjective point of view. This literary dearth is the impetus for the ensuing remarks. Even the redoubtable reflex hammer remains unraised and idle among the other medical tools in the following consideration. This is strictly the view from the inside out.

A facet of my drive to thrive has been a search for the facts of my case as I reconnoitered the lacks and losses resultant from my trauma. My allegiance to the established theory of the involvement of the hypothalamus and contiguous basal brain structures[4] in such injuries has grown stronger as I sought to understand my injured self. Brief comments concerning this conviction, clearly causative conjectures, are appended to this discussion in a rather cavalier display of speculation which may strike some as disagreeably doctrinaire. Subjective clinical data here predominates, however. Supporting evidence for my surmises does exist, but must bide its time for debut in another place where it can fully command the presentation. It is alluded to here at all solely because the accumulation of pieces of the puzzle is an integral part of the process under discussion.

That my deliberation must emanate from my mind, the tenant of the damaged organ under surveillance, my brain, may interest my medical colleagues. I have previously thoroughly conveyed my general impressions of this event in my life.[5, 6] I have also sought to dissect the related affect from my hit-on-the-head, in which anosognosia/denial was prominent.[7] Now, beyond these introductory remarks, lies a neurological view from within which will hopefully be useful to physicians caring for brain-injured patients.

Physicians whose function has been compromised by disability have before shared the experience with their fellow clinicians, and the laity, as well, through the documentation and subsequent dissemination of their own description of their malfunction.[8, 9] This exercise is useful to physicians sometimes, affording them the opportunity for new insight into conditions which they traditionally view exclusively through examination of externally perceived and evaluated evidence. Such accounts have intrinsic weaknesses, however, as does my own.

Subjectivity yields knowledge from within the inner shell, but is sometimes deceptive and fallible. Opinion, inference, and speculation are essential and inescapable aspects of it. The physician orientation of the discussant makes his discourse unlike that of an individual not medically trained; some of his responses are inapplicable to the mass of men with the same disorder. A further limitation to this investigative approach is steadfast concentration on only the manifestations of the subject case; a 'series' of one case is suspect.

Only the belief that some of these liabilities are, paradoxically and simultaneously, assets outweighing their imperfect aspects propels this scrutiny of self. An advantage of the physician scribe over his lay counterpart is that he can exploit the natural curiosity of the afflicted by pondering his circumstances from a more knowledgeable posture. It can be argued that it would be difficult to find one

better motivated, more endowed with enthusiasm, and more capable of fruitful systematic inquiry of a given medical entity than a physician harboring it. The revelation of his thoughts and feelings may even become an obligation to the rest of us. The physician is trained to identify factors of significance not heeded by the untutored. The physician's insides are at least as reliable as those of the medically unschooled patient; and the whole of the science of symptomatology is based on the subjective impressions of the untrained. We daily see successful therapeutic regimes commenced on the basis of symptoms alone, testifying to our usual faith in the validity of the verbal reports of others. We derive truth from clinical confidence in our ability to know how to weigh one utterance against the other, a skill that will of necessity have to be used in the appraisal of my remarks.

The chronology of cases such as mine is not well recorded, likely because it is so variable. Yet, he who moves headlong into trouble wants and needs an estimate of many aspects of his morbidity. Times referred to herein provide, I realize, only another rough rule-of-thumb that is not universally relevant. A crude gauge may emerge as a tool for doctors.

Thirty-three months ago, I was involved in a one-car automobile accident. The scene of the accident was familiar to me. I had known the road for ten years, since it was a lonesome gravel trail. The pebbled path had recently gained sophistication when a new airfield emerged from the wheat fields at its side. It was undergoing change and its novelties were my undoing. My survival was fortuitous, my vehicle coming to rest athwart my prostrate form. My chance position in a niche in the debris makes this composition possible. My head was subjected to the sudden application of extrinsic force of sufficient magnitude to render me wholly unconscious for a few hours and unaware for just over three weeks. I retain a nearly total amnesia for the eight-hour period just preceding the wreck and for the twenty-five days immediately following it. My memory resumes on the twenty-sixth post-trauma day, this temporal hiatus in recollection being largely spent in hospitals, much of which time I was reportedly in a state closely resembling awareness, especially toward the end of this time. Apparently my lack of memory during and for this period of simulated awareness is the essential attribute which distinguished this automatism from its directly succeeding state of mind. I 'awoke ' gradually over the next three days to find myself impaired, recalling this thirteen weeks after the brain injury when I first recorded my feelings.

My feeling was that I had been converted, in one fateful moment, from a vigorous and productive man into a stumbling, exhausted, incoherent, incontinent derelict. I was crippled, dysphagic, gluttonous, eunuchoid, weak beyond comprehension, and incapable of the most elementary pursuit.

I had dextrad lateralizing motor signs. This was an accurate view, as attested by other professionals.

Certain facts of my injury and my subsequent behavior have hopefully contributed to the authenticity of my present judgment of it. The clinical picture has not been as severe in my case as it might have been, or as that of many cases recorded in the literature. I did not have cerebrospinal fluid under increased pressure or of unusual composition. my EEG spoke normally. I am an enthusiastic journal keeper and preserved my impressions at intervals during the recent months of reconstitution, thereby compiling records that are now useful. Then, too, my injury was thirty-three months ago; persisting brain damage has reached a point of diminution permitting me a clearer view, no doubt. My prior medical and my subsequent psychiatric orientations have probably yielded some accrued benefits, such as a different slant or greater insight.

By the time I was brought home, all concern for my general condition had abated, of course. My pulse and blood pressure had been among the matters, for instance, that had seen me moved to the intensive care unit of the hospital.

I recall very real anger at the least, or no, provocation when I first came home, little furies that seem now to have been un-provoked. My injury had been the frequent sire to ire which was not at all appropriate to the mild excitation spawning it, this lasting one month. But I contend that 'sham rage' is a myth. This sham lies in unsuitable semantics. I can vividly recall instances of my intense anger. It was no sham; the emotion was there! I was irate! The causes now seem unrealistic, but the feelings were real, just the same. 'Unprovoked fury' is how I shall ever think of this from now on. And, I think the furious feline or the enraged rodent would, if he could, agree. The cat and the rat and I feel, if I may speak for them, that our experiences are analogous, and we prefer the newer term over the wobbly words of yore!

A related subject of mild controversy is whether or not an animal jabbed in the ventromedial nucleus of the hypothalamus has 'increased appetite' or 'hunger'. May I again venture that a fat rat or a fat cat would, if he could, testify to 'hunger'. I was hampered by no academic semantic confusion; it felt that way to me.[10–13]

Thirteen months post-trauma, I happily found that I could limit my food intake without feeling unduly weak. Within six months of that time, I had readily dropped off thirteen pounds that had frustrated all my efforts since the accident. Prolonged and really painful endeavor over that year had seen me shed but eleven pounds of the excess which I gained after an initial period of weight loss which had at first been present despite my beginning omnivorous hyperphagia. I became a permanent sympathizer with the incorrigibly obese who must diet or die. My total weight loss was finally one-sixth of my present weight, the last half of which was easy. I began this monotonous marathon of weight moderation worrying over the *emotional* compulsion that must be driving me, and ended it convinced that the other incorrigibles and I must share *organic* bases for our mutual problem. The basic fuel of the brain is glucose, and I was driven to incorporate it. I ate with gusto and satisfaction, but early adopted the habit of drinking gallons of apple cider, as well, thus satisfying my excessive needs for sugar and fluid simultaneously. This had measureable effects which were both subjective and objective. I felt restored; my fatigue lifted; my slurred speech became coherent; numbness in my right hand lessened. The quadrad of signs and symptoms just listed served as my personal early warning system in diminishing degree until very recently, presaging imminent fatigue when I had exceeded my limitations. Present for up to thirty months, it was ever very responsive to food, especially sugar, or rest, departing quickly after but a little of either.

I had learned to crudely draw my signature by dint of much tedious effort by the time I could again hold forth in my medical office at ten weeks. The motions of this and other routine and habitual sequences of letters were not nearly so elusive as random script, which is only now acquiring some polish. My hand is still labored, tires easily, and does not well withstand the fatigue. It is nearly illegible after too rapid use or in the evening when I am tired. I have great difficulty in keeping pace on paper with an ordinary conversation. Writing has been a slow skill to return, presumably because it is a very intricate fine motor activity enlisting and coordinating diverse functions of the central nervous system. I have improved with practice, which I pursue at every opportunity. Refusing to be seduced from this resolve by confiding my affairs to a recorder has at times been trying.

Encopresis was virtually a past humility by six months. It had been an utterly frustrating occasional occurrence until then, for my preliminary defecatory urge had been gone. The return of this ordinary signal of need was a minor glory. I now get ample warning, also, when my detrusor urinae entertains a contractile urge. I can drink before I retire without fear of spontaneously saturating the sheets. The opposite was the case for the first year.

Seven months saw the return of a significant aspect of myself that I welcomed home, my sexual drive and ability. That this is a significant part of one's identity is clearly apparent to me. Until it returned, I adroitly denied its departure. Both my enabling mechanisms and my libido are back; all systems are 'Go'. I again find myself trading on my French surname in mock seriousness in appropriate social situations, even though the English corrupted my family name long ago. I routinely looked past a well-turned ankle before, but now take a customary male pleasure in spotting a decolletage at a hundred yards.

My former cataclysmic lassitude persisted for nine months. Until then it was an exasperating and unassailable problem. When I felt the need before, it was an immediate one which I learned to heed. The alternative was to turn into an ineffectual pumpkin. It has greatly diminished to the present, no longer being insurmountable and incontestable. Like the abruptly felt need for nourishment, it has waned.

Midday lethargy stalks me yet to some extent. It is two-edged. I find that the postprandial hyperglycemia with its accompanying languor which is a common experience is often now a more adroit thief of time than I recall, as well. A hearty meal is utterly incompatible with vigilance immediately thereafter, though I am shortly visibly restored still by a reasonable snack. I still prudently relax after lunch when circumstances permit. If I am able to be somnolent for twenty minutes, I can arduously pursue routine activities until I retire at night.

In another week, at nine months and six days after my blow on the head, I felt able to begin the resumption of a routine of body conditioning exercises which I had maintained since my army parachutist indoctrination in calisthenics two decades ago. I recall the combination of triumph and chagrin with which I undertook push-ups. I was just able; exhausting effort resulted in but five repetitions. At that, I was doing little more than writhing in sagging lordosis on the floor. It took nine more months to attain my previous prowess, sixty push-ups and 150 sit-ups, for example. However, I managed this by prevailing in this activity every other day, and it had mixed benefits for me. Persevering gave me an objective index or retrieved function, a very soothing psychic salve as well as a physical source of gratification. Seeing is believing; performing is knowing. I evaluated myself with some extrinsicality as I merrily monitored my mounting muscle power.

Every disabled patient needs this. If he fails to adopt his own realistic program of physical therapy, one should be compelled by his physician. Some activity allied to previous behavior, adapted in the interest of practicality, is likely best; it needs to be a program the patient can·be expected to prosper in. In my own case, compromise and adaptation was essential. I had to realize and accept the fact that my muscles are ignorant and unappreciative of heroic efforts. I had to abandon at first a traditional measure of physical fitness and comparative excellence among men, namely, the number of consecutive sequences of a given exercise performed. I was too feeble for robust performance. I convinced myself that it was quite all right to do a few exercises several times a day, rather than an exhausting number at once. My muscles saw virtue in this. Their tonus increased proportionate to the total effort, however fragmented.

I danced in my antiquated ballroom style at thirteen months and ten days, any sort of fluid total body movement being until then beyond me. I had long been capable of the 'jerk' and some of the other hyperkinetics popular with my adolescent sons, for such was my way in all things for a while. No doubt the casually observing teen-agers of our neighborhood were curious as to why I 'danced' up my front walk from my car every night! At about this time, I perceived that numbness that had persisted until then in my right foot had vanished. Nor could splinters any longer invade my right hand unheeded. Since then my right hand has not merely hung on my arm like an insensitive glove.

At eighteen months, I bid farewell to a paresthesia that had until then plagued me. It was literally and figuratively a pain in the buttocks, which jabbed me with seeming malice at times. It was especially intrusive when I sat without stirring for relatively long intervals, as on a two-hour drive.

My position sense, its departure early appreciated through my deficit in equilibrium, had largely returned after a year and a half also. I no longer had trepidation about swimming, for instance, an activity I had until then found impossible due to poor ability to maintain my head upright in the water. I no longer wallowed drunkenly in the pool, and have recently splashed my way through thirty laps. I could climb hills with disdain again, whereas before, the straight and narrow on the level had been my limit. I could close my eyes and tilt my head about while taking a shower without falling out of the bathtub.

The sneaky sting of an insect on my right cheek was again noticeable and objectionable at twenty months. I had theretofore had to depend on observes to caution me to discourage mosquitoes drilling my skin. My dysarthria subsided almost entirely at the same time, an objective fact that I could quickly ascertain when I could again say, 'statistics', for which I had learned to use, 'figures'. It was a landmark of retrieved function only equalled by my tongue's earlier coup in singing a 'tra-la-la'.

My need for inordinate insulation on balmy days subsided after two years. I had until then always gone about more heavily attired than others. A mountain sunbath with a snowbank at my feet is again a luxury.

My stamina and endurance have progressively increased. I strive actively to augment this, taking advantage of and trying to enhance the neurological betterment. I refuse elevators, shoulder my golf bag, and park a few blocks from my destination nearly always. Skiing was a problem at fifteen months, but less of one at twenty-seven, the season just past. My right leg descended the mountain at variance with my left last year. I could control it only by observing it constantly and using the snowplow technique. I must have looked like a tent toiling tediously through the snow. My style was dazzling. I wore a hard hat to protect my head, on the recommendation of my physician. I dressed like Mercury and moved like a snail. My children delighted in the spectacle of a 'racer', the illusion such a helmet sometimes fosters, surmounted by his brain bucket and being overtaken by every arthritic old lady on the hill. I must have looked like I was intent upon peering at a barrel clutched between my ankles. But I was at twenty-seven months post-trauma this year, and determined not to be the clown prince of snow. My right leg was less autonomous and I was not torn between mountains. My slats behaved as if they were kin, or even twin.

Feats of about the same time were tying a tie and buttoning a shirt, my dexterity finally reaching that stage. For six months, I have been able to introduce a button into its thread-bound foramen again, and twist a cravat into an acceptable knot around my neck! And I no longer found it necessary to place my foot on my car's accelerator under direct vision. I had previously found myself sometimes with an unresponsive automobile, only to discover my errant foot struggling valiantly to indent the floorboard.

Running was difficult for thirty months. Its return is an advent of three months ago. For months I managed reasonably well if I accelerated and decelerated cautiously. Gross movements were more easily accomplished. Galloping was simpler than cantering. I will never again be a sprinter, but I am not now a frenzy of flailing limbs either.

After two and a half years, I could also again light a lady's cigarette. Prior to then, it had been an intricate social procedure, so burdensome that I avoided it and suffered the possible condemnation. I had to strike while my match was hot, otherwise. If I required my victim to nurse fire from a feebly glowing coal, the ready fatigue of my outstretched arm soon provided her with such a dancing target that she was seldom agile enough to score. Her lunges at an ember with widely convergent eyes were embarrassing to us both.

The here and now is much improved over the there and then. Relatively inconsequential residuals remain. One practical thing I am unable to do is to use my right hand to evaluate my whiskered face when shaving. Its fine touch sensation is not so fine. Nor can that hand juggle a full cup of coffee from room to room without inundating the intervening carpet. Its proprioception is also laggard, like my right foot. It does not know straight up from over, and inevitably sags the cup to overflowing unless it is under direct vision.

Vestiges of my initial ophthalmoplegia remain, complicating some activities. My sight was never compromised by premature retinal retirement, this established by actual performance test. Slightly more than ordinary superimposition of images occurs on extreme lateral gaze, as when I glance over my shoulder. I try to face things squarely. While driving my car, for instance, I turn bodily in my seat to securely survey the rear at crucial points, as at the confluence of acutely merging lanes of traffic. Shaving brings another vexation to the fore, when my focus is just beyond my fovea. I close one eye to enable me to discern but a single image squinting back at me from the mirror. When I blow out the match that has just ignited my cigar, I as often as not direct my gale above it. And an inexplicable blister that recently surmounted my proboscis got there after I aimed at a carefully preserved carcass of cigar and lit instead the end of my nose. Presently is the first I have been able to confront the summer sun without it offending my eye. In reading, the same line parades by me now but rarely, when I am fatigued. And this is generally true of the tombstones of my infirmities; the ghosts ride the skirts of lassitude.

My confidence in my vision, my coordination, and my total self had been immeasurably augmented by chance at fourteen months. While returning from a deer hunting adventure on the Continental Divide with my three sons, a trek which had necessarily seen me remain ensconced behind the steering wheel of my Jeep almost consistently, we had not sighted an antlered head or a cloven hoof. When we happened upon a lazy marmot draped across a pile of rotting mine timbers sixty yards off the road, the boys cajoled me to shoot him. My arrow, finally loosed after ample hesitation to allow the varmint to save my face by vacating, pierced the animal. The fortuitous flight of that single shaft helped shatter and dispel the image of the invalid daddy, a circumstance I had devoutly wished.

My right platysma is still lethargic when I jut my chin, producing less of a webbed neck than on the left. My gourmet's sapidity is settling back into the tongue from which it had decamped; foods are no longer tasteless substance. My facial muscles make the right side of my face an inscrutable mask but rarely now; there is a little drooping of my vesper visage sometimes. I have recently regained the ability to close my right eye tightly enough that face soap does not invade and irritate my eye.

Until very recently, I had to chew primarily on the left side of my mouth before guests to avoid embarrassment. I otherwise soon looked like a squirrel with a cached cud of goodies, for food collected in the flaccid side of my face. The next step, swallowing, is almost entirely uncomplicated by choking now. I need no longer masticate every morsel to microscopic maceration to get it beyond my mouth, the previous situation which has steadily improved to the present.

Smell is still an insensitive sense, although I now seldom smell odors and aromas not smelled by others. My memory is much more retentive than it was, probably due to both the neurological restoration of its circuitry and to less distraction with the trauma and its aftermath. But I find myself reading again things that I have spent ample time on in the past without registering a permanent memory trace. Such things do not now go in one eye and out the other.

Thus has been my return. It has etched a permanent swath across my life, the neurological and psychological scarification of which has persisted beyond my hope and expectation. But it has diminished markedly, and continues to do so. My current fantasy is that I shall, with the continuing help of others, view my situation as realistically as we are able. If disabling residuals persist, in either realm of the brain's function, I am determined to see them gone.

I have attempted to highlight my restoration here for the perusal of my fellow physicians, with the thought that such information will serve them in clinical medical practice.

COMMENT

The moorings and mechanisms of the malfunctions of the mind and its matrix in closed brain injury may be succinctly summarized in support of the hypothalamic hypothesis with contiguous basal bailiwicks of the brain brought similarly to account. A cursory countdown from front to rear with allusion from my own experience follows. Not every charge can be leveled, for thorough indictment is impossible in this preliminary hearing.

Forward on the keel of a bruised brain is the olfactory system; my aberrations of olfaction come to mind. The preoptic nuclei stand accused of implication in the distraction of my thermostat. Up for several counts are the median eminence-pituitary axis and the supraoptic and paraventricular nuclei, namely, food and water intake, escalating body weight, and lethargy, to name some.

The amidship hypothalamic aggregations do not avoid censure. Little furies have their origin in the dorsal, ventral, and lateral areas. Guilt for lazy libido and erratic emotions is assumed to be that of the second named. The latter is thought to share blood pressure responsibilities with the posterior areas, these last remaining fixed in accusatory gaze with the ascending reticular formation for their involvement in consciousness-awareness. The mammillary bodies protrude in the midst of the memory maze at this point, as well.

The genua of the internal capsules clasp the hypothalamus firmly to the third ventricle, their sturdy knock-kneed strands proceeding as compact cables to create the bulk of the cerebral peduncles. These structures stand accused of massive traumatic indolence, with many motor and sensory modalities idled.

Such is but a partial list of allegations.

REFERENCES

1. National Academy of Sciences, National Research Council: Accidental Death and Disability (1966). *The neglected disease of modern society*, Washington, DC.
2. Caveness, W. F., and Walker, E. A. (ed.) (1966). *Head injury conference proceedings.* Lippincott, Philadelphia.

 3. McLaurin, R. L. (1966). *Clin. Neurosurg.*, **12**, 143–60.
 4. Walshe, F. M. R. (1952). *Diseases of the nervous system*. Williams and Wilkins, Baltimore.
 5. LaBaw, W. L. (1966). *Med. Times*, **4**, 407–14.
 6. LaBaw, W. L. (1967). *Res. Physician*, **3**, 149–60.
 7. LaBaw, W. L. Subjective experience with denial. *Psychiatry*, in press.
 8. Grotjahn, A. (1929). *Aertze als Patienten*, Georg Thieme, Liepzig.
 9. Pinner and Miller (1952). *When doctors are patients*. Norton, New York.
10. Magoun, H. W. (1963). *The waking brain*, (2nd edn). Charles C. Thomas, Springfield, Il.
11. Hetherington, A. W. and Ranson, S. W. (1940). *Anat. Rec.*, **78**, 149
12. Hess, W. R. (1963). In D. E. Wooldridge. McGraw-Hill, New York.
13. Hess, W. R. (1954). Diencephalon, autonomic and extra-pyramidal functions, *Monographs in biology and medicine*, Vol. 3. Grune & Stratton.

(LaBaw 1968)

COMMENTARY

LaBaw incurred his head injury in 1964, and he wrote this account almost three years later. His account is remarkable for the richness of the language. While it suggests that he suffered little in the way of significant expressive dysphasia as a result of his head injury, the prose occasionally comes across as rather 'flowery', and parts of it may in fact represent a subtle semantic memory impairment. He offers an interesting note of caution relating to self-reports after brain injury. Firstly, he makes the general point that subjective knowledge may be deceptive and fallible. Second, he notes that comments from a physician may tend to have a particular bias due to the medical background of the individual. Third, being a single-case study the account may not be representative of other cases. Despite such limitations, LaBaw admits that 'it would be difficult to find one better motivated, more endowed with enthusiasm, and more capable of fruitful systematic inquiry of a given medical entity than a physician harboring it . . . The physician is trained to identify factors of significance not heeded by the untutored' (p. 299).

As a result of his head injury, LaBaw was unconscious for several hours and he appeared to have a post-traumatic amnesia of around three and a half weeks. He also had a pre-traumatic amnesia of eight hours. These data would appear to suggest that he suffered quite a severe head injury. LaBaw kept a diary record of some of his observations during the recovery phase of his head injury—he noted being converted from 'a vigorous and productive man into a stumbling, exhausted, incoherent, incontinent derelict. I was crippled, dysphagic, gluttonous, eunuchoid, weak beyond comprehension, and incapable of the most elementary pursuit' (p. 300). For the first year, LaBaw had urinary incontinence and for the first six months he had faecal incontinence. These deficits suggest that during his first year he may have had a significant degree of damage to frontal lobe or related structures.

During his first month at home, he suffered a shortness of temper—he notes that this was not 'sham rage' in the sense of his feelings not being genuine. He admits that, when he looks back, the reasons for his being provoked now appeared unrealistic. He also had a voracious appetite, and he attributes this to hypothalamic damage caused by his head injury. He had difficulty in writing, especially writing notes at speed, and he resisted the temptation to use a tape recorder. His sexual drive and sexual ability returned after seven months—this he recognized as 'a significant part of one's identity', but one that is often ignored in discussions of the after-effects of head injury (cf. Griffith *et al.* 1990). His increased tiredness lasted for nine months post-injury, and even after this period he continued to feel the need for a rest or a quick nap after lunch.

Prior to his injury, LaBaw had been very fit, having trained as an army parachutist. After his head injury, he practised press-ups and push-ups every other day, and by eighteen months post-injury he was capable of performing at his pre-injury schedule. He noted that doing this activity gave him an objective index of improvement and resultant self-confidence. LaBaw recommends that such a routine should be incorporated into all therapy programs for head injury patients: 'Some activity allied to previous behavior, adapted in the interest of practicality, is likely best; it needs to be a program the patient can be expected to prosper in' (p. 302). The overall pattern of LaBaw's deficits, and in particular the ways in which subtle neurological deficits affected his social adjustments, brings home the importance of a holistic approach to the assessment of psychosocial adjustment, one that takes account of cognitive, 'executive', emotional and physical deficits (Lezak 1989).

REFERENCES

Griffith, E. R., Cole, S., and Cole, T. M. (1990). Sexuality and sexual dysfunction. In *Rehabilitation of the adult and child with traumatic brain injury* (2nd edn) (ed M. Rosenthal, E. R. Griffith, M. R. Bond, and J. D. Miller), pp. 206–24. F. A. Davis, Philadelphia.

Lezak, M. (1989). Assessment of psychosocial dysfunctions resulting from head trauma. In *Assessment of the behavioural consequences of head trauma* (ed. M. Lezak), pp. 113–43. Alan Liss, New York.

Cerebral concussion

Lawrence R. Freedman

Lawrence Freedman was a professor of medicine at the time of his injury.

A little over two years ago I set off for a usual day at the hospital. After breakfast I put on my bicycle helmet and gloves and started off for my five-minute refreshing ride in the cool morning air. About 200 yards from my home, passing a construction site, I noticed a small truck emerging from an alley . . .

I learned much later that someone had called the paramedics, who found me on the ground and brought me to the hospital where I was admitted with the diagnosis of cerebral concussion. I have no memory of the event or of the subsequent six-day hospitalization. I am told that I was confused and disoriented, but not unconscious. It was not until three days later that I easily recognized my family. I am told that I complained of considerable headache during the first days after the accident, that my appetite was poor, and that I suffered from severe shoulder pains. Since there were no fractures, the pains were attributed to the fall.

A CT scan of the brain upon admission to the hospital revealed a small amount of intracerebral blood, which resolved by the time I was discharged. Yet, since there was no reliable information about how my accident had occurred, a cerebral angiogram was performed to rule out aneurysm as the precipitating cause. The angiogram was negative. I have no recollection of any of the procedures or of any of the events in the hospital, even though I am told by my family that I seemed to participate appropriately in the consideration of what was done and signed the required permission forms. I probably looked better than I actually was since I also recognized visitors by name but had no recollection of their visits even a few minutes after they left.

I was on a neurosurgical service where my management consisted of close observation and two prophylactic medications—one to assure the stability of my blood pressure and the other to prevent the possibility of convulsions.

It is hard to be precise about when I began to realize that I had a bicycle accident and had been hospitalized for a week.

The first clear memory I have, and treasure, dates to the early days at home when my daughter talked me into going for a walk around the block. I was anxious about the walk—I wondered if I would be able to maintain my balance walking down the front steps. I wondered whether it was as safe outside as I felt it was indoors, at home. Going down the steps turned out to be quite easy, and it felt wonderful to be outdoors. The weather was good, the air was delicious. Still, I was very pleased when we arrived back home. Exhausted, I went directly to bed.

My daughter told me later that when we had gotten halfway around the block, I wanted to turn in a direction that, she explained to me, was the wrong way. She seemed so sure! I told her that exceptionally I would go her way, but that I would bet her a million dollars that we wouldn't arrive home that way. I still owe her the money!

An early memory is of the worrisome fatigue that had me spending a good part of the day in bed. Taking a shower was particularly tiring; doing anything was, in fact, exhausting. Even food had lost its attraction.

Another early memory dates to about three weeks after the accident when I awoke with generalized teeth-chattering shaking chills that lasted over an hour. My wife, worried, called my internist, who came over as soon as he could. He and I both concluded that I was probably having a reaction to the blood pressure medication. My other medication, an anticonvulsant, had already been discontinued before I left the hospital because of my developing a generalized skin rash. I was now medication-free. Within 24 hours my shoulder pains disappeared, my appetite improved, and I was no longer enveloped by the cloud that contributed so much to my fatigue. I continued to feel very good being at home. I became aware of a resting, recuperating process within me to which I abandoned myself completely.

There was one thing I noticed in the early days at home that disturbed me greatly—I was no longer interested in listening to music. I heard the music, I knew it was music, and I also knew how much I used to enjoy listening to music. It had always been the primary unfailing source that nourished my spirit. Now it just didn't *mean* anything to me. I was indifferent to it. I knew something was very wrong.*

The realization that something was wrong was the major issue I had to struggle with during the months that followed. I felt that I had been far, far away and had now 'returned', that I was now doing and experiencing things that I knew and understood from a distant past but had not done for a very long time. The sight of trees and flowers was spectacular—colors were delicious and exciting.

Along with the excitement of discovery there was the fear and anxiety of what seemed uncertain or unknown. After not having driven an automobile for a month, I was suddenly not sure that I knew how to drive or how to deal with traffic and was not sure that I was capable of doing any sport. I was uncertain of my ability to move quickly and appropriately.

I was pleased to have visitors, but I didn't mind when they left, and I wondered when I would regain the full pleasure of being with people.

Professionally, I had similar anxieties when I returned to work part time after six weeks at home. I was concerned about seeing patients, making rounds, and working with students and residents. I felt the need to be particularly attentive in the hospital to even

---

* I have since spoken with two people, both musicians, who had the same experience after a head injury. They were greatly reassured by hearing of the complete restoration of my 'musical connection'.

routine matters. This must have contributed significantly to my fatigue.

The first talk I had to give, about three months after the accident, was accompanied by a lot of anxiety. I took a long time in preparing it and worried about the most unlikely aspects of it. When the talk went easily and well, I realized that the main difficulty at this point was most likely due to the uncertainty and anxiety related to the thought of doing something, rather than an inability to actually do what I contemplated doing.

Guessing the probable source of my difficulties did little to help resolve them. I realized that my physicians had not addressed the psychological consequences of my injury, nor had they prepared or advised my family of the inevitable anxiety that would accompany recovery. I felt intensely alone with my worries, too frightened, too protective, and too insecure to do anything but worry more. A potential vicious circle was at hand that made our family life gloomy and tense. My wife and my daughter helped me to decide to consult a psychiatrist in an effort to bring some relief and attend to the escalating doubts and anxieties. In retrospect I realize that the more I recovered, the more frightening and shaking the whole event seemed and the more I worried. My meetings with the psychiatrist were fascinating but, more importantly, were immensely helpful and, in fact, constitute one of the important gains that this accident carried with it.

The early period of recovery at home was, in a sense, reexperiencing childhood. I was told what I could and could not attempt, I was cared for, I slept a lot, and there were few demands put on me; I had no responsibilities other than to 'emerge'. I can best characterize this as a time of infantilization.

Coincident with feeling infantilized, I was gradually naggingly aware of having passed a period of time when I had existed but about which I had no memory. The thought that there was a time when I might have been dead occurred often.

The image that I still retain of this early time after my accident is that of being enveloped by combined feelings of uncertainty and constraint—as in childhood, coming immediately up against the anticipated uncertainties and constraints of aging and the void that may be death. It was as if the inner devices, which normally kept my early experiences separated from concerns of future dependence by a 'healthy' distance, weren't working properly. Life events, fears, and memories seemed linked when, in fact, they were far apart. I searched to find my proper place in my present three-dimensional landscape, which, although familiar, needed a readjustment of scale. I felt as if I were looking through a powerful telescope that brought vaguely perceived objects too near. In one's 'normal' adult state, the memories of childhood and the unknowns of aging are generally perceived through the wrong end of a telescope—both extremes of life are vague and seem a long way off. The accident had somehow turned the telescope around.

Professionally, these experiences gave me a vivid insight into the complex human issues that loom so large in caring for the aged, to whom childhood seems near and who, at the same time, struggle with feelings of loss of competence and increasingly dependent needs.

On still another personal level, feelings of this early period after the accident required that I focus attention on my relationships with my wife of over 30 years and my children. For me to have become 'the child' in a setting where I had been the parent and husband and then to return to the latter status required devoting considerable thought and feeling to my place within the family. This effort was, of course, essential to my personal sense of identity but was even more rewarding on an inner level for all of us.

What did I miss most as a patient recovering from a cerebral concussion? I wanted my physicians to talk to me; I needed them to talk to me, particularly as I improved and knew what I wanted to discuss and was able to retain more of what was being said. As I look back, I know that I was unaware of this need at the time and was, therefore, incapable of expressing it. Yet I believe I would have benefited enormously from regular meetings with my physician, especially during the

first few months after being discharged from the hospital.

I would have wanted to hear about the experiences to be anticipated after such an injury, about their evolution, about their impact on me personally and professionally. I would have benefited from the identification of any signs of progress and encouragement as to the probability of full recovery.

In this regard, it had been particularly satisfying for me to see the relief of the two musicians (described earlier) with whom I spoke after their cerebral injuries, when I described my difficulty in 'connecting' with music and the recovery from it after my accident. This was an experience that was troubling to both of them—indeed, so troubling that they did not/could not bring it up in conversation with me.

I would have benefited from the opportunity to express concerns and ask questions. It is clear to me, however, that I would not have gotten to personal issues without having first developed a relationship of trust with my physician, and such relationships take time to develop.

I realize, as I write, that I sound like the army of patients who have expressed and continue to express these sentiments. But why is this dimension of care so lacking? Several reasons come to mind. Perhaps one important reason is that physicians are poorly compensated for their time unless they carry out well-codified, remunerative procedures.

Another reason is that the human aspects of illness and medical care are not infused with the attention and emphasis that they deserve. In the physician, human understanding and involvement is presumed to be inborn and then enhanced by experience—and sometimes it is. But 'sometimes' is not enough and, most important, is unpredictable. The reality is that such care requires instruction and guidance—elements that are conspicuously absent from our traditional formal medical teaching. I hope the current effort of the American Board of Internal Medicine to focus on 'humanism' will require that attention be directed to this vital dimension of medical care.

However, it is not at all certain that identifying the need to consider the human aspects of illness and addressing them in the curriculum will be sufficient. After all, Dr. Kübler-Ross began her pioneering work on death and dying about 20 years ago, and, despite her accomplishments and the development of hospice as a care unit, the usual professional response to terminal illness, still today, is withdrawal. The human aspects of the care of patients with nonterminal illness also have broad implications. The subject matter will require definition, and medical student and house staff instruction will require that both faculty and students explore personal feelings and attitudes about not only death, but also about illness in general, and personal vulnerability. These issues are, perhaps, brought into particular focus in caring for a colleague.

It is surely the human aspects of care that patients are looking for when they search for practitioners of 'holistic' medicine. I suspect that patients are driven to practitioners of a variety of 'paramedical' practices because traditional physicians seem so unavailable to attend to nonbiological aspects of illness.

In my experience and for my family, it was the nurses who were most alert and sensitive to our needs for both human and biological dimensions of medical care. The nurse was the major conveyor of information and feelings, the translator, the interpreter of questions and answers between the patient, his family, and the physicians—in all directions. This is a major component of care that does not receive the acknowledgment and respect it so richly deserves. The role of the nurse should be accorded the most careful attention and nurture, particularly at this time of rapid change in the organization of medical care.

As I reread my discussion of the human aspects of medical care, I feel that it is incomplete because I know that these issues have been raised many times in the past and yet the general dissatisfaction with care continues. Indeed, there are many who believe that we physicians are less effective in providing this human dimension of care today than we were in the past, when we could do little to influence the biology of disease but when we could at least talk, listen, reassure, and comfort.

Recent comments by Oliver Sacks pertain directly to that aspect of care which is lacking today.[1] Sacks has called attention to the reaction of an individual affected by illness 'to restore, to replace, to compensate for and preserve his identity'. He suggests that it is 'an essential part of our role as physicians' to study or influence the means by which individuals react, no less than it is our responsibility to direct attention to the primary illness or injury.

Somehow, coincident with the spectacular advances in science and medicine in recent years, the physician is perceived as being less aware of/competent to manage the human aspects of medical care. We can perhaps be aided in our efforts to incorporate this responsibility into our general understanding of medical care by referring to the means by which mankind has responded generally to change.

Arthur Schlesinger, Jr. has estimated recently that more change has taken place in the past two lifetimes of man than occurred in the first 498. He went on to observe that whereas 'science and technology revolutionize our lives, memory, tradition and myth determine our responses'.

I would like to suggest that this idea is transposable to what I have been referring to as the biological and human aspects of medical care. The biological dimension of care is easily seen in terms of the science and technology that revolutionize our lives, and I believe that the human aspect of care is inseparably intertwined with the memory, tradition, and myth of the patient and the society in which he lives.

Schlesinger's use of the word *response* to characterize the relation of memory, tradition, and myth to science and technology brings to mind the principle established by Newton's third law of motion, that 'for every force acting on a body, the body exerts a force having equal magnitude in the opposite direction along the same line of action as the original force'.

Applying Newton's law, memory, tradition, and myth become the means by which the individual exerts a force of equal magnitude and in the opposite direction along the same line of action as the original force, science, and technology. In medical care terms, the human responses to illness generate an equal force in a direction opposite to the force of the biological consequences of illness.

In other words, what traditionally has been referred to as the dissociation between the attention directed to the biological and that directed to the human consequences of illness is, perhaps, more easily understandable as conflict, since the human aspect of care would address powerful forces that have arisen in opposition to the biological forces requiring attention and care. The physician, in directing his attention primarily to the biological forces responsible for illness, becomes inevitably linked to these forces. It is not surprising, therefore, that he would be viewed as inadequate to deal with the patient's human needs. In order to address the human aspects of care and illness, he would also have to direct his efforts in opposition to the biological aspects of illness with which he has become identified.

There is another dimension to the dissociation/conflict between the biological and human aspects of medical care. Perhaps the youth of science and technology generates a pressure to struggle against the power of memory, tradition, and myth, which, after all, have been around for a long time and which have a firm hold on the attitudes and behavior of mankind. perhaps science has understood, as did Robert Pirsig,[2] that 'there are human forces stronger than logic'. In other words, perhaps scientists and technologists, with all of their spectacular achievements, feel that they must struggle to achieve dominance over those powerful archaic forces—forces that are still stronger than logic—which continue to maintain their power.

It is not difficult to understand the profound personal conflicts generated in patients by scientific triumphs such as blood transfusions, artificial organs, organ transplantation, artificial insemination, surrogate motherhood, and still others. Yet the meaning of these advances is rarely considered in the light of memory, tradition, and myth. If my hypothesis offers a valid explanation for the conflict between the biological and human aspects of illness and care, we are not likely to reduce this conflict until we start learning how to talk about it. I suggest that the first step would be to encourage physicians to begin questioning themselves about their personal views and then to encourage their talking about them with each other. Ultimately, it will require skill and sensitivity to learn how to incorporate this understanding of human aspects of illness and care into the traditional educational programs of students and physicians.

I remember when, during the recovery from my concussion, I realized that I no longer understood or felt music. it was then that I knew something was wrong with me. As I reflect upon the emphasis in medicine today and the forces pushing it in the direction in which it is evolving, I no longer understand the music; I know something is wrong.

REFERENCES

1. Sacks, Oliver (1985). *The man who mistook his wife for a hat*, p. 4, Summit Books, New York.
2. Persig, Robert M. (1974). *Zen and the art of motorcycle maintenance*, p. 17. Bantam, New York.

(Freedman 1987)

COMMENTARY

The duration of Freedman's post-traumatic amnesia appears to be around a week, perhaps slightly longer, and this would put his concussion into the category of a severe head injury. Freedman's amnesia for the early post-traumatic period, during which he could identify visitors by name and could carry on normally in a number of activities, is a commonly reported experience of head injury patients. His spared ability to name visitors during the period indicates that Freedman's 'semantic memory' for pre-injury knowledge was largely intact, whereas the 'episodic memory' that governed the laying down of new memories was severely compromised. The fact that he could not recollect visits by visitors, even a few minutes after they left, attests to the severity of his memory impairment during this early stage of his recovery.

He suffered the fatigue that is common to many neurological conditions. The fact that he had difficulty in finding his way about, and the fact that he had great difficulty in finding meaning in music, point to some right hemisphere dysfunction. It was the latter musical deficit that brought home to Freedman that his brain had been significantly altered by his head injury.

From the management point of view, Freedman remarks on the lack of knowledge about what to expect in the various stages of recovery, and he also devotes much of his discussion to the humanistic aspect of dealing with patients' impairments. He found meetings with a psychiatrist to be very helpful. He also has praise for the nurses who looked after him, since they were often the ones to whom he could express his concerns. He describes the first few weeks/months of recovery as a period of 'infantilization', during which he felt as if he was being treated as a child, and where he consequently had to re-evaluate his role within the family. It is often forgotten that head injuries, perhaps more so than other forms of brain injury, affect the family as much as the individual, and that therapies sometimes need to be tailor-made along specific lines (Muir *et al.* 1990).

REFERENCES

Muir, C., Rosenthal, M., and Diehl, L. N. (1990). Methods of family intervention. In *Rehabilitation of the adult and child with traumatic brain injury* (2nd edn) (ed. M. Rosenthal, E. R. Griffith, M. R. Bond, and J. D. Miller), pp. 433–448. F. A. Davis, Philadelphia.

Neurosurgeon as victim

Lawrence F. Marshall and Ronald M. Ruff

Lawrence Marshall was a practising neurosurgeon at the time of his injury. (R. M. Ruff is a neuropsychologist).

There has been a surge of interest in the morbidity of mild head injury. From the pioneering works of Gronwall and Wrightson (1974, 1981), it became apparent that mild head injury was associated with objective disturbances of cognitive function, particularly in the area of memory, information processing, and attention. Confusion has arisen regarding the length of time that these sequelae persist. An initial report by Rimel et al. (1981) suggested that recovery was, in fact, delayed in many instances and that a significant number of patients had long-term sequelae. A more recent cooperative effort by Levin et al. (1987) indicates that most of the cognitive sequelae of head injury have abated by three months but that there are occasional patients who do not recover fully.

Because one of us (L.F.M.) was a victim of minor head injury, it seems appropriate to relate his experiences following the injury.

CASE REPORT

This 42–year-old moderately coordinated neurological surgeon was in Vail, Colorado in 1984, for a meeting of the National Traumatic Coma Data Bank. Following the morning meeting, he spent the afternoon touring the mountains of Vail, and while descending one that had only a modest incline, he lost his balance and fell, striking his head. He was rendered immediately unconscious for a period of a few seconds—certainly no more than 10–15. Upon awakening, the world appeared upside down, with the sky below and terra firma above. This condition cleared, but a very modest vertigo persisted. This did not interfere in any way with descent from the mountain, and in fact did not interfere with further skiing activities. Neuropsychological testing was soon recommended by the neuropsychologists at the meeting, but was respectfully declined.

Upon returning home, the neurosurgeon noted that he was a bit more distractable than was his norm and that he had a great deal of difficulty remembering recent events, including particularly the location of objects necessary for work, such as a dictaphone, briefcase, and keys. List making in order to recall meetings scheduled and tasks to be performed became necessary, whereas they were not necessary before. Referencing articles from memory storage was difficult; authors were frequently transposed and dates incorrectly recalled. Information processing did not appear to be affected, but the ability to attend to a task required a higher level of energy expenditure than previously. These symptoms persisted, but they improved gradually over a period of approximately 18 months, and by the fall of 1985 they appeared to have reached their asymptote. Modest improvement in information storage retrieval has continued, indicating that neither Alzheimer's nor a presenile dementia was revealed by the head injury. Function as judged by others remains good, but is not optimal.

DISCUSSION

The above description is an accurate recollection of the events that occurred, given the recent memory disturbance that accompanies this condition. What does such an injury illustrate? It illustrates first that recovery from mild head injury is a *gradual* process which, although it has a much steeper curve or slope initially, continues for many months. Second, in each instance, measurement against the individual's previous performance would be ideal but is usually unobtainable. The neurosurgeon in question here is certain, however, that had he been tested within one week of his injury, performance would have exceeded at least the average for national controls, if not for local controls in San Diego. Thus, frustration would have set in because clearly the individual was not functioning at this level after the injury.

This is a modest illustration of the need for physicians and neuropsychologists to listen to their patients when they describe symptomatology that cannot be detected by neurocognitive testing. The problem with testing performance in a laboratory setting is that the individual gears up or increases the level of intellectual energy expenditure to function, just as I do in an attempt to maintain a rather busy work pace. In addition, the introduction of significant distractors—for example, someone talking in the background —which had never been disturbing before, now became a major burden. Music on the other hand, which used to interrupt performance, seemed to have no effect. This clearly cannot be captured in a neuropsychological test mode, and I am not suggesting that it should. Rather, we need to think about the consequences of our conclusions when we indicate to the subject that everything is fine—when the subject continues to maintain that things are *not fine*.

For those who function at above-average levels of intellectual performance, neurocognitive testing is likely to leave significant unanswered questions. Perhaps the strategy of asking the patient to judge his or her performance, if and when the test results are also normal, might be a useful one. In such a strategy if the patient claims that his or her performance is normal and the test results support that, then one can assume that the patient has completely recovered. Thus I would not have been convinced if Dr. Ruff or his colleagues had told me that my performance was normal, because I knew that in fact it was *not normal*, and it now continues to be minimally impaired, although it has improved. The latter point is important, because one can begin to blame all dysfunction of recent memory on the aging process, whereas in my case, although it may have played a minor role, it certainly was not the major factor.

Has this discussion from a minimally brain-injured neurosurgeon been of any value? It is probably only of very limited

value, but it does serve to make the point that perceptions of a disease by one who has not had the disease as a patient tend to be modestly inaccurate. Recovery from head injury appears to be a prolonged process, one requiring innumerable strategies for compensation. Neurocognitive testing will indicate part of the story *only* if the results are abnormal; it leaves something to be desired in predicting levels of performance for those who are adequate competitors in a modern society.

COMMENTS BY A NEUROPSYCHOLOGIST

The insightful reflections of the neurosurgeon expressed here suggest a variety of conclusions regarding the sensitivity, if not validity, of neuropsychological assessment in those individuals who function somewhat above average. Although one might agree that conventional memory tests do have a ceiling effect, the neurosurgeon's challenge to the neuropsychologist should not go without reply. It is possible to develop memory measures that would more closely match individual potential as it is presently conceptualized in intelligence tests. Even for those who function at a superior level, anterograde memory can be assessed at an upper threshold. For example, one could determine the individual's span for immediately recalling words; that is, a word span for an individual could be established. In a second step, the lists to be learned could be double that of the individual's word span so that, for example, a patient who could recall only four words would have to learn a list of eight, whereas an individual who could immediately recall 12 would now need to recall 24 words.

Neuropsychological testing, therefore, could be made more sensitive to individuals who function at the higher level of performance if test measures were individualized with no absolute fixed end point. It is true, however, that such test batteries do not, in general, exist and would need to be developed and normed.

The neurosurgeon here also noted that referencing articles of scientific merit for testing remote memory was difficult. To some degree, recall of remote memory relies primarily on information stored prior to the minor head injury. However, retrograde memory measures are typically not standardized or clinically useful. However, Squire and Slater (1978) have described an empirically developed test to measure interference with retrograde memory in a more sophisticated fashion, and such a test might be applicable here.

The ability to focus on a task, the ease with which one is distracted, and alterations in specific features of attention have not received much investigation when one assesses minor head injury. Neuropsychological testing typically has lagged behind the more sophisticated investigations that are done, for example, in the selection of astronauts or pilots. In simulator environments, such individuals are asked to process multiple tasks—often four or five—concurrently, by selectively attending and prioritizing their information processing. Thus, similar to anterograde memory, attention measures need to be devised which can be individualized and which do not have ceilings.

The neurosurgeon who suffered this minor injury estimated that the duration of recovery was approximately 18 months, in spite of the fact that a variety of compensatory mechanisms, such as list making and an increase in the level of energy expended (using the term 'energy' in a very global fashion) in order to improve function, were employed. In the absence of normative data, one could plot

attention and memory recovery for such an individual. The availability of norms would be useful in teasing out the learning effect from repeated testing, and perhaps this brief chapter has adequately demonstrated the need for developing such norms.

What this case report illustrates is that individuals do in fact suffer long-term residua from head injury, and that it is dangerous to conclude from the recently completed group study that cognitive recovery per se occurs entirely within three months (Levin et al., 1987). In these group studies, the minor head injury subjects were matched to local control groups, and thus the comparisons merely take into account significant differences between the groups. Thus, if an individual were to have functioned at the 95th percentile level prior to injury and, as a result of the accident, dropped to the 60th percentile rank, the use of such group comparisons would be relatively insensitive, and conclusions based on them would in fact be misleading. However, if longitudinal testing were performed using instruments that had relatively high ceilings of performance, one could then argue that recovery or compensation for the injury is taking place.

This description of the course of head injury by a person who has had some experience in the field serves to emphasize the need for a continued search for test measures that not only describe reliably the varying aspects of brain function, but also relate closely to the day-to-day experiences of the individual patient.

REFERENCES

Gronwall, D. and Wrightson, P. (1974). Delayed recovery of intellectual function after minor head injury. *Lancet*, **2**, 605–9.

Gronwall, D. and Wrightson, P. (1981). Memory and information processing capacity after closed head injury. *J. Neurol. Neurosurg. Psychiatry*, **44**, 889–95.

Levin, H. S., Mattis, S., Ruff, R. M., Eisenberg, H. M., Marshall, L. F., Tabaddor, K., *et al.* (1987). Neurobehavioral outcome following minor head injury: a three-center study. *J. Neurosurg.*, **66**, 234–43.

Rimel, R. W., Giodani, B., Barth, J. T., Boll, T. J., and Jane, J. A. (1981). Disability caused by minor head injury. *J. Neurosurg.*, **9**, 221–8.

Squire, L. R. and Slater, R. P. C. (1978). Anterograde and retrograde memory impairment in chronic amnesia. *Neuropsychologia*, **16**, 313–22.

(Marshall and Ruff 1989)

COMMENTARY

Marshall suffered what appeared to be a mild head injury. Duration of coma is given as 10–15 seconds at the most. No duration of post-traumatic amnesia is given, though the patient appears to recollect much of what happened afterwards.

He found himself with significant memory symptoms after the injury, and these recovered over a period of 18 months. Both the retention of new information and the accurate and fast retrieval of past stored information was difficult for him. Marshall notes the importance of considering the patient's premorbid level of cognitive functioning, obviously very high in this case. He also points to the underestimation of deficits that may result from cognitive testing (e.g. the role of distracting activity is seldom examined in test settings, the subject is trying to perform at his very best, etc.). Therefore, he emphasizes the importance of listening to the symptoms of patients. He also points out that with elderly patients who suffer a minor head injury, there is the need to distinguish any deficits from those associated with ageing.

The neuropsychologist author of the paper, Ruff, points to the importance of developing attention and other measures that are sensitive to minor head injury (e.g. multiple task performance, effects of distraction, etc.). There is clearly a practical need for a number of 'management tools' to help the care of patients with minor head injury:

1. Neuropsychological assessment procedures that are sensitive enough to elicit subtle but significant deficits in patients with mild head injury. Such procedures would also be of help in cases of more severe head injury where the patient had a very high premorbid level of cognitive functioning prior to a head injury.

2. Measures that will help to distinguish cognitive changes that are due to cerebral pathology from those that are due to what has been termed the 'post-concussional syndrome', where cognitive symptoms may be regarded as non-specific and secondary to anxiety, depression, etc.

3. Techniques for managing such patients, especially those who have persistent psychological and physical symptoms that are not directly related to a distinct physical pathology.

Some of these and related topics are discussed in a special issue of *Seminars in Neurology* (Packard 1994), and also in a recent review paper (Alexander 1995).

REFERENCES

Alexander, M. (1995). Mild traumatic brain injury. *Neurology*, **45**, 1253–60.
Packard, R. C. (ed.) (1994). Mild head injury. *Seminars in Neurology*, **14**, 1–92.

What does it feel like to be brain damaged?

Frederick R. Linge

Frederick Linge was a clinical psychologist at the time of his injury.

INTRODUCTION

It is generally accepted that people working with individuals who have any type of handicap, should have a certain amount of empathy with their clients and should strive to understand how their clients feel and think. People working with those who are brain damaged have a particularly difficult time doing so. One can have some understanding of what it means to be blind simply by closing one's eyes; yet how can a normal person understand what it feels like to be brain damaged?

I am in the unusual position of being a trained clinical psychologist who suffered brain damage and who has slowly recovered most of my faculties. In other words, I have been on the outside looking in, and also on the inside looking out of the world of the brain damaged person. At this point in my recovery, I have a foot in both worlds, for I can remember what it felt like to be completely normal intellectually, and also what it felt like when loss of function was at its worst.

Perhaps this informal and very subjective narrative may be of some help in assisting normal people to empathize a little better with the brain damaged individual. For, unfortunately, most brain damaged people are unable to explain precisely how they feel; those who have been brain damaged since birth, of course, have never had the experience of functioning normally and thus have no standard of comparison of their present state with that of others.

At age thirty-nine, I was an exceptionally healthy male with a keen interest in outdoor sports such as skiing, canoeing, and swimming. I had been a clinical psychologist for sixteen years and was married to a social worker; we had three children. I was active intellectually, reading a great deal both in and outside my field, and enjoying classical music and playing the piano.

THE TRAUMA

I have no memory of the head-on automobile collision that took place one spring evening. I have driven the same stretch of road innumerable times since then, listened to the testimony of witnesses, even examined official photographs of the wrecked vehicles, but nothing triggers any memory or emotional responses. Hospital records indicate that I was admitted in critical condition, with a broken neck, fractured skull, broken jaw, broken ribs, multiple fractures of the right arm, splintered left leg and ankle, broken hip, internal injuries and numerous abrasions and contusions. The brain damage, which could be only partially assessed at first, was severe enough to render me totally unconscious for almost a week. I was paralyzed on the right side and showed no response to visual, auditory or other stimuli. Heroic surgical procedures and the use of life-support machinery kept me alive the first few days, but I was given little or no chance of surviving and it was thought that if I did survive, I might well do so as a 'human vegetable'.

I have no memory of the first few weeks in the hospital's Intensive Care Unit. My wife was with me almost around the clock for the first two weeks and for several hours per day thereafter until I was discharged. She tells me that, even when seemingly unconscious, my body was constantly in motion, tugging at the traction, trying to move limbs immobilized by casts, testing out my limits of movement. On some level, it would seem that my body was fighting on its own even when my brain was unable to function.

EARLY COMMUNICATION ATTEMPTS

As the profound coma lifted towards the end of the first week, my first response was to recognize, by smiling, familiar figures such as my wife, the children, and other relatives. At this time, my wife thinks that I had regressed emotionally to almost an infantile state, wanting to touch her and the nurses, wanting to hold onto her hand and becoming agitated if she had to let it go for even a moment.

At the same time I showed a great deal of agitation and rage. Frequently, I would fight desperately to be free of the traction and would hit out angrily at those around me. When, somehow or other, I managed to roll completely out of bed and land on the floor, cast, traction, broken neck and all, I was placed in a straitjacket and wrist restraints, and these added greatly to my emotional distress.

My family recall that I seemed quite desperate to communicate and my failure to do so infuriated me as much as the physical immobility. I would try to write, but the script was almost illegible. Many letters were reversed; syllables were repeated over and over; and the meaning was garbled and incomprehensible. I am told that I would become so frustrated at people's inability to understand me that I would stab the pencil through the paper, crumple it up, or hit out at those around me. Speech was, of course, out of the question since I had had a tracheotomy and was also on a respirator. I can only guess at the fear and confusion that must have filled me during those long, pain-filled weeks during which I was unable to move and unable to communicate in any way. Perhaps it is as well that I have no memory of them.

It was only with the removal of the tracheotomy tubes and the restoration of my speech, that my confusion and agitation began slowly to subside. I have some hazy memories of this time. My first memory is of the plastic surgeon removing wires from my jaws that had held them in place while the fractures healed. The intense pain seemed to jolt me into some contact with reality. I remembered seeing the doctor as a gigantic, looming figure, although in reality he is quite a slight person.

TIME AND REALITY ORIENTATION

During this period I had no awareness of time. I existed in a world of the here and now. I was not even aware that such a concept as 'time' existed. I knew who 'I' was, but I did not think of myself as being a child, a boy, or a man. My wife and my mother (who had died some years previously) were both present in my thoughts and were indistinguishable to me. The staff of the hospital were also interchangeable, shadowy figures. I remember feeling passive, accepting, acquiescent. People came and went, did things to me: I did not question them. I am told by my wife that during this period I was less physically agitated: calm, often dreamy; and seemed happy in a childlike sort of way, smiling frequently and making few demands.

On the day that I regained some consciousness, my wife constructed a large homemade calendar, which she placed beside my bed in clear view. On each visit, she would make a point of drawing my attention to the day of the week, the date of the month, and the year; as well as the time displayed on the large wall clock near my bed. This seemed to have no effect at first. I would repeat information after her but forget it immediately. It had no meaning for me.

One day, however, my 'mental clock' began ticking again and the concept of time began to become significant. Somehow, I assimilated the fact that eight o'clock meant the end of visiting hours and my wife's departure, something I hated to have happen. One morning, I remember becoming quite agitated as the clock drew towards eight. 'Why isn't my wife here? It's almost eight and visiting hours are ending'. When she laughed at me and informed me that it was eight in the morning, not eight in the evening, I remembered feeling foolish and embarrassed, and covering up as best I could: 'Oh, yes, of course, you're right'. From that time onwards, I began to orient myself in time, frequently becoming confused, but making steady progress. It was in the area of daily time that I first began to realize that I had a deficit within myself, since those around me were clear-headed and confident about the facts and I was not.

As the sequence of night and day became clearer, the larger chronological picture began to come into focus, though with difficulty. Looking back, I know that while I was in the early stages of recovery, I 'lost' about ten years of memories. At first, this did not matter to me, since past, present and future were all combined into one seamless here and now.

Nor was there a boundary between reality and fantasy. I cannot myself remember, but I am told that during the first weeks I was delusional and hallucinatory at times. A nurse's gown hanging behind the door would become an intruder, ready to attack. Some delusions obviously served as an escape mechanism from the everpresent pain and physical restriction, or served to explain to me why I was in the position that I was. For example, I am told that I thought for some days that I was on an ocean liner with my wife, bound on a pleasure cruise. Observation windows in the intensive care unit became portholes, nurses became stewardesses, and so on, and my cubicle was a stateroom. Or, I would imagine that I was on a desert island, surrounded by lapping waves.

Gradually, as I became more oriented, and more aware that 'something had happened to me', the split between reality as seen by those around me and as I interpreted it, became more painful. I would argue with those around me in defence of my fantasies. Gradually, most of these died away, but the fantasy persisted that I was in the Kamloops hospital, where I had spent some months as a teenager, and that my parents were still alive and living in the family home near Kamloops, where I had grown up. I see now that this was my way of coping with the ten-year gap in my memory, a gap that I simply could not admit to myself at that point in my recovery.

The first breakthrough towards acceptance of reality came in a particularly poignant form. I had been asking with increasing vehemence for some days why my mother had not been to visit me, and harassing my wife with demands that she do something about it. Too tender-hearted to confront me with the fact that my mother was long dead, my wife tried to fob me off with various excuses. Quite suddenly, one day, I looked up at her and said in surprise and grief: 'What are we arguing about? My mother can't come to see me. She is dead'. I began to weep. Traumatic though this reliving of the grief of her death was, it was the beginning of a new stage of progress. From that moment on, I knew roughly where I stood in the stream of time. I had some grasp of the continuum of life and death, youth and age, childhood, parenthood and adulthood.

STEP-BY-STEP RECOVERY

It was at that time also that I bean to wish with great intensity to get out of the hospital. Moving to the Rehabilitation Ward was a positive step for me and my memories shift in sharper focus at this time. Getting out of bed and into a wheelchair, moving around the ward, socializing with other patients, and eating my meals in a communal dining room, all helped me to get back into the world of reality. Staff members became individuals instead of interchangeable, but there was still a degree of fuzziness about my perceptions of people and things at that time. Returning for further surgery months later, when I had regained a much greater degree of functioning, I was astonished at how worn the ward was, housed as it was in the oldest wing of the building: details which had completely escaped my attention before.

It was then, also, that I started to use my adult qualities of judgement for the first time since my accident. Wanting desperately to get out of the hospital, I made a conscious decision that I would 'play the hospital game' in whatever way was necessary to get out. I made sure, for example, that before my doctor's visits I carefully noted the date, day and time, so that I could answer his questions. I ate all my meals, I spent hours exercising and practicing with my crutches, I worked hard at physiotherapy, and I refused sleeping pills and painkillers at night so that there was no danger of sleeping too soundly and wetting the bed.

All of this paid off, for after having spent only two months in the hospital instead of the eighteen months that had been anticipated, I was allowed to go home. I have to confess that until I saw the inimitable silhouette of the Okanagan Lake Bridge at Kelowna etched on the horizon, I secretly cherished the last of my delusions (that I was still in Kamloops).

The car ride is sharply delineated in my memory. I had great difficulty in visually 'tracking' sights as they whirled past the windows. I felt dazed and stunned by the kaleidoscope of sights and sounds. It felt strange to drive along the streets, unable to remember what came around the next corner, yet knowing as soon as I saw it that it was familiar. I have never felt so intensely what it was like to be poised on the knife-edge between the known and the unknown, with strangeness turning into familiarity as the road unreeled before my eyes.

MEMORIES RETURN

The most intense moment came when we drove into our yard. I had wanted ardently to 'get home' while in the hospital, but 'home' was just an emotional feeling, I had no idea what it looked like. Suddenly, there it was, in all its loved reality, with a homemade sign my son had made: 'Welcome Home Dad' flapping from the porch. As I hobbled in, a huge chunk of memories fell into place, intact: but these were not just memories of the physical layout of the house, where things were, and so forth, but also the feelings and emotions that went with them. When I saw the sign,

for example, I knew that my son had made it, that 'Dad' was me, and that I was an adult and a father.

For the next eight months, I recuperated at home before returning to work. Looking back, I see that I had three problems to deal with. First of all, there was the physical rehabilitation: learning to cope with casts and crutches and when these were eventually discarded, learning to cope with the permanent disabilities that remain. Secondly, there was the task of assessing the brain damage, and learning to live with and work around the deficits. Thirdly, there was the process of emotional or psychological healing: building up sufficient confidence in myself to be able to discard the role of 'handicapped person' and reassume the full load of responsibility at work and at home. I had to keep working on all three of these areas at the same time, for lack of progress in one area slowed down progress in the others, and vice versa. For example, an arrangement of stout knotted ropes enabled me to pull myself up out of bed, and the purchase of an electric coffee maker permitted me to get up at my preferred early rising hour and make my own morning coffee, rather than lying helplessly in bed waiting for my wife to wake up and haul me to my feet. This gave me a great psychological 'lift' and spurred me on to other steps to independence. Learning to manoeuvre safely on crutches led to being able to go shopping, to church, or to friends' homes, all of which provided mental stimulation and promoted a return to normalcy.

Learning to live with the brain damage was, for me, the major area of challenge and still is. The diagnosis, after extensive testing, was damage to the left temporal lobe of the brain, several cranial nerves and lesser damage to the right parietal area.

IMPLICATIONS

The results of this damage were: lack of taste and smell, impaired short-term auditory and visual memory, lessened emotional control, and a greater tendency towards depression.

It has been found that damage to the right temporal area of the brain very often leaves the sufferer blissfully unaware that there is any deficit, even when it is quite obvious to those around him. Damage to the left temporal area, however, often allows the individual to be keenly aware of his deficits. It is thought that this is why this type of damage predisposes the sufferer to depressions. In my own case, I initially denied that I had any deficits at all, and it was only after the process of physical and psychological healing was well under way that I could accept that I had damage in some areas and begin to cope with it. For example, for weeks I denied that I had any loss of taste or smell, yet these senses were, in fact, totally absent for over a year and have only partially returned even two years later.

My short-term visual and auditory memory was severely impaired for a long time. Here again, I initially denied this and it was quite frustrating for my family to tell me things, which I would forget immediately, later on insisting vehemently that I had not been told anything in the first place. Again, I would meet a person for the first time and, seeing them an hour later, fail to recognize them. Or, I would read a simple paragraph in the newspaper and by the time I got to the last sentence, have no recollection of what the first one was.

Having been a highly self-controlled person all my life, I found myself with a hairtrigger temper and labile emotions. It is theorized that this state is due to CNS irritation or else that some part of the brain, which is responsible for 'braking' the mental motor, is dysfunctional after brain damage has occurred.

A corollary of this deficit is the perseveration frequently displayed in brain damaged people, and which I recognize in myself. I realize that I have much more of a 'one track mind' than I used to, and my thinking tends to proceed along linear lines. Possibly, this is due to the deficit in the mental 'braking' process, discussed above. When once embarked on a train of thought, I find it very hard to stop, deal with a side issue, and then return quickly to the original theme. Distractions, either external or internal, are hard to handle, and I find myself most comfortable in dealing with clear-cut issues, where I can reason in a straightforward fashion.

COPING NEEDS

In learning to live with my brain damage, I have found through trial and error, that certain things help greatly and others hinder my coping. In order to learn and retain information best, I try to eliminate as many distractions as possible and concentrate all my mental energy on the task at hand. A structured, routine, well-organized and serene atmosphere at home and as far as possible at work, is vital to me. In the past, I enjoyed a rather chaotic lifestyle, but I now find that I want 'a place for everything and everything in its place'. When remembering is difficult, order and habit make the minutia of daily living much easier.

Coping is also easier in the milieu that is free of emotional tension, competitiveness, anxiety, and pressure. I see all of these as 'distractions' that lessen my ability to learn, just as surely as do noise, chaos, and change in the physical setting. I find it hard to absorb and retain new information in a meeting with people who are new to me and where there is a constant interchange of ideas and personalities. Yet, in a one-to-one situation with a familiar client, or working in my office with colleagues whom I know and trust, in an orderly and systematic fashion, I can retain far more and function far more effectively. In other words, simplification of the external situation, both physical and emotional, assists me to master new information. The more complexity around me, the less able am I to cope.

I also find that physical fatigue cuts down my concentration and so I now try to tackle new tasks in the morning, when I am physically fresh. I resort to extensive note-taking on professional matters as well as carefully recording all appointments, financial details and so forth at home. In mastering new information, I go over the subject matter many times, using all possible sensory input channels: reading it, writing it down, repeating it aloud, and having someone re-read it to me.

These ways of modifying the external environment will, I am convinced, assist any brain damaged person to learn better. From a purely internal point of view, however, I feel that other, psychological factors are extremely important.

UNDERSTANDING THE BRAIN DAMAGED PERSON

First of all, any brain damaged person is going to feel some degree of anger, denial, and depression as his deficits become apparent. These have to be dealt with if the individual is to succeed in using his fullest potential and coping with the real world.

For example, as I have mentioned, for many weeks I denied that I had lost my sense of taste and smell. I never mentioned the loss to anyone while I was in the hospital and it was only on the 'safe ground' of home that I took the first steps towards admission of the deficit. This was to complain to my wife that food 'tasted funny'. I accused her of having added something strange to it; then I theorized that she had bought food that wasn't fresh or that had gone bad. Finally, when I was able to accompany her to the store, buy the food myself and be assured of its quality, and do the actual cooking myself, I had to admit that the fault was not in the food itself but in my own senses. The same process had to be gone through in other areas of deficiency, mental and physical, as I denied the deficits, came up against the hard edge of reality, and finally accepted them.

Anger and depression inevitably accompany the final admission of such deficits, sometimes separately, sometimes together. I remember periods of intense depression during which I would retreat to the bedroom for hours on end, covering up my true feelings by saying to myself that 'the noise of the children was too much for me'. I was also subject to fits of rage and had a hairtrigger temper that could be ignited instantly by the smallest incident. This all became so difficult for my

family (themselves under great stress) that my wife finally insisted that we see the psychiatrist who had worked with me while I was in the hospital.

Almost immediately that the interview began, he recognized and pointed out my extreme depression. I broke down and began to weep, and it was then that I was able to recognize my feelings for what they actually were. Talking with this understanding doctor, who was familiar with the medical and neurological background to my situation, was of great help in 'working through' my depression. Medication was of help as well, but the important part was seeking help, being able to understand my feelings, and being able to talk about them and express them, in tears if appropriate.

My intense anger was dealt with in the same way. I talked about it with my doctor and my family, and we discussed what situations were most likely to trigger off an explosion and how to avoid these situations or defuse them. Medication eased the process, and gradually, the anger dissipated.

I have had to recognize, however, that a problem still remains in this area. I cannot cope with anger as well as I was able to do before my accident. Rage, related to my losses, does not lie just under the surface waiting to explode as it did earlier in my recovery. Yet, like any other person living in the real world, situations arise which make me justifiably angry. Before my accident, it took a lot to make me angry, and I am still, today, slow to anger. The difference is that now, once I become angry, I find it impossible to 'put the brakes on' and I attribute this directly to my brain damage. It is extremely frightening to me to find myself in this state, and I still have not worked out a truly satisfactory solution, except insofar as I try to avoid anger-provoking situations or try to deal with them before they become too provoking.

REGAINING INDEPENDENCE

In the final analysis, though, the problem was greatly alleviated by my taking on gradually increasing responsibilities, first at home, then at work. Each step in this process gave me a sense of accomplishment and self-confidence. It is salutary to accept one's losses, but there comes a time when one must reaffirm what remains and even begin to explore previously-untapped potentials.

In this vein, I have mentioned already that being able to get out of bed unassisted and make the morning coffee was a great step forward for me in the direction of full recovery. Next, I took over the planning and organization of the family's meals, shopping lists, and some limited cooking. As time went on and I grew stronger, I took over all of the housework, cooking, cleaning, laundry, and so forth. I enjoyed doing these things but at first they were quite an ordeal for the family. A shopping trip that would have taken my wife an hour would occupy an entire morning, with me making laborious lists, checking and rechecking, let alone the problem of getting me in and out of the car, manoeuvering up and down the aisles with crutches, casts and shopping cart to be taken into account.

Yet, looking back, I realize how vital it was for me to feel that I was no longer totally dependent, that I had certain responsibilities and tasks within the home that were mine alone, and that I was to some degree at least justifying my existence.

My family were most supportive but I remember having to push hard at times against their tendency to overprotect me and treat me as a fragile invalid. In fact, at times I lost confidence in myself because they didn't think I could do something. This is a sensitive area and one that probably presents the greatest difficulty for the families of brain damaged people. Most people have reserves of compassion and protectiveness that they can draw on in dealing with a hurt member. Supporting the injured one is not hard: it is the letting go that is difficult. It takes a great deal of sensitivity and courage for a family member to change roles at the appropriate time and let the handicapped person 'go it alone'. At times, it may take the intervention of an outsider (doctor, friend, colleague) who is not so emotionally involved, to nudge the family into their new role and allow the handicapped person to take the next steps on the road to recovery.

In my case, this happened when I had to make the decision to resign from my job. I had no confidence in my ability to handle the work again and my wife accepted this. I felt that it was only fair to my clients and colleagues that I resign and allow my job to be filled, so with much sadness I sent in my letter of resignation.

My director, backed by the rest of the staff, then did something that took courage and perception. She refused to accept my resignation and after a long emotional session, somehow gave me the confidence and courage to return to work on a part-time, trial basis. Her confidence was not misplaced: I found that I could handle the work, and thanks to her, retained my job.

I would say that it is imperative that brain damaged people (especially youngsters who have no previous achievements to fall back upon) be provided with challenges and responsibilities. What is the point of struggling to learn, to absorb, and to achieve on an intellectual level when one is not allowed to exercise one's new powers in the real world? Such a person is, literally, 'all dressed up with no place to go'.

No matter how 'hard' it is for family members, teachers, and others to let the brain damaged person 'do it on his own' . . . no matter how much 'easier' it would be to take pity on him and to do it yourself . . . no matter how long it takes or how messy the job when done . . . the brain damaged person must keep moving towards the fullest development of his potential. In my own case, without that gradual buildup of confidence in small matters, starting with making that first cup of coffee on my own, I would never have been able to take the final step of going back into full-time employment.

CONCLUSION

In brief then, I have found that internal and external factors must mesh smoothly in order for the brain damaged person to reach his fullest potential and cope with his disabilities.

An accurate diagnosis of the deficits must be made and must be understood and accepted. by the individual and by those closely involved with his rehabilitation. The individual and his family must be motivated to pursue the fullest development of his potential. Challenges and responsibilities must be provided as he progresses, permitting a growing sense of self-worth and involvement in the real world. Environment at home and at school or work must be structured to maximize learning.

One last word. No one really knows just how great an individual's potential is. In my own case, I was given a slender chance of survival and it was thought that I would be a human vegetable if I did live. Instead, I am living a full and productive life and in fact, can say quite honestly that I enjoy it more than I did before.

People close to me tell me that I am easier to live with and work with, now that I am not the highly self-controlled person that I used to be. My emotions are more openly displayed and more accessible, partially due to the brain damage which precludes any storing up of emotion, and partially due to the maturational aspects of this whole life-threatening experience. I have come through this crisis in my life with more respect for myself and more trust in others. My new openness of feeling makes it easier for me to communicate with others and for others to understand me. People know 'where they stand' with me at all times and trust me more.

Furthermore, my blood pressure is amazingly low! My one-track mind seems to help me to take each day as it comes without excessive worry and to enjoy the simple things of life in a way that I never did before. As well, I seem to be a more effective therapist, since I stick to the basic issues at hand and have more empathy with others than I did previously.

I do not bewail what I have lost because I am at peace with myself.

I have fought a hard battle, given it my best, and won far more than I or anyone else ever thought I would. I ask only that other brain damaged people be given the chance to fight their battles, too, and to find out for themselves what their potential is.

(Linge 1980)

Faith, hope, and love: nontraditional therapy in recovery from serious head injury, a personal account

Frederick R. Linge

Twelve years ago, I survived a serious head injury. In the second it took for my car to crash head-on, my life was permanently changed, and I became another statistic in what has been called 'the silent epidemic'.

Twelve years ago most people with injuries as serious as mine did not survive. I am one of the few who did, although I was living in a rural area where no advanced medical care or equipment was available. Later, I joined an even smaller group of survivors when, despite an utter lack of formal rehabilitation of any kind, I was eventually able to return to my previous practice as a clinical psychologist and to attain a reasonable quality of life.

The past decade has seen much progress in the treatment of head injury, especially with improved ambulance and emergency room techniques. It is apparent even to a cursory observer that there are now many more survivors of head injury than 10 years ago. I need only look around my own family to see this for myself. My wife's teenage nephew has been in coma for the past $1\frac{1}{2}$ years. My younger brother and my daughter-in-law are both survivors of serious head injury, are on permanent disability pensions, and must take anticonvulsant medication. Again, in my practice as a community psychologist, I now regularly assess and counsel other head-injured people, whereas a decade ago I had no such clients.

Obtaining precise statistics on head injury in Canada is a complicated and difficult challenge.[1] Classification methods used on admission or death vary from hospital to hospital and province to province. An extrapolation from head injury statistics of the United States, taking into account American and Canadian 1988 census figures, gives a conservative estimate of 2100 deaths from head injury per year in Canada. Another 15 600 persons per year require hospitalization as a result of the trauma. Most of this group recover (are able to return to work, re-integrate into family and social milieu, and manage personal and financial affairs), but up to 2030 per year are permanently disabled and unable to resume a normal lifestyle.

Even minor to moderate injuries may leave people with chronic problems which disrupt their lives on the job and at home. Of the estimated 14 400 cases of minor to moderate head injury in Canada per year, nearly all resume normal life within 6 months, but one third continue to experience problems for years.

The price to society is reflected in the fact that more than two thirds of survivors with serious head injury and permanent disability are under 30 years of age. Not only are these young people's contributions to society lost and their families disrupted, but each severe head-injury survivor requires several million dollars for a lifetime of care. Head injuries cause more loss of working years than cancer and heart disease combined, are the leading cause of epilepsy, and are the leading cause of death for people under age 34. And, sadly, it is estimated that 95% of all marriages break down following a serious head injury to one of the spouses.

These numbers become even more staggering when one realizes that many survivors will not recover completely and disappear from the statistics. Typically, a survivor of serious head injury requires from 5–10 years of intensive rehabilitation and lifetime follow-up, forming the apex of an ever-growing pyramid of those living on and facing permanent impairments. The magnitude of the problem is compounded by the fact that despite the achievements of the last 10 years, only about 10% of head injury survivors (even those with serious and easily recognizable impairments) receive adequate diagnosis and rehabilitation.[2]

I am one of the minute group of people who have not only survived a serious head injury, but have maintained an intact family and have been able to return to their former employment. To do this, however, has meant that my life for the past 12 years has been a highwire balancing act requiring constant effort and vigilance to get from each day's beginning to its end.

My new clients probably don't notice anything unusual about me. Long-term clients realize that I am a bit forgetful, that I have to take a lot of notes, and that if I see them unexpectedly in another context than the office (at the supermarket, for example) I may not recognize them.

Colleagues know that I am not much good in a group discussion where there is much bouncing around of ideas and switching from the main issue to side issues and back again. My secretary knows how dependent I am on my routines, how carefully I must plan ahead, how important aids such as planning diaries and report formats are, and how easily I am derailed if something out of the ordinary occurs. I must keep physically fit and keep a constant balance between work and relaxation if I am to avoid mental fatigue and do my job properly. Alcohol and many medications create problems, and I must avoid them.

Adjustments, too, have had to be made in my personal life. My sense of smell and my sense of direction have been impaired. I have to be careful not to hike or ski alone, and I

---

[1] Personal communications from Ministries of Health in all 10 provinces, the Yukon, and the Northwest Territories.

[2] All statistics courtesy of the Canada Head Injury Association, Statistics Canada, and the National Head Injury Foundation (U.S.A.).

have trouble finding my way around a new city. Once spontaneous and freewheeling, I have become a person of habit and routine in my daily life. To conserve my mental energy for my job, I now leave much of the family finances and scheduling to my wife. Social events tend to tire me, and I try to limit them; I find myself most comfortable with old friends rather than new acquaintances. Emotional lability is still a problem to be reckoned with, as are anxiety and depression.

THE INJURY

At the time of my accident in 1977, I was 39 years old and had been married for 15 years to Angela, a social worker. We had three children: David, aged 14, Rachel, aged 12, and Winnie, aged 7. I was physically active, enjoyed classical music, played the piano, and read a great deal.

I was admitted to hospital with a broken neck, fractured skull, broken ribs, multiple fractures of the right arm, a splintered left leg, broken hip, and abrasions and contusions. The brain damage, which could be only partially assessed at first, was severe enough to render me unconscious for 2 weeks. I was paralyzed on the right side and showed minimal response to visual, auditory, or other stimuli.

For the first few days, I was kept alive only by heroic surgical procedures and the use of life-support machinery. I was given little chance of survival, and my family were warned that if I survived at all, it probably would be in a vegetative state.

Since I had been taken to a small-town hospital near where my accident occurred, neither specialists nor specialized equipment were available until I could be moved to a larger hospital 2 weeks postinjury. My broken neck was not diagnosed for several weeks, during which time I was constantly at risk every time I thrashed around in bed or was moved by the staff.

The initial assessment by a neurosurgeon showed severe cerebral contusion, cerebral haemorrhaging, a fractured skull, and a right-sided hemiplegia. These were of grave and immediate concern; unseen, yet just as serious in terms of long-term consequences, was the microscopic disruption of nerve connections caused by the shearing and tearing of the tissues at the moment of impact.

Four months later, a neuropsychological assessment pointed to maximum involvement of the left temporal lobe, pronounced short-term memory deficits, and severe impairment in concentration. A retest 6 months later commented tersely: 'Some improvement'. Unfortunately, none of this information was available to us at the time of the injury, and it was only years later that more bits and pieces of information came our way. For example, when our local hospital acquired a CAT scanner, it was found that there was significant calcification in the basal ganglia and mid-brain areas and dilation of the ventricles. I also found out, eventually, that there had been damage to several cranial nerves, including the optic and olfactory nerves.

By the end of the second week, the deep coma began to lighten, and the beginnings of consciousness and of primitive emotions began to appear. Weeks of confusion followed, of which I have only the vaguest memories. I could not talk because I was on a respirator, and I was immobilized by the various casts, traction, halo, and restraints. I had no idea of who I was, who other people were, and what was real and what was not. I was desperate to communicate, but when I tried to write, all I could produce was gibberish.

With the removal of the tracheotomy tubes, the restoration of my speech, and the removal of the wrist and head restraints, my confusion and fear began slowly to subside. I began to see that family, friends, and hospital staff were individuals, not just shadowy, interchangeable figures. I began to realize that there was a separate person: 'I', although I did not know who 'I' was. The delusions and hallucinations I had experienced faded when I realized that others did not share them. Time began to have some meaning instead of past, present, and future being combined into one seamless whole. Memories began to come back, although at first I had 'lost' about 10 years of my life. I began to want to get out of hospital and to get home, although home was just a word, an emotional feeling, and I had no idea what it meant.

I had begun to suspect, even in the hospital, that 'something had happened to me'. I knew that I was not perceiving, thinking, and remembering the way everyone else was. Yet my doctors acted as if the head injury did not exist and as if I had sustained solely physical injuries. A conspiracy of silence seemed to surround the topic, and I was too fragile physically, emotionally, and intellectually to demand some answers.

RETURNING HOME; BEGINNING THE REAL WORK OF RECOVERY

As my family helped me out to the car to begin my journey home, I was a virtual skeleton, having dropped to only 112 lbs. from a preinjury weight of 155 lbs. One arm and one leg were in full casts, my neck was in a brace, and I was so weak that I found great difficulty in holding up my head at all. I could not get out of bed or even rise from a chair without help. I had very little bladder capacity or control, which meant that my wife had to wake up many times each night to help me out of bed to urinate. I had poor resistance to infection and, in fact, lost 15 pounds following a bout of flu shortly after my arrival home.

I well remember my closest male friend saying to me a day or so later: 'Now the hard part is just beginning'. At the time, I did not understand what he meant, but I realize now that his words were both prophetic and accurate. I had no idea that the struggle to cope with the deficits caused by my brain damage would be far harder than the business of physical survival. I thought that when I left the hospital I was ending my journey. I did not realize that it was just beginning.

Once home, I began the real work of rehabilitation, which is simply trying to live as normal a life as possible. During this entire process, there was no help of any kind for the

head injury other than the simple kindness of family and friends. As I have said there was no diagnosis, no information, and no support. This was not due to any neglect on the part of my physicians, but because support groups, associations, programmes, resources, and treatment centres for head-injured survivors and families did not then exist.

During the next months, my family and I began to understand something of the reality of the experience of head injury. I had to begin the painful task of recognizing and accepting my physical, mental, and emotional deficits. I couldn't taste or smell. I couldn't read even the simplest sentence without forgetting the beginning before I got to the end. I had a hair-trigger temper that could ignite instantly into rage over the most trivial incident.

Accompanying these rages were periods of depression, withdrawal, and paranoid notions. Because of my brain damage, I could not process data from the outside world correctly. The computer adage, 'Garbage in, garbage out', described my situation. For example, because I could not taste or smell, I imagined that Angela must have put some sort of poison in the food.

The family faced problems which were as great as mine. Because no professional help was available, my family had to assume the role of therapists themselves. They were without guidance or information. They did not even know that books had been written on the subject of rehabilitation. Thus, they had to use their imagination and gut-level feelings to help me, literally having to 're-invent the wheel' and finding out by trial and error what worked and what did not.

We know now, years later, that most of what they did instinctively at the time was right. For example, from the first day my wife spent as much time as she could at my bedside. She talked to me, hugged me, kissed me, brought the children, family, and friends to see me. She put a small radio beside my bed to play news, weather, sports, and music. As soon as I began emerging from coma, she hung up a big calendar in my room and began telling me what day, month, and year it was. She brought a felt board with felt letters so that I could make words on it when I was unable to talk because of the respirator. She brought a picture that I had loved as a little boy and hung it up where I could see it, plus any other familiar objects that would make me feel more at home.

She knew intuitively that the sooner I could be in familiar surroundings, the more chance I would have, and so she supported the doctors' plan to send me home, fragile though I was. She recalls being so naive that she actually thought, when I was discharged 2 months postinjury, that sending me home must be part of a carefully laid-out treatment plan! It was only later that she realized that, in fact, no plans whatsoever had been made, and that I was being sent home to 'wait and see' what spontaneous recovery might bring about.

She says now that the fact that we had no diagnosis and no treatment had one good effect, which was that she was optimistic almost from the start. She took it for granted that, since no one had said anything to the contrary, it was to be assumed that I would get better.

When I came home, like many head-injured people, I had very serious memory and concentration problems as well as a hair-trigger temper and tempestuous emotions. Angela did not know what to do about the emotional storms, but she decided to try to help me with the memory and the concentration. She had enjoyed teaching our children to speak, to read, and to reason, and she tried out the same methods on me. She had a completely free hand, so she simply went ahead and tried different things until we found what was comfortable and what worked best.

To help me to read and remember, she dug out some of our children's *Rupert Bear* comic books. They were big, colourful books that had an action-packed story-picture on each page. At the top of each page was a one-sentence, very simple summary of the action on that page at the level of a first-grader, such as RUPERT BEAR GOES TO THE OLD MILL AND SEES A GHOST. In addition, underneath the pictures was a much more detailed and complex summary of the action, at about a sixth-grade reading level.

Angela began by having me look at the pictures while she explained the story to me. After some weeks, she had me read out the one-sentence simple headings and then repeat back to her, in my own words, what the sentence had said. We kept at this daily for months until I could tackle the complex and longer sentences and repeat the sense of them back to her. If I forgot, I could always look at the simple sentence or the picture to jog my memory.

While working on the cognitive aspects of rehabilitation, I also began taking small steps in other areas. For example, one of my brothers, Pat, visited us and rigged up some stout knotted ropes over our bed, anchored to the wall with eyebolts. Using my one good arm, I was able to pull myself up out of bed instead of lying there helplessly waiting for Angela or David to haul me to my feet. This had immediate positive ramifications, for it meant that I could now get to the bathroom on my own instead of Angela having to wake up many times per night to assist me.

A further step came when Angela suggested our buying an electric coffeemaker. I was too weak to lift a heavy kettle, but Angela could fill the coffeemaker at night so that all I had to do was switch it on in the morning. I still remember the simple joy of being able to get out of bed on my own, at the early morning hour I have preferred all my life, to make my own coffee. These were small steps and small victories but to me they provided an immense psychological lift.

Another step in my rehabilitation came when I was left alone in the house to shift for myself. At the end of my first month at home, Angela had to go back to work and the children to school. There was no choice in the matter. If she didn't work, we didn't eat, and on her small salary there was no money to hire a care attendant for me even if such an idea had been suggested by my doctors. This was stressful for her, for she had to leave for work in the morning, 8 miles away, afraid all day that I might fall or burn or injure myself in some way.

I certainly am not recommending that people with recent serious head injuries be left at home alone all day, but for some reason it turned out to be the right thing for me. Left alone, I had to become more independent. With no one to do things for me, I began, step by step, to take over the running of the house. Beginning with that first cup of coffee, I progressed to planning and organizing the family's meals, making up shopping lists, dishwashing, and some limited cooking. Since I was alone most of the time, it did not matter how long I took to complete a task or how many mistakes or messes I made. After 8 months of convalescence, I had taken over the housework completely.

Becoming more independent and taking responsibility was very important for my recovery. It put me in touch with reality in a familiar and nonthreatening setting.

It was excellent physical therapy too. I can remember Angela coming home from work to find that I had solved the problem of getting the laundry basked up and down the basement stairs when I needed both arms for my crutches. I ran a rope through the handles, tied the rope to my belt, and dragged it up and down that way.

Taking on responsibility was also good for my memory and reasoning ability and helped with the emotional problems. I did not feel so powerless and helpless when I was able to feel that I was taking some of the load off Angela, that I had my own responsibilities, and that I was pulling my weight.

Part of the reason my homemade rehabilitation worked was that Angela responded so warmly to my efforts. During the first few months, she was exhausted by the weight of stress and responsibility. She recalls coming in at night carrying groceries, looking down at her shoes, and literally wondering whether she had the strength to put one foot in front of another. Anything that I could do, no matter how small or how poorly done, was welcomed with delight by her, which of course provided additional incentives for me.

Emotional problems had to be addressed while I was working on the cognitive and physical ones. The main difficulties were my hair-trigger temper, turbulent emotions, and deep depression. During the first year, I could not take too much stimulation from other people. My brain would simply overload, and

I would have to go off into my room to get away. Noise was hard for me to take, and I wanted the place to be kept quiet, which was an impossibility in a small house with three youngsters in it. Angela spent much of her time trying to keep the children quiet or calming me down when I began to yell at them.

In those early months, I tried to make some sense out of the chaos in my mind by attempting to order the outside world. I remember laying down some impossible rules for all of us, which contributed to the resentment of the children. For example, I made rules that everybody had to be in bed by 9:30 p.m., that all lights had to be out, and that no noise of any kind was permitted after that time. No TV, radios, or talking was allowed, and even the sound of one of the children turning over in bed would be enough to make me erupt.

Angela is an easy-going person, and she went along with this for a while, trying to persuade the children to be more tolerant, but eventually the whole family was in an uproar. In desperation, she made an appointment with a psychiatrist to discuss what was happening. Because no one had told her what to expect when I got home or even put a label on what had happened to me, Angela had no words to describe what was going on. She could only say over and over: 'Something is happening in our family! Something is happening in our family!'

I finally saw the psychiatrist as well. He did not talk much about the head injury, but he did help me to recognize that I was extremely depressed and angry. He put me on antidepressants for a short time, but the important thing was that he got me talking about the problems and worked with me at avoiding situations that triggered my anger, or at least defusing it before I exploded.

Another very real problem during that first year was the question of our sex life. I was unable to resume marital relations for a full year after my accident. This was hard on my wife, because in our small house, she could not retreat to another bedroom even if I had let her. I wanted her there in our bed to cuddle and cling to, especially at first. I needed nurturing and mothering, which she felt comfortable with at first while I was physically fragile. As I became stronger, she no longer felt this was appropriate and wanted to be my wife again rather than a nurse or a mother. Angela remembers feeling irrationally angry at me, feeling I was deliberately denying myself to her, and she had to work hard at concealing these feelings from me. She is a persistent person, and she does not give up easily. Constant physical contact, lots of affectionate gestures and encouragement, time, and my increasing robustness eventually led to the resumption of normal marital relations and another step forward for us toward a normal life.

Rebuilding my personality was a giant task in itself, for I realize now that many of the unique qualities that made me myself were effaced by the injury. I use rather a homely analogy when thinking in retrospect about this job of rebuilding my self. It was like putting the layers of a flower bulb back together, building from the inside out. One by one, these delicate membranes had to be placed smoothly and symmetrically into position. Sometimes the old layers did not fit or were damaged beyond repair, and I had to discard them and create new ones. My family were aware on some level of this process, for I remember one of my daughters dreaming at this time that I had been ground to a powder, and that she was trying to mix water into this dust and knead and mold it into some semblance of my former self.

RETURNING TO WORK

The final stage in rehabilitation came when, after a year's absence, I returned to part-time work. I could not have done this without the courage of my Director at the Mental Health Centre, who took the bold gamble of refusing my resignation. She made this decision without having access to any medical or neuropsychological assessments or prognoses, but judged, instead, on the basis of her frequent visits to me in the hospital and at home. Not only did she encourage me to try a return to work, but she ensured that major modifications were made to my work programme. She arranged that I would start by

working a few hours only, and she made sure that I was assigned tasks that used skills I had learned previously.

Still in the earlier stages of recovery, I could not concentrate for more than a few hours without becoming exhausted. I could not sustain attention unless in a one-to-one situation, I could only retain the gist of a few simple paragraphs at a time, and my memory was extremely poor. I remember with embarrassment an incident which happened almost a year after returning to work. I had spent several hours interviewing a woman about family problems. She forgot her handbag and came back unexpectedly an hour later. I had completely forgotten who she was and stared at her as if she were a stranger!

Looking back, I am amazed at my Director's courage in entrusting the responsibility for these patients to me when I was so fragile myself. Psychology is both an art and a science, involving many levels of the mind, spirit, and personality, and all three had been damaged by my injury. Neither Angela nor I had the firm conviction that I could work as a psychologist again, but others did. I can only say that it was because of the faith, hope, and love of my Director, my colleagues at work, and my patients that I managed to return to work; and it was they who bore me up for the first grim months until I could carry the load on my own.

THE SEARCH FOR MEANING: LOOKING OUTWARD

Two years after my injury, I wrote a short article 'What Does It Feel Like to be Brain Damaged?' At that time, I was still intensely focussing on myself and my own struggle. (Every head-injured survivor I have met seems to go through this stage of narcissistic preoccupation, which creates a necessary shield to protect them from the painful realities of the situation until they have a chance to heal.) I had very little sense of anything beyond the material world and could only write about things that could be described in factual terms. I wrote, for example, about my various impairments and how I learned to compensate for them by a variety of methods.

I did have some intuitive feeling, even then, that there had been gains, but I could recognize only very superficial ones. I spoke, for example, of the greater access that I had to my emotions, of my more relaxed attitude toward life, and my lower blood pressure. I also spoke about the maturational aspects of the experience and the fact that others found me easier to work with. Even then, I was beginning to grope toward a realization and there was something more when I wrote: 'It is salutory to accept one's losses, but there comes a time when one must reaffirm what remains and even begin to explore previously untapped potential . . . No-one really knows just how great an individual's potential is.'

By the third year post-injury, I had begun to move beyond simple healing and gratitude at being able to enjoy ordinary daily activities. I began to ask more profound questions than just 'Why me?' I began to look outward, away from myself and my own personal struggle against my own limitations, to make some larger sense out of my own experience.

At this point in my life, I began to involve myself with other brain-damaged people. This came about in part after the publication of my article. To my surprise, it was reprinted in many different publications, copied, and handed out to thousands of survivors and families. It brought me an enormous outpouring of letters, phone calls, and personal visits which continue to this day. Many were struggling as I had struggled, with no diagnosis, no planning, no rehabilitation, and most of all, no hope.

FAITH, HOPE, AND LOVE

Two themes emerge from all these letters, phone calls, and visits. One is the loneliness which is so much a part of head injury. We are social beings, and when we are in extremis we desperately need to share our feelings and to be comforted by others. To be unable to do so compounds our suffering. The poet John Donne understood this when he wrote

As sickness is the greatest misery, so the
  greatest misery of sickness is solitude . . .
Solitude is a torment which is not threatened
  in hell itself. (Meditation V)

The other theme is the need for hope. Every family I have ever met who has been touched by serious head injury has asked me, 'Is there any hope?' Hope is a primary necessity for rehabilitation; it sustains survivor and family for the long journey that lies ahead.

Under this tidal wave of fellow survivors my personal barriers fell, and in reaching out to others I began to grow again and to feel a need for more spirituality in my life. At first, this need grew slowly, but over the last years there has been a flowering of spiritual life and a revelation of new horizons. These gains, to me, outweigh the losses that I have sustained, and I do not regret undergoing the experience of head injury.

I judge the quality of life in a very different way now than I did before my own injury. When I meet a person with brain damage, I do not look first at the medical history or the testing that has been done. I look first for the presence in them or their family of a quality that could be called guts, the fighting spirit, or faith. With it, we have a foundation on which we can build. Without it, full return to productive, giving, growing personhood is slower or impossible.

Sadly, I meet some people whose brain damage is minimal, yet who lack this spirit and who cease to grow. Perhaps this is because the faith they had was extinguished at the beginning, or perhaps because their families' motivation to help was also snuffed out.

On the other hand, I know many people, such as my brother, Raymond, whose brain injury is severe, who also suffer permanent physical handicaps. They display unquenchable courage and faith and continue to grow, to give, and to explore new areas of potential even though other areas may be closed.

I heard an anecdote recently that immediately made me think of my brother. When Alexander Alekhine, the Russian chess master, was playing a chess game, someone pointed at him and said 'You have a poor position, there'. Alekhine snapped back: 'Position? What does the *position* matter? It is my *will* that counts!'

When I meet a new patient with brain damage, I also look for another element that is vital to full recovery: hope. Hope is the longing for better things and the small flame that comforts in the darkness. One might think that hope is the most evanescent of all expressions of the person, as delicate and as easily crushed as a butterfly's wing. I have not found this to be true. On the contrary, I have found from my own experience and the shared experience of others that hope is tough and tenacious, like one of those common flowers that forces its way up through bricks or concrete toward the light.

I often think of Freddie Prinze, the young comedian who killed himself some years ago. He 'had everything' the world could offer: money, celebrity, and success. Moments before he shot himself, he turned to his friends and said some of the saddest of words: 'Is this all there is? Is this *all* there is?'

If Freddie Prinze, who 'had it all', had no hope, how much harder the loss of hope is to bear for someone who has suffered head injury! Often, if a person lives a purely materialistic life and then is injured in mind or body, he feels that his entire world is destroyed. However, if he sees that there are other dimensions, new worlds that he can strive towards and reach out for, there is once again hope, meaning and purpose. As Browning wrote:

Ah, but a man's reach should exceed his grasp,
Or what's a heaven for?

Faith and hope are vital, but the mightiest impetus to healing is love. Love rekindles courage, nurtures hope, and conquers loneliness. If one can give nothing more to a head-injured person than love, one has given the greatest of all gifts. St. Paul summed this up when he wrote:

If I speak with the tongues of men and of angels and have not love, I am become as sounding brass . . . and if I . . . should know all mysteries and all knowledge; and if I should have all faith, so that I could remove mountains, and have not love, I have nothing . . . And now these remain, faith, hope, and love, these three: but the greatest of these is love.

These three elements—faith, hope and love—are inextricably linked. In my experience, their presence is the best indicator of whether an individual is going to come through the experience of head injury with gains that outweigh the losses. I would rather look at these and not set any limits on what they and their family can achieve together as they begin their shared journey.

In the early years, I had nothing to offer other survivors except myself, because programmes and resources did not exist in my part of the world. I could offer only faith, hope, and love. Years later, I still put these three things first, although I can now refer clients to support groups, residences, and various programmes in our area. I have heard other colleagues hesitate, saying that they are '. . . afraid of raising false hopes that are doomed to disappointment', but I have never regretted instilling hope in a family nor have I ever been reproached for it by one.

Greater experience over the past decade, based on millions of head injuries, has provided more accurate ways of predicting and planning the course of rehabilitation. Sometimes, however, these predictions can be used with a harmful rigidity. It saddens me to see families crushed and despairing when they are told: 'This is all you can expect. You will go no further.' These are only predictions, based on statistics, but there is something about the human spirit that allows it to evade the rules.

I will not destroy hope. I will not tell anyone, 'This is the end of your journey', for I have seen too many miracles in the past 12 years. They do not happen in every case of head injury, but they do happen sometimes. I have seen people awake from coma who were supposed to be permanently brain-dead. I have seen people making slow but noticeable gains 25 years after severe head injuries. I have seen people who had been on a recovery plateau 8 or 9 years postinjury suddenly begin to flourish and blossom.

OTHER CASES: THREE
SURVIVORS' STORIES

I would like to mention three people whom I know personally, whose stories illustrate what I have just said. In each case, each individual had faith, hope, and love in full measure from supportive families and friends. The first, a professor at a British university, sustained a severe head injury when he was 39. Three years later, he wrote to me as follows:

My speech was jargon . . . at the same time I can't write more than a word and none grammar. Often I called my wife as 'the man' and all people as 'mummy and daddy' . . . I want to say something, but the subjects are gone before I can get the words together . . . I had to resign my job because after two years sick leave I couldn't talk and write which is my job.

Statistically, this man could be expected to remain permanently at this level of recovery and had 'gone as far as he could' in the 3 years postinjury. His letter went to my heart, and we wrote to each other for a couple of years. Then, last summer, I received another letter which I could hardly believe was from the same man:

Dear Fred,

Thank you for the letter and the maps. This is a quick note to say that my colleague, with whom I will be staying for two nights at——, said we would be leaving for Vancouver via Penticton on Friday, 1st July. He estimates that it will take about eight hours to reach Penticton and wonders if I would be able to visit you on Saturday morning. So, I hope that I will be able to see you on that morning. I am sure that we can find your house from the maps. I, my colleague, his wife and young son, are all going to the International Congress of——at Vancouver. When I get into——, Wednesday 29th June, I will phone you to see if everything is OK.

Best wishes,

He had experienced a breakthrough, a leap forward to another level of recovery. He was back at work at the university, had written a paper, and was presenting it at an international conference. We had the opportunity of meeting and spending a week together, and I found a man of courage and dignity, a man with a sweetness of spirit and a humble acceptance of still-existing impairments in speech: in short, a man who had *gained* from his experience.

My second example is my own daughter-in-law. Gail was severely injured 10 years ago and was in a coma for several months. She had no rehabilitation other than for her physical injuries and, when our son David met her 3 years ago, was living at home with her parents after some troubled years trying to live independently. She was on a permanent disability pension, had a serious thought disorder, spoke in a bizarre and disjointed fashion, slept much of the time, was withdrawn and depressed, and was unable to complete most of the tasks of daily living.

She and David fell in love, married 2 years ago, and have just become the parents of a healthy baby girl. Gail has made amazing progress in the past 3 years. With David's constant loving presence, with the stimulus of having her own home and her own responsibilities and status as a wife, she is a happy, robust, outgoing young woman who is enjoying motherhood. The bizarre speech and thought patterns have vanished, and the only signs of the injury that remain are that she is still more emotionally labile than most people and needs more rest and less stress. Gail has such a sweetness of spirit and a spirit of love and joy that we are honoured to have her in our family. She has given more to our son and to us than we have given to her. She, too, is someone whose journey was supposed to end years ago, but did not.

Sometimes these breakthroughs do not happen for the injured person but for a family member or helper. Some years ago, I met a woman whose husband received terrible injuries in a car accident. He has been in a vegetative state in an extended care hospital for years. She is in a happy second relationship, but she still cares for her husband, visits him frequently in hospital, and acts as his advocate and guardian. In addition, she has been deeply involved in the local, provincial, and national head-injury movement from its inception.

It takes courage and tenacity to be a survivor of a survivor, like this woman. She did not walk away from the challenge, thereby losing forever the chance to grow more, to love more, and to give more. She told me that for a long time after her husband was injured, she prayed for a miracle. The miracle did not happen for him; but she told me that after some years she realized that it had happened for her. She found that she was a stronger, more compassionate, and more loving person than she had ever dreamed was possible.

CONCLUSION

Survivors of head injury, families, and professionals have much in common. We are part of a growing movement to inform, to support, and to help head-injured people to attain their potential. But there is also a movement in our society, fuelled by economic considerations, to place the containment of health costs ahead of the best interests of the individual. Priorities are being set and distinctions made regarding the availability of scarce treatment resources, based on arbitrary standards regarding the individual's 'quality of life' or 'usefulness to society'.

We survivors of head injury are especially vulnerable because of our large numbers and the high costs of rehabilitation, and because when we are most in need of help, we cannot ask for it. Our common cause must be based on rigorous respect for life and an equally vigorous rejection of any *apartheid* approach that would separate disabled people from others. It is imperative that we look beyond our individual struggles, allying ourselves with the larger movement which seeks to bring all disabled people into the mainstream of society. This endeavour, to my mind, represents one of the finest flowerings of our society and of our age, far more so than the space programme or the computer revolution.

It has been 12 years since my head injury: for me, 12 years of suffering, of challenge, and of personal growth. Above all, I have learned that there is no limit to the power of faith, hope, and love. With these, I made the journey out of the shadows into a larger, brighter world than the one I had left behind before my injury.

The far-ranging effects of head injury on the survivor's life and that of his or her family cannot be overemphasized. In my own case I realize that it was for me the single most significant event of my lifetime. The catastrophic effect of my injury was such that I was shattered and then remoulded by the experience, and I emerged from it a profoundly different person with a different set of convictions, values, and priorities. From this tremendous experience I came to a bedrock of conviction, a place where, like Martin Luther, I could say 'Here I stand!'

I believe that there is hope, even for the severely head-injured person such as myself. In so saying, I am at risk of sounding like a facile Pollyanna, but I speak as one who has experienced the reality of head injury to its fullest, not only as a survivor but as a family member and as a therapist.

I no longer measure the worth of my life or that of others by standards such as money or appearance or even by usefulness to society. I believe that all life is worthy of respect and is precious. I no longer evaluate a victory in terms of power and prestige. In the eyes of society, the daily struggles, defeats, and successes of a survivor may be trivial, but to me now, they are greater than the televised victories of a professional athlete. And finally, I believe that it is the struggle itself that gives life dignity, at the last.

(Linge 1990)

COMMENTARY

As a result of his injury, Linge had severe cerebral contusion, cerebral haemorrhage, a fractured skull, and a right-sided hemiplegia. He indicates that there was
focal cerebral contusion in the left temporal and right parietal regions. He was in
coma for the first week, and he appeared to be semi-conscious or very confused for
several weeks afterwards. He himself reports that he has no memory for the first few
weeks that he spent in the hospital's intensive care unit, and so it seems that the
duration of his post-traumatic amnesia (often used as an indicator of severity of a
head injury) was at least four weeks. Linge's two articles provide such a detailed
account of so many aspects of head injury that it is worth commenting separately
on particular features of his accounts.

1. Early recovery and retrograde amnesia.   The word 'home' had little real meaning
for him in the early phase of his recovery. He was very much aware that he was
'not perceiving, thinking, and remembering the way everyone else was' (p. 327).
During his initial hospital stay, his wife brought him familiar items such as photographs, and also items that enabled him to communicate and know what was
going on around him. She herself seemed uncertain about what to expect in terms
of future recovery, and retained an optimistic view that his current difficulties were
only temporary. In view of Linge's left temporal lobe damage, it is not surprising
that there appeared to be significant semantic memory loss, in terms of loss of
knowledge that he had acquired before his injury. One of the head injury patients
studied by colleagues and myself suffered severe left temporal lobe pathology and
was left with marked memory loss for pre-injury events (Kapur *et al.* 1996*a*). In the
early stages of the head injury, her mother indicated that this patient had a loss of
knowledge retrieval in respect of common words (e.g. she had to relearn the names
of everyday objects such as knives, forks, clothes and colours, and she had considerable difficulty in understanding written words).
    Linge makes a number of interesting comments in relation to his loss of memory
for pre-injury events. His pre-traumatic amnesia for events that occurred just
before the injury was total and irreversable—even with many prompts, such as
returning to the scene of the accident, looking at photographs of the cars, and hearing witness testimonies. In the early stages of the injury, he had 'lost' around ten
years of his life. He thought his mother was still alive, when in fact she had died a
number of years earlier. At a conscious level, he did not appear to be fully aware or
concerned about this gap—for him past, present, and future seemed to merge into
one. However, at another level his brain was trying to come to terms with this gap
in his past, and one of the results of this endeavour were 'delusions' that went
unchecked—he thought that he was in another hospital, one closer to his early
family home, and that his parents were still alive. His 'delusion' could be seen to be
a severe form of confabulation, and also a form of coping strategy. The scenario
could be as follows. A patient such as Linge tries to make sense of what to him are
distressing and puzzling circumstances, he partly relies on information that is still
intact, usually from many years earlier, and he constructs a story that he believes is
true and which can account for the situation in which he finds himself. He does not
have the benefit of numerous checking mechanisms—such as concordance with

recent information and events, logical status of his account, etc.—that normal individuals take for granted, and this helps to maintain the delusion for a number of days.

Linge had to go through a grieving process again when he realized that his mother was dead. Being unaware of the deaths of loved ones is an overlooked but relatively common feature of patients who suffer an acute brain illness/injury that results in a significant period of retrograde amnesia. One case whom several colleagues and I studied (Kapur *et al.* 1966*b*) suffered an episode of transient global amnesia (TGA). Her dog had died the week previous to the TGA attack. As she was recovering from the attack on the evening of the same day, she suddenly remembered that her dog had died and she became very upset about it. Observations such as these led me to develop a test of retrograde amnesia, the Dead-or-Alive test (Kapur *et al.* 1989), which we have found to be useful in clinical and research work. In this test, the subject is shown names of famous personalities and has to indicate whether they are dead or alive, how they died, and when they died.

The severity of an initial period of retrograde amnesia after severe head injury, and the spontaneous shrinkage of such memories, has been described in a number of articles (Benson and Geschwind 1967; High *et al.* 1990), but it remains a poorly understood set of phenomena. Perhaps it was the continuous argument with his wife over his false belief relating to his mother, and why she was not visiting him in hospital, that somehow triggered the return of Linge's memory for his mother's death. A further, fairly sudden return of memories occurred when he returned home after being discharged from hospital—on the way home, he could not anticipate the next place along a particular road, but when he encountered the place it was familiar. When he was outside his house 'a huge chunk of memories fell into place' (p. 320)—one could argue that his associative memory for elements of a spatial map was faulty, but that familiarity recognition of the elements themselves was intact. It is quite likely that the severity of Linge's retrograde amnesia related to the left temporal and additional diffuse pathology that was present on his brain scan. The 'falling into place' of past memories as a result of exposure to specific cues is in contrast to what is seen in some cases of persistent, focal retrograde amnesia—one of the cases that we studied (Kapur *et al.* 1992) did not recover lost memories even when she was specifically taken by her family to visit places with which she had been familiar prior to her head injury.

Related to Linge's dense retrograde amnesia was his lack of awareness of time, with little differentiation between past and present, and also within past and present time intervals. Neuropsychologists sometimes talk of the 'stream of consciousness', to indicate the automatic time-keeping mechanism that helps us keep the present within the context of the recent past. It seems that this stream no longer existed for Linge in these first few months of recovery from his head injury. He also admitted to a lack of differentiation amongst people, including himself—he knew who he was, but he could not ascertain if this person was a child, a boy or a man; his wife and mother were indistinguishable for him; and hospital staff all seemed the same. When some level of differentiation did return, he magnified particular individuals in his mind—he saw his doctor as a gigantic, looming figure when in reality he was in fact a slight person. Recovery of orientation for person, time and place was studied in a group of severely head injured patients by High *et al.* (1990).

They found that 10% of patients did not know their name at some point during their recovery (although High *et al.* did not report how many cases were due to a dysphasia or to a problem in articulation). In most patients, the sequence of recovery consisted of orientation for person, then for place and then for time.

2. Temperament, personality, and behaviour.   Linge confessed to having a difficulty in 'putting on the brakes' when he lost his temper. It would seem that he had lost some of the inhibitory mechanisms that we all take for granted in such situations. It is difficult to suggest a remedy for such a complaint—distracting attention towards some other topic may sometimes work, but the advice mentioned by Linge of trying to avoid potential triggers in the first place is perhaps the best one. A further example arose where it helped to avoid provoking situations or to defuse events in the early stages. Linge found it difficult in the first year to take too much stimulation from other people, finding it more comfortable to be alone. Similarly, noise was more stressful to him than to others. He and his wife saw a psychiatrist, and they found it helpful to talk about his temper and intolerance.

The first year also saw a loss of normal sexual activity. This gradually improved over that year: 'Constant physical contact, lots of affectionate gestures and encouragement, time, and my increasing robustness eventually led to the resumption of normal marital relations and another step forward for us toward a normal life' (p. 330). He compares the rebuilding of his personality to the delicate rebuilding of a flower bulb from the inside out.

In addition to his cognitive handicaps, Linge initially had one arm and leg in plaster cast, his neck in a brace and he had little control of his bladder. This resulted in demands on his wife, (e.g. she had to wake up many times each night to help him urinate). He also had poor resistance to infection, and had lost around 40 lbs (18 kg) from his pre-injury weight. 'I had no idea that the struggle to cope with the deficits caused by brain damage would be far harder than the business of physical survival' (p. 327). In the early stages of recovery after he returned home, Linge indicated that he only had help and support from family and friends, with no formal rehabilitation being offered. At that time, 1977, there was little in the way of specialist rehabilitation services in the area where he lived. In the early recovery phase, he had to 'begin the painful task of recognizing and accepting my physical, mental, and emotional deficits' (p. 327). He had lost his sense of taste and smell. He had difficulty remembering what he had read a few sentences earlier. He had a 'hair-trigger' temper, that was accompanied by times of depression, withdrawal, and paranoid delusions—because he could not taste nor smell, he imagined that his wife was putting poison in his food. Such delusions are a rare occurrence after severe head injury, although they have occasionally been reported to occur (Lishman 1987). It would appear that in Linge's case, they resulted from a specific combination of sensory and emotional changes that resulted from his head injury—either of the changes alone would not have resulted in the delusions.

His wife found it easier to handle his memory and concentration difficulties than his temper outbursts. In order to improve his concentration, she used techniques similar to those that she had tried when bringing up their children. She would show him a page showing pictures and related sentences, and he would be required to repeat back to her what the sentences said. The page title and the pictures were used as cues to help if he forgot. Linge probably benefited from the non-verbal, pictorial cues in view of the relative sparing of right hemisphere functions.

3. Long-term rehabilitation. Both Linge and his family improvised with therapy aids to help his mobility and self-reliance. Being able to do things such as make his own coffee in the morning were 'small steps and small victories but to me they provided an immense psychological lift' (p. 328). Often being alone at home, he had to make constant efforts to do things by himself, such that after eight months of convalescence he was relatively self-reliant for many household duties. He himself would improvise for tasks such as getting the laundry basket down a flight of stairs. He enjoyed the responsibility of doing things for himself, and the confidence that it gave—it also helped to take some of the work load off his wife.

Linge (1990) succinctly states some of the sequelae with which he is still afflicted—forgetting faces that are not in the context that he originally saw them, difficulty in taking part in a group discussion where there is bouncing back and switching between major and minor issues; a reliance on routines, habits and memory aids; a tendency to tire more easily; some emotional lability that includes anxiety and depression; organization of his work load so that some areas of mental activity such as family finances are left to his wife; limitations in the number of social events he attends—due to their fatiguing effects; and a difficulty in learning to find his way around unfamiliar places. The number and variety of such deficits point to the importance of drawing up a careful balance when planning the re-entry of head injury patients into the community—a balance that incorporates the use of spared functions to the maximum, that limits demands on fragile or lost functions, and that allows for physical and emotional changes when planning cognitive activities in everyday settings (Kreutzer and Wehman 1990).

Linge was fortunate that, when he returned to work a year post-injury, he had a very understanding boss who arranged that he should initially work a limited number of hours and on tasks that used well-learned skills that were still spared after his head injury. His capacity for sustained concentration and his memory were still significantly impaired. On one occasion, he did not recognize the face of a patient with whom he had spent several hours just one hour earlier. It would be highly unusual if he did not have some familiarity recognition for the face, and it is more likely that he could not recall the name of the patient or the context in which he had seen the face. Linge had sympathetic and supportive colleagues and patients during these early months back at work, and this probably made all the difference to his successful readjustment.

Linge offers some useful hints for those who have residual handicaps from a severe brain injury:

(1) eliminate as many distractions as possible and concentrate on the task at hand;
(2) try to create a structured, routine, well-organized, serene atmosphere at home and at work;
(3) there should be 'a place for everything and everything in its place';
(4) tackle new tasks when you are feeling fresh and have plenty of energy, such as in the mornings;

(5) use a note-book extensively and systematically, rehearsing the material a number of times and in varied ways;

(6) talk to others about your feelings and concerns;

(7) avoid situations that will lead to losing control of your temper.

Linge does talk about the few *gains* his traumatic experience has had for him—a greater access to his emotions, a more relaxed attitude to life, a lower blood pressure, the maturing effects of his experience, and the fact that others now found him easier to work with. Similar observations of paradoxical benefits from a severe head injury have been noted by researchers. For example, Bond (1984) reported the case of a 62-year-old salesman who, prior to a severe head injury, was a heavy drinker and abusive to his wife. After his injury, he was left with a minor physical handicap and marked memory impairment, but his wife indicated she was pleased that, as a result of his injury, he remained at home, was not abusive or irritable and had developed a good sense of humour!

The publicity that Linge had for his head injury, as a result of articles that he wrote, brought him into contact with many other brain injured people. In his words, this brought home to him the loneliness that accompanies afflictions such as brain injury; the hope, faith, and fighting spirit which is necessary in the early stages; the enhancement of spiritual life that he felt; and the love of others that was also a vital ingredient of his recovery. It is always difficult to be certain about the precise role that such factors play in improvement in severe head injury, over and above spontaneous recovery mechanisms, and there are no doubt individual differences in premorbid personality and support structures that are important.

Linge ends his 1990 article with an eloquent summary of what he has learned from his experience: 'I no longer measure the worth of my life or that of others by standards such as money or appearance or even by usefulness to society. I believe that all life is worthy of respect and is precious. I no longer evaluate a victory in terms of power and prestige. In the eyes of society, the daily struggles, defeats, and successes of a survivor may be trivial, but to me now, they are greater than the televised victories of a professional athlete. And finally, I believe that it is the struggle itself that gives life dignity, at the last' (p. 334).

REFERENCES

Benson, D. F. and Geschwind, N. (1967). Shrinking retrograde amnesia. *Journal of Neurology, Neurosurgery and Psychiatry*, **30**, 457–61.

Bond, M. (1984). The psychiatry of closed head injury. In *Closed head injury* (ed. D. N. Brooks), pp. 148–78. Oxford University Press.

High, W. M., Levin, H. S., and Gary, H. E. (1990). Recovery of orientation following closed head injury. *Journal of Clinical and Experimental Neuropsychology*, **12**, 703–14.

Kapur, N., Young, A., Bateman, D., and Kennedy, P. (1989). Focal retrograde amnesia: a long-term clinical and neuropsychological follow-up. *Cortex*, **25**, 387–402.

Kapur, N., Ellison, D., Smith, M., McLellan, L., and Burrows, E. (1992). Focal retrograde amnesia following bilateral temporal lobe pathology: A neuropsychological and magnetic resonance study. *Brain*, **115**, 73–85.

Kapur, N., Scholey, K., Moore, E., Barker, S., Brice, J., Thompson, S., *et al.* (1996a). Long-term retention deficits in two cases of disproportionate retrograde amnesia. *Journal of Cognitive Neuroscience*, **8**, 354–72.

Kapur, N., Abbott, P., Footitt, D., and Millar, J. (1996*b*). Long-term perceptual priming in transient global amnesia. *Brain and Cognition*. In press.

Kreutzer, J. S. and Wheman, P. (ed.) (1990). *Community integration following traumatic brain injury*. Edward Arnold, Sevenoaks, Kent.

Lishman, W. A. (1987). *Organic Psychiatry* (2nd edn). Blackwell, Oxford.

Brain injury: a personal view

Andrea E. Ostrum

Andrea Ostrum was a clinical psychologist at the time of her injury.

Psychological effects of severe brain damage have often been attributed primarily to physical causes. Because most brain-damaged patients have neither the training nor the capacity appropriate for this kind of analysis, the literature about brain damage has been written by the able-bodied. This author is paralyzed below the neck as a result of severe injury to the brain stem suffered during an automobile accident. She is also a trained psychologist with a Ph.D. from Columbia and 6 years of postdoctoral work in the NYU postdoctoral program in clinical psychology. This presents a unique opportunity for the blending of three viewpoints. First, there is the viewpoint of a badly disabled person. Second, there is the viewpoint of a trained psychologist. Third, there is the contribution of clinical psychology which has been de-emphasized in favor of neurology, psychiatry, and neuropsychology, all of which tend to be physically oriented.

The most severe physical disability is paralysis of the entire body. This can be caused by an injury to the brain or spinal cord, a tumor, a disease, an operation, a birth defect, and a multitude of other things. Whatever the genesis, some psychological factors are the same. The overriding factor with total paralysis is complete helplessness and dependency on others for everything and the concomitant absence of control. When one is dependent on others to such a degree, that dependency makes others very powerful and they are perceived that way. The distortion is so great that it outweighs the most obvious contradictory factors. Voices actually become louder and people seem taller than they really are. One tends to attribute to them magical things of which reason in any normal situation would say they were incapable. Because of this dynamic, home health aides who do not occupy a powerful

socioeconomic position are perceived as very powerful by the paralyzed person, and doctors whom society endows with omnipotence can be seen as being potential saviors. The self-image is filtered through the body-image. When one is not able to do the things one used to be able to do with ease, one sees oneself as totally incapable. There is, therefore, a discrepancy between how one sees oneself and the effect one has on others. The result may be interpersonal disturbances and sharply lowered aspirations. One may behave in either of two extreme manners—both distortions. Either one can be overly docile as a reflection of one's physical weakness or one can overcompensate by behaving in a way that makes up for the physical helplessness. Either way, the behavior does not correspond to the reality of the situation and will take the recipient by surprise.

With other people perceived as so powerful because of the paralyzed person's dependency on others, there is an extraordinary pull to suppress and internalize anger. This, if it is allowed to continue uninterrupted, can cause physical ailments, sleep disturbances, and inappropriate outbursts that disrupt social relationships. These are some of the factors that are currently attributed to physical causes. The other possible outcome is acute depression that mitigates against the motivation to work and not only condemns the person to paralysis for life but also deprives society of whatever contribution he or she could make.

The lack of control has equally profound effects. When a person loses control of his or her body, he or she loses not only self-esteem but also all sense of having any control in the world. Because of this, the paralyzed person may issue a flurry of directions in an effort to make herself or himself believe that he or she has some control. This attempt is ultimately

self-destructive because it leads to disorganization and, if not understood, to anger on the
part of the listener, whether family, caregiver, friend, or employee. Repeated repetitions that until now have been seen as
physical in cause can, from this perspective,
be understood as a magical attempt to regain
the lost control. Everything is affected by the
lack of mobility. Because of this, the paralyzed person is forced to get closure verbally
and the most important thing becomes being
sure that something will get done. Due to these
concerns, social manners are of secondary
importance and relationships may suffer.

These are only some of the psychological
ramifications of complete paralysis. It is
hoped that this note will be of help to both

families of, and people who work with, the
paralyzed by helping them to understand
their world so that they can better understand their behavior. Many people who work
with the brain-damaged regard them as a
species apart—some kind of 'pet'. Perhaps it
is an attempt to put as much distance as possible between themselves and the brain-damaged person to try to avoid the fact that
'there but for the grace of God go I'. It could
happen to anyone and it is most people's worst
nightmare. Regardless of the cause, however,
it still hurts. Brain-damaged people should be
treated as individuals, not textbook cases.
After all 'if you prick us do we not bleed'?

(Ostrum 1993)

The 'locked-in' syndrome—comments from a survivor

Andrea E. Ostrum

In this day and age of denial of sustenance for 'coma' victims, the description of a psychologist's own travail with the 'locked-in' syndrome is very
pertinent. There is a real chance of an inexperienced physician mistaking
the 'locked-in' syndrome for 'coma' or the 'vegetative syndrome'. People
with a pure brainstem lesion can be in real coma for a long time and still
have a chance of waking up and be in a state of 'locked-in' syndrome which
would superficially look like a vegetative state. These people are completely
aware of what is going on, but may not be able to move, breathe, talk or
swallow. With rehabilitation they can live a useful life. One of my patients,
like Dr Ostrum, lives independently, works and has the same intelligence as
before the accident. We must be very aware of this syndrome and prevent
these people from being starved to death by a court order.

(Henry Stonnington)

PREFACE

Dr Ostrum is unique in my clinical experience. Locked-in syndrome is itself rare and Dr
Ostrum is the only one of traumatic aetiology
whom I've treated. Although I first examined
her in her contractured, spastic, ataxic and
dysarthric states in November of 1988, she
had written me innumerable letters during
the many months prior to this consultation
detailing the horror of her situation, railing
against the medical system, and anticipating

full recovery once she was admitted to my
rehabilitation unit. Clearly, she was a woman
with cognitive and behavioural problems
when I finally saw her during November of
1988—with her flailing gesticulations, yell-
ing, interrupting, demanding demeanour
and uncooperativeness. I was certain I was
dealing with a 'classic' head injured, cogni-
tively and behaviourally impaired person.
But that was fallacious as the reader can tell
from the intelligent, articulate and accomplished person presented in her article.

I embarked upon a personal and professional adventure that will be with me all my days and that I recount to house staff and new colleagues regularly. I have travelled with her through the depths of bitterness, depression and fatalism, because of the crushing realities of life as a physically challenged person, to the heights of excitement and accomplishment, because she could wash her own hair or stand unsupported. I was not a believer in the beginning, but that changed rapidly and Andrea has become an inspiration. Her accomplishments have continued to beat the odds. She has evolved from unrealistic expectations of herself and others to acceptance of neurological limitations and the lack of superhuman powers in those who care for her.

Denial and unrealistic optimism have their places in healing, both physically and psychologically. Patients must be kept out of the pit of despair while you, the clinician, hold the reins on their search for the Holy Grail. Physicians caring for people like Dr Ostrum need to be good listeners, as well as advisors. You need to be an anchor from which possibilities can be explored, providing a safe harbour to which to retreat. This certainly does not sound like the traditional medical model of patient care. But rehabilitation medicine is well known for breaking that mould.

People like Andrea struggle all their lives to be accepted for whom they are, not for what their bodies appear to be. To 'judge a book by its cover' is unfair, but it happens all too often. One of our jobs as rehabilitation clinicians is to recognize the contents of the book, understand the complexity and uniqueness of the prose within and convince others to read it too.

JOSEPH CARFI
Great Neck, NY, USA

INTRODUCTION

The most important thing to know about me is that my injury magnifies every sensation, so that I feel every little thing—even the food moving through my intestines. It is impor-tant to not let anything touch me hard. Second, my damage is bad but it is all physical. My mind isn't affected at all. Finally, I am not as helpless as I look. The following is an account of what I do.

CASE STUDY

I used to be on life support.

I could not talk comprehensibly until $2\frac{1}{2}$ years ago. Now I can talk to strangers on the telephone, and my doctor says that I am often 90% intelligible. I also wrote this myself on my own computer. I can eat and drink anything. I feed myself with a regular fork and spoon and off a regular plate. I drink unaided. I cut my food and write notes, wash myself, get dressed and undressed, and when brushing my teeth I can take the cap off the toothpaste, squeeze the tube, and return the cap. I can turn all the way round; I can stand up, and I have even done this without leaning on anything. I have taken a step, balancing on my therapists. I can sit at a desk on an office chair and answer the telephone, open the drawers, drink, ring a bell and more. I eat, drink and write at a regular chair and table. I can stand at the parallel bars alone. I have a bank account and I sign and endorse cheques at the table.

I live without my family. I transact my own business and run my own household, although I cannot do the actual physical labour. I am writing a book about my rehabilitation experience, and a film, for which I am to be a consultant, is also being made. I am working with the New York State Committee on Rehabilitation Technology, and I am trying to get funding for a research study I designed. I am also sponsoring an independent research project under the auspices of the Centennial Scholar Program of Barnard College. An article that I wrote appeared in *Longevity* magazine. I run a private consultation business in rehabilitation psychology from my home for which I use a computer. I am on the supervisory staff of the Institute for Contemporary Psychotherapy, a psychoanalytic training institute, and I write magazine articles.

In June 1985, as I was on my way, with my companion, to our country house near Albany, I drove our car into a tree. My companion, who was in the passenger seat, sleeping, was killed on impact. I was found 6 hours later, lying in a ditch, alive but in a coma. I was in the coma for months; my son says 6, my Doctors say 13. One thing is certain: I was conscious long before I could let anybody know. I was aware of everything that was going on around me. I even have memories that are as clear as if it were yesterday, although it was more than 5 years ago. I was unable to let anyone know because the accident left me paralysed below the neck, unable to signal in any way, and all the technology showed damage so extensive that nobody with that much damage could possibly survive and be aware.

Eventually, the fact that I was out of the coma was discovered by an experienced doctor and gifted clinician, Dr D. Levy, then of New York Hospital, when the court required an evaluation before my feeding tube could be removed. I was saved from death, but then entered a nightmare that was to last 5 years.

Unbeknownst to me at that time, what distinguishes traumatic brain injury (hereafter called TBI) from other forms of brain damage is the impairment of cognition and emotional expression.[1]

The impaired cognition can be as localized as to affect only specific functions such as memory or analytic ability, or it can be so general that a person may not know whether or not she or he has ever seen someone before. The emotional impairment can take the form of a lethargy so deep that the person will not initiate anything or even stir themselves at all. Conversely, it may take the form of an impulsivity so extreme that the person can be barely controlled. In my case this meant that for 3 years, until I was living in my own apartment, I was surrounded by people the likes of whom I had only seen on television. Once a man came into my room and began shaking the bars of my hospital bed uttering loud, wordless moans all the while. I was petrified and thereafter closed my door. It meant that I was surrounded by constant screaming and by people who had repeated fits of temper.

If I thought that was bad, a nightmare that was worse was beginning, and it was to go on for years. The nightmare was that although I had injured my brainstem in the automobile accident and, technically, therefore, fell under the rubric of 'TBI patient', I did not conform to the other distinguishing textbook characteristics in any way, for although the damage was severe, it was all physical. In every other way, in my thoughts and my core identity, I was my old self. It was all inside and you couldn't see it. Now, because I was trapped in a badly injured body and because the medical books said it was not possible, I no longer existed. For 3 years, I was addressed by every new person as if I weren't in my right mind; I knew immediately by the voice that was used—kind of like the voice that someone who doesn't know any better uses with a 2-year-old. I soon came to call that 'the hospital voice'.

After people had got to know me for a week they knew my thinking was intact, but emotional damage was to be a lot harder to disprove, and for 5 years my very words were used against me. I have always been by nature blunt and confrontative. What before had been accepted as a personality trait and even admired by some was now used to prove I was emotionally injured, and whenever I protested that I was just being myself it was taken as further proof and called denial. I eventually began to feel like a rat trapped in a maze. The harder I tried to make people in the hospitals accept that I was my old self inside, the more I felt as if I were a rat running in circles chasing my own tail.

Even in physical tasks I do not follow the textbook. I can do more than other paralysed people. Doctors have called me 'the miracle worker'. It may sound as if I am blowing my own horn, but I cannot even recount how much I despaired whenever (and it happened all the time) I wanted to learn how to do something I knew I could do and can do today only to be refused and told it was impossible and I was 'denying'. It was no miracle, but a lot of hard work and pain.

After coming out of the coma (from which every doctor said I would never emerge) I was completely inert, with tubes to eat and eliminate. Now I am living without my family, directing my medical care, transacting my business and even earning money. After the accident, in the name of being therapeutic they wanted to change my personality—the very thing that has made my recovery possible.

Angry? Sure I was angry. An accident over which I had no control, which was completely random, had permanently and irrevocably altered the course of my entire life—whether for better or for worse only time will tell—but life is already more difficult and painful. And how much longer will it be? It has already been $7\frac{1}{2}$ years, and in some ways I have come far but in other ways not at all. I have to remember that the things other people take for granted, I cannot, and I have to measure my progress in teaspoons. Every time I get a spoon of food in my mouth or drink something without coughing, that is a victory, and I have to put everything else out of my mind in order to do the most simple things. There was a time when I had to deny how badly I was hurt. If I had not, I would have given up. I did not understand why in every hospital I was in I was always put in the room for the worst patients, and I couldn't understand why if I said I was the same inside everyone treated me differently. Thank goodness for that drop of denial when I needed it.

I can see myself very clearly now. In fact, that picture never leaves my mind. It is always a prod to keep myself working to be different. One thing I can take comfort in: nobody else will have to go through what I did. Thanks in part to my experience, David Levy and others discovered more about the kind of coma with which I was afflicted—'the locked-in syndrome'.

REFERENCE

1. Kay, T. and Lezak, M. (1987) The nature of head injury. In *Rehabilitation of traumatic brain injury* (2nd edn), (ed. Institute on Rehabilitation Issues). Research and Training Center, University of Wisconsin DK—Stout.

(Ostrum 1994)

COMMENTARY

Ostrum's head injury resulted in brainstem damage that led to total paralysis below the neck. It would appear that she has few cognitive problems. Her main comments relate to the major physical and associated psychological disabilities that have resulted from her injury.

In her 1993 article, Ostrum notes the dependence on others, and the fact that this leads to other people appearing much greater in stature—both physically and socially. A consequent reduction in self-esteem and internalization of feelings of anger can result in inappropriate compensation strategies that may in turn lead to feelings of depression or psychosomatic symptoms. Loss of control is also a major difficulty that has to be handled, and efforts to compensate for this may also lead to problems in relationships with others. The author ends with a plea for patients like her to be treated as human beings rather than textbook cases.

In her 1994 article, the nature of her 'locked-in' syndrome is more clearly outlined. Her account is a graphic illustration of the problems faced by a patient who has severe handicap and who also has severe communication difficulties. Her account itself suggests the presence of good reasoning, language and memory skills ('my mind isn't affected at all', p. 343), and also excellent ability to perform many self-care and work duties. If, as Ostrum indicates, the duration of coma was between 6 and 13 months, then it is all the more remarkable that cognitive functions have remained relatively preserved. Her 'blunt and confrontative' nature was immediately presumed to be a sequel of her head injury, since impulsivity and increased irritability is often associated with such a condition. However, her own observation—that she was always like this—suggests caution in immediately regarding such changes as pathological. It seems that improvement of function continued for a long period in Ostrum's case, seemingly up to a period of 7–8 years. This may be related to the severity of the injury and the major readjustments and learning in the use of aids that took place. Ostrum also points to denial as sometimes being a useful coping strategy—denying how badly she was hurt seemed to help give her the optimism and motivation to go on (cf. Caplan and Schechter 1987).

REFERENCE

Caplan, B. and Schechter, J. (1987). Denial and depression in disabling illness. In *Rehabilitation psychology desk reference* (ed. B. Caplan), pp. 133–70. Aspen, Rockville, MD.

Epilepsy 8

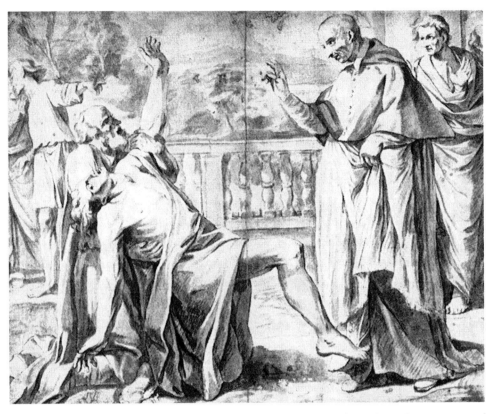

Figure 12. An epileptic man being restrained by another man, and being brought to a priest to be blessed.

INTRODUCTION

Epilepsy is estimated to affect one in every 200 people. Epilepsy is not a disease process, rather the clinical manifestation of an abnormal and excessive discharge of a group of neurones in the brain. The occurrence of epileptic fits or seizures may be one of the consequences of specific brain pathology, such as a stroke or brain tumour, or it may reflect some inherent imbalance within brain tissue, perhaps present from birth, that results in the abnormal electrical activity which contributes to the occurrence of seizures. Seizures are generally classed into 'partial' seizures and 'grand mal' seizures, and a diagnosis of epilepsy is generally based on the occurrence of a fit on at least two separate occasions.

Focal or 'partial' seizures result from the involvement of a focal area of brain tissue, usually an area of the cortex, and they may not necessarily be associated with any loss of consciousness. There is often a warning of an impending epileptic fit. Where partial seizures involve discrete sensory or motor symptoms, they are often referred to as '*simple* partial seizures'. Where there are also more significant changes in psychological functioning, with deficits such as amnesia, dysphasia, behavioural changes, or loss of consciousness, then the term '*complex* partial seizure' tends to be adopted. Complex partial seizures may often be followed by 'automatic' actions outside the person's control (e.g. chewing movements, and also a period of 'confusion' for which the person will later have no memory). While any area of the cortex may be susceptible to the development of epileptic activity, the temporal lobes—and in particular medial temporal lobe structures such as the hippocampus—are a particularly important locus for the occurrence of abnormal electrical activity that results in the occurrence of complex partial seizures.

Grand mal seizures, on the other hand, involve a more widespread disturbance of the brain, often as a result of an abnormality in deeper structures such as the thalamus or brainstem. Such seizures are usually associated with loss of consciousness and with the absence of any warning. A further category of seizure, also presumed to be subcortical in origin, is that known as 'petit mal' seizure or 'absence attack', where there is loss of responsiveness for a short time, due presumably to a short burst of abnormal electrical activity that results in a brief period of generalized cerebral dysfunction.

The pattern and severity of psychological impairments that are associated with epilepsy are due to a number of factors, including the type of epilepsy, the locus of any focal lesion, the number and severity of seizures, and the duration of the epilepsy. Other factors that need to be borne in mind include lack of oxygen to the brain during status epilepticus (a prolonged period of unconsciousness due to the continuous occurrence of multiple seizures), and the side-effects of anti-convulsant medication.

Of the cases that are reprinted, four are examples of epilepsy that appear to be related to the presence of temporal lobe pathology (**Hughlings-Jackson's** two cases; **Morris; Lisyak**). In the remaining four cases (**Darling; Anonymous 1952; Anonymous 1977; Kaufman**), there is less certainty as to the nature of the epilepsy that is present. The lesions in two cases (**Lisyak; Darling**) were in the right cerebral hemisphere. The symptoms in one of the cases (**Anonymous 1977**) points to a left hemisphere locus to the lesion, and in one of **Hughlings-Jackson's** cases

(**Hughlings-Jackson 1898**), there was definitive post-mortem evidence of a left medial temporal lobe lesion.

FURTHER READING

Bennett, T. L. (ed.) (1992). *The neuropsychology of epilepsy*. Plenum, New York.

On a particular variety of epilepsy ('intellectual aura'), one case with symptoms of organic brain disease

J. Hughlings-Jackson

Both of J. Hughlings-Jackson's cases included in this extract, Quaerens and Patient Z, were doctors, and one (Patient Z) appeared to be a general practitioner.

I have notes of about fifty cases of the variety of Epilepsy I am about to speak of. I have seen very many patients with symptoms of local gross organic brain disease (optic neuritis, &c.); in many of the latter, as subsequent necropsies showed, there was intracranial tumour. But one of the cases (Case 1, p. 191) I am about to relate and remark on (I have referred to it briefly, Bowman Lecture, 'On Ophthalmology and Diseases of the Nervous System', *Trans. Ophth. Soc.* vol. 6), is the only one I have seen in my own practice in which this variety of epilepsy was found associated with marked symptoms of local gross organic brain disease.[1] Although necropsy was forbidden, the case is of great clinical importance. The variety of epilepsy alluded to is one in which (1) the so-called 'intellectual aura' (I call it 'dreamy state') is a striking symptom. This is a very elaborate or 'voluminous' mental state. One kind of it is 'Reminiscence'; a feeling many people have had when apparently in good health (see p. 184, the case of Quaerens and that of Dr. Ferrier's patient, Case 3). Along with this voluminous mental state, there is frequently a 'crude sensation' ('warning') of (*a*) smell or (*b*) taste; (or, when there is no taste, there may be movements, chewing, tasting, spitting, *implying*(?) an epileptic discharge beginning in some part of the gustatory centres), or (*c*),

the 'epigastric' or some other 'systemic' sensation. The wording of this statement implies, at any rate it is meant to imply, that the 'dreamy state' sometimes occurs without any of the crude sensations mentioned, or movements supposed to imply discharges of gustatory elements, and that sometimes those crude sensations and movements occur without the 'dreamy state'; this will be exemplified in cases shortly to be given for incidental illustration.

I have been struck by certain non-associations. In my experience vertigo, in the sense of external objects seeming to move to one side, rarely occurs with the 'dreamy state'. In this paper I have to state exceptions (see Case 2) to this. The other variety of vertigo, that is, the feeling of the patient himself turning, does not so rarely occur with the 'dreamy state'. Again, I have no account of crude sensations of sight (colour projections) associated with the 'dreamy state', but I have notes of one case in which the patient, *at other times*, had migrainous paroxysms with visual projections. In cases of epilepsy beginning by colour projections, the much less elaborate mental state 'seeing faces', is not uncommon. I have thought that crude sensations of hearing are not associated with the 'dreamy state'. Until recently I have known of no exception, but I shall have to relate one in a case, the notes of which are supplied to me by Dr. James Anderson. Auditory sensation-warnings are not rarely followed by 'hearing voices' (really words as if spoken to the patient), a less elaborate state than the 'dreamy state'. I now return to the variety epilepsy with the 'dreamy state'.

There is not always *loss*, but there is, I

---

[1] Since this was written I have had a necropsy of a woman who had had paroxysms with the 'dreamy state', and crude sensation 'warnings' of smell. She had left hemiplegia and double optic neuritis. I can now only say that there was a tumour in the right temporo-sphenoidal lobe. My colleague, Dr. Beevor, who sent the patient to me, has kindly undertaken the examination of the specimen; on receiving his report I shall publish the case.

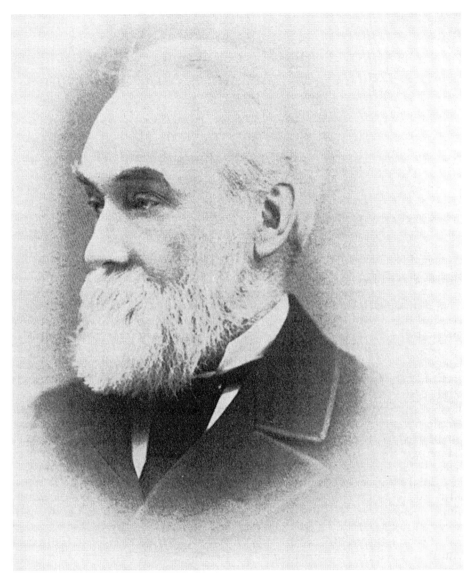

Figure 13. John Hughlings-Jackson, pioneering nineteenth century physician who worked at the National Hospital for Neurology and Neurosurgery, London.

believe, always, at least *defect*, of consciousness co-existing with the over-consciousness ('dreamy state'). *After* some paroxysms in which consciousness has been lost there are exceedingly complex and very purposive-seeming actions during continuing unconsciousness; in a few cases the actions appear to be in accord with the 'dreamy state'.

It will have been seen that I do not consider the 'dreamy state' to be a 'warning' ('aura'), that is to say not a phenomenon of the same order as the crude sensations of smell, &c. Hence my objection to the term 'intellectual aura', and adoption of the less question-begging adjective 'dreamy', one which is sometimes used by the patients. It is very important in this enquiry to distinguish mental states according to their degree of elaborateness—from crude, such as the crude sensation-warnings of smell, &c., to the vastly more elaborate, such as the 'dreamy state'—in order that we may infer the physical condition proper to each. The crude sensations are properly called warnings; they occur during *epileptic* (sudden, excessive and rapid) discharges; the elaborate state I call 'dreamy state' arises during but slightly raised activities (slightly increased discharges) of healthy nervous arrangements.

I have previously considered this variety of epilepsy, *Med. TImes and Gazette*, Dec. 2nd, 1876, and Feb. 1, and March 1, 1879; *Brain*, July, 1880. These papers have attracted very little attention; they have, however, been referred to by Dr. Mercier; by Dr. Beevor, in his important article On the Relation of the 'Aura' Giddiness to Epileptic Seizures, *Brain*, January, 1884, p. 488; and by Dr. James Anderson (*vide infra*, p. 182). The following quotation is from a lecture I published, *Med. Times and Gazette*, March 1, 1879, p. 224;— 'I think it will be found that in many, I dare not say in most, cases the voluminous mental ["dreamy"] state occurs in patients who have at the onset of their seizures some "digestive" sensation—smell, epigastric sensation, taste, or, in cases where there are movements implying excitations of centres for some such sensations, such movements as those of mastication'.

Under the name 'intellectual aura', the 'dreamy state' has long been known to occur in epileptics. The case of Quaerens (*vide infra*, p. 184) is, so far as I know the first definite case of epilepsy with that phenomenon published in this country. Dr. Joseph Coats, *Brit. Med. Journal*, Nov. 18, 1876, has recorded a very important case of an epileptic whose fits, with few exceptions, were preceded by giddiness and a 'peculiar thought'. 'Sometimes the fit only consists of the aura [the thought], followed by a peculiar feeling in the abdomen which passes up to the head and back to the abdomen, when vomiting results'.

Dr. James Anderson has recorded a case of this variety[1] of epilepsy in which, from symptoms, ocular and cerebral, detailed in his report, he correctly predicated tumour, and its position. This case has several important bearings, but for my present purpose it will suffice to say, that the patient's 'dreamy state' was associated with a rough 'bitter sensation' in his mouth. It is the only case published which I know of in which a necropsy has been had revealing any local morbid changes in a case of the variety of epilepsy mentioned. Dr. Anderson refers to a case, closely like that of his own patient, recorded by Mr. Nettleship, *Trans. Ophth. Soc.* vol. iv. (Necropsy by Dr. Sharkey). In the report of that case, however, the 'dreamy state' is not mentioned; there was a crude sensation warning in the patient's fits, 'a sudden feeling of suffocation in the nose and mouth'. I think it not impossible that the 'dreamy state' was present in the slight seizures (the patient did not always lose consciousness). I doubt not that I have in former years disregarded this important symptom. I have suggested (Bowman Lecture, *op. cit.*) that ophthalmic surgeons who see very many cases of optic neuritis (that is, cases in most of which there is local gross organic intracranial disease, such as tumour) should minutely investigate any paroxysms, however slight and transient, their patients may have, especially when there is any kind of defect of smell or taste. Just as the most exact knowledge we

---

[1] On Sensory Epilepsy. Case of Basal Cerebral Tumour, affecting the left Temporo-Sphenoidal Lobe, and giving rise to a Paroxysmal Taste-sensation and Dreamy State: *Brain*, Oct. 1886.

have of the seats of 'discharging lesions' in different epilepti*form* seizures is from cases of gross local organic brain disease, so no doubt our most exact knowledge of the seats of 'discharging lesions' in epilep*tic* seizures will be obtained from cases of such kind of disease. Some preliminary remarks on *slight* epileptic fits are necessary. I mean fits commonly called attacks of epilepsy proper.[2]

The slighter paroxysms are, the more deserving are they of minute and precise investigation, both for the patient's sake and for scientific purposes; for the patient's sake since, unless we give most careful attention to the details of them, we shall sometimes altogether overlook epilepsy; for scientific purposes, because the analysis of slight seizures is more easy and fruitful than that of severe ones. It often happens that a patient has sometimes slight seizures of the variety of epilepsy under remark, and at other times severe seizures; and not rarely he has no 'warning', in any sense of the term, of the latter. Obviously the clue to the seat of the 'discharging lesion' is only given definitely by the 'warning' (such as the crude sensations mentioned); so that of the patient's slight seizures we may learn much, of the severe ones without warning very little that is definite.

---

[2] Using the colourless word 'fits' generically, I make three classes of fits (see *Brain*, April, 1886): (1) Ponto-Bulbar; (2) Epileptiform; (3) Epileptic (Epilepsy proper of nosologists). As the name implies, (1) depends on discharges beginning in bulbar and pontal centres (laryngismus stridulus, certain uraemic fits(?) and asthma? and I imagine some fits *called* epileptic). I have published (*Brit. Med. Journ.*, Nov. 20, 1886) the case of a boy who had fits started by touching his head, a case analogous to fits artificially produced in guinea-pigs (Brown-Séquard), and due, I presume, to abnormal changes in the ponto-bulbar region. Class (2) is of fits depending on discharge beginning in some part of convolutions of the so-called 'motor region'. I imagine that (3) is owing to discharge beginning in some part of convolutions of the cerebrum other than those of the 'motor region'. Both (2) and (3) are to my mind 'cortical', although that term is commonly given to (2) only. I think it most likely that migrainous paroxysms are 'fits' which are the (chiefly) sensory analogues of (2) epileptiform seizures. I feel confident that (3), epilepsy proper, will have to be subdivided very considerably, and possibly some seizures we call epileptic will have to be classified apart. I hope the above classification will be useful provisionally.

I urge strongly that the great thing as to the diagnosis of epilepsy is not the 'quantity' of the symptoms, nor the severity of the fits, but paroxysmalness. Again, *loss* of consciousness is not essential for the diagnosis of epilepsy; there may be *defect* of consciousness only; and, as we have been saying, there may be 'over-consciousness' ('dreamy state') co-existing with the defect of consciousness; with defect of consciousness as to present surroundings there may be a rise of consciousness as to some other and often quasi-former surroundings ('dreamy state'); the latter may attract exclusive attention, the co-existing defect of consciousness being ignored. The most seemingly trifling symptoms, when occurring paroxysmally, deserve careful analysis in proportion to their paroxysmalness; suddenly 'coming over queer' for a moment or two, may be a slight epileptic attack and the forerunner of severe attacks. Of course it is a very old story that veritable epileptic fits may be very slight indeed, and, often enough, so slight and transitory that bystanders do not notice them; but there are particular reasons for insisting on this point with regard to cases of the variety of epilepsy the subject of this paper. I particularly wish to remark that, in many of them, the slight seizures are so very slight, that the patient unfortunately disregards or underrates them until a severe fit comes and declares their evil significance. As bearing closely on this neglect, I here say that such slight seizures are not always disagreeable, but sometimes positively agreeable. I have heard patients say that they used to 'encourage' the feeling, before they knew what it meant. The day I write this, a patient told me that he used to try to bring the feelings on when he first had the attacks; they are now disagreeable. The symptoms often seem to be so fanciful to the patients that they may reckon them for a time as mere oddities. Even when they have found out the bad meaning of their slight attacks, they are often seemingly unwilling to give any details of the 'dreamy state'. Dr. James Anderson's patient 'showed some reluctance to talk about the scene'. They and their friends do not seem to care for questions as to movements of chewing, smacking the lips, &c., thinking, probably, that such little things have no real bearing on a serious condition. I would go further and say, that some medical men seem to think questionings on the 'dreamy state', enquiries about spitting, champing movements, &c., are unpractical. I now stay to illustrate some of the preceding remarks.

One of my patients (*vide infra*, Case 5), a medical man, had seizures of this variety of epilepsy in so slight degree at first, that he took no more notice of them than to make them a subject of joking (to use the words from the report he made of his own case, he 'regarded the matter playfully, as of no practical importance'). He now has severe as well as slight fits. I refer also to the case of a medical man who reported it himself under the pseudonym Quaerens (*Practitioner*, May 1870, p. 284). The title is, A Prognostic and Therapeutical indication in Epilepsy. When he consulted me, Feb. 1880, he had had eighteen severe fits (loss of consciousness, convulsion, tongue biting), and had had 'many hundreds' of slight attacks. The *slight* attacks which he still had when I first saw him, were so slight that strangers noticed nothing wrong with him; he is never quite unconscious in them; the severest of these slight fits only 'bemaze' him for a minute or two; he can go on talking. Here are epileptic attacks with defect ('bemazement'), but not with loss of consciousness. A medical friend who sees much of Quaerens observes a little flushing of the patient's face, that he is 'as if considering something', but only to his intimate friends is it known that he has any kind of seizure. The only local symptom I heard of is a peculiar feeling in the right hand. In each slight fit he has that variety of the 'dreamy state' which I call Reminiscence; this peculiar feeling occasionally occurs in many people who are supposed to be healthy.

. . .

CASE V.—SLIGHT ATTACKS OF EPILEPSY WITH THE 'DREAMY STATE' FOR SOME YEARS BEFORE SEVERE ATTACKS—MOUTH MOVEMENTS—AUTOMATIC ACTIONS DURING UNCONSCIOUSNESS (WHICH CONTINUED AFTER THE SLIGHT FITS).

The following is a very important case. It is that of a highly educated medical man, who reports it himself. Names of places are omitted or altered from his original report, the alterations being endorsed by the patient; the alterations make no difference in the medical import of the case. He had first very slight attacks, then severe attacks at long intervals also. I shall comment on the slight attacks only.

What he calls 'recollection' is what I have called 'reminiscence'. I retain his term 'aura', putting it between commas, although I do not use it myself for any form of the 'dreamy state'. The report shows clearly that he has some attacks without *loss* of consciousness (see his remarks on reading poetry and on his glacier expedition). In other attacks he had loss of consciousness, and during unconsciousness continuing after them he acted automatically. The actions related in the closing paragraphs show very complex, special, &c., actions after a fit which was presumably slight. I may refer to remarks on this matter in my part of the discussion on Dr. Mercier's paper on 'Inhibition', which will appear in some future number of this Journal.

He had no crude sensation, but the words I have italicised in his account of his physical state, p. 204, during the slight paroxysms imply, I consider, discharge of cortical elements, serving during taste. (The report was finally sent in July 1888.)

I first noticed symptoms which I subsequently learnt to described as *petit mal* when living at one of our Universities, 1871. I was in very good general health, and know of no temporary disturbing causes. I was waiting at the foot of a College staircase, in the open air, for a friend who was coming down to join me. I was carelessly looking round me, watching people passing, &c., when my attention was suddenly absorbed in my own mental state, of which I know no more than it seemed to me to be a vivid and unexpected 'recollection';—of what, I do not know. My friend found me a minute or two later, leaning my back against the wall, looking rather pale, and feeling puzzled and stupid for the moment. In another minute or two I felt quite normal again, and was as much amused as my friend at finding that I could give no distinct account of what had happened, or what I had 'recollected'.

During the next two years a few similar but slighter attacks occurred, involving mental states which struck me as like to the first and to each other, but of which I can now recollect no details. I asked medical advice, but gathered no explanation, received no treatment, and regarded the matter playfully as of no practical importance. I have been in the habit of dreaming very little all my life, but during these years noticed a few occasions when I woke in the night with an impression that I had succeeded in recollecting something that I wanted to recollect, but was too sleepy to give any attention to it, and had no definite idea of it in the morning. These feelings were slightly uncomfortable, and usually, I think, accompanied by a slight involuntary escape of saliva found on the pillow in the morning, and once or twice by a soreness of the edge of the tongue, due, I should presume, to its having been slightly bitten. They did not recur after about 1875.

In 1874 I first had a *haut mal*, preceded by the mental condition I had felt in *petits maux*, and after medical advice from a physician in London learnt the nature of the disease, and began to attend a little more carefully to the symptoms, which interested me more, as I had then begun to turn my attention to medicine.

I had a severe attack of pneumonia with pleurisy, and perhaps empyema, beginning in October, 1875, and during slow convalescence (Dec. 1875–March 1876) was more frequently affected. The character of the *petits maux* gradually became more stereotyped, and during the period 1876–1886 varied only within comparatively narrow limits. I will attempt to describe the features which I think were common to all, or nearly all.

Mental Condition.—In a large majority of cases the central feature has been mental, and has been a feeling of Recollection, *i.e.* of realising that what is occupying the attention is what has occupied it before, and indeed has been familiar, but has been for a time forgotten, and now is recovered with a slight sense of satisfaction as if it had been sought for. My normal memory is bad, and a similar but much fainter feeling of sudden recollection of a forgotten fact is familiar. But in the abnormal states the recollection is much more instantaneous, much more absorbing, more vivid, and for the moment more satisfactory, as filling up a void which I imagine at the time I had previously in vain sought to fill. At the same time, or perhaps I should say more accurately in immediate sequence, I am dimly aware that the recollection is fictitious and my state abnormal. The recollection is always started by another person's voice, or by my own verbalised thought, or by what I am reading and mentally verbalise; and I think that during the abnormal state I generally verbalise some such phrase of simple recognition as, 'Oh yes—I see,' 'Of course—I remember,' &c., but a minute or two later I can recollect neither the words nor the verbalised thought which gave rise to the recognition. I only feel strongly that they resemble what I have felt before under similar abnormal conditions. I re-enter the current of normal life, as a rule, quickly—sometimes, as far as I can judge from my own movements or other people's evidence, within ten or fifteen seconds; there is never, however, as sudden a rush of returning normal consciousness as there has been on incipient abnormal consciousness; it is more gradual, and it is hard to say when it is complete, as it almost always leads up to a passive and non-critical mental attitude, in which I feel no originative mental impulse. One point which I almost always feel a tendency to avoid, though I am generally dimly aware of a previous wish to attempt it, is to go over my previous abnormal mental state critically and to give my attention to all its details. But attention seems not to be completely under my control; I sometimes put it off, and delude myself with the impression that remembrance will be just as complete after another five minutes, sometimes let it slip with a feeling of indifference, and sometimes, if I am in company or in any active employment, I have no distinct recollection of any desire for self-criticism or analysis. Accompanying this want of control over reflection I often notice a temporary loss of memory for habitually familiar names or faces, which lasts a minute or two, or sometimes more, after my consciousness seems otherwise normal. This may co-exist, indeed, with so normal a state of consciousness, that I can hardly believe I shall find any difficulty in saying what I want to say, and so I fall now and then into the mistake of beginning without hesitation a sentence which I cannot finish. I have found myself just after a *petit mal* at a London Railway Booking Office, meaning to go to K—, and asking without hesitation for 'Second return to—to—that school, don't you know—' (or some such words) and being a good deal startled at my forgetfulness.

A *petit mal* has two or three times come on when I have been reading poetry aloud—the line I am reading or just going to read seems somehow familiar, or just what I was trying to recollect, though I may never have seen or heard it before. I recognise my morbid condition and stop, though I have generally sense enough to finish the line or even sentence, and remain silent for a minute or so; then go on again where I left off, recovering my sense of rhythm and metre sooner than my capacity of giving attention to or understanding the words. I do not remember to have made any deliberate effort to go on reading aloud, *coûte que coûte*, throughout a *petit mal*. I have made several rude attempts to go on writing, and have kept four or five specimens of what I have written. They were made in very slight *petits maux*. The writing was done slowly and in a fairly normal hand. I was in the main occupied with the usual impression of recollection, but was dimly aware that I was morbid, and attempted to criticise what I was writing. My impression at the time that I was writing was that the words and sense were quite reasonable, and that I had kept within very familiar and prudent limits of expression. I had found, I thought, just the words I was seeking for. A minute or two later I could see that some of the words were grotesquely *mal à propos*, though I think the grammatical forms of sentence were always preserved. I could not trace any undercurrent of thought or recollection from which the irrelevant words had come.

Physical Conditions.—As to the physical conditions accompanying these mental states I can gather a little from my own consciousness, and have learnt a little more from friendly observers. At the onset I can rarely notice any physical change in myself, my attention being chiefly occupied with my mental condition; but once or twice when I have been standing near a mirror I have noticed pallor of the face, and I have learnt from others that this is common, and that my eyes have a somewhat staring vacant look as if they were not directed at anything near me, or indeed taking notice of anything particular. In this condition I am told, and in fact occasionally remember, that I often say 'yes', with an air of complete assent to any remark made to me, whether it is a pertinent answer or not; and further, that I occasionally make a slight half-vocalised sound, whether addressed or not. This latter, I have been told, *is somewhat like a modified and indistinct smacking of the tongue like a tasting movement, and is generally accompanied by a motion of the lower jaw*, and sometimes by some twitching of the muscles round one or both corners of the mouth or of the cheeks, but

by no sense of taste in my recollection. I have no clear evidence that one side of the face is affected more than the other, and no clear evidence against it; from what little I can learn, if it is at all unilateral it is rather more on the right side than the left; but the evidence is very scanty. I never notice it myself. I also never notice myself, but learn from others, that sometimes, especially if sitting, I give one or two light stamps on the floor with one foot; and in the only cases where this has been accurately observed it has been with the right foot.

With the returning normal consciousness I generally feel some superficial flush over the skin, especially over the face, and a slightly quickened and more thumping heart-beat which does not go beyond causing me very slight *malaise*. A very constant symptom is increased urinary secretion, which sometimes makes itself felt in as short a time as five or ten minutes, but usually after a longer interval. The water, if soon passed, is very light in colour, of low specific gravity, once or twice as low as 1005, and contains no albumen.

The *petits maux* have not been accompanied or followed by hallucinatory sensations of sight, sound, taste, smell or feeling. There has been, I think, no loss of balance. I well recollect in 1878 running across a Swiss glacier, and jumping across many small crevasses when the initial stage of 'aura' came on, and a reflection shot through my mind, that if ever I was likely to pay dearly for the imprudence of going on, it would be then. But I had insufficient control to stop myself and felt no fear, but only a slight interest in what would happen. I went through the familiar sensations of *petit mal* with such attention as I had to give concentrated on them, and not on the ice, and after a few minutes regained my normal condition without any injury. I looked back with surprise at the long slope of broken ice I had run over unhurt, picking my way, I know not how, over ground that would normally have been difficult to me. In the same way a *petit mal* when I was playing lawn tennis did not in the opinion of my adversary make my strokes or judgment of pace and position of balls to be struck any worse than normal. I had no recollection of the strokes during a minute or two.

I had no *haut mal* before 1874, and since then such attacks have recurred mostly at long intervals, sometimes of as much as eighteen months; during slow convalescence from pneumonia, however; in 1875–6 I had as many as seven or eight in two months. The 'aura' of recollection has preceded all of them, more or less, but is less vivid in my subsequent memory than after a *petit mal*. My evidence as to the subsequent phenomena of the *haut mal* is very incomplete. My loss of consciousness has not seemed longer to those who watched me more than five or ten minutes as a rule, but my loss of memory has been longer and my return to consciousness more gradual. I have not heard that there has been any epileptic cry; the muscular spasms have been variable but generally slight, and not specially localised (except that once I was told of a constant grasping motion of my right arm and hand). In one or two cases the spasms have not been noticed, and the state has been at first supposed to be one of syncope; but some snoring has almost always been noticed before recovery. My subsequent mental condition has been one of indifference and a sense of fatigue; my bodily sensation is, as a rule, of having been lightly bruised all over.

During the past year (1887), and more especially during the last four months, there has been some change in the symptoms of the *petits maux*, which may be shortly summed up by saying, that there has been less vivid sense of recollection and there have been longer periods of automatism without memory. I think I had best attempt to explain what I mean by two or three instances.

(1.) In October 1887 I was travelling along the Metropolitan Railway, meaning to get out at the fourth station and walk to a house half a mile off. I remember reaching the second station, and I then recollect indistinctly the onset of an 'aura', in which the conversation of two strangers in the same carriage seemed to be the repetition of something I had previously known—a recollection, in fact. The next thing of which I have any memory was that I was walking up the steps of the house (about half a mile from the fourth station), feeling in my pocket for a latch-key. I remembered almost at once that I had had a *petit mal* coming on at the second station, and was surprised to find myself where I was. I recollected that I had meant to reach the house not later than 12.45, and had been rather doubtful in the train whether I should be in time. I looked at my watch and found it within a minute or two of 12.45. I searched my pockets for the ticket, which was to the fourth station, found it gone, and concluded that I must have passed the third station, got out at the fourth, given up my ticket and walked on as I had previously intended, though I had no memory of anything since the second station came ten or twelve minutes previously. I imagine that I had carried out my intention automatically and without memory.

(2.) Again, in November 1887, after dark— about 6 P.M.—I was walking westwards in a London street, when I felt a *petit mal* coming on of which I can remember no particulars. My intention was to walk westwards for about half a mile; my thoughts were occupied with some books I had been reading in a house which I had just left. With my return of memory (which was incomplete and indistinct) I found myself in a street I did not at first recognise. I was somewhat puzzled, and looked up at the street corners for information as to the name of the street. I read the name 'P— St.' which crossed my path at right angles, and with some difficulty realised that I was walking not westwards, as I had been intending, but eastwards, along the street by which I had come, and had, in fact, retraced my steps some three hundred or four hundred yards. I felt no purpose in doing this, no aim at going anywhere in particular, and to save further difficulty, and because I was puzzled, I got into a hansom which was standing still close by me. I have no recollection of giving the driver any orders, and was in a very unreflective state. My impression is that the cab-driver drove quickly to the right house, and I distinctly remember some slight surprise I felt at his knowing the house, and at finding myself giving him a shilling, when I doubt if I could have explained where he came from. Immediately after entering the house I realised tolerably distinctly what had probably happened, and looking at my watch, I calculate that I had not lost more than five minutes by this, if so much.

(3.) About a fortnight later I was walking by the same route about 10.30 P.M., and again felt a *petit mal* at a point within a hundred yards or so of the one described above. I cannot be certain that a memory of the previous attack recurred to me, but I think it is very probable. My memory again was a blank until I found myself facing eastwards and looking up at the name 'P— St.' Then the memory of the previous retracing of my steps recurred to me at once. I more quickly than before gathered together full consciousness, felt a cab unnecessary, walked home, and had no difficulty in writing steadily for about three hours without fatigue.

In the earlier of this pair of cases (2 and 3) I had no thought whatever of going back to the house where I had been reading, or to any point in that direction; but I believe I am correct in saying that I was thinking of what I had just been reading there. As far as I know, this is the first instance of changing my intended action *ex proprio motu* in a mental state of which I have no memory. In the companion case (3) I cannot feel sure how much I was influenced by recollection in the earliest stages of the *petit mal*.

(4.) A fourth occasion is perhaps worth record. I was attending a young patient whom his mother had brought me with some history of lung symptoms. I wished to examine the chest, and asked him to undress on a couch. I thought he looked ill, but have no recollection of any intention to recommend him to take to his bed at once, or of any diagnosis. Whilst he was undressing I felt the onset of a *petit mal*. I remember taking out my stethoscope and turning away a little to avoid conversation. The next thing I recollect is that I was sitting at a writing-table in the same room, speaking to another person, and as my consciousness became more complete, recollected my patient, but saw he was not in the room. I was interested to ascertain what had happened, and had an oppor-

tunity an hour later of seeing him in bed, with the note of a diagnosis I had made of 'pneumonia of the left base'. I gathered indirectly from conversation that I had made a physical examination, written these words, and advised him to take to bed at once. I re-examined him with some curiosity, and found that my conscious diagnosis was the same as my unconscious,—or perhaps I should say, unremembered diagnosis had been. I was a good deal surprised, but not so unpleasantly as I should have thought probable.

(Hughlings-Jackson 1888)

A prognostic and therapeutic indication in epilepsy

Oft o'er my brain does that strange fancy roll,
  Which makes the present (while the flush doth last)
  Seem a mere semblance of some unknown past,
Mixed with such feelings as perplex the soul
Self-questioned in her sleep; and some have said
  We lived, ere yet this robe of flesh we wore. COLERIDGE

Moreover, something is or seems
That touches me with mystic gleams
Like glimpses of forgotten dreams—

Of something felt, like something here;
Of something done, I know not where;
Such as no language may declare. TENNYSON

We have all some experience of a feeling which comes over us occasionally, of what we are saying and doing having been said or done before, in a remote time—of our having been surrounded, dim ages ago, by the same faces, objects, and circumstances—of our knowing perfectly what will be said next, as if we suddenly remembered it! *David Copperfield*

Last year I had the misfortune to become, for the first time in my life, subject to occasional epilepsy. I well remember that the sensation above described, with which I had been familiar from boyhood, had, shortly before my first seizure at a time of over-work, become more intense and more frequent than usual. Since my first attack, I have had only few recurrences of the feeling in question. On two occasions, however, it was followed next day by an epileptic seizure, and I have since treated its occurrence as an indication for immediate rest and treatment.

There seems to me a twofold therapeutic interest in this experience. First that, whatever pretty suggestions Coleridge and Tennyson may make to account for it, and however universal its occurrence may be regarded by Dickens, it probably ought to be regarded as showing disturbance of brain-function; and that, perhaps, its recognition and removal might sometimes prevent the development of a more important disorder. Secondly, that inquiry in cases of epilepsy may detect a something of this sort, put aside as not being of sufficient consequence to speak of; and yet in truth being a minimised form of *petit mal*, warning to precautions against a larger seizure.

('Quaerens' 1870)

Case of epilepsy with tasting movements and 'dreamy state'—very small patch of softening in the left uncinate gyrus

J. Hughlings-Jackson and Walter S. Colman

PART I[1]

In this article are given further particulars of a case of epilepsy which I published[2] about ten years ago. I will call the patient Z. There was in this patient's slight attacks the 'dreamy state' (commonly called 'intellectual aura'). With at least some of his seizures there were certain movements of the mouth and tongue, tasting movements; these were, I suppose, the indirect 'reflex' results of an epileptic discharge beginning in gustatory elements of a certain region of the cerebral cortex—(Taste region of Ferrier.) After Z's slight attacks, or after some of them, there were very elaborate actions during 'unconsciousness'. The patient died, January, 1894, from an overdose of chloral. Dr. Walter Colman found at the necropsy a very small lesion of the left uncinate gyrus. A report of Dr. Colman's examination of the brain will be found in the second part of this article.

History of the case of Z

I first saw the patient, a medical man, whom I call Z, in December 1877. He was then 27 years of age. He began to have slight epileptic attacks in 1871; they were so slight at first that he, to use his own words, 'regarded the matter playfully and as of no practical importance'. In 1874 he had a *haut mal*, and then for the first time knew the evil meaning of the slight seizures he had disregarded. He afterwards wrote out for me an account of his

---

[1] This part is written by J. H. J.
[2] *Brain*, July, 1888. On a Particular Variety of Epilepsy (Intellectual Aura); one Case with Symptoms of Organic Brain Disease. Case V. of that paper, p. 200, *et sq.* is the case of Z.

case, which, with his consent, I published (*Brain*, Part XLII, July, 1888, p. 201 *et seq.*). I may remark at once that there were no such signs of local intra-cranial gross organic disease (such disease as tumour, I mean) as optic neuritis and severe headache in any part of the patient's illness. I now give some details I obtained from Z in 1877.

He had that variety of the dreamy state I call 'reminiscence'; he called it 'recollection'. In his slight attacks there was, he told me, a sentence in his mind which was as if well remembered. For example, if anyone was at the time speaking to him it would be as if he (Z) were trying to remember it, as if it were familiar, but yet he could not remember it. Again, he said—I give the words I hastily wrote in my case book, here intercalating other words in square brackets—'Attending to what was going on in [my] mind because [it was] interesting, and dim to what [was] going on outside'. He could not, on recovery, remember what the 'interesting matter' was. (*See Brain*, July, 1888, pp. 202–3, for further particulars of his dreamy state.) According to a report Z gave me in 1890, the reminiscence had disappeared, and from this report I gathered that he had had another kind of dreamy state with the reminiscence, and that this other kind occurred in his later fits. After the severe fit in 1874, in which he bit his tongue, he was subject both to slight and to severe attacks.

There was no evidence of any crude sensation warning of smell, taste, hearing or sight, nor did I ever afterwards hear of any; there was no epigastric sensation. There was no vertigo. Although there was no crude sensation warning of taste at any time, there were certain movements which, I think, imply an epileptic discharge of gustatory elements of the cortex cerebri. I did not, when I first saw the patient, obtain any information as to such movements. He wrote of them (*Brain, op cit.*, p. 204) as being, he had been told, '*somewhat like a modified and indistinct smacking of the tongue like a tasting movement, and is generally accompanied by a motion of the lower jaw* (italics in original), and sometimes by some twitching of the muscles round one or both corners of the mouth or of the cheeks, *but by no sense of taste in my recollection*'. (My italics.)

I ought here to say that several observers, one of them a highly accomplished medical man, who saw many of Z's attacks, never noticed any such movements as I have mentioned. They were very slight; in an attack (*vide infra*) which I witnessed, the noise made was only just audible. That they occurred in at least some of Z's slight attacks I do not doubt, because of the observation I made, and because he reported (*Brain, loc cit.*, p. 204) that some others had noticed them. It may be that the patient had, during the period this medical man knew him, ceased to have such movements. Z wrote to me, May, 1890, a report in which, among other things, he says, comparing with previous years: 'Although I have often asked observers to describe such a sound as I have made, and which in former notes [those published, *Brain*, July, 1888, p. 204] I described as a smacking of the tongue like a tasting movement, I have not found it so described, but rather as some indistinct attempt to speak'.

He had a slight feeling of dread. It was not a fear of the fit; the dread came first and then the fit, or rather the rest of the fit.

He said the fit seemed somewhat within his control; he made a rule when it set in to try to do something definite, for instance, to speak. He gave, as another example, that he once made an excuse to pick up a ball. In August, 1880, he was still subject to slight fits. When a clinical clerk, he would have them in the wards of the hospital, but they were so slight that no one noticed anything particularly wrong. One medical man observed something peculiar, and so did several friends. Z was told that he appeared anxious to answer, but seemed to have lost the drift of

the conversation—used in the connection some wrong word, and yet appeared to search about for another word. This is not very definite, but serves to show how slight the slight attacks were at the time.

In the remainder of this article, I shall speak only of Z's slight seizures. I witnessed but two of them, and these I saw years after his first visit to me. In one he stopped talking to me, remained standing, and made slight, very slight, just audible (*vide supra*) smacking movements of his lips. I have no further details of this seizure; it occurred at the meeting of a Medical Society, and I had no opportunity of watching him throughout the attack. I knew that he was quite safe; no one but myself noticed anything amiss with him. On another occasion he was sitting in a room consulting me; he stopped talking—I have no remembrance of any smacking movements of his mouth on this occasion—his head was bent forward, but in a second or two, the paroxysm being then, I suppose, over, he looked up, and next (post-paroxysmal stage of actions) he leaned over one arm of his chair and felt about on the floor as if searching for something; next he did the like on the other side. Shortly, having a pin in his hand (how he got it I know not, perhaps from the floor) he made a feint of pricking my hand; the action was as if in fun, for he stopped well short of my hand and was smiling. This little affair was exactly after the manner of joking with a child, as if one said playfully to a child, 'Now I'm going to prick you', and smilingly pretended an attempt to do so. Z, however, did not accompany his playful-seeming feint by words. Soon, perhaps a minute, afterwards, his actions, or I should say the irrelevant-seeming actions, ceased; he replied correctly to simple questions, and told me that it was not necessary for me to go home with him. He, however, looked confused and seemed strange. When we got to his house a few yards away, I thought he was fully recovered, and, as I was thinking of making another room on the ground floor of my house, I took the opportunity of speaking to him about a third room there was on the ground floor of his house. Among other things he said he used to breakfast there. I was surprised when he afterwards, next day, told me that he remembered nothing from the time of being in my room consulting me (before the fit) to a little time after I left him at his own house.

These post-paroxysmal actions during what we clinically call unconsciousness were as elaborate and purposive-seeming as any of those of his normal self; such post-paroxysmal actions are very important in a medico-legal point of view. On another occasion there were post-epileptic actions by Z during 'unconsciousness', of a kind which in a man fully himself would be criminal, and must have led to very serious consequences had not, fortunately, his condition been known. What he did was overlooked by those concerned.

In Z's report of his case (*Brain*, July, 1888, p. 206, paragraph 4), he speaks of examining and prescribing, when temporarily unconscious after an attack, for a patient. I now give a specimen of what he wrote—notes of a patient's case—in such circumstances. The words I have put in curved brackets were crossed out by Z; those in square brackets are my words. 'For six or seven (years) weeks he has felt very discomfort of the throat and also for the swelling of the throat and (legs) arms and —' [The word for which I have put a mark signifying a blank I cannot decipher]. Here is another specimen: 'For the last few days his beginning (starting to walk?) is more difficult for his tenderness of speechlessness and quick power of talk light swolleness of feet last three days'. The words 'starting to walk' in the square brackets were inserted later. Here is another specimen with Z's remarks on it: 'I had written the above [i.e., he filled up the form for name, age, &c., of the patient] correctly and ascertained that the man had had gradually increasing œdema of the legs lately, when a *petit mal* came on with no overpowering impression, or indeed any distinct impression that I can recollect. I wrote the words below [below the heading] slowly and with difficulty, wishing to be correct; on reading them over they seemed to me correct; but I could not go on; I turned over the page and tried to describe the man, stared at him and felt too undecided to write more

than "A rather";—could easily copy what I saw before me written down over the man's bed already as to the urine. Altogether it took two or three minutes. I remained undecided and disinclined to write, but able to talk for five minutes more'. This is what Z wrote on this occasion: 'For about the last fortnight about the legs are about the gradual for several debts of the' (Z adds, 'no connection in thought traceable for the word "debts"').

Still one more specimen of Z's writing. He wrote the following in a state, which at the time, he thought was full consciousness: 'There [then a word obliterated] was constant repetition of sickness for the last twenty-four hours. Abdomen [this word crossed out]. The sick [a word like "neck", joined to sick, crossed out] on the grateful rightnessness has felt a large knowfulness'. Z wrote down when well what he thought this should have been: 'The sickness has left a painful feeling on the right side; she has felt much fulness there'.

The following specimen of Z's writing (it was written as notes of a case) was not corrected: 'For the last 18 mos [mos, no doubt, is for months] years there has been some decided indefinite on R. side in dress circle'. Moreover in the heading of the case in the part for occupation he made a mistake—'Hairdressship' for, I presume, 'Hairdresser'. The patient was a woman, but this may have been for her husband's occupation.

For localisation of the lesion I relied entirely on Ferrier's researchers. I say this not only because credit should be given to the right man, but also because, having said what I have said, I can without immodesty put some facts more strongly than I otherwise should like to do. Let the following four statements be considered.

(1) Ferrier found that certain movements of the lips, tongue and cheek-pouches follow on artificial excitation of a certain region of a monkey's cortex. From the nature of these movements he inferred that that region contains gustatory nervous elements—that the movements were 'reflex' consequences of the artificial excitation of those elements. (2) I suppose that similar, or analogous, movements in human beings subject to certain

epileptic fits, as in the case of Z, at the onset of their seizure, are 'reflex' effects of epileptic discharges beginning in some gustatory elements of that cortical region which, according to Ferrier, is for taste. (3) I begged Dr. Colman to call on me before he went to make the necropsy on Z, in order to ask him to search the taste region of Ferrier on each half of the brain very carefully. (4) Dr. Colman (see Part II) found a very small focus of softening in that region (in the uncinate gyrus) of the left half of the brain.

There was no trustworthy evidence to point to the half of the brain affected. Z wrote (*Brain*, July, 1888, p. 204): 'I have no clear evidence that one side of the face is affected more than the other, and no clear evidence against it; from what little I can learn, if it is at all unilateral it is more on the right side than on the left; but the evidence is very scanty. I never notice it myself. I also never notice myself, but learn from others, that sometimes, especially if sitting, I give one or two light stamps on the floor with one foot, and in the only cases where this has been accurately observed it has been with the right foot'.

There are many points for comment in Z's case. I refer to Lectures on Epilepsy, *Medical Times ad Gazette*, vol. i., 1879; *Brain*, July, 1880; *Brain*, July, 1888, for remarks on the group of cases to which this case belongs. In those papers I consider the Dreamy State in its association with crude sensations of smell and taste, and with the epigastric sensation and with chewing and tasting movements. In *Brain*, October, 1889, Dr. Beevor and I record a case of epileptic attacks with a crude sensation of smell and a dreamy state; there was tumour of the right temporo-sphenoidal lobe. in that paper Dr. Beevor refers to cases previously recorded of epileptic attacks with warning of smell. In the *Lancet*, January 14, 1899, I published a note on what I call the Uncinate Group of epileptic fits. I there consider the asphyxia in slight fits of some cases of this group, and suggest, having regard to some researches of Mr. W. G. Spencer (*Transactions of Royal Society*, vol. clxxxv., 1894, B, pp. 609 to 657), that the asphyxia may be owing to inhibition of the respiratory

(medulla) centre by discharge spreading from a discharge lesion of the uncinate gyrus to the cortical centre for arrest of respiration; this arrest centre is close in front of the uncinate gyrus.

PART II[1]

Pathological report

The autopsy was made thirty hours after death. The weather was very warm and damp. *Post-mortem* lividity was extreme, and decomposition was rather advanced.

Examination of Head. The scalp was unusually thick, and firmly bound down to the periosteum. The *skull cap* was natural except for two symmetrical, flat, rounded elevations about half an inch in diameter situated on the outer table, on each side of the bregma. The *dura mater* was unusually adherent to both parietal bones, but not elsewhere. The surface of the pia-arachnoid was normal, except beneath the bony prominences at the bregma, where there was some adhesion. Pacchionian bodies were large and numerous in this region, but inconspicuous elsewhere. There was no adhesion between the pia mater and the surface of the convolutions at any part.

Both hemispheres were fully convoluted, especially in the frontal and occipital regions, the convolutions following the usual arrangement. Their surface was perfectly normal in appearance, and the consistence of the brain was natural except in the left uncinate gyrus, where it could be felt that there was a patch of softening beneath the surface. The position of the softened patch is shown in fig. 1, which is drawn from a tracing of the brain after hardening in spirit. On a section being made through the patch it was found to be a small cavity, collapsed and almost empty, with indefinite walls, situated in the uncinate gyrus, 5/8 inch below the surface just in front of the recurved tip of the uncus (*see* figs. 1 and 2). The existence of the patch and its position were verified in the fresh specimen by Dr. Hughlings Jackson, Dr.

[1] This part is written by W. S. C.

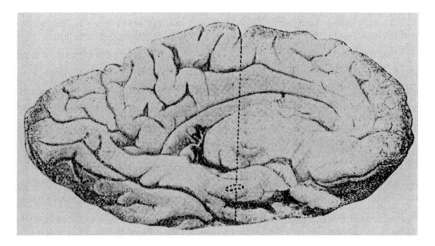

Figure 1. Drawing of internal surface of left hemisphere (case of Z). The black ring corresponds with the position of the cavity found, which is shown in section in Figure 2.

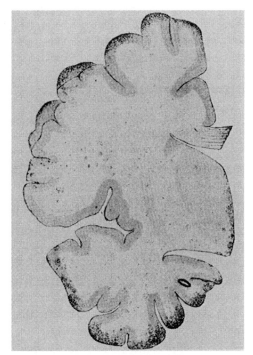

Figure 2. Vertical section of left hemisphere (case of Z, from a tracing). Site of small cavity apparently due to softening, shown by black ring.

Dawtry Drewitt, Dr. James Taylor, and Dr. Guy Wood. The cavity was like those seen long after softening from thrombosis or embolism; there was no surrounding inflammation nor any indication that it was of recent origin. Search was made for an occluded artery in the neighbourhood, but without success. The other vessels of the brain did not show any signs of atheroma to the naked eye.

Unfortunately the uncinate region became so soft and friable during the hardening process that it was impossible to make satisfactory sections, and the microscope did not throw any further light on the cause of the lesion.

The urine contained a small amount of albumen, and there were early interstitial changes in the cortex of the kidneys.

There were many pulmonary infarcts apparently produced during the prolonged coma which was present for twenty-four hours before death, and the lungs themselves were extremely oedematous.

With these exceptions the organs were healthy.

A localisation of the lesion in this situation had been suggested by the presence of the 'dreamy state' or 'intellectual aura'. In a paper read before the Medical Society of London in 1889 and afterwards published in Brain, Drs Hughlings Jackson and Beevor published the case of a woman, 53 years of age, who had a tumour, the size of an orange, at the anterior extremity of the temporal lobe. During life she had numerous fits, with an intellectual aura and with 'a horrid smell'. A very instructive case recorded by Sander[1] is quoted in the paper by these authors. The patient had fits which were preceded by the warning of a 'dreadful disagreeable smell', and he then had *'chewing movements of the jaws, and spitting of saliva'.* Later on he had convulsions about the face, but not in the limbs. He became very dull mentally, so that few subsequent observations on his sense of smell or of taste could be made. On *post-mortem* examination a gliomatous tumour the size of half a large apple was found on the under surface of the brain, at the junction of the left frontal and temporo-sphenoidal lobes. Half the growth involved the anterior part of the temporo-sphenoidal lobe, the other part reached across the fissure of Sylvius involving the lower convolutions of the frontal lobe. Inwards the growth reached the middle line.

(Hughlings-Jackson and Colman 1898)

---

[1] Sander, Epileptische Anfälle mit subjectiven Geruchs Empfindungen bei Zerstörung des linken Tractus olfactorius durch einen Tumor. *Archiv f. Psych.*, iv., 234.

COMMENTARY (Hughlings-Jackson, Quaerens, Hughlings-Jackson and Colman)

The two articles by Hughlings-Jackson mainly deal with Patient Z, but they also make reference to a patient who used the pseudonym of 'Quaerens', and who wrote a brief note relating to his epilepsy. The case of Patient Z is a fascinating account of the subtle cognitive manifestations of epileptiform activity. There are a number of issues raised by these three articles, and I will consider each of the issues in turn in the light of recent research findings. These issues relate to: (1) déjà vu episodes; (2) transient amnesic episodes; (3) clinical/diagnostic issues; and (4) awareness of memory loss.

1. Déjà vu episodes

Memory-related experiences in epilepsy, which may also be induced by electrical stimulation of areas in the temporal lobes, are now accepted as reflecting abnormal discharges from the hippocampus, amygdala, and related structures (Halgren *et al.* 1978; Fish *et al.* 1993), rather than the neocortex, as originally proposed by Penfield (Penfield and Perot 1963). A number of the 'dreamy states' or 'intellectual aura' described by the patient and discussed by Hughlings-Jackson were characterized by feelings of déjà vu—in this case, they were feelings of 'realising that what is occupying the attention is what has occupied it before, and indeed has been familiar, but has been for a time forgotten, and now is recovered with a slight sense of satisfaction as if it had been sought for' (p. 356). It is of note that Fish *et al.* (1993) found a greater right hemisphere focus for déjà vu episodes, whereas patient Z's lesion was in the left uncus. This may be explained by the fact that the actual subjective experience of déjà vu may take the form of familiarity misrecognition for the visual environment, or it may have a more general/verbal nature. In the case of the Fish *et al.* (1993) study, the emphasis was probably on the visual manifestations of déjà vu, whereas for patient Z the content of the déjà vu experience seemed to be related to thoughts and verbal statements (e.g. when he was reading poetry and found the lines to be familiar).

Patient Z's illusion of familiarity was often quite dramatic: '. . . the line I am reading or just going to read seems somehow familiar, or just what I was trying to recollect, though I may never have seen or heard it before' (p. 357). While such phenomena have frequently been described in cases of temporal lobe epilepsy, both in terms of spontaneous experiences and those induced by brain stimulation, there appears to have been little attempt to dissect the cognitive components of such experiences. An interesting, related observation that has recently been reported in the experimental psychology field is that of false memories—these are induced by asking subjects to recall word-lists where a target word (e.g. sleep) is missing, but their high-associated words (e.g. bed, rest, awake) are present (Roediger and McDermott 1995). In the laboratory setting, subjects will not only recall the target words (in this case 'sleep'), but in recognition memory tests they will make false-positive responses to these words, indicating that they were present in the original word-list. It would be interesting to see if patients with temporal lobe epilepsy, who may be susceptible to feelings of déjà vu, and also those amnesic patients who show an increased tendency to produce confabulatory responses, would demonstrate a greater degree of false-familiarity effects in paradigms such as those used by Roediger and McDermott.

2. Transient amnesic episodes

The term 'transient epileptic amnesia' (Kapur 1993) may usefully classify some of the attacks shown by patient Z, especially those that were observed by colleagues and where no other abnormality of behaviour was apparent apart from memory loss. It is important to distinguish such episodes from post-ictal confusional states, where behaviour may appear to be quite normal for a period of time and where there is no subsequent recollection for the behaviour in question—it is quite possible that the epileptic event of patient Z that was observed in detail by Hughlings-Jackson himself (pp. 362–3) did represent a case of post-ictal confusion or 'unconsciousness' after an attack, the term 'unconsciousness' being one adopted by Hughlings-Jackson. Hughlings-Jackson makes the interesting comment: 'On another occasion there were post-epileptic actions by Z during "unconsciousness", of a kind which in a man fully himself would be criminal, and must have led to very serious consequences had not, fortunately, his condition been known' (p. 363).

Cases of transient epileptic amnesia (TEA) may be manifest in a variety of forms, but typically the episodes are shorter and more frequent than transient global amnesia (TGA). The degree of anterograde memory impairment (inability to retain new information) is more variable than in TGA with some cases only manifesting some degree of retrograde amnesia. There is also a tendency for TEA attacks to occur more frequently in the morning. Although I found (Kapur 1993) that in three cases of TEA, out of a sample of four cases, there was a greater left temporal lobe focus to the EEG abnormality, bilateral medial temporal lobe abnormality has also been implicated in these types of amnesia (Palmini et al. 1992). Here again, it is of interest that the abnormal focus in patient Z was found in the left uncus. It needs to be borne in mind that more sophisticated neuropathological examination might have yielded evidence of right hippocampal/parahippocampal abnormality, and that in any case spread of seizure discharge to contralateral medial temporal lobe structures may have resulted in effective bilateral abnormality (Halgren et al. 1991).

TEA itself is best conceived of as a term to describe a type of attack that may occur in temporal lobe epilepsy, rather than a disease classification. It is therefore important to be sure that the amnesic episodes are not post-ictal confusional states related to simple or complex partial seizures, and that they do not reflect petit mal/'absence' attacks. The following format may be of practical help in the diagnosis of the condition. Where transient amnesic episodes may be classified as TEA, the clinician should ask the following questions:

1. Are there instances of memory loss for established knowledge (facts, personally experienced events, etc.) or for retaining new information? Patient Z refers to episodes where he noticed a 'temporary loss of memory for habitually familiar names or faces' (p. 356). In the case of past memory loss ('retrograde amnesia'), it is useful to note the temporal features of any such amnesia (how far did it go back?), together with information on how quickly this amnesia resolved or 'shrunk'.

2. Apart from the memory loss, was the behaviour of the patient abnormal during the episode? Important features include any disorganized behaviour, incoherent or repetitive speech, etc. Patient Z clearly had some abnormality in behaviour during certain episodes for which he had complete amnesia (e.g. there were errors in his written notes made during a consultation, for which he subsequently had amnesia, p. 363).

3. Are there witnessed descriptions of the amnesic attacks (to be certain that they were instances of pure memory loss with no other clinical or behavioural impairment)? Witnessed information is important in order to get an accurate description of the behaviour of the patient during the attack, and in particular to confirm the absence of motor or other physical manifestations of epilepsy. In the case of patient Z, some attacks were witnessed, although the only witnessed account that was published relates to Hughlings-Jackson's own observations. Hughlings-Jackson (1898) notes that a number of patient Z's attacks were observed, some of them 'by a highly accomplished medical man', and that this particular observer did not find evidence of the minor changes (grunt sounds, lip-smacking movements) that seemed to accompany some attacks.

4. Does the patient have subsequent amnesia for the episode in question? It is important to realize that in some cases of epilepsy-related transient amnesic attacks, the behaviour of the patient may have been quite normal during the episode in question, without any abnormal behaviour or impairment in recalling old memories/retaining new memories, but that at a subsequent time the patient will show amnesia for the period in question (Palmini et al. 1992; Kapur 1993). In some cases, the patient will suddenly find himself/herself in a different location, and realize that there is a gap in their past that they cannot account for. However, in other cases there may be no spontaneous awareness of an episode of amnesia. Such episodes of 'subclinical amnesia' may never come to the notice of the patient or anyone else, unless a subsequent discussion or event somehow relies on memory of this 'missing period'. By their very nature, these particular episodes are notoriously difficult to document.

5. Is there evidence of an epileptogenic lesion—classical epileptic seizures, spike waves on EEG recording, brain imaging evidence of temporal lobe pathology, or reduction of frequency/severity of attacks after the introduction of anti-convulsant medication? Some forms of transient epileptic amnesia could be seen to be a type of 'Todd's paralysis' (Morrell 1980). (In Todd's paralysis, a minor seizure involving the motor cortex results in transient motor weakness.) One might argue that, where the clinical manifestations of a complex partial seizure are very subtle, it may never be possible, without depth electrode recordings from limbic structures and video monitoring, to be certain that a case of TEA was not one of post-ictal amnesia.

Where there is no witnessed information, or where there is no firm evidence of an epileptogenic lesion, but where the attacks are strongly suspected of being instances of TEA, then I would recommend a diagnosis of *presumed TEA* be made. Where there is a wide range of supportive evidence, then I would suggest that a diagnosis of *established TEA* be made.

3. Clinical/diagnostic issues

The feeling of dread noted by patient Z (p. 362) is a common accompaniment of temporal lobe epilepsy, and probably relates to the involvement of the amygdala (Fish *et al.* 1993). Patient Z uses the term 'petit mal' to describe some of his attacks, but they would probably be classed as 'partial seizures' in current terminology.

From the clinical point of view, some of the attacks that patient Z suffered vividly bring home the diagnostic dilemma when a clinician is faced with minor behavioural changes, but where there is no physical or laboratory evidence of structural brain abnormality. When he first experienced his attacks, patient Z 'regarded the matter playfully and as of no practical importance' (p. 356). It was three years before he had a grand mal seizure (what Hughlings-Jackson calls a 'haut mal'). Just as Alzheimer's disease is often a purely neuropsychological diagnosis, with no reliable biological market currently available to help in the clinical decision process, in a similar fashion some forms of epilepsy can only be diagnosed on the basis of careful neuropsychological interviews of the patient and a close observer, followed up by detailed neurospychological testing. This needs to include, if possible, assessment of very long-term retention and performance on tests of retrograde memory (cf Kapur *et al.* 1996).

4. Awareness of memory loss

From the theoretical point of view, transient amnesic episodes such as those experienced by patient Z provide a dramatic illustration of the disconnection that may occur at different levels of the memory awareness system. Purposeful, coherent activity may appear to take place—with no awareness of any abnormality on the part of the patient or a close observer—but significant errors may be present in parts of the performance of the individual (e.g. Z during his consultation with a patient, when his subsequent notes were found to contain semantic/grammatical errors). At a further level, normal activity may appear to take place, this time without evidence of any performance errors, but the individual may have no sub-sequent recollection of the period in question. In a sense, this is little different from what may pertain for a number of sample behaviours of a patient with a classical amnesic syndrome—it may be possible to have a normal conversation with the individual or for that person to perform a number of everyday tasks without error, but there will be no subsequent recall of events that took place during that period of time. In one form of these attacks of 'subclinical amnesia', the dissociation between awareness and amnesia is complete and absolute, with the individual having no conscious awareness that memory processes have returned to normal or even that anything abnormal ever took place. In another form of the attacks, there may be a sudden realization of a memory gap—this may be precipitated by, for example, the individual finding himself/herself in a different location to one where he/she was at the beginning of the period of subclinical amnesia. In this case, there is awareness that the 'stream of consciousness' has been broken. At each of these levels of awareness and disconnection, it would seem that normal neural feedback/loop mechanisms are at fault—this may be due to disturbance of an overall executive/control mechanism, perhaps located in the frontal lobes, or it may represent the involvement of one or more connections between discrete processing centres which give the individual continuous feedback with regard to the integrity of cognitive functioning. If one postulates that there are at least two universal, continuous 'streams of consciousness', one for awareness of time and the other for awareness of place, then the evidence from phenomena such as those shown by patient Z would seem to suggest these levels of consciousness can be disconnected from the mecha-nisms governing the consolidation of more discrete events into long-term retention (see also case 2 of Palmini *et al.* 1992). This level of disconnection is seldom seen in the classical amnesic syndrome, and TEA episodes may be one of the few handles with which to examine such dissociations.

REFERENCES

Fish, D. R., Gloor, P., Quesney, F. L., and Olivier, A. (1993). Clinical responses to electrical brain stimulation of the temporal and frontal lobes in patients with epilepsy. *Brain*, 116, 397–414.

Halgren, E., Walter, R. D., Cherlow, D. G., and Crandall, P. H. (1978). Mental phenomena evoked by electrical stimulation of the human hippocampal formation and amygdala. *Brain*, 101, 83–117.

Halgren, E., Stapelton, J., Domalski, P., Swartz, B. E., Delgado-Escueta, A. V., Walsh, G. O. *et al.* (1991). Memory dysfunction in epilepsy patients as a derangement of normal physiol-ogy. In *Advances in neurology*, Vol. 55. (ed. D. Smith, D. Treiman, and M. Trimble), pp. 385–410. Raven, New York.

Kapur, N. (1993). Transient epileptic amnesia: An update and a reformulation. *Journal of Neurology, Neurosurgery and Psychiatry*, 56, 1184–90.

Kapur, N., Millar, J., Colbourn ,C., Abbott, P., Kennedy, P., and Docherty, T. (1996). Very long-term amnesia in association with temporal lobe epilepsy: Evidence for multiple-stage consolidation processes. *Brain and Cognition*, in press.

Morrell, F. (1980). Memory loss as Todd's paralysis. *Epilepsia*, 21, 185.

Palmini, A. L., Gloor, P., and Jones-Gotman, M. (1992). Pure amnestic seizures in temporal lobe epilepsy. *Brain*, 115, 749–69.

Penfield, W. and Perot, P. (1963). The brain's record of auditory and visual experience: a final summary and discussion. *Brain*, **86**, 595–6.

Roediger, H. L. and McDermott, K. B. (1995). Creating false memories: Remembering words not presented in lists. *Journal of Experimental Psychology: Learning, Memory and Cognition*, **21**, 803–14.

The story of my epilepsy: the fortunate fate of a stubborn fool

John P. Darling

John Darling initially trained in surgery, but then moved into pathology after the onset of his epilepsy.

This autobiography does not attempt to prove anything. It tells only how one patient discovered and controlled, during more than nine years, numerous ostensible causes of his convulsions and consequent difficulties. Growing health and very modest professional success have resulted.

Jenner applied in his vaccination against smallpox an age-old principle. The human body, when subjected to harm it can withstand, develops ability to tolerate even greater amounts of similar harm. That principle should be applied to epileptics. This is the story of a post-traumatic epileptic who fought for that principle, and succeeded.

Once upon a time, long, long ago (1941), in a land (Des Moines, Iowa) beyond a wild sea (epilepsy), opportunity smiled. Marital happiness, professional success, friends, seemed there for the taking. I decided to work until I dropped. I did. But the floor did not break my fall. When, figuratively speaking, I picked myself up, my friends told me to change my specialty, to quit medicine, to retire to a farm, to avoid heavy physical work, and to take dilantin to obliterate chemically convulsions which were due to a brain tumor (oligodendroglioma or meningioma) beneath the center of the right side of my brain. They told my wife to watch me for signs of growing blindness. They tested my intelligence because pressure from growth of the tumor might already have impaired my ability to think. Six years later they told one of the staff of a hospital where I sought employment, that they were not sure I was strong enough to do the pathology work which comes to such a hospital. My specialty has been pathology since the onset of my convulsions.

Nine years (1941–1950) were filled by a fight. The fight was all-encompassing for me, and, insofar as my success may have made it possible to help others, the original misfortune may have been worth while. Life in 1951 seems very good to me, in spite of occasional convulsions, which are still decreasing in frequency, and allow me most privileges, except, for instance, driving an automobile.

Individuals or groups many times kept opportunity open—and so hope alive—for me. What that meant each time, can be fully appreciated only by others who have felt they were being excluded from the practice of their profession—probably permanently. The gratitude the patient feels when helped is a tribute very much greater apparently than the helper realizes.

Dr. D. J. Glomset, Sr. referred me to Dr. Peter Bassoe, who had been my neurology teacher in Chicago. Fortunately, he was willing to meet the challenge when I begged for 'clinical judgment' rather than more tests. He wrote Dr. Glomset that I was more likely suffering from regeneration and calcification of the brain than from brain tumor. Dr. Glomset gave me the letter.

That letter was probably one of the biggest helps I have ever received. At least now I knew there was disagreement among those who condemned me to a bad future. Now I could publicly demand with some semblance of authority a chance to prove a third, my own diagnosis, which was full of hope. I thought the convulsions were due to my recent, nearly fatal, basilar skull fracture and the subsequent strain. I came to the end of the customary period for training in surgery. From those in charge, I asked that the last three months of my training be postponed one year so that, if free of convulsions for a year, I could for three months test my ability to withstand the strain of surgery. The chief threatened that if I kept on trying to get back into surgery, my teachers would not recommend me to future potential employers or appointments. Fortunately the power of the American public's sense of fair play apparently was on my side. Previous legal consultations had made my intentions obvious. I threatened in my turn to make the biggest possible public stink unless I was given a chance to recover. My request was granted.

A pathologist is a medical specialist who works closely with surgeons as well as other doctors. Training in pathology was suggested as the best supplement for that which I had had in surgery. I found it thrilling—and a pathologist subject to convulsions might be acceptable. The year passed. My three teachers in pathology sent me back with the recommendation that I be given surgical training again. The supervisor of the men taking training told me that I had had a convulsion in his office. I was brokenhearted. Time passed, however, and America went to war (1941). The shortage of doctors due to the war—or some other fate—left me still working in pathology. As if some benevolent deity had so willed it, an article in *Science News Letter* pointed out that friends should avoid talking to neuropsychiatric war casualties about their war experiences. Such conversation too often precipitated a recurrence of symptoms. I felt understanding and hope again. Now I knew why I had had that strange, fatalistic attack in the office of the chief who had been urged to return me to surgical training. Also clinical texts mentioned 'conditioned epilepsy', convulsions occurring immediately after some superficially harmless but really meaningful stimulus, like the blowing of a particular whistle. Obviously it was necessary to anticipate and avoid such stimuli, or to get set for them in advance.

As time passed, it was first apparent that many of my attacks came from the same causes. Then it gradually became possible to tolerate most of those causes. One particular cause was a stimulation demanding rapid

recall of material only partially recallable. Examinations, or the sudden meeting of an old, partially-forgotten friend are examples. Excessive confidence is my greatest danger. I fail to protect myself enough.[1]

The next lease on life was given me by my teachers in pathology, Drs. MacDonald, Parkhill, and Broders. Dr. MacDonald told me that I had been appointed a 'first assistant'. That meant everything, I thought. Immediately I had a convulsion. The sudden release of happy emotion caught me off guard. There were several convulsions during the first few weeks of this first assistantship. My teachers were so wise and kindly that they rightly ascribed them to my new responsibility, and waited for me to become accustomed to the new job. The future now really seemed encouraging, regardless of the floods of ominous predictions. At least I was getting unusually good training in a useful specialty at which many men are happy to spend their entire lives.

Incapacitating troubles still lay ahead. When my first assistantship came to the customary end, the war was over. Officials, entrusted with appointments for physicians in training, refused to allow me the training in clinical pathology which is vital to a pathologist seeking appointment in a hospital not large enough to support two pathologists. In a way I had come to the end of the road again, although now qualified in one field. One morning I was at work two doors away from the surgical operating room; a pain hit my abdomen as though a mule had kicked me. The surgeon opened my abdomen from top to bottom, cleaned up the inside, and sewed shut the hole in my stomach from a perforated ulcer that worry had caused.

Permission was granted that I obtain the

[1] It is only reasonable that the reader should know all the many ways in which medicine and surgery can benefit epileptics. The possibilities are so great that it may not seem practical to consider them in a personal account such as this. I still take dilantin three times a day. I used to take it four times a day, and the benefit it gives to many patients is great. It never gave me complete relief of symptoms, and it was toxic for me. Tridione did me harm. Nevertheless this paper is intended only to supplement other forms of treatment, not to detract from any.

vital training in clinical pathology. Apparently the devastating effect of refusing permission caused some change in the minds of those in authority. Not much later I received from the American Board of Pathology a certificate stating that I was eligible for examination both in pathological anatomy and clinical pathology. That meant I could prove my training was equal to that required by the highest authority.

There was still trouble ahead. The American Board of Pathology examinations were too much of a strain for me. They required uninterrupted hours of maximum effort. I flunked repeatedly.

At my suggestion, Dr. E. J. Boyd of the State University of Iowa, and Dr. F. C. Coleman at Mercy Hospital in Des Moines made a special arrangement for me, two new practice examinations for each month of the year. The monthly trial examinations did more than give me confidence and training for the Board examinations. At first, a convulsion followed the examination each month. Gradually the convulsions disappeared. I became desensitized to that strain. Finally I was able to pass the American Board of Pathology examinations in anatomy and, warned by past experience, avoided having a convulsion when the good news came.

The Park Hospital Clinic in Mason City, Iowa, wanted me as their pathologist on the same basis as other new members of the staff. Heaven seemed at hand. I could do the work. The staff doctors were thoughtful and understanding, not only in tolerating my convulsions, but also in positive diagnostic and therapeutic suggestions. After two years (1949) they voted me the right to buy a partnership like the others of the staff.

In 1950 in Mason City, Mercy Hospital needed a pathologist. Mercy and Park Hospitals co-operated so that it was possible for me to be responsible for the pathology at both hospitals. Many others helped out so that I could do in less time by proxy much that I had done previously on my own. It was a thrill to know and learn with the physicians at both hospitals. The additional responsibility for six months pleased me especially, because in 1947 those who were supposed to

know had said that they were not sure that I was strong enough to do the pathology at one hospital. What a contrast with the days when I used to look at various things in the library to make sure there were still no signs of oncoming blindness!

The following findings turned up during the years in which the above described progress was made. They were essential to understanding and controlling my convulsions. Each as it appeared seemed a triumph. They were each like a new part of an antagonist wrestler, to be grabbed as hard, fast, and skillfully as possible, always with the hope of immediate victory. The antagonist wrestler was my epileptic self. Each time he found a way to break the grip my nonepileptic self had on him. Only now the attacks come infrequently, and on occasions not too embarrassing. They seem like typographical errors. Complete freedom from convulsions seems to depend on training myself to apply better what I know, rather than on discovering important new things.

My convulsions began when I was subject to very great strain. It seemed only reasonable to try to identify, evaluate, and eliminate or control the essentials of strain. That would first give me relief, and then train me to endure easily, enthusiastically.

The essential strains were of two kinds: those which affected the brain (central nervous system) directly, and those which affected its circulation directly and indirectly. This discussion makes no effort to emphasize either as more important or fundamental, and separates the two and their components to facilitate understanding. The two are as important to each other as are a horse and its rider. The circulation provides the brain with energy (food) for thinking, and the brain unconsciously and consciously controls circulation.

The essentials of strain were six: three follow the patient like his shadow; two are usually at home; and one is on the calendar. The first three, the ubiquitous triad, were 'posture', 'temperature', and 'effort' (the job in hand). The two usually at home were food and sexual stimulation. The sixth was the next date marked on the calendar.

Long ago attacks obviously occurred often early in the morning, between awakening and finally getting to work at my office after breakfasting and doing the other things people routinely do when arising in the morning. At first a cause of convulsions as simple as *assuming the erect posture* apparently did not occur to anybody. Later at a Mayo Clinic conference, post-mortem examinations were reported on six epileptics. They all had waterlogged (edematous) brains. Many of the causes of edema can be controlled. It was only sensible for me to eliminate that as a possible factor in my case. Studying circulation as a cause of brain edema, disclosed how assuming the erect posture could cause convulsions and showed many other circulatory factors. One of these was decreased blood pressure in the vessels of the brain. When one gets up after a night's sleep, the blood tends to run out of the brain into the feet, until one's blood vessels in the lower part of the body narrow their openings. In that way they milk blood up to the heart and brain. I now wait first for the veins to narrow their openings, as shown by their shrinking, and then sit up till thoroughly awake before rising to my feet. This seems to have *eliminated my early morning attacks*. The veins dilate and shrink alternately as I oscillate between supine and sitting postures.

The effect of *temperature and weather* on circulation has been studied by many. Cold winter nights gave me a convulsion when I rose the next morning. Now I sleep safely in a warm bed with an electric hot pad. Walking into cold basements has given me convulsions. Dr. Horton and his associates demonstrated my *allergy for cold*, which gives me hives, and knocks down my blood pressure. The fall in blood pressure in the brain in my case causes convulsions much as did rising in the morning, for mechanical reasons.

Heat may cause convulsions, but has been more useful than harmful. For the most part, it increases circulation, and protects against the effect of cold. A hot bath when I rise in the morning seems to awaken my circulation to care for my brain. Warmth and sitting down seem an effective treatment when, during the strain of the day, my hands get cold and so

give me warning of threatened general circulatory exhaustion and falling blood pressure.

Heat can cause convulsions in two ways: Extremely prolonged, high, humid heat of summer may exhaust in part the circulation, which is a cooling mechanism as well as other things. Sudden, excessive heat on the head, particularly in combination with other predisposing factors, may cause convulsions by increasing excessively the blood flow to the head. I avoid a hot shampoo at bedtime or before breakfast. A bath which is too sudden, too hot, or too deep is dangerous.

Strain due to effort (nervous or muscular) is of three kinds: direct; confusing; or sentimental. It causes convulsions by increasing the brain's need for blood above the amount the circulation can provide. The reverse may be true at the sudden termination of excessive strain. Expert athletes, although not subject to convulsions, terminate their strain slowly.

Type 1: Sudden, severe, prolonged, uninterrupted effort and particularly an abrupt cessation of severe effort, are the most dangerous direct strain.

Type 2: Unexpected demands, and problems, requiring complete memory of only partially recallable material, illustrate the second type of strain causing convulsions. Doctors with proper equipment can record from the scalp under such circumstances kappa waves, which are specific electrical responses of the brain to such conditions.

Type 3: Events reminding the patient of past events which caused great emotion or strain may also cause convulsions.

Examinations have exemplified Type 1 for me; suddenly meeting partially forgotten but important friends, Type 2, and the convulsion which kept me from returning to surgery exemplifies Type 3. It was precipitated by conversation which reminded me of the emotions I felt when they first told me that a brain tumor was the cause of my symptoms.

Sexual stimulation may be very important, even a fundamental cause of convulsions. It may be both a circulatory and a nervous strain, particularly if natural impulses are interfered with unwisely, no matter how ideal the motive. It has been commented that this or that elderly person who married a mate much younger, might die of a 'stroke' (sudden disruption of the circulation of the brain) because of the unusually great sexual strain occasioned by the marriage. Le Mon Clark in his book, *Emotional Adjustment in Marriage*, points out that prolonged frustration in sexual intercourse often causes neuroses (sickness due to abnormal thoughts and emotions). Gradually my postcoital attacks disappeared. Circulation in the sexual organs seems much more closely associated with the circulation and function of the brain and other organs than suspected. Distention of the veins in one organ seems to spread to other organs.

Food caused many of my most embarrassing convulsions. Often many people were at the table at the time. By relaxing thoroughly for perhaps fifteen minutes before meals, and by eating slowly, not too much, especially not bulky hot food, I now avoid the effect of food most of the time. A small drink of cold water seems to counteract, somewhat, bulky hot food. *Constipation* used to increase, without bringing itself to my attention until a convulsion occurred. That cause of my seizures has been eliminated by regular defecation. *Water* as well as food can be an important cause of convulsions. Some patients are completely relieved of attacks by limiting sufficiently their fluid intake.

The calendar and clock help me fight convulsions. A diary has taught me to expect some regular increases in my tendency toward convulsions. So I know best when to take extra care. A diary proves I am getting better, and how fast. It also sets for me a definite objective, a certain frequency of convulsions which I must decrease like others in the past. Diaries and clocks also suggest possible causes of convulsions, because at least the patient can study what he was doing at the time of and before the convulsion. Finally, and this is vital, a diary warns me of my insidious but human tendency to neglect prevention the longer I had gone without attacks. I must learn to live with a partially petrified brain without convulsions just as one learns to walk with a wooden leg without falling. The tricks to learn are new, but

not more numerous for getting along with a partially calcified brain.

These six causes of convulsions have each been identified here as yet only by a conspicuous characteristic of each. All had many aspects and applications. Unsuspected combinations of these six causes still catch me off guard. As time passes, however, more and more of conscious self-protection becomes automatic, unconscious, reflex. It is like the co-ordinated motion of many muscles involved in walking when consciousness is almost wholly absorbed in interesting conversation with a friend. As convulsions decrease in frequency, the *signs* of a possible convulsion become more important. Then the patient controls the causes of convulsions to increase personal efficacy rather than to prevent convulsions; but knowledge of the danger signs also makes prevention of convulsion much easier.

Danger signs in me are these four: tension, apathy, error and deceleration. Tension is apparent inside, outside, and in my face. Internal tension includes five abnormal conditions: obstruction of my nose on the right side; a throat full of 'frogs'; a tongue pressed out against closed teeth (tooth imprints are often seen on it in the mirror); breath (yawning, sighing and halitosis); bowel (constipation, hemorrhoids, and prolapsed hemorrhoids).

The clot of blood in the veins at the base of the right side of the brain interferes with the exit of blood from that side of my head. So the right side of my *nose* swells shut much more than the left side, and serves as a measure of dangerous congestion in the brain. Intense, thought-provoking reading will fairly rapidly close the right side of my nose, and redden the right side of my right eye. The cure is easy: rest and walking. I can rest by doing other work. Resting suddenly, completely, especially standing, is somewhat dangerous. Like good automobile drivers, I decelerate and accelerate slowly whenever I can.

In my *throat*, 'frogs' or dryness like that of a man about to make a speech, suggest that I must reduce a little whatever strains are wearing at me, or take them more philosophically. Unconsciously people, particularly Americans, seem inclined to become stiff because of their great effort to do well. A free-and-easy swing helps a golfer, and similar grace and apparent ease help us all in many activities, including the prevention of convulsions.

If my *tongue* is tight against closed teeth, I need the same treatment. Especially helpful is work or play with objective, absorbing, pleasant, routine, mechanical jobs. They are as different as possible from the situations or ideas which cause such a tongue. Frustrating, confusing, verbal problems, especially old ones, seem to make one's tongue strain against set teeth, as though unconsciously trying to talk. The patient can see in a mirror that his tongue is a perfect cast of the inside of his teeth, and so has their imprint on its edge.

Halitosis suggests constipation (discussed previously).

Abnormal yawning suggests abnormal circulation in one part of the brain, the part which makes us yawn. This abnormality is very often true of the circulation in the rest of the brain, where it may cause a convulsion, unless corrected. I yawn after swimming in ice-cold water. The yawning warns me of falling blood pressure in the brain, even if I disregarded the warning in the cold.

The lowly *rectum* can be a friend indeed. Constipation is one warning it gives. Another may be internal piles which have fallen out through the anus, and so cause discomfort. They suggest the homely slang expression, 'My tail is dragging'. They demand correction both of constipation and the exhaustion or excessively prolonged standing which has caused rectal symptoms, and may cause convulsions. Even pure psychological depression can be apparent through rectal symptoms.

External danger signs also force themselves on my consciousness to warn me. They are six in number: twitching right eyelid; a neck which grated when I turned my head as if to say, 'No'; hands cold, blue, unsteady, tremulous; posture stooping; toes, wet with cold sweat, and with blistered, macerated skin; tumescence. A tremor of the right *eyelid* was years ago an ominous sign of a coming convulsion, inevitable as far as I knew. Now it warns me to be careful, especially of sudden

change of posture, but also in other ways. Formerly almost always, now only sometimes, blowing my nose causes the right-eyelid tremor immediately, once for each forcible expiration. Apparently raising the air pressure in my chest to blow my nose, blocked momentarily the blood flowing from brain to lung, and so caused a miniature convulsion, that is, one of the eyelid alone. Lying down too long is still prone to cause a convulsion, probably for a similar reason, interfering with the return of blood from the brain, in this instance by means of the force of gravity. Now I nap at noon rather than sleep (lie down) too long at night, if I have lost sleep.

My *neck* grates for an hour or so after I get up in the morning if I turn my head side to side as if to say, 'No'. It offers some measure both of the effect of lying down, and of early adaptation to an erect posture.

Cold hands are one of the best measures I have of deficient adaptation to an erect posture. They also show the effect of cold, nervous exhaustion, confusion, emotion, and food sometimes. The slang expression 'I have cold feet', meaning fear, shows how natural it is to see meaning in hands or feet.

A sagging, relatively lifeless *posture* is usually an early sign of most of the exhaustion and other things which cause internal hemorrhoids to sag out of the anus. Posture-consciousness helps both to alert against a potential convulsion and to correct the important deleterious effects of bad posture on circulation, bowel, and mental attitude. The importance of posture and daily normal bowel motion have long been recognized in hospitals.

The corpora cavernosa have been one of the most recent 'finds' for me for prevention of convulsions. When they are contracted before I rise in the morning, I avoid most of my remaining convulsions which occur when I rise. Apparently dilated corpora cavernosa indicate abnormally great pooling of blood in veins, probably especially veins in the internal organs. Then the brain lacks blood when an erect posture is suddenly taken. Waking thoroughly, rolling over, warming the rest of my body with a hot pad, and avoiding sexual stimulation at the moment, help contract the corpora cavernosa, and so presumably the other veins of the internal organs.

Toes are useful, somewhat like hands. These perhaps show some circulatory changes especially soon because they are more subject than other areas of the body to the weight of the blood in the body above. Also, even shoes which are not unusually tight may tend to restrict circulation in the toes. My toes get varying degrees of blister formation in the skin after unusual mental strain.

Warnings I can sometimes see in my face, if I have a mirror, are sweat, pallor of the forehead, reddening of the right side of my right eye, bags under both eyes, loss of the skin crease which normally runs from the right edge of the nose to the right edge of the lips, tooth indentations on the edge of the tongue (noted previously). I look in a mirror occasionally usually when reading and thinking intensely very long. Reddening of the right side of my right eye seems most important, and a 'cold' sweat and pallor, next most important.

'Apathy' struck me as the loss of the usual evidence of abundant energy and enthusiasm, loss of smiles, loss of spontaneity.

'Error' meant both in sensation and in action, particularly so-called 'stupid', 'absent-minded' errors. In sensation, 'error' meant excessive narrowing of the normally wide zone of surrounding things apparent to me even when I was not looking at them. Certain jobs were especially effective for detecting tendency to error.

Error, apathy, and various signs of tension are not only an efficient check list for minimizing predisposition to convulsion. They also can help the patient evaluate his faulty or improving specific construction abilities.

The foregoing are the barest instructions for eliminating post-traumatic convulsions of at least one patient. In retrospect, the most important lessons I have learned are unconscious adaptations to unconscious reaction. Each lesson I learned many ways, but finally well enough so that I do the right thing most of the time almost instinctively, instantly, accurately and forcefully. It seems only natural to sense almost simultaneously all of whatever strains I am subject to, and to perceive likewise simultaneously most of the signs I show of predisposition to convulsion, even though minimal. These habits help my personal efficiency even when there is no danger of convulsion. May many epileptics be spared fear, confusion and ostracism! May they all have health, wealth and happiness!

(Darling 1952)

COMMENTARY

Darling's article illustrates the stigma that can be encountered when trying to follow a career while having the label 'epilepsy'. It brings home the frequent observation that epileptic seizures are more frightening to non-sufferers of epilepsy than to the sufferers themselves, and that one of the major obstacles to the everyday adjustment of people with epilepsy is the attitude of the public, employers, etc. Darling provides a detailed account of his epilepsy, in particular the factors that appear to contribute most towards the occurrence of convulsions and how these factors may be controlled. Darling did not have the benefit of a firm diagnosis of his condition— it was initially thought to have been a right hemisphere brain tumour, but a subsequent opinion thought it may be atrophy/calcification of the brain.

The idea suggested by Darling of some fits being 'conditioned' to occur in certain situations finds echoes in some of the research literature. Forster (1977) used the term 'reflex epilepsy' to include people whose seizures were induced by higher cognitive functions. More recently, Antebi and Bird (1992) reviewed case reports that included a range of seizure precipitants, such as reading, mental arithmetic, etc. While 'conditioning' is typically used to describe the association of a small number of specific stimuli to certain reflexive behaviour, Darling covers a range of potential precipitants (e.g. posture, temperature, effort, food, sexual activity, etc.). It is interesting that Darling also found one of his 'triggers' to be 'stimulation demanding rapid recall of material only partially recallable. Examinations, or the sudden meeting of an old, partially-forgotten friend are examples' (p. 373). His search for, and discovery of, a range of triggers almost reached obsessional proportions and this level of interest and concern is something that is often shown by people with epilepsy in the early stages after diagnosis of their condition.

While cognitive stimulation has now been shown in a number of studies to trigger the occurrence of epileptic seizures (Helmstaedter *et al.* 1992), their occurrence in this type of recall setting is rather unusual. In a number of places throughout his description, Darling notes that stresses of various forms contributed directly or indirectly to the occurrence of fits. In my experience, this is often reported by people with epilepsy. Although it has been well documented in the literature (Lishman 1987), the precise neural mechanisms underlying this relationship remain a mystery.

REFERENCES

Antebi, D. and Bird, J. (1992). The facilitation and evocation of seizures. *British Journal of Psychiatry*, 160, 154–64.

Forster, F. M. (1977). *Reflex epilepsy, behavioural therapy and conditioned reflexes*. Charles C. Thomas, Springfield, IL.

Helmstaedter, C., Hufnagel, A., and Egler, C. E. (1992). Seizures during cognitive testing in patients with temporal lobe epilepsy: Possibility of seizure induction by cognitive activation. *Epilepsia*, 33, 892–7.

Lishman, W. A. (1987). *Organic psychiatry* (2nd edn). Blackwell, Oxford.

Epilepsy

This anonymous author worked as a district midwife.

I

Epilepsy is defined in the dictionary as the 'falling sickness'. I do not propose to enter into an academic discussion concerning types, characteristics, and causation of such seizures; I will tell quite simply what happens if I have a fit.

It starts with a peculiar sensation in my chest, but before I can do anything about it I am unconscious. I know and feel nothing. On recovery, I have a feeling of extraordinary well-being: wherever I happen to be lying, whether on a couch, the floor, or even the roadside, it is as if I were lying on the most comfortable bed. I may hear voices asking if someone has injured herself and I wonder of whom they are talking. If I notice someone looking down at me with evident concern, I wonder at the anxiety shown. After a few seconds, I am completely awake; I find that I am lying on the floor, remember the aura, and know that I must have had another fit. I feel myself gingerly to make sure that I'm whole, get up, and that is all.

That is my version of the event, but what do spectators think? Perhaps I have been talking to them a few moments previously, I utter a cry and fall to the floor. My arms and legs jerk convulsively, my lips are covered with saliva, and my breathing is stertorous. After a very short interval these movements cease and I lie still, but my face remains pale and my eyes are open and appear vacant. It is a shock to whoever is present; they feel baffled and helpless. They wish to help, but there is little to be done: the interval during which I lie inert seems interminable, and because there is nothing much they can do their imagination becomes active. The person with me wonders what would have happened if the fit had occurred a few moments earlier when I might have been with a patient, or an hour later when I might have been alighting from a bus in a busy street, and determines that I must not run such risks in future.

These two opposing viewpoints magnify the difficulties which we epileptics have to overcome. There must be a compromise between the epileptic, who regards an attack as a 'bolt from the blue', a rather unreal hazard; and the non-epileptic, who dislikes these dramatic happenings and regards them as an ever-present source of danger.

I started to have fits at the age of 30. It is easy to describe one's physical and emotional reaction to a single fit, but the mental attitude adopted by an epileptic is not easy to define. Diagnosis of a chronic ailment is rarely made in a flash, so that one has often accepted the physical conditions before the 'label' is attached. For about a year I must have had nocturnal attacks at intervals of 2–3 months: after each of these I awoke with a headache and a bitten tongue, and an attack of vomiting followed; I had no suspicion of the underlying cause. Intermittently, during the daytime, I had the symptom which I recognise now as an aura, and at times a more disturbing sensation, as if I had received an electric shock to the base of my skull. The culmination was a daytime fit, which was not recognised by those who saw it but which gave me the clue to these strange events. I then sought medical advice. Fortunately the doctor whom I consulted was sympathetic and advised me to carry on as long as possible, and to keep my own counsel.

When I knew that I was an epileptic, my first reaction was one of surprise: I had thought of this as a terrible complaint and was amazed to find it entailed very little physical discomfort. Its social significance was not brought home to me for some years. I continued with my work as district-nurse-midwife. It was war-time, and even in country areas we were too busy to worry needlessly. After five years the strain of repeated night calls for midwifery proved too great, and fits occurred during the day. These could not be hidden, so adjustments had to be made. Because I had a good record, and because nurses were in demand, I was allowed to continue, but only in a casualty department among people who were not in the strict sense of the word 'sick people'.

I did not take kindly to this ultimatum, perhaps because of the manner in which it was issued. For the first time I realised something of the barrier which exists between the epileptic and the non-epileptic. There was an implication that there was no future in nursing for me, and that I had been guilty of a grave misdemeanour in having hidden my handicap. Although, in my new post, I met with kindness and consideration from the medical officers under whom I worked, I cannot describe the mental anguish which I suffered. It is better to forget this period; it was dominated by feelings of frustration, guilt, fear, and loneliness. For two years I was 'unstable', but then I began to adopt a more reasonable attitude. I realised that if as an epileptic one cannot do the work of one's choice one must make the best of the work one is allowed to do, and interest in it will develop.

Besides making adjustments to the work one can reasonably be allowed to do, one must learn to live with people who do not want to have the embarrassment of an epileptic thrust on them in their leisure hours. To do my job I must live away from home. I find the best way of managing is to take a furnished room and be independent of outside help. It is often wiser to keep one's secret, and to move to other rooms if trouble arises with the landlady; although sometimes an unexpectedly helpful attitude is shown. Household tasks—cooking, cleaning, mending, and shopping—occupy several evenings usefully and happily. An occasional meal in a restaurant, a visit to a cinema or theatre, provide diversion. The natural anxiety which my parents felt for my safety had to be allayed. My own powers of persuasion proved inadequate, but they agreed with my views more readily after reading some of the booklets published by the American League Against Epilepsy.

The solution of such problems is an individual matter, but epileptics who have met with much social frustration would welcome the advice of a social worker. I realise that the rather placid life which appeals to me, a woman of 40, would not satisfy an adolescent. I have talked to many epileptics, some of them young men and women on the threshold of life, eager for companionship and adventure. I have been impressed with their good sense, and their desire to help each other. Perhaps the social problem could be solved by the formation of an association for epileptics: such an association would help us to learn more about each other, and would teach us that we face a common difficulty. It would serve an excellent purpose if it became the channel through which the simple truth about the condition could be made known to the general public

Some of the ideas which I have held have helped me; some have proved fallacious. One should not generalise from a single instance, but an analysis of some of my hopes, doubts, and fears may be useful to others. The conviction that an attack would never occur when I was actually doing a job has been my safeguard. It has proved true. Daytime attacks have invariably come on when I have been trying to do two things at once—I may have been awaiting the arrival of a patient and worrying over a private matter such as the illness of a relative or a love affair not progressing well. It would be interesting to verify this from the experience of others. Investigation might embrace not only the frequency and the time of day at which attacks occur but what the person was actually doing, and his state of mind at the time. Considering the insecurity of employment of many epileptics, it is likely that anxiety is ever-present in their minds, preventing proper concentration.

Medication is the responsibility of the physician, and its purpose is too seldom understood by us patients. The physician who will devote time to discussing it, and will emphasise that a more hopeful prognosis is possible with the aid of modern drugs, will gain the intelligent co-operation of his patient, without which the optimum dose and drug will not readily be found. We epileptics know that many of our fellows are in the wards of mental hospitals; we know that the drugs used are also given to neurotics; hence the fear that the tablets are only 'dope', and that we may some day be inpatients. It cannot be said too often that, with modern medication, the outlook is more hopeful, that the number of fits will decrease, and that age as well as medication improves the chance of stabilisation.

Since fits are not unpleasant to the sufferer the fuss which the onlooker makes appears to us unreasonable. But we do shock their aesthetic senses. We would gladly hide away for a time and emerge with the fit over, but the peculiar nature of the disease rules out such a course. We can only reiterate that we do not suffer during attacks, and if our fellows will allow us to lead normal lives these embarrassing events will occur less and less often.

Although a fit is not unpleasant, the aura which precedes it is: it is a sensation which cannot be described, and will persist after fits have been 'controlled'. There must be many individual manifestations of the symptom. I have learned from experience that there are variations in its intensity—a violent aura will be followed immediately by a fit; a milder one may occur several times a day, for two or three days, without an aftermath. One never feels completely confident on such days, but the repetition of this cycle over many months without harmful effect dispels some of the alarm originally caused by this strange phenomenon.

In short, we epileptics are ordinary people to whom occasionally something 'strange' happens. We do not want to make a fuss about it, and we do not want other people to do so. If we could find a method whereby the public could be educated on this subject: if, too, we could tell those in charge of industry the plain facts about the ailment and convince them that potential manpower and womanpower is running to waste, so that they would employ epileptics with confidence, perhaps making a minor adjustment in working conditions to suit each individual case, most of our difficulties would be solved. Perhaps the medical profession will lead us in this matter and help us to establish a realistic and rational attitude to epilepsy in the public mind and help ourselves to a fuller life.

(Anonymous 1952)

COMMENTARY

This article also brings home the social consequences of a diagnosis of epilepsy and of the occurrence of fits in public—it offers credence to the truism that epilepsy affects non-epileptics more than it affects the sufferer. The article was written when the British Epilepsy Association was just being formed, and when some epileptics were treated as inpatients in mental hospitals, and it provides an interesting historical perspective to the way that epilepsy was viewed and treated. The author points to the possible role of stress, and having to do two things at once, in bringing about fits. If such emotional and cognitive overload is indeed a common trigger factor in cases of epilepsy, it highlights the need for counselling/behaviour therapy that focuses on reducing this overload, perhaps by changes in the person's work-style, use of compensatory cognitive aids, etc.

The author appears to have gone through three stages in coming to terms with her epilepsy, and these may well apply to most other cases:

(1) a general disregard for the condition as a major problem;

(2) feelings of frustration, guilt, fear, and loneliness—these are largely brought about by the reactions of others, such as employers; and

(3) an acceptance of a changed life-style and differing social expectations.

The author vividly demonstrates in her article that it is others, such as family members, work colleagues, the general public and even health care workers, who need educating about epilepsy more than the patient himself/herself. It could be argued that all brains are susceptible to the occurrence of epilepsy and will display seizure activity given the appropriate stimulus. In the author's words, 'we epileptics are ordinary people to whom occasionally something "strange" happens' (p. 382). Perhaps the label of epilepsy, when it is used to describe a chronic predisposition, should be replaced by the term 'prone to intermittent seizures', or some other more neutral term, if only to reduce its fatalistic connotation and to emphasize that for most of the time the person may be no different to those without such a predisposition.

Epilepsy

This anonymous author initially studied medicine, but switched to zoology after the onset of his epilepsy.

Twenty years ago while a student doing 2nd M.B. I had a 'grand mal' epileptic fit. Now, the fact that I had flooded my room with D.D.T. in an attempt to rid myself of bed-bugs may, I consider, have been a contributory cause, but at the time all that I could think of was hard work and a hereditary contribution in the shape of a female second cousin with chorea and epilepsy.

One Saturday afternoon I was walking from Shoreditch to London Bridge to meet a friend when, by Shoreditch Church, I felt that the buildings around were unreal facades as in a theatre, that the people walking by were puppets and that I was the only living creature around. I knew that the feeling was ridiculous but could not throw off the depression of dread. At this point the quality of my thinking began to deteriorate for if I kept moving I felt that I should be 'all right'.

As I continued to walk, the white disc of my consciousness began to be cut into by a segment of darkness that increased in size with each heart-beat. Like a drunk I began to think that if I got to the next lamp-post I should solve all my problems. I do not remember walking much further but when I got to the police-station opposite Liverpool Street Station a policeman saw me weave out in front of a trolley-bus, fall and go into a kind of convulsion. I have a vague memory of a policeman stuffing a splintering pencil between my teeth and nothing more until I woke up feeling very refreshed in Bart's. I had been taken there in an apparently obscure state of awareness and answered all the questions asked of me as if I was sixteen years old. I was just twenty one but looked much younger. I lost consciousness a second time and this awakening I remember. As I came to there was a slight semen ejaculation so that there may have been accompanying convulsions. The fact that I had holes in my socks made me rather worried, more so than

the fact of the fit. It was about four o'clock so that the whole episode must have taken about three hours. On the following Monday an emminent neurologist examined me and I was put on phenobarbitone. This interfered with subtle thinking but I was able to carry on with my course.

My biggest fear was the possibility of a series of fits progressively depressing my intelligence. At the time I was referred in Physics 1st M.B. and failed it a little later. I was asked to leave before sitting 2nd M.B. The neurologist insisted that there had been no intellectual deterioration but I became more and more withdrawn over the next few months, maintaining contact only with my family during the vacation and with the 'crammers' when I worked at Physics. I passed both Conjoint and 1st M.B. Physics but the hospital would not accept me back. Withdrawal became more complete and I stayed in my room for weeks at a time.

Although there was no intellectual deterioration (my I.Q. is supposed to be in the top 3%) I feel that there was at this time, quite a coarsening of my emotional fibre. The memory trace of the 'viva' the morning before and of events two days before that remained hazy even now. I applied to other medical schools but was of course rejected. I took various temporary jobs and about two years after the first fit I finally came to accept that even with the support of the neurologist I would not be allowed to continue medicine. I switched to Zoology instead.

One of the features that I most dreaded was the look that came into the eyes of any group interviewing me when I mentioned epilepsy. (This may be a delusion but I don't think so.) In the public mind there is still I feel, a superstitious tie-up with 'possession by the devil', even amongst the enlightened. Since I changed the disease to a respectable 'rheumatic fever' there has been no trouble in obtaining posts.

In the examination after the fit, old right rectus weakness and slight spasticity of the right arm were confirmed. They may have been caused by a forceps delivery or a bad attack of measles in infancy. In childhood I had experienced myoclonic twitching when riding a bike past a sunny hedge and disorientation of space in nightmares. After the fit I occasionally got (and still get) bouts of shaking that last for about half a minute and then pass off but nothing else of diagnostic importance except that writing this now in my forty-second year makes me very depressed indeed.

(Anonymous 1977)

COMMENTARY

The anonymous contribution notes that the major fear of the writer when he first found himself afflicted with seizures was that continued epilepsy might depress his intelligence and therefore hinder his career. The fact that his epilepsy started during his medical student days, and that he subsequently failed his exams on a number of occasions and had to abandon medicine, suggests that his cognitive functioning was affected to some extent, either by the epileptogenic lesion or indirectly by the occurrence of the fits. His reference to spasticity in his right arm suggests the possibility of a left hemisphere lesion, and this may have contributed to verbal memory difficulties. In addition, he was prescribed phenobarbitone, a drug that is known to have adverse side-effects on memory functioning (Thompson 1992). The author admits to periods of withdrawal/depression during this time, and to a 'coarsening of his emotional fibre'. This probably combined with his cognitive symptoms to produce problems in coping with his medical course and exams. This writer of the article appeared to have encountered some discrimination when applying for jobs, with the label 'epilepsy' resulting in looks of dread amongst some of his interviewers. One point of neuropsychological interest is that during the recovery phase of one of his fits, the author appeared to have a retrograde amnesia of five years, answering questions as if he were 16 years of age. Retrograde amnesia can sometimes occur during, and as a consequence of, seizures (Kapur 1993, 1997), though in this case it is difficult to be more certain of its type and extent in view of the sole observation of age-disorientation.

REFERENCES

Kapur, N. (1993) Transient epileptic amnesia: an update and a reformulation. *Journal of Neurology, Neurosurgery and Psychiatry*, 56, 1184–90.

Kapur, N. (1997). Autobiographical amnesia and temporal lobe pathology. In *Classic case studies in the neuropsychology of memory*, (ed. A. J. Parkin). Lawrence Erlbaum, in press.

Thompson, P. J. (1992). Anti-epileptic drugs and memory. *Epilepsia*, 33(Suppl. 6), S37–S40.

My life with epilepsy

Cathy Morris

Cathy Morris is a doctor who was a medical consultant to the magazine where this article appeared.

I had my first fit—a 'grand mal' seizure—when I was 13. My head started spinning and I yelled as I cartwheeled through the floor. After a period of darkness, I came to, in bed. Parents, doctor and neighbours leaned over me, but I had no idea what had happened.

Epilepsy involves an electrical fault in the brain, in my case in both temporal lobes, each side of the head. Anyone can have a fit given the stimulus, but some of us inherit or acquire a lower threshold for blowing a fuse. An aunt and some cousins of mine have epilepsy, and it's possible that stress, and the hormones of puberty, may have played a part in triggering the first fit.

I treated the experience with adolescent arrogance and flushed away the phenobarbitone tablets because they made me drowsy. I'm glad I did, as these pills can interfere with learning. But though my studies didn't suffer, late night cramming for exams, and early morning music practice provoked more fits—which left me bruised, broken and even burnt. I insisted the fits didn't trouble me. I camouflaged black eyes with outrageous make-up and a floppy hat, and hid battered legs under trousers. I misdirected my rage against the dentist who was trying to repair my broken teeth, and discharged myself prematurely from hospital.

At the time I knew nothing of my parents' anguish. They both channelled their concern into visits to neurology clinics, adhering strictly to the specialists' exhortations that I should 'live normally'. It was spelt out to me that epilepsy didn't mean I would become mentally handicapped. Some handicapped people have fits as one manifestation of a damaged brain, but the majority of people with epilepsy have normal intelligence. Nor is it a form of insanity, though those who suffer from it have a higher-than-average risk of becoming mentally ill. My parents never let me think that epilepsy carried a stigma, and we treated it as a very trivial part of my life.

I didn't see a 'grand mal' fit from the outside until I was a medical student, years later, I heard the scream, witnessed the twitching, clenched limbs, frothing mouth and the incontinence. I was shocked, but still avoided seeing my epilepsy from another's viewpoint. Fortunately my attitude of denial didn't prevent me from undergoing tests and taking medication to minimise the risk of injuries, or of prolonged fits leading to brain damage. Ordinary X-rays of the skull rarely show up the source of epilepsy, and until recently, the most helpful test was the electroencephalograph (EEG). Wires are glued to the scalp to sense the brain's electrical activity which is then recorded on rolls of paper. It's painless, and often shows an abnormality which indicates where the damage lies. But many people with epilepsy have normal EEGs and here CT (computer tomogram) scans are more likely to identify abnormalities. Lying in the long tube while being scanned was claustrophobic, but it was fascinating to be shown pictures of my brain and good to hear I had no tumours. Tumours rarely cause epilepsy though, most sufferers are classed as 'idiopathic'—which is jargon for an unknown cause.

For some years I took the drug phenytoin (Epanutin), which reduced the frequency of my fits to a tolerable two or three a year. It caused me less drowsiness than phenobarbitone, though my hair thinned and my gums swelled. My oral contraceptive had to be a high-dose one, as phenytoin increases liver activity and reduces the effectiveness of the Pill. It also interacts with alcohol, so my teenage experiments with drink were risky.

Drugs minimised the physical problems, and everyone I met was so enlightened that the question of discrimination did not arise. Contemporaries in the psychedelic Seventies made me feel that I was privileged to experience altered states of awareness, and academics at school and college cited Julius Caesar, Dostoevsky and Van Gogh as fellow sufferers. I was accepted into medical school without trouble. There was some dismay that I was a woman, but my epilepsy wasn't mentioned!

Some years later, the situation changed. I was so punch drunk with the life I'd let myself in for, it took me months to notice I was having more fits. I'd taken on a punishing job which deprived me of sleep and replaced meal-times with raids on the chocolate machine. My personal life was a mess, and I'd moved hundreds of miles away from my family and friends. Despite taking a cocktail of three drugs, I was having more and more fits—I even had one while taking a blood sample from a patient. Usually my fits 'wait' until moments of concentration are past, but at that time, I even lost the 'auras' which signalled that a seizure was on its way. I simply blacked out without warning and came round howling, at work, in the street, or in ambulances. And on top of all this, I had a full-blown eating disorder.

I lived with the minor injuries and the attitude of an ostrich. But, for my husband, there was the distress of witnessing the fits, sometimes twice a day, and the fear and sheer inconvenience of being called to casualty. He told me how joyless it was for him to endure the hours I spent sleeping after each fit, and the dullness that affected me for days afterwards. I decided to ask for help.

I underwent tests and hoped for an operation. Unfortunately, both my temporal lobes were affected and it's important to leave one side to preserve memory. My neurologist suggested a series of drugs, one at a time. So I tried clonazepam (Rivotril) which affected my memory and made it hard to study. I then took carbamaxepine (Tegretol) until I felt cross-eyed and came out in a rash. I tried sodium valproate (Epilim) which made my hair curl, but increased my appetite.

It was the sodium valproate which gave me the best control of the fits with the least side effects. Other changes also led to a dramatic improvement. I moved to a more specialised field of medicine which allowed me more sleep, I sought help with my eating problems—and I finally acknowledged that I wanted a baby. For years I'd watched my body revolt against me, so it was an immense joy to experience immediate fertility, a blooming pregnancy and swift, natural labour. Anticonvulsants may increase the risk of deformities in the unborn child, but we felt the risks of uncontrolled epilepsy were far greater. My daughter Alice is now 5, and she is perfect, though she does run a slightly increased risk of suffering from epilepsy. I've had no more fits since her birth, and I'm now pregnant for a second time. Respecting my own stress threshold, and paying more attention to sleep, food and medication seems to have made it less likely that I'll blow a fuse. I still have to take tablets twice daily as even after several years without fits, stopping drugs could provoke a recurrence.

The future holds exciting prospects. Highly sophisticated scanning techniques such as positron emission tomography (PET) scans and magnetic resonance imaging (MRI) should allow very precise surgery for more sufferers. Meanwhile, pharmacologists are exploring GABA and glutamate, two natural brain substances which affect the excitability of nerve cells, and two anticonvulsants to control them: lamotrigine and vigabatrin. Psychological advances in the management of epilepsy are valuable too, as counselling can help to control it by identifying the triggers and by specific relaxation techniques.

My own attitudes have advanced too. I don't regret having epilepsy. Not because I regard it as trivial, but because it's been so important in shaping the person I have become. This I accept.

(Morris 1991)

COMMENTARY

Morris' account points to the delicate balance that has to be maintained with a potentially serious condition such as epilepsy—trying to lead as normal a life as possible, and often ignoring the presence of the disease, while at the same time leading a life-style that does not precipitate acute disturbances associated with the disease. Early on in the diagnosis of her condition, Morris found it reassuring to be given clear information that epilepsy did not mean she was going to decline intellectually or become insane. The attitude of her family and others in key positions was helpful and supportive: 'My parents never let me think that epilepsy carried a stigma, and we treated it as a very trivial part of my life (p. 386) . . . Everyone I met was so enlightened that the question of discrimination did not arise. Contemporaries in the psychedelic seventies made me feel that I was privileged to experience altered states of awareness, and academics at school cited Julius Caesar, Dostoevsky and Van Gogh as fellow sufferers' (p. 387). These observations highlight the role of counselling of the individual with epilepsy, and the importance of understanding shown by those close to the individual. Despite the relatively poor control of her seizures, the probable bitemporal lobe abnormality, and side-effects from medication, it is of interest that Morris was able to pass her school and university examinations without major problems. This point brings home the self-limiting nature of some forms of epilepsy. Morris appears to have had evidence of bilateral temporal lobe abnormality, and this would have been a contra-indication to surgery. She does not, however, mention any specific cognitive symptoms that interfered with her work, apart from those that were occasionally associated with the side-effects of her drugs or that followed a major fit.

It appeared that stress and eating habits interacted with her form of epilepsy to exacerbate problems relating to control of seizures. She faced the dilemma about going through pregnancy, with the contrasting risks of possible effects of anticonvulsants on her unborn fetus, and the risks of poorly controlled epilepsy that could have resulted in a major seizure. Here one sees an example of a sex difference in the effects of a neurological illness, something that is seldom apparent for other illnesses reviewed in this book (although it should be pointed out that most of the articles have been written by, or about, men with a brain illness/brain injury).

Epilepsy in my life

John Lisyak

John Lisyak is a retired general practitioner.

My own diagnosis of complex partial seizures (temporal lobe epilepsy) was not made for over a year, despite characteristic complex partial seizures. Several times a day I experienced the sensation of an unusual smell, or had feelings of déjà vu. Later on I also experienced 'absences' when for a few seconds I was not aware of what I was doing.

Such seizures are fairly common in this form of epilepsy. However, what prevented me from making such a diagnosis, and what must have confused the specialists whom I saw, were the 'feelings' that accompanied my seizures. It was the 'feelings' that I was most aware of. I wasn't even aware of my absences, and my wife who had noticed them, thought that they were just an exaggeration of being easily distracted, which I always have been.

The déjà vu experiences were not a simple awareness of something seen before, but a feeling of something strange happening to me, as though for a moment I became part of my surroundings. As I got out of the car, on my general practice call, I became acutely aware of the shadows and the winter sun and the cold air. They reminded me of something from the past and stood out vividly. Similarly with the 'funny' smell, reminiscent of satay chicken. The thing that made that experience worse was again 'the feeling'. Each occurrence made me restless and fearful that something dreadful was about to happen to me. Eventually I did suffer a major tonic-clonic convulsion, which occurs if minor ones remain untreated. That convulsion made the diagnosis of epilepsy obvious. Further investigation showed a scarring in my right temporal lobe, probably the consequence of a difficult birth.

Mixed up with the above phenomena was the feeling of helplessness caused by a difficulty with my memory. The memory problem seemed to be getting worse and worse, until I reached the point of having to work out my calls with a street directory, in spite of having worked in the area for some 15 years. Treatment led to an improvement but left me with pockets of memory deficit, which interfered with my ability to recall diseases and their treatments. Because I was already in my sixties I decided to retire.

KNOWING SET ME FREE

It has been said that happiness is a good anti-convulsant. I am convinced that understanding is also a good anticonvulsant and that the two go together. Prior to my knowledge about my epilepsy I can't say that I had had an unhappy life. I had succeeded in a number of fields and enjoyed a happy married life. I was always aware, however, of something missing, something that seemed impossible to define. It wasn't discontentment. It was lack of fulfilment, but why or because of what shortcoming, I could not tell.

All failure was devastating to me. Being a perfectionist even the most understandable lack of success produced feelings of hopelessness, which I had to learn to control—by means of self-suggestion, through positive thinking, and by various methods of deep relaxation and meditation. I know that my interest in psychiatry came from that search.

Understanding does not necessarily change the reactions but it makes a difference to their severity. When it was decided that I go off the tablets because I had no fits for over three years, I was all right for a few weeks and then suffered another tonic-clonic convulsion. That was followed by the usual depression. However, because of the knowledge I had gained this depression was not accompanied by the feelings of hopelessness.

And even the 'funny smell' that returned together with the emotional dread, wasn't nearly as disturbing because I understood what was happening.

'YOU'RE NOT LIKE THE OTHERS'

Most people who suffer from epilepsy start having convulsions early in life and become aware of being different from an early age. The late Manning Clark, a noted Australian historian, suffered from complex partial seizures and had his first convulsion when he was 14. His mother, however, noticed differences much earlier.

'Each night my mother clings to me: sometimes I think she is crying, and I wonder why. I look up at her from my bed, and see tear drops on her cheeks, and she says to me, "I worry sometimes, Man dear, what's going to happen to you. You're not like the others".'[1]

I have no such memories of my mother, but I do have memories of not being able to do what other children could. The village fair that filled everyone with wonder and excitement made me feel uneasy, and I was never happy to go on the ferris wheel. And in December, on St Nicholas night, I hid under the bed.

These early memories help to explain the uncertainty that I felt about myself and how I happened to be searching for answers. This search became all the more acute when I came to Australia, at the age of 12. Not knowing the language I couldn't understand or properly relate to other children. Our situation and status changed. In Yugoslavia, in the village, everyone knew us and respected my family because my grandparents had been mead-makers. In Sydney, in 1936, apart from a few people we had contact with through the Yugoslav Club, no-one knew us.

'LIBERATION THROUGH ILLNESS'

Such experiences are not unique to those with epilepsy. Any chronic illness or chronic stress changes our lives and causes unpleasant symptoms. It may also make us develop capacities that remain undeveloped in other people. Roslyn Woodward, a psychologist, explains, '. . . chronic illness just actually means you have a chance to reflect, and gain insights and wisdom and knowledge and humour that many people who are fit and healthy don't have a chance to develop'[2]

Professor Oliver Sacks believes that people suffering from illness or handicap can reorganise their lives in order to find undeveloped potential within them (*Further reading*). There are many epileptics throughout history who achieved not just ordinary success but an extraordinary one. People like Alexander the Great, Dante, Leonardo da Vinci, and Alfred Nobel, who must have come to that understanding through their own intuitive powers, or through someone's guidance. Manning Clark's parents were given such advice in 1929. Their doctor told them that his was 'a form of epilepsy which was a common affliction for those with extraordinary imagination, stormy temperaments, and strange insights into human behaviour. I should think of it not as a badge of infamy, or a handicap, but a gift which I must treasure, and turn to advantage'.[1]

Repeatedly I hear from members about the special feeling that they have towards people who suffer. Dostoyevsky, the great Russian writer who suffered from epilepsy, is known for his uncanny insight into the minds of the mentally disturbed, or those leading wretched lives. Such affinity, such empathy could surely be directed into work involved in helping others.

I found much fulfilment in my medical career. Major and urgent decisions were stressful to me, as were irregular hours. However, the opportunity that treatment gives in bringing two people into a positive relationship is unique. Apart from the satisfaction that a successful outcome brings, there is the potential for reaching and influencing another human being, at a most crucial time. To help someone gain insight, to see change coming about, to be part of that change, and part of that very human interchange, is extraordinarily uplifting, and a source of personal growth.

This leads me to agree with Rosey Gold, 'artist-in-residence' at Sydney's Children Hospital in 1989. She wrote, 'I don't like chronically ill kids being told to aim for a so-called normal life, to be like other children'[3] How can you be like others when you're different? How can those with epilepsy model themselves on the 'normal' when they experience 'blackouts' that completely disrupt their lives, stop everything that's going on, and alter life patterns?

Even between the fits there is a difference—in moods, in feelings of dread and feelings of exhilaration, and wouldn't it be more sensible to help sufferers recognise these and adjust to them, understand that there are handicaps, but potentials as well?

Rosey herself suffered from 'chest problems' as a child, but did not feel deprived or less capable. Her mother 'romanticised illness'. 'She talked about the Brontes and convinced me that people who were ill were truly dignified.'

How can we tell a child, or anyone, that illness is not a bad thing and that there might even be some good in it? How can we, when the only value in life seems to mean plenty of action and plenty of participation?

Is there another way? Is Professor Sacks right in saying that there is a positive side of illness? Can we lead a full life without frenzied activity of the 'normal'? Can we be different or must we all be 'normal'?

WHY SUPPORT GROUPS?

One of the best ways of obtaining better understanding of one's handicaps and coming to terms with them is to share experiences with people with similar handicaps. No professional advice, no intellectual discussion or textbook description can give the same immediacy, the same day-to-day detail, or the same feeling of conviction. Those involved with counselling can often acquire special feeling for the sufferer's plight. However, there is a barrier between the professional and the one suffering from illness.

There is nothing more liberating than to be able to talk freely and openly about things that at other times might be considered silly or trivial and might not be understood. At the end of a good group meeting there's enthusiasm and goodwill all-round and people are exchanging ideas and suggestions on all sides. There's fluency with words and acuteness of ideas, and there's liveliness and joyfulness that make you feel that real human existence was always meant to be like that.

I joined the group to learn more about myself because I could not understand why I should have so many personality traits in common with others with epilepsy, and I could not understand why so many of my interests should be similar. Why should interests in philosophy and cosmology be the same? And how was it that preference for written expression was so common in epilepsy that it has been labelled 'hypergraphia'? Is there an epileptic personality, or what has been called 'interictal behaviour syndrome'?

The suggestion is that certain traits go with complex partial seizures and from my observation I would agree, even though it is too early to give a definite view. There are many such aspects of epilepsy that are begging further answers. For instance some of our members have developed ways of controlling their fits:

'. . . I had an episode while driving on Parramatta Road I pulled over—engine off, hazards on, and a combination of prayer to the Sacred Heart of Jesus and the exertion of willpower, mindpower, whatever, I refused to lose consciousness. I didn't.'[4]

Another member finds that activity, such as an exercise bike, stops her fits.

Apart from giving me new understanding the support groups have shown me the positive side of epilepsy. In spite of inadequacy of treatment in the past many sufferers learnt to adjust. Our oldest member, now in his 70s, has had tonic-clonic (grand mal) epilepsy from the age of nine, and managed to keep a horticulturist job throughout his long working life. Like so many he has proved that epilepsy is not a sentence. It is another way, with certain limitations and certain potentials as well.

REFERENCES

1. Clark, M. (1989). *The puzzles of childhood*. Penguin, Ringwood, Vio.
2. Woodward, R. (1992). The management of chronic fatigue syndrome. *Me and you*. Sept.
3. Gold, R. (1989). A healthy dose of imagination. *Observer Fortnightly*. 7 July, 60.
4. Newsletter. Nepean Support Group (1992). Bridget's story. Oct., 2.

FURTHER READING

Sacks, O. (1986). *The man who mistook his wife for a hat*. Picador Pan, London.

(Lisyak 1994)

COMMENTARY

Lisyak had symptoms of déjà vu and the sensation of an unusual smell, these symptoms preceding more obvious clinical manifestations of epilepsy. He had absences, of which he was not aware, and which were passed off by his wife as being reflections of his distractibility. He also had a feeling of something strange happening to him, as though for a moment he was becoming part of his surroundings. It is interesting to speculate why, in the presence of all of these symptoms, it still did not 'click' to Lisyak, with his medical background, that something serious was amiss. A simple form of denial may be a likely explanation. Alternatively, it could be a reflection of some problem in judgement, in collating information into short-term or 'working' memory, that may in fact have been a very symptom of the disease process itself.

Lisyak noted that his memory symptoms included finding his way about familiar places—this is something that would be consistent with the right temporal focus of his lesion (Habib and Sirigu 1987). He also found that he was left with 'pockets of memory deficit', which interfered with his ability to recall diseases and their treatments. This would imply more widespread pathology, with probable involvement of the left temporal lobe, contributing to difficulties in knowledge retrieval.

Lisyak found that having a better understanding of his illness and his symptoms did go some way to helping his emotional status, and in particular his occasional bouts of depression. He came to cope with an aura of fear, something that can naturally be distressing to individuals with epilepsy—to understand that such feelings represent a seizure can help them re-label the feelings, and therefore reduce their general feelings of psychological distress. Counselling to patients with epilepsy may therefore be very worthwhile, if—as in this case—enhanced knowledge about symptoms reduces the likelihood of irrational fears, etc. Lisyak also comments on the positive side of having epilepsy, and the famous individuals who have been reported to have suffered from the illness. It is heartening to see Lisyak emphasizing this side of his condition.

Lisyak also comments on the so-called 'epileptic personality', one that is associated with temporal lobe epilepsy. A particular personality type associated with temporal lobe epilepsy, one that includes circumstantiality, reduced sexual drive ('hyposexuality'), and emotional intensity, has been termed the 'Geschwind syndrome' (Benson 1987), named after the famous American neurologist Norman Geschwind. There remains some controversy about this. While some formulations suggesting that behavioural changes associated with temporal lobe epilepsy are associated with a consistent set of traits, including the two symptoms mentioned by Lisyak—intense interest in philosophical issues and hypergraphia, others have pointed out that features such as hypergraphia are only found in a small number of cases of temporal lobe epilepsy (Davey and Thompson 1991).

Finally, the question of control over the occurrence of epileptic seizures is a fascinating one. Lisyak mentions some second-hand reports of such control. In recent years, such evidence has been more systematically documented (Mostofsky and Loyning 1993; Thompson and Baxendale 1996). Presumably only certain types of seizures, and certain types of individuals, would lend themselves to self-control of fits, but this remains an area that is wide open for systematic research.

REFERENCES

Benson, D. F. (1987). Epileptic personality disorder: The Geschwind syndrome. In *Behavioural disorders in epilepsy—Course 219*. (ed. D. F. Benson), pp. 77–98. American Academy of Neurology, Minneapolis.

Davey, D. and Thompson, P. (1991). Interictal language functioning in chronic epilepsy. *Journal of Neurolinguistics*, 6, 381–9.

Habib, M. and Sirigu, A. (1987). Pure topographical disorientation: A definition and anatomical basis. *Cortex*, 23, 73–85.

Mostofsky, D. I. and Loyning, Y. (ed.) (1993). *The neurobehavioural treatment of epilepsy*. Lawrence Erlbaum, Hillsdale, NJ.

Thompson, P. J. and Baxendale, S. (1996). Non-pharmacological treatments. In *The treatment of epilepsy* (ed. S. D. Shorvon, F. E. Dreifuss, D. F. Fish, and D. G. T. Thomas). Blackwell, Oxford.

Life with epilepsy: 1960–1992

Kenneth R. Kaufman

Kenneth Kaufman is a practising physician.

Too often epilepsy is viewed simply as a neurological process with the complicated psychosocial elements ignored. Sadly, when the seizures are controlled, the psychological problems may persist. It is critical for the clinician to appreciate such, for the pressures from these problems could result in recurrent seizures as well as seriously influencing the patient's life in a very negative manner.

This autobiographical poem depicts how epilepsy affected one patient's education, careers, relationships and even child rearing. It is hoped that this forceful description will enlighten clinicians such that they can be better advocates for their patients and educators to the community of what the true havoc of epilepsy might be unless the whole is treated.

(Seizure)

What is a seizure?
Why should it matter?
Only a little electrical activity,
Yet all is changed.

That young boy so erect and proud
Suddenly becomes confused, nauseous,
     unconscious
But with involuntary muscle movements;
To think hepatitis was a desired misdiagnosis.

To be twelve and witness the shutters of one's
     life close;
How cruel, how real when labeled epileptic.
Couldn't control come faster?
Didn't doctors know the effects?

Secondary schools refused entrance to science
     laboratories,
Was that fair?
To date, to socialize, to tell the truth—
All limited by societal invalidism.

When secondary school becomes college,
Better it must be whether controlled or not;
For obviously the faculty and students are more
     mature.
Or are they?

A seizure in the chemistry building
Bouncing down two flights of marble steps
Black and blue but less than four weeks from
     graduation
Suddenly threatened with expulsion.

He joined the elite in graduate school;
Though seizures persisted still he fought on.
This time a smoking muffin at home
And the landlady confronted the chairman.

How can you have an epileptic at university?
Will he explode your building?
Three Nobel Prize Laureates decide—
Take English not chemistry for your degree!
Again he must fight.
How dare you crush his plans, his dreams.
That resourceful boy now eighteen saw adult
     truths;
Age would not prevent further wounds from
     childhood.

Synthetic, even instrumental organic
     chemistry they refused;
English, please, they presumed.
Another argument and finally compromised—
Theoretical organic chemistry had a doctoral
     candidate.

But dreams and faith once shattered are gone.
An audited sociology of medicine course
   opened new eyes.
Perhaps there is a field without prejudice?
Perhaps he should try!

AB, AM, summa cum laude—what do they mean?
'No epileptics please', the medical schools did
   say.
The chairman of neurology at one school
   prevailed regardless.
'If he's gone this far, give him his chance'.

So off he went to a brand new school.
With seizures still present,
What could he do—
Research at best.

As years did pass, the episodes became less;
One professor commented clinical is best.
Residency, not research, was the next step;
Yet socially withdrawn he did remain.

Patients' problems were puzzles he could solve
His own an impasse hard to resolve
His seizures a stigma difficult to explain
And what was a car he did complain

His research was varied
His clinical expertise did grow
His seizures were less
Could he dare fly?

From research fellowship to professorship
From one school to the next
He finally felt free
Part of the rest.

Seizures were rare
Relationships were made
He could share his condition
Without any shame

Then in his thirties a more confident he
Did marry a beauty without pretense.
She knew of his epilepsy but alleged did not
   care.
Would true love be his emotional/societal
   panacea?

Intermittent battles did ensue
Professionals tried to block his progress
'No privileges for epileptics' was heard
For each battle won new wounds appeared.
But the marriage shone brightly:
A wife, four children
What more could he ask
If only the present could last?

Yet was the present so bright?
Had the wife unvoiced fears?
Did she invalid?
Was he truly free?

Thirteen years, four children and only three
   seizures later
She filed for divorce.
She demanded monitored visitation
For his epilepsy makes him unsafe!

Thirty-two years by now have flown
But the present remains the past;
Education, careers, relationships and child
   rearing—
All once and still affected by epilepsy.

                   (Kaufman 1994)

To not be afraid

The psychological aspects of epilepsy are lifelong. To maximize a healthy life, it is critical that the patient with epilepsy not view such illness as a stigma. During the Twentieth International Epilepsy Congress, the author presented an autobiographical poem entitled: 'Life with epilepsy: 1960–1992'. The following poem represents his feelings following the presentation, and his underlying fear of rejection even by educated colleagues.

                   (Seizure)

It is over now;
The poem shown and read.
Wherein have I changed—
Sharing openly with my peers.

But, haven't you done such before?
Don't your friends know?
Why this sudden relief?
Was I afraid of rejection?

To allow professional colleagues to see your life
How frightening if not responsive.
You never hid; you never lied.
Still, they rarely knew.

Now they do and do they care?
Of course not!
If anything, they are proud of the courage—
Pleased with the greater understanding of complex issues.

Now I truly am free.
I go with a clear heart.
I may never be whole
But I am happy with who I am.

(Kaufman 1995)

COMMENTARY

Dr Kaufman's poems have three main, practical take-home messages:

1. Epilepsy is often a chronic condition, and the stigma of it is always there to some extent. There remains considerable prejudice against people with epilepsy, even in the academic world.

2. Many people with epilepsy can function very well, and even above average, in scholastic and career settings. The prognosis for some cases of childhood epilepsy may therefore be very good.

3. In spite of excellent academic/career progress, social relationships and emotional adjustment may remain affected to some degree in people with epilepsy. Coping with the fear of being rejected or being poorly understood by friends/colleagues is an important part of such emotional adjustment.

PART III

Overview

Overview 9

OVERVIEW

It's not what happens to you that's important. It's how you take it.
(G. R. Girdlestone in the preface of *Disabilities and how to*
live with them, 1952, *Lancet*)

Doctors and other health care workers are no less mortal than the rest of the population. When they fall ill, however, they provide a rare instance of an encounter
between two sets of knowledge and experience—that of the healer, and that of the
person to be healed. I will consider three general issues that arise from this
encounter: (1) the management of patients; (2) the training of medical staff; and (3)
our understanding of recovery of function after brain injury.

In this final chapter, I will also draw on other published self-report articles that
provide data of relevance to these issues.

1.   PATIENT MANAGEMENT

Awareness/acceptance of diagnosis of brain abnormality

Does having a medical or scientific background result in quicker/more accurate
diagnosis and management of a brain disorder? One might expect this to be an
unequivocal 'Yes', but the answer is, 'Yes, but not necessarily'. Quite often it
appeared that having a medical background simply made the patient more aware
of a wider range of possible aetiologies, thus lending more confusion than clarity to
the clinical picture. Thus, the doctor with a pituitary cyst (**Anonymous 1977**), continued to carry out operations while having symptoms that were misdiagnosed as
being due to viral or inflammatory disease, rather than due a brain tumour. **Dr X**,
who had normal pressure hydrocephalus that was eventually found to be due to a
midbrain tumour, went so far as to remark that 'my medical training did not help
me understand my illness and those around me did not perceive its nature either'
(p. 38). In this case, both **Dr X**, who was a consultant psychiatrist, and also his consultant colleagues, thought that he was suffering from a stress-induced depressive
illness rather than a neurological condition! Even when symptoms such as ataxia
appeared, the detailed medical knowledge of the patient/his colleagues pointed
them in the direction of a rare, but documented, side effect of the anti-depression
medication he was taking, rather than the more likely cause of cerebellar
dysfunction.

A feature that may perhaps be more common in medical personnel who suffer an
illness is that of denial of the illness itself. This was apparent in a number of the articles in the book, and it related both to the perception of symptoms that occurred as
the first signs of a slowly progressive illness (e.g. brain tumour, Parkinson's disease)
and also to disabilities that were present after an established brain pathology was
evident. Denial itself may be due to a number of mechanisms:

(i)   Lack of awareness that results from specific types of brain pathology, as is
      presumed to occur in some instances of right hemisphere damage (Bear 1983;
      Bisiach *et al.* 1986) and frontal lobe damage (Stuss and Benson 1987), for

example, **Dr X**, thought that his 'hydrocephalus had leuctomised me, sparing me from such appropriate worry' (p. 38).

(ii) A consequence of cognitive deficits such as memory loss, whereby the patient may not have available the full sets of information with which he/she can be fully aware of the symptoms that are present;

(iii) Psychogenic mechanisms, whereby denial is seen as a form of coping mechanism with a conscious or unconscious attempt to play down the presence or significance of certain symptoms, due to the threat and related stress that they pose to the individual.

One doctor, suffering from motor neurone disease, explicitly declared that he would 'vow denial to the strength sapping saprophytes of depression, despair, frustration, and fear' (Worthen 1987, p. 1225). In the case of brain disease, there is the added complication that many of the early symptoms of brain pathology are psychological changes—these of course carry their own stigma, and for a number of authors in this book it seemed as if the diagnosis of a neurological illness almost came as a relief, and that the denial may have in part been an attempt to repress the presence of a psychiatric condition. As Richards (1989) pointed out, doctors may be quite willing to seek an opinion from a colleague with respect to physical symptom, but may be reluctant to seek advice with respect to what appear to be purely psychological symptoms.

Denial itself may vary in its totality, and in the particular ways in which it is manifest. In its psychogenic form, denial may be present both on the part of the doctor-turned-patient, and also on the part of the colleague who has been asked to examine the patient. It is possible that in doctors' minds there is the 'It could not happen to me' reaction when symptoms first appear. Doctors may also be inclined to give themselves the automatic reassurance reaction that they are accustomed to offering to patients or to members of their family. There may also be a reluctance to appear to be neurotic, or a desire to appear to be brave, that comes with the image of being in a position of medical authority. In this respect, doctors may form a special breed of patient—one surgeon, writing about coming to terms with a diagnosis of AIDS, remarked: 'Medical doctors make bad patients. Surgeons are probably the worst—I'm sure glad I never had to look after a patient like me. We're used to making decisions for others but we're not good at letting others decide for us' (Messenger and Messenger 1995, p. 79). Whatever is the case, there would certainly be opportunities for research into whether doctors or other clinicians are different in the ways that they perceive and respond to symptoms—the fact that many doctors leave diagnosis until it is too late has major implications not only for the health of doctors but also for the patients with whose care they have been entrusted. Recent years have seen an impetus to recognize this situation (Pfifferling 1980; Lancet Editorial 1993; Donaldson 1994; Brandon 1995), but there is scope for further research to be carried out and for additional resources to be made available in this field.

At the practical level, early warning systems should be in place in health care organisations, such that the doctor or other health care worker with symptoms of brain failure can seek advice and support from relevant professionals (cf. Gooddy 1994). It is imperative that there is adequate communication between parties involved—the patient, his own specialist/GP, his supervisors at work, personnel officers, the patient's spouse, relevant professional/legal bodies, etc. It is also important that informed decisions are made on the basis of hard evidence—thus, there is clearly a need for the early involvement of a clinical neuropsychologist in the case of a doctor with suspected or established brain pathology. Evidence from a clinical neuropsychologist will help to substantiate any observations in work settings relating to functional competence, will help to provide an objective and impartial view with regard to cognitive symptoms, and will provide an opportunity for therapy/counselling to be offered at a stage where it may relieve some of the symptoms of brain pathology and prevent coping difficulties in work settings. These types of measures will help to ensure that the self-respect and mental well-being of the patient are maintained, and that matters such as career development, financial affairs, etc. can be discussed on a rational basis.

Doctor–patient communication

An issue that holds for most of the articles in this book relates to the communication of information by clinical staff to a patient. Such information may relate to clinical diagnosis, treatment/rehabilitation, long-term prognosis, or more general advice relating to everyday adjustment. The time that a patient is first told a diagnosis, especially where this is life-threatening and where the diagnosis itself is unexpected, can be a shattering time for the patient. On the one hand, the information given at the time of diagnosis may be so new and meaningful to the individual that every word could well be retained. On the other hand, the shock associated with the news may induce such a state of anxiety that information passes through one ear and out the other. It is wise for clinicians to allow for the latter, and to use measures that will aid understanding and retention of what has been told to the patient (Ley and Llewelyn 1995). These measures include repeating the information at the end of the consultation or on another occasion, ensuring that a spouse/carer is also given the information, and putting down in a clear, written form critical items from the consultation. Freedman (1993), on the basis of his experience of being treated for myasthenia gravis, a neuromuscular disease, offers a couple of simple rules: 'always listen to the patient; don't underestimate the patient's intelligence or talk down to him or her' (1993, p. 306). Items that are put in writing may include information such as the diagnosis, treatment options, possible course of recovery, and everyday limitations that may occur, especially in so far as they relate to loss of independence and economic hardship for the patient and his/her family. From the practical point of view, it would probably not be feasible to have individually prepared written notes—pre-set information leaflets may often suffice, either prepared by the physician himself/herself or of the type drawn up by pharmaceutical companies.

At a more specific level, it is worth bearing in mind that most of the authors of articles in this book probably did *not* have one of the major difficulties inherent in a patient–doctor consultation, namely differences between patient and doctor in the use of clinical terms. Hawkes (1974) noted that while lay patients and neurologists agreed on terms such as 'blackout' and 'paralysis', other terms tended to be interpreted differently, including the terms 'numbness', 'headache', and 'dizzy turns'.

Rabin *et al.* (1982), in the light of the experience of a physician who suffered from motor neurone disease, offer three specific bits of advice for the doctor who has to treat a doctor. 'First of all, do not ignore your colleague. Greet him. Inquire about his health. Offer him support if he is physically handicapped. Don't assume that he prefers seclusion. Ask to visit him. Don't hide behind the false morality of "respecting his privacy"; if it is inconvenient, he will tell you. Secondly, be conscious of the family and extend your support to them. Make a point of asking how your colleague's spouse is feeling and how he or she is coping. The spouse and children are suffering at least as much as the victim and need support, encouragement, and acknowledgement of their travail. Do not expose the wife to the "premature-widow syndrome", as some physicians do who encounter my wife and never mention my name or inquire about me at all. Thirdly, bear in mind that the absence of a magic potion against the disease does not render the physician impotent . . . Fundamentally, what the family needs is the sense that people care. No one else can assume the burden, but knowing that you are not forgotten does ease the pain' (1982), pp. 508–9).

Veith (1988), a medical historian who suffered a stroke, made the interesting point that, had she fulfilled her early pressures and ambitions to become a violinist or surgeon, her career would have been even more devastated by her stroke and its accompanying hemiplegia. Being a medical historian by career meant that she could carry on with some of her work. Perhaps those who have a career that is critically dependent on intact motor skills, such as surgeons, should also develop a related area of endeavour which, if not bringing in income, will at least help to keep them stimulated should a major illness strike. Since many of the authors of the articles were playing active professional roles at the time of their brain damage, they were understandably more concerned with losing their independence rather than the specific disabilities associated with their condition. This is something that is worth bearing in mind by doctors when they are faced with neurological or other conditions that may have a major impact on their patient's everyday adjustment. Perhaps every doctor should ask his patient with a significant medical condition, 'How has your independence been affected?' Likewise, perhaps every patient should ask his doctor when discussing his/her illness or before a course of major treatment, 'How will this affect my independence?'

Practical aspects of medical and nursing care

A number of authors in this book, such as **Moss**, complained bitterly of the lack of appropriate care, counselling, and support after they had been discharged from hospital. The concept of community psychiatric nursing is now well-accepted in the field of psychiatry, but it would seem that there is an equally pressing need for a post of *community neurological nurse* to be established, someone who has been specially trained to give advice and support for everyday difficulties that brain-injured patients face once they have been discharged from hospital and are trying to re-adjust to life in the community. This person should have relevant training in areas relating to occupational therapy, physiotherapy and clinical neuropsychology, rather than only nursing, as it is these areas where patients and their families probably have the most pressing needs (Kreutzer and Wehman 1990).

In the case of in-patient care, there are also changes that are worth considering.
Medawar, on the basis of his own experience as a neurological patient, pulls no
punches in how he thinks that patient care could be improved in British hospitals.
Later in the same chapter of *Memoir of a thinking radish*, reproduced on pages
283–7, he gives a series of aphorisms on life in hospital. The 13 aphorisms are
reproduced here; most of them probably apply to other health care systems:

1. *Where to be ill.* Large teaching hospitals are recommended. Unless privacy is of overriding
importance or you really dislike your fellow-men don't go into a private ward. The nursing
won't be better than in a public ward, and may easily be much worse. Besides, in a public
ward you will be entertained all day by the unfolding of the human comedy and by contem-
plating what literary people call the Rich Tapestry of Life.

2. *Long stays in hospital.* Lying in bed for any length of time is itself a weakening process, as
you will soon find when you try to get up. In adequately staffed hospitals, however, physiotherapists will keep your muscles and joints in working order.

An analogous treatment is necessary for the mind. It is a natural tendency of the mind to
come to and remain at a complete standstill. This is a principle of Newtonian stature. Prolonged disuse of the brain is also bad for you. Try therefore to think or converse about something other than the exigencies of hospital life and your own piteous plight. Guests come in
useful here (see below: *Visitors*) and so do books.

3. *Books.* If you are well enough to read books, they are crucially important for entertainment and keeping the mind in working order. Some serious works should therefore be
among them. Remember, however, that if you didn't quite follow Chomsky when you were
well, there is nothing about illness that can give you an insight into the working of his mind.
Do not read a genuinely funny book within a week of having had an abdominal operation.
So far from giving you stitches, it will probably deprive you of them. Books should never be
so heavy as to impede the ebb and flow of the blood. A slender anthology of selected English
aphorisms is strongly recommended. Ten aphorisms are normally reckoned to be equivalent
to a quarter of a grain of phenobarbitone, so never take more than twenty aphorisms except
under medical supervision.

4. *Sleep.* If you sleep all day you must not be aggrieved if you don't sleep all night. If wakeful
don't clamour for sleeping draughts, but take ten selected English aphorisms with a cup of
warm milk (see above: *Books*).

5. *Food.* The food in hospitals is surprisingly good, but was not intended for people with
dainty or fastidious appetites. Be warned that if you eat all day you will become disgustingly
obese and thus very properly an object of derision to your friends. Desist, therefore, and give
those chocolates to the nurses.

6. *Radio.* It is traditional for hospital beds to be equipped with radio outlets that don't work.
Test the radio at the earliest opportunity, complain as soon as possible, and go on complaining until somebody does something about it. When the radio works see that kind friends
bring in the *Radio Times*. Then you won't have to reproach yourself for missing that talk on
the vegetation of Boolooland. Small transistor radios are fine, provided they have an ear
monophone attachment.

7. *Sister.* Your ward sister—the head nurse of your ward—is well worth knowing and trying to make friends with, because she is an unusually capable and intelligent woman, which
is just as well because she is nurse, teacher, administrator, psychotherapist, and everybody's
confidante. You are doing well if you manage to make friends with her.

8. *Nurses.* The qualities of character that induce young ladies to enter this overworked and
underpaid profession are such as to make them specially likeable people. You will almost cer-

tainly want to do something to show your appreciation of them. Flowers and profuse gratitude are not very imaginative. It is a fact, however, that nurses are often ravenously hungry after a long day's duty on the wards or soon after coming on duty after a characteristically inadequate breakfast. A supply of biscuits and cheese may be more acceptable and will certainly be more digestible than a pot of hothouse blooms. Another trait which nurses find agreeable is to be visited by a stream of handsome and preferably unmarried sons, cousins, or brothers.

9. *Visitors.* Some visitors come because they love you or are genuinely concerned for you, and these you will generally welcome. Others come because they feel they ought to or to indulge their *Schadenfreude.* The latter should be got rid of as quickly as possible. This can be done only by prior arrangement with Sister, who is adept at making unwanted visitors feel, as well as merely being, unwelcome.

10. *The bodily motions.* In some wards the nursing staff give the impression of regarding it as a personal affront if the entire great bowel is not evacuated daily. They attach considerably more importance to this than you need (see Ritual purgation, by Professor L. J. Witts in the *Lancet,* 20 February 1931).

It is a rightly humiliating thought that, in spite of man's ability to reach the moon, no-one has yet designed a bedpan which is not physiologically inept, uncomfortable, and somewhat obscene. The main factor in making physiotherapy supportable is the feeling that ultimately it will equip you to get out of bed yourself and look after your own needs.

11. *Hospitality to guests: drinking.* It has been said that the Middlesex Hospital will do anything for you except allow you to park in the forecourt, and in general the great teaching hospitals were erected at least half a mile from anywhere it is possible to park a car. This means that your visitors when they arrive will be harassed and exhausted and must be offered the drink which (if they have any sense) they will have brought with them. They will probably offer you a drink at the same time, but as the words 'Thanks, I don't mind if I do' rise to your lips, remember the medical staff may easily mind quite a lot. They certainly will if you are suffering from a serious liver disorder. If your complaints are merely orthopaedic they are not likely to object at all. But here again consult with the ward sister. Tell her, if need be, that you get a funny sort of dizzy swimming feeling in the head if you don't have a drink at six o'clock.

12. *Serious illness: the will to live.* A well-known public figure who has taken it upon himself to become the Conscience of the World has objected to organ transplantation as an unnatural and somewhat unwholesome method of prolonging life. But before they insist too vehemently upon the Right to Die, such people should remember that a very decided preference for remaining alive has been a major motive force with human, as with all animal evolution. The firm determination to remain alive has a mysterious therapeutic effect which helps to promote that very ambition.

13. *The National Health Service.* Don't run down the National Health Service which, in spite of faults which are inevitable in any man-made scheme, represents the most enlightened piece of social legislation of the past 150 years. If you think you can do better as a private patient attending private clinics, then good luck to you. You may need it.

Neurological rehabilitation

In the case of specific rehabilitation procedures, the papers in this collection suggest that we should be more innovative and creative in our thinking about possible techniques that may improve functioning after brain damage. A number of the articles in this book point to a range of everyday 'compensatory' aids that would be useful in specific settings to help with a particular disability. It is important to develop a rational framework for viewing such compensatory behaviour, so that rehabilitation procedures can be developed on a more solid basis (Dixon and Bäckman 1995).

Those who suffer disability as a result of a neurological illness are more likely than other patients to have a significant handicap that will not only limit their functional independence but also mean that they are at greater risk for accidents such as falls. This may be because vision or balance have become impaired as a result of the neurological illness. Wilson (1982, p. 35) offers some sound practical advice in this regard, based on her experience of looking after her doctor-husband who suffered from motor neurone disease:

(a) Provide a rubber-tipped walking stick.

(b) Fix hand supports in appropriate places around the home, particularly in the bathroom and lavatory.

(c) Train the patient to fall correctly to avoid breaking bones (a physiotherapist can help with this).

(d) After a fall, always allow the patient time to collect himself, then help him up by using graduated heights—books, stools, chairs.

(e) Always be on hand to guide limbs into the position desired by the patient—as in getting in and out of bath.'

While the general dictum has been that practise in a cognitive task will not *per se* result in a general improvement in neuropsychological functioning (Riddoch and Humphreys 1994), it may be fruitful to look more closely at what happens after task-specific improvements in cognitive performance. In the Chapter on memory disorders, the article by **Meltzer** reported him as saying that he found playing bridge an important part of his rehabilitation. 'Like muscles are strengthened by exercise, the brain must be stimulated, and there is nothing more stimulating than duplicate bridge' (p. 12). In the Chapter on language disorders, **Rose** reported that memorizing large amounts of poetry and text appeared to improve his speech expression skills. Visual defects in primates can be made to shrink significantly with specific forms of retraining that appear to 'stretch' the capacities of alternative, subcortical visual pathways, and it appears that similar effects can be found in human patients (Zihl 1980). It may also be worth exploring whether, as appears to be the case in the motor domain (Jeannerod and Decety 1994), imagery-based practice in the cognitive domain has the same effects as reality-based practice. Perhaps we should look again at the effects of repeated practice on cognitive tasks, and reconsider whether there is a role for some forms of such practice in certain types of cognitive rehabilitation. Recent research on the neural correlates of practice in sensory-motor tasks points to specific forms of reorganization of brain function, with 'plastic changes' such as enlargement of the neural representation of particular body parts (Ramachandran 1993) and changes in patterns of blood oxygenation (Karni *et al.* 1995). A coalescence of clinical and imaging data on the effects of task practice may help provide clues to specific rehabilitation procedures that may benefit neurological patients.

2. TRAINING OF MEDICAL STAFF

There are three broad sets of implications for the training of health care professionals that emerge from the evidence in this book.

Firstly, clinical staff need to be trained to be more aware of the patient's perspective (and to some extent that of the patient's family). Hahn (1985) has given some vivid examples of doctors—such as Oliver Sacks (1984)—who gained significant insights into their professional skills after having sustained a major medical condition that required them to assume the role of a patient. Such awareness could be taught in a number of ways. One way is for medical education to incorporate role-play situations, so as to give the prospective health care worker an idea as to what it is like to be a neurological patient. The ability to see symptoms from the patients' point of view varies considerably between doctors, as does the ability to communicate effectively to patients and to be a good listener. 'The caregiver will do well to remember that warmth and the ability to convey a sense of understanding of what the person in pain is experiencing are as therapeutic as any medicine and surgery', comments a nurse who suffered from trigeminal neuralgia (McConaghy 1994, p. 89). In a similar vein, is a comment by El-shunnar—a neurosurgeon who suffered from Guillain–Barré syndrome, a peripheral neuritis that left him paralysed for a period of time: 'Being on the other side has certainly given me a first hand experience of the mental and physical suffering of the patients I deal with every day and made me more compassionate towards them' (1991, p. 1474). These qualities are all the more important in the case of brain-damaged patients, since such patients may lack the ability to provide a clear and full set of symptoms because of specific cognitive or other deficits that arise from the brain injury itself. Some of these skills are best taught in role-play formats, preferably with video-feedback.

A second way in which medical education could be improved is for students to be taught how to cope with their own limitations, should they suffer an illness that results in cognitive or other symptoms. It would seem that, as a mechanism to cope with symptoms, denial may be more prevalent amongst health care staff such as physicians. It is possible that current forms of medical training indirectly encourage traits that contribute to such denial, and it would seem appropriate for medical and other health care students to at least be given the opportunity to consider such issues and be given advice on how to deal with such situations, if they were to arise. It is important that such interventions occur both at the undergraduate and post-graduate level, especially in view of the work pressures that continue to be present throughout the career of a health professional, and which some might argue have become more acute with resource and organizational pressures in many health care systems.

A third, general factor that should be incorporated into the medical curriculum is an emphasis on functional disability. Standard medical education has tended to concentrate on diseases, their diagnosis and the elimination of the pathology that forms the basis of the disease. The questions of functional disability of the patient has tended to figure much lower down in the trains of thought that guide doctors in their interactions with patients. DeWitt (1981, p. 458) put this succinctly when he noted the attitude of opthalmologists to his blindness: 'We are interested in vision but have little interest in blindness'. Two of the authors of the self-report articles in this book also made similar comments. **Meltzer** noted: 'Of little help were the two neurologists I saw. Both suggested that I just relearn what I had forgotten, but they didn't recognize or appreciate the learning problems that I had, and they were unable to suggest strategies for relearning' (p. 14). Likewise, **Moss** remarked in a later section of his book, not reprinted here: 'As I have come to recognize, neurosurgeons are a specialized breed, whose main interest is in neurology quite removed from the behavioural issues. They are interested in the 'dynamics' of the circulatory system (why it was that my collateral circulation was so great), quite removed from my psychological dynamics. I have come to accept that their interest was restricted to my nervous system and was not in me as a human being' (1972, pp. 182–3). My plea is not necessarily that doctors become experts in assessing and treating functional disability. Rather, that they remember to ask the patient and his/her family about this aspect of the illness and that they channel the person to suitable colleagues or resources who may deal with the functional disabilities in question. Such an approach will also help to make patients feel that their doctor really understands and cares for their condition and circumstances.

3. RECOVERY OF FUNCTION AFTER BRAIN INJURY

Consciousness/awareness

There have been interesting swings of the pendulum in psychology and in medicine on the importance of mental events, and phenomenological experiences based on those events, as a means to understanding how the brain works. William James, one of the great psychologists of the 19th century, gave considerable importance to such events. Freud was, of course, instrumental in making them of prime importance in the clinical sphere. Experimental psychologists in the first half of the 20th century, from Hull to Skinner, somewhat belittled their value. In recent years, however, there has been a major revival of interest in 'consciousness', which itself is an all-encompassing concept that has resulted in a birth or re-birth of a wide range of topics related to phenomenological aspects of cognitive functioning (Marcel and Bisiach 1988; Prigatano and Schacter 1991).

Can the self-report articles in this book shed light on the nature of 'consciousness', 'free will', and the 'soul'? While it is tempting to speculate along the lines of Crick (1994), there is little clear agreement as to how such terms may be defined, and it is unlikely that they are unitary concepts. In the case of consciousness, I am inclined to agree with Minsky (see Davidson 1993) that consciousness is 'one of those words we have for things we don't understand'. If 'consciousness' is defined as awareness of particular sets of knowledge, then it is clear from research in clinical neuropsychology that it can be readily dissociated from other aspects of cognitive functioning. For example, a neurological patient in the early stages of recovery after a brain injury may be conscious of his surroundings, be aware of time and place, and yet on a subsequent occasion he may be unaware of memory for events that took place during the earlier recovery phase. Conversely, a neurological patient may display lack of awareness for events in his environment, yet on a subsequent occasion he may display behaviour that indicates processing and retention of information during this earlier phase—an extreme example of this is where, during anaesthesia, information is presented to the unconscious patient but where there is evidence, some time after recovery from anaethesia, for enhanced processing of that information when it is presented again (Jelicic *et al.* 1992).

In the case of awareness of the self, which is sometimes equated with consciousness, one of the closest accounts of the loss of self is the description by **Meltzer** of how he felt at the early stages of his recovery from amnesia due to cerebral hypoxia. Commenting on his loss of memory for whole areas of factual and personal knowledge related to everyday activities, he concluded, 'I felt to some extent that I had lost my identity' (p. 8). A further way in which consciousness may be disturbed is awareness of the self in relation to time and place. Such a disturbance was most dramatically shown in the transient global amnesia (TGA) patient described by **Klawans.** The perplexed nature of the patient's repeated questioning is of course a classical feature of TGA, and highlights the fact that the stream of contextual consciousness is something we take for granted, that is, we are normally continually aware of the temporal, action, and spatial context of our current behaviour (e.g. what day it is, how our present actions relate to our earlier actions in the previous few days/weeks/months, and where we are now in relation to where we were in the hours and days previously). During the TGA attack, it is as if the tap that supplies this stream of consciousness is suddenly turned off, denuding the present of its past. These two examples from articles in the book would appear to indicate that consciousness and memory are closely inter-twined—this hearkens back to Minsky's own definition that, 'When somebody says they are conscious, what they are saying is I remember a little bit about the state of my mind a few moments ago.' (Davidson 1993, p. 26). Conscious awareness is, however, only one part of the brain's understanding of itself, and it is best to retain some humility as to our ability to obtain measures of such understanding and our ability to map their representation in the brain.

Individual differences in recovery of function

The articles in this book have highlighted individual differences that occur in the level of final recovery of function after brain injury. Perhaps one (hitherto relatively unexplored) avenue to gain information on the nature of such individual differences is to consider in detail those brain damaged patients who show 'spectacular recovery' after what appeared in the initial stages to be a very severe brain insult with major physical and cognitive deficits. Clinical and research studies have for understandable reasons tended to focus on patients with deficits, those who have fared poorly, and tended to ignore those who have made spectacular recoveries, 'against the odds'. Yet most clinicians know of at least a few neurological patients who demonstrate a degree of recovery of function that was totally unexpected in the light of the known variables about the brain insult (cf. Minematsu *et al.* 1992). A few cases in this book, such as **Meltzer** and **Moss**, could be seen to fall into such a category of recovery. By the detailed study of such individuals, it may be possible to gather clues as to the role of genetic, biochemical, cognitive, psychosocial, and other variables that influence outcome after brain injury. How can we best explain such variability? In addition to factors that are particular to the specific function in question (e.g. primary visual functions and a recently learned cognitive skill have quite different acquisition characteristics), there are a number of clinical/neural factors that may play a major role in determining the level of recovery of function that takes place. These include:

1. The intensity of the cerebral insult—this may be related to a number of other parameters such as lesion size, acute versus gradual onset of the lesion, disruption of cerebral blood flow, disruption of flow of cerebrospinal fluid, adverse effect on neighbouring or connected structures, extent to which neuronal tissue is directly involved (as in intrinsic versus extrinsic tumours), hypoxia resulting from the lesion, release of toxic substances as a result of the lesion, etc.

2. The number of cerebral insults.

3. The spacing of cerebral insults.

4. The age of the brain at the time of the insult.

5. The premorbid cognitive status of the brain.

6. The extent to which the function is not rigidly associated with particular brain regions and can be subsumed or 'taken over' by another brain area (e.g. right hemisphere mechanisms have been implicated in recovery of language function after left hemisphere stroke, Nagata et al. 1994)

7. The integrity of the remaining parts of the brain and, in particular, the presence of related or unrelated brain pathology, such as brain irritability (usually in the form of susceptibility to epileptic activity), cerebral atrophy, etc. (Levine 1994).

8. Specific individual idiosyncrasies in structural or vascular architecture, and in neurochemical and hormonal make-up—these idiosyncrasies may be related to particular genetic or non-genetic factors.

9. More general factors such as emotional/motivational changes after the brain insult, the methods used to test for the functional recovery in question, time since occurrence of brain insult, amount of rehabilitation in the intervening period, etc.

A considerable amount of research needs to be done to ascertain the contribution of each of these variables, and also the importance of interactions between such variables.

On the basis of the study of his father, who suffered a brainstem stroke, Bach-y-Rita (1980) reached several conclusions (this remarkable study had the benefit both of observations in natural settings and post-mortem examination of brain tissue):

(i)   'unmasking' of pre-existent neural pathways may play a critical role in recovery of function;

(ii) motivation and concentration are important factors in promoting recovery of function;

(iii) rehabilitation programmes should incorporate real-life activities and pre-lesion interests; therapy from family and friends, additional to formal therapy in clinical settings, should be attempted.

In the case of the latter, it is worth recalling a useful definition of occupational therapy given by a sufferer of motor neurone disease: 'Anything that requires your concentrated attention in order to achieve a pleasurable and satisfying result is occupational therapy' (Woodcock 1985, p. 1044). The incorporation of such activities into everyday domestic settings should be an important part of the overall rehabilitation strategy for the patient, bearing in mind that the activities should be enjoyable and should not strain the physical and mental resources of the patient.

Assessment of recovery of function after brain injury

A number of the articles in this book, such as those of **Brodal, Linge, Kolb, Moss,** and **Dr X,** point to two distinct phases underlying recovery of function after brain injury—an acute phase, that includes recovery during the initial few days/weeks/months, and a chronic phase that takes place over a period of months or years. The severity of the insult to the brain will probably play a major part in determining the temporal parameters of these two stages of recovery. Some of the articles in this book point to recovery of function taking place beyond the normal two-year cut-off point that is often quoted as the period after which recovery plateaus, and the observations in these articles are reinforced by similar findings in recent studies of recovery of function after brain injury (Sbordone *et al..* 1995). There remains uncertainty as to the precise mechanisms underlying the two phases, but there is evidence that the acute phase may relate to rapid changes in brain metabolism, cerebral blood flow, cerebral oedema, neurochemical changes, etc., and that the chronic phase may entail processes such as unmasking of previously inactive neural pathways, sprouting of fibres from surviving neurones to form new synapses, and use of alternative brain regions as substitute, compensatory mechanisms for performing a particular task (Kertesz 1993; Lee and Van Donkelaar 1995). While it has traditionally been assumed that psychological factors will mainly influence recovery in the second, chronic phase, some of the self-report papers pointed to a major awareness of, and need for, psychological stimulation during the more acute period of recovery, and this would appear to be an area of research that is worth exploring.

An important thread that has run through many of the articles in this book is that brain damage will usually result in a range of functional deficits, that cross general domain boundaries, and that proper management of the neurological patient requires a recognition of the overall profile of deficits, even where rehabilitation itself may only be geared to a particular problem area. Thus, as Lezak (1994) has clearly pointed out, a number of types of brain pathology, such as stroke and Parkinson's disease, will result in changes at the purely cognitive level (e.g. memory, language, perception, etc.), changes at the level of emotional adjustment, and alterations at the level of 'executive functioning', whereby it may be more difficult for the patient to plan and control his/her behaviour, to be aware of the severity of his/her deficits, etc. To treat one of these domains in isolation, without being aware of the possible effects of the other two domains, will inevitably result in difficulties in achieving an accurate understanding of recovery of function after brain injury.

A number of articles in the book allude to difficulties that brain damaged patients have in performing more than one task at a time. We take it for granted that we can perform an over-learned skill, such as walking, and at the same time another over-learned skill, such as listening to a conversation. For an individual with a compromised brain, this automaticity of dual-task performance cannot be taken for granted. Difficulties become all the more evident when one of the skills is not as over-learned as walking/listening, where there are significant information demands within one or more of the skills (e.g. listening to a conversation involving several people discussing a complex topic), or where there may be additional tasks or background distraction. Goldsmith (1952), a sufferer of multiple sclerosis (but where there was no 'hard' evidence of cerebral involvement, since the article was written many years before the advent of brain scanning), reported that if he was walking and someone asked him a question, he had to stop before he answered—the mere effort to walk demanded concentration, and effectively barred any other activity. It would seem that, in some neurological conditions, activities that were previously 'automatic' have now come under 'conscious cortical control', perhaps regulated by frontal lobe mechanisms. It is possible that this is equivalent to the active use of a 'working memory system', and that in such patients having to perform another activity at the same time mimics dual-task performance in an experimental setting. Another explanation is to ignore the possible involvement of a 'supervisory' or 'executive' system, and instead to view the brain as a 'mass action' system, whereby a cognitive or motor activity uses up a general reserve of brain capacity, in addition to particular demands on specific structures—the more tasks that are performed at any one time, the greater that such a general reserve neural capacity gets utilized. Whatever the precise neural mechanisms involved, some of the articles in this book, such as the one on the effects of a mild head injury (**Marshall and Ruff**), highlight the need for neuropsychologists to develop measures of cognitive dysfunction that will be sensitive to subtle sequelae of brain injury, and those measures that incorporate a dual-task performance component will probably be particularly useful in this regard.

4. POSTSCRIPT

The one enduring impression that emerges from the various contributions in this book is how the doctors/scientists-turned-patients were inspired by their illness to seek new insights into the human condition, and in many cases to achieve a paradoxical enhancement of the quality of their life. William James (1901), the famous American psychologist, alluded to this nearly a 100 years ago when he noted in his book, *The varieties of religious experience*: 'Few of us are not in some way infirm, or even diseased; and our very infirmities help us unexpectedly'. More recently, his sentiment found echoes in the experience of a doctor who found himself disabled with multiple sclerosis: 'A healer who has personally experienced the grip of the Gods and the unfairness of fate can be a healer with increased powers' (Burnfield 1985, p. 169; cf. Burnfield 1989).

This philosophy can also be seen in several self-reports of patients who suffer from motor neurone disease, a particularly debilitating neurological condition which results in motor paralysis, but which usually spares the brain. In the case of Justice Sam Filer, a judge suffering from motor neurone disease, his illness meant that 'I am not living with a life-threatening disease, but rather a life-enhancing condition' (Greenblatt 1993, p. 379). In a similar vein, Woodcock (1985, p. 1045) commented on the heightened awareness that resulted from her encounter with motor neurone disease: 'Thus, sunrise and sunset, moon path across water, finches frolicking in our bird bath, tuis [a tui is a New Zealand bird] talking in our trees, the moods of the sea from our window, scent of roses, the infectious laughter of children at play, my kind of music, faith in God—these are but a few of the things that give my life a new perspective. It is not that they are new discoveries, but rather that they have new dimensions of length, breadth, height and depth that add volume to appreciation of life'.

Perhaps I may be permitted to leave the final words of this book to my mentor, Nelson Butters, who died of motor neurone disease in 1995, aged 58 years, and who showed a determination and a pragmatism that was admired by all of us who knew him. 'I decided years ago that if I ever developed a chronic disease I would try to make the process of dying an opportunity for growth, closure and resolution' (Butters 1994, p. ix).

REFERENCES

Bach-y-Rita, P. (1980). Brain plasticity as a basis for therapeutic procedures. In *Recovery of function: Theoretical considerations for brain injury rehabilitation* (ed. P. Bach-y-Rita), pp. 225–63. Hans Huber, Berne.

Bear, D. M. (1983). Hemispheric specialization and neurology of emotion. *Archives of Neurology*, 40, 195–202.

Bisiach, E., Vallar, G., Perani, D., Papagno, C., and Berti, A. (1986). Unawareness of disease following lesions of the right hemisphere: anosognosia for hemiplegia and anosognosia for hemianopia. *Neuropsychologia*, 24, 471–82.

Brandon, S. (1995). The national counselling service for sick doctors. *British Journal of Hospital Medicine*, 54, 545–7.

Burnfield, A. (1985). *Multiple sclerosis: A personal exploration*. Souvenir Press, London.

Burnfield, A. (1989). Multiple sclerosis: an aid to maturity? *Clinical Rehabilitation*, 3, 75–78.

Butters, N. (1994). Foreword. In *Neuropsychological explorations of memory and cognition. Essays in honor of Nelson Butters* (ed. L. Cermak), pp. ix–xi. Plenum, New York.

Crick, F. (1994). *The astonishing hypothesis. The scientific search for the soul*, Simon & Schuster, London.

Davidson, C. (1993). I process therefore I am. *New Scientist*, 137, 22–6.

De Witt, S. (1981). Coping with blindness. *New England Journal of Medicine*, 305, 458–60.

Dixon, R. and Bäckman, L. (ed.) (1995). *Compensating for psychological deficits and decline*. Lawrence Erlbaum, Hillsdale, NJ.

Donaldson, L. J. (1994). Sick doctors. A responsibility to act. *British Medical Journal*, 309, 557–8.

El-shunnar, K. (1991). Guillain–Barré syndrome: a neurosurgical experience. *British Medical Journal*, 302, 1473–4.

Freedman, S. (1993). Six weeks in limbo. *British Medical Journal*, 306, 1421.

Goldsmith, N. (1952). Multiple sclerosis. In *When Patients are doctors*, (ed. M. Pinner and B. Miller), pp. 157–68. W. W. Norton, New York.

Goody, W. (1994). Brain failure in private and public life: a review. *Journal of Neurology, Neurosurgery and Psychiatry*, 57, 377–80.

Greenblatt, D. (1993). A life-enhancing condition: The honourable Mr Justice Sam N. Filer. *Seminars in Neurology*, 13, 375–9.

Hahn, R. A. (1985). Between two worlds: Physicians as patients. *Medical Anthropology Quarterly*, 16, 87–98.

Hawkes, C. H. (1974). Communicating with the patient—an example drawn from neurology. *British Journal of Medical Education*, 8, 57–63.

James, W. (1960). *The varieties of religious experience*, p. 45. Collins/Fontana Library, London. (Original work published 1901).

Jeannerod, M. and Decety, J. (1994). From motor images to motor programs. In *Cognitive Neuropsychology and Cognitive Rehabilitation* (ed. M. J. Riddoch and G. W. Humphreys), pp. 255–43. Lawrence Erlbaum, Hove, UK.

Jelicic, M., De Roode, A., Bovill, J. G., and Bonke, B. (1992). Unconscious learning during anaesthesia. *Anaesthesia*, 47, 835–7.

Karni, A., Meyer, G., Jezzard, P., Adams, M. M., Turner, R., and Ungerleider, L. G. (1995). Functional MRI evidence for adult motor cortex plasticity during motor skill learning. *Nature*, 377, 155–8.

Kertesz, A. (1993). Recovery and treatment. In *Clinical neuropsychology* (3rd edn) (ed. K. Heilman and E. Valenstein), pp. 647–74. Oxford University Press, New York.

Kreutzer, J. S. and Wehman, P. (1990). *Community integration following traumatic brain injury*. Edward Arnold, Sevenoaks, Kent.

Lancet (editor) (1952). Disabilities and how to live with them. *Lancet*, London.

Lancet (editorial)(1993). The doctor is unwell. *Lancet*, 342, 1249–50.

Lee, R. G. and Van Donkelaar, P. (1995). Mechanisms underlying functional recovery following stroke. *Canadian Journal of Neurological Sciences*, 22, 257–63.

Levine, D. N. (1994). The influence of brain atrophy and irritability on right hemisphere stroke syndromes. In *New Horizons in neuropsychology* (ed. M. Sugishita), pp. 185–96. Elsevier, Amsterdam.

Lezak, M. (1994). Domains of behaviour from a neuropsychological perspective: The whole story. In *Integrative views of motivation, cognition and emotion* (ed. W. D. Spaulding), pp. 23–55. University of Nebraska Press, Lincoln.

Ley, P. and Llewelyn, S. (1995). Improving patients' understanding, recall, satisfaction and compliance. In *Health psychology. Process and applications*, (2nd edn) (ed. A. Broome and S. Llewelyn). Chapman & Hall, London.

Marcel, A. J. and Bisiach, E. (ed.) (1988). *Consciousness in contemporary science*. Oxford University Press.

McConaghy, D. J. (1994). Trigeminal neuralgia: A personal view and nursing implications. *Journal of Neuroscience Nursing*, 26, 85–9.

Messenger, O. J. and Messenger, D. R. (1995). *Borrowed time. A surgeon's struggle with transfusion-induced AIDS*. Mosaic Press, Oakland, Ontario.

Minematsu, K., Yamaguchi, T., and Omae, T. (1992). Spectacular shrinking deficit: rapid recovery from a major hemispheric syndrome by migration of an embolus. *Neurology*, 42, 157–62.

Nagata, K., Kawahata, N., Yokoyama, E., Sato, Y., Watahiki, Y., Yuya, H., *et al.* (1994). Evolution of cortical metabolism and blood flow during recovery from aphasia. In *New horizons in neuropsychology*, (ed. M. Sugishita), pp. 55–70. Elsevier, Amsterdam.

Pfifferling, J. H. (1980). *The impaired physician*. Health Sciences Consortium, Chapel Hill, North Carolina.

Prigatano, G. P. and Schacter, D. L. (ed.) (1991). *Awareness of deficit after brain injury*. Oxford University Press.

Rabin, D., Rabin, P. L., and Rabin, R. (1982). Compounding the ordeals of ALS. Isolation from my fellow physicians. *New England Journal of Medicine*, 307, 506–9.

Ramachandran, V. S. (1993). Behavioural and magnetoencephalographic correlates of plasticity in the adult human brain. *Proceedings of the National Academy of Sciences*, 90, 10413–20.

Richards, C. (1989). *The health of doctors*. King Edward's Hospital Fund, London.

Riddoch, M. J. and Humphreys, G. W. (1994). *Cognitive neuropsychology and cognitive rehabilitation*. Lawrence Erlbaum, Hove, UK.

Sacks, O. (1984). *A leg to stand on*. Summit Books, New York.

Sbordone, R. J., Liter, J. C., and Pettler-Jennings, P. (1995). Recovery of function following severe traumatic brain injury: a retrospective 10-year follow-up. *Brain Injury*, 9, 285–99.

Stuss, D. T. and Benson, D. F. (1987). The frontal lobes and control of cognition and memory. In *The frontal lobes revisited* (ed. H. Levin, H. Eisenberg, and A. Benton). Lawrence Erlbaum, Hillsdale, NJ.

Veith, I. (1988). *Can you hear the clapping of one hand? Learning to live with a stroke.* University of California Press, Berkeley.

Wilson, B. (1982). Battling with motor neurone disease. *British Medical Journal*, 284, 34–5.

Woodcock, D. V. (1985). Motor neurone disease. *New Zealand Medical Journal*, 98, 1043–5.

Worthen, D. M. (1987). Inside the diagnosis. *Journal of the American Medical Association*, 258, 1225.

Zihl, J. (1980). 'Blindsight': improvement of visually guided eye movements by systematic practice in patients with cerebral blindness. *Neuropsychologia*, 18, 71–7.

Acknowledgements of sources

The author and publisher are grateful for permission to include the following published material in this volume. The numbers in square brackets represent the pages in this volume where the article appears.

ARTICLES

Andrewes, F. W. On being bereft of speech. *St. Bartholemew's Hospital Journal*, October 1931, 3–5. [53–6]

Anonymous. Cerebral tumour. In *Disabilities and how to live with them*. © The Lancet Ltd. 1952. Reproduced by permission of the publisher. [220–3]

Anonymous. Epilepsy. In *Disabilities and how to live with them*. © The Lancet Ltd. 1952. Reproduced by permission of the publisher. [380–2]

Anonymous. Epilepsy. In *Sick Doctors*. (ed. R. Greene), pp. 115–16. Heinemann, London, 1977. [384–5]

Anonymous. Parkinsonism. In *Disabilities and how to live with them*. © The Lancet Ltd. 1952. Reproduced by permission of the publisher. [169–71]

Anonymous. Pituitary cyst. In *Sick Doctors* (ed. R. Greene), pp. 205–6. Heinemann, London, 1977. [224–5]

Arthur, L. An astrocytoma. *Lancet*, 1 (7 April), 786–7. © The Lancet Ltd. 1984. Reproduced by permission of the publisher. [226–7]

Ashcraft, M. H. A personal case history of transient anomia. *Brain and Language*, **44**, 47–57. © 1993 by Academic Press, Inc. Reproduced by permission of the publisher and the author. [104–10]

Boles, D. B. Visual field effects of classical migraine. *Brain and Cognition*, **21**, 181–91. © 1993 by Academic Press, Inc. Reproduced by permission of the publisher. [154–61]

Brodal, A. Self-observations and neuroanatomical considerations after a stroke, *Brain*, (1973), **96**, 675–94. Reproduced by permission of Oxford University Press. [251–67]

Buck, M. The language disorders. *Journal of Rehabilitation*, **29**, 37–8. © National Rehabilitation Association. 1963. [246–9]

Coubrough, F. On the receiving end. *Nursing Times*, **88**, 28–9. © Macmillan Magazines. 1992. [290–2]

Darling J. P. The story of my epilepsy: The fortunate fate of a stubborn fool. In *When Doctors are patients* (ed. M. Pinner and B. F. Miller), pp. 328–41. WW Norton & Co, New York. 1952. [372–8]

Doe, J. Alleviation of severe emotional symptoms by Carbidopa-Levodopa, MSD, in a Parkinson's patient: A personal report. *Journal of Nervous and Mental Disease*, **197**, 185–6. © Williams and Wilkins. 1987. Reproduced by permission of the publisher. [177–8]

Dr X. Busman's holiday. *Psychiatric Bulletin*, **19**, 571–2. © Royal College of Psychiatrists. 1995. Reproduced by permission of the publisher and the author. [38–9]

Freedman, L. R. Cerebral Concussion. In *When doctors get sick*, (ed. H. Mandell and H. Spiro), pp. 131–8. Plenum Medical Book Company, New York. © Plenum Publishing Corporation. 1987. Reproduced by permission of the publisher and the author. [307–11]

Goldberg, D. My experience had a famous name. *British Medical Journal*, **306**, 216. © BMJ Publishing Group. 1993. Reproduced by permission of the publisher. [276–7]

Guss, L. B. Parkinson's disease. In *When doctors get sick*, (ed. H. Mandell and H. Spiro), pp. 123–7. Plenum Medical Book Company, New York. © Plenum Publishing Corporation. 1987. Reproduced by permission of the publisher. [181–3]

Hackel, D. B. Parkinson's disease. In *When doctors get sick* (ed. H. Mandell and H. Spiro), pp. 119–21. Plenum Medical Book Company, New York. © Plenum Publishing Corporation. 1987. Reproduced by permission of the publisher. [179–80]

Howell, T. H. How my teaching about the management of stroke would change after my own. *British Medical Journal*, **289**, 35–7. © BMJ Publishing Group. 1984. Reproduced by permission of the publisher and Prof. Eleanor Peel on behalf of the late Trevor Howell. [272–5]

Hughlings-Jackson, J. On a particular variety of epilepsy ('intellectual aura'), one cause with symptoms of organic brain disease. *Brain*, (1888), **11**, 179–85 and 200–7. [351–9].

Hughlings-Jackson, J. and Colman, W. S. Case of epilepsy with tasting movements and 'dreamy state' – very small patch of softening in the left uncinate gyrus. *Brain*, (1898), **21**, 580–90. [361–6].

Kaufman, K. R. Life with epilepsy: 1960–1992. *Seizure*, **3**, 77–8. © Academic Press. 1994. Reproduced by permission of the publisher and the author. [394–5]

Kaufman, K. R. To not be afraid. *Seizure*, **4**, 145. © The British Epilepsy Association. 1995. Reproduced by permission of the author. [395–6]

Klawans, H. L. 'Did I remove that gallbladder?' In *Toscanini's fumble* (ed. H. L. Klawans), pp. 9–28. Contemporary Books, New York. © 1988 by Harold Klawans, MD. Reproduced by permission of the publisher and the author. [21–30]

Kolb, B. Recovery from occipital stroke: a self-report and an inquiry into visual processes. *Canadian Journal of Psychology*, **44**, 130–47. © Canadian Psychological Association. 1990. Reprinted with permission. [138–51]

Kyle, D. Personal view. *British Medical Journal*, 10 April, 895. © BMJ Publishing Group. 1976. Reproduced by permission of the publisher. [270–1]

LaBaw, W. L. Thirty-three months of recovery from trauma, a subjective report.

Closed brain injury. *Medical Times*, **96**, 821–9. © Resident Staff and Physician. 1968. Reproduced by permission of the publisher. [298–305]

Lashley, K. S. Patterns of cerebral integration indicated by the scotomas of migraine. *Archives of Neurology and Psychiatry*, **46**, 331–9. © American Medical Association. Reprinted with permission. [121–7]

Linge, F. R. What does it feel like to be brain damaged? From *Canada's Mental Health*, Vol. 28, No. 3, Health Canada, September 1980. Reproduced with permission of the Minister of Supply and Services, Canada, 1996. [317–24]

Linge, F. R. Faith, hope, and love: nontraditional therapy in recovery from serious head injury, a personal account. *Canadian Journal of Psychology*, **44**, 116–29. © Canadian Psychological Association. 1990. Reprinted with permission. [324–34]

Lisyak, J. Epilepsy in my life. *Australian Family Physician*, **23**, 1951–6. © Australian Family Physician. 1994. Reprinted by permission of the publisher and the author. [389–92]

McCool, J. A. In memory of a brain tumour. *British Medical Journal*, **290**, 296–7. © BMJ Publishing Group. 1985. Reproduced by permission of the publisher and the author. [228–31]

McCool, J. A. Brain tumour. In *When doctors get sick* (ed. H. Mandell and H. Spiro), pp. 277–86. Plenum Medical Book Company, New York. © Plenum Publishing Corporation. 1987. Reproduced by permission of the publisher and the author. [231–7]

Mainwaring, C. Life without a cerebellum. *British Medical Journal*, **301**, 447. © BMJ Publishing Group. 1990. Reproduced by permission of the publisher. [238–9]

Mainwaring, C. Life without a cerebellum: update. *British Medical Journal*, **307**, 1570. © BMJ Publishing Group. 1993. Reproduced by permission of the publisher. [240–1]

Marshall, L. F. and Ruff, R. M. Neurosurgeon as victim. In *Mild Head Injury* (ed. H. S. Levin, H. M. Eisenberg, and A. L. Benton), pp. 276–80. Oxford University Press, New York. 1989. [313–5]

Medawar, P. *Memoir of a thinking radish*. © Peter Medawar 1986. Reproduced by permission of Oxford University Press. [283–7]

Meltzer, M. Poor memory: a case report. *Journal of Clinical Psychology*, **39**(1), 3–10. © Clinical Psychology Publishing Co. Inc. 1983. Reproduced by permission of the publisher. [8–15]

Mize, K. Visual hallucinations following viral encephalitis: a self report. *Neuropsychologia*, **18**, 193–202. © Elsevier Science Ltd., Pergamon Imprint, Oxford, England. 1980. Reproduced by permission of the publisher. [129–37]

Morgan M. J. Looking after a patient with Alzheimer's disease. *British Medical Journal*, **299**, 1606–7. © BMJ Publishing Group. 1989. Reproduced by permission of the publisher and the author. [35–7]

Morris, C. My life with epilepsy. *Good Housekeeping*, April issue, pp. 103–5. ©

National Magazine Company. 1991. Reproduced by permission of the publisher and the author. [386–7]

Moss, C. S. *Recovery with aphasia.* University of Illinois Press, Urbana. © University of Illinois Press. 1972. Reproduced by permission of the publisher. [82–101]

Moss, C. S. Notes from an aphasic psychologist, or different strokes for different folks. In *Neurolinguistics,* Vol. 4, *Recovery in aphasics* (ed. Y. Lebrun and R. Hoops), pp. 136–45. Swets & Zeitlinger B. V., Amsterdam. © Swets & Zeitlinger B. V., Amsterdam. 1976. Reproduced by permission of the publisher. [76–81]

Ostrum, A. E. Brain injury: a personal view. *Journal of Clinical and* Experimental Neuropsychology, 15(4), 623–4. © Swets & Zeitlinger B. V., Amsterdam. 1993. Reproduced by permission of the publisher. [341–2]

Ostrum, A. E. The 'locked-in' syndrome—comments from a survivor. *Brain Injury,* **8,** 95–8. © W. W. McKinlay. 1994. Reproduced by permission of the publisher and the author. [342–5]

Quaerens. A prognostic and therapeutic indication in epilepsy. *The Practitioner,* (1870), **4,** 284–5. [360]

Riese, W. Auto-observation of aphasia. *Bulletin of the History of Medicine,* **28,** 237–42. © John Hopkins University Press 1954. Reproduced by permission of the publisher. [71–5]

Rose, R. H. A physician's account of his own aphasia. *Journal of Speech and Hearing Disorders,* **13,** 294–305. © American Speech Language and Hearing Association. 1948. Reproduced by permission of the publisher. [59–70]

Smithells, P. A. personal account by a sufferer from a stroke. *New Zealand Medical Journal,* **87,** 396–7. © Southern Colour Print, Dunedin. 1978. Reproduced by permission of the publisher. [279–80]

Thompson, A. W. S. *On being a Parkinsonian.* Rumford, Rhode Island. 1989. Reproduced by permission of Mrs J. Thompson. [185–98]

Todes, C. Inside Parkinsonism . . . A psychiatrist's personal experience. *Lancet,* 977–8. © The Lancet Ltd. 1983. Reproduced by permission of the publisher and the author. [172–4]

Todes, C. Somatopsychic. In *Shadow over my brain,* pp. 152–5. The Windrush Press, Glos. © Cecil Todes. 1990. Reproduced by permission of the author. [174–6]

Williams, J. *Parkinson's disease: Doctors as patients.* Parkinson's Disease Society, London. © The Parkinson's Disease Society. 1992. Reproduced by permission of the publisher and the author. [200–10]

FIGURES

Figure 1   Reproduced by permission of Barbara Wilson.
Figure 2   Reproduced by permission of Mrs M. J. Morgan.
Figure 3   From *Images of mind* by Posner and Raichle. © 1994 Scientific American Library. Reproduced by permission of Marcus E. Raichle MD, Washington

University of School of Medicine, St. Louis, Missouri and W. H. Freeman and Company.

Figure 4 From *Royal Society Obituary Notices* Vol. 1 (1932–35); reproduced by permission.

Figure 5 Peabody Picture Vocabulary Text—Revised © 1981 by Lloyd M. Dunn and Leota M. Dunn, American Guidance Service, Inc. 4021 Woodland Road, Circle Pines, Minnesota, 55014-1796. Reproduced by permission of the authors. All rights reserved.

Figure 6 Courtesy of the Harvard University Archives; reproduced by permission.

Figure 7 Attitude et Facies, a statuette by Paul Richer, PP3137C; reproduced by permission of the British Library.

Figure 8 Reprinted from Kapur, N., Thompson, S., Cook, P., Lang, D., and Brice, J. (1996). Anterograde but not retrograde memory loss following combined mammillary body and medial thalmic lesions. *Neuropsychologia*, **33**, 1–8. © 1996, reproduced by permission of Elsevier Science Ltd.

Figure 9 Reproduced by permission of Professor Rentschler.

Figure 10 © Sydney Weaver/Medical Research Council.

Figure 11 Reproduced with permission from Damasio, H., Grabowski, T., Frank, R., Galaburda, A. M., and Damasio, A. R. (1994) The return of Phineas Gage: Clues about the brain from the skull of a famous patient, *Science*, **264**, 1102–5. © 1994 American Association for the Advancement of Science. Reproduced by permission of AAAS and Dr H. Damasio.

Figure 12 Reproduced by permission of the Wellcome Institute Library, London.

Figure 13 Reproduced from *Selected writings of John Hughlings Jackson, Vol 1 On epilepsy and epileptiform convulsions* (ed. J. Taylor) (1931), Hodder and Stoughton Ltd., London.

Figure 14 Reproduced by permission of Professor J. P. W. F. Lakke.

Index

Authors of original articles are indicated in *italics*. Page numbers of principal sections relating to a particular topic are indicated in **bold**.

occipital lobe 138–53
oedema (peripheral), after stroke 274
oligodendroglioma 372
on–off symptoms in Parkinson's Disease 172–6
Ostrum, Andrea E. 341–5

parietal lobe 91, 279
Parkinson's disease **165–215**
  and anal sphincter control 208
  and breathing habit 191
  and clumsiness 191–7
  and control mechanisms 213–14
  and dementia 210–12
  and depression 187–8, 204
  and emotional changes 173, 177, 200, 202,
    212–13
  and memory disorders 190, 196
  and salivation, excessive in 170, 187, 201, 203,
    208–9
  and sexual functioning 208
  and singing, impairment in 206
  and sleeping difficulty 190, 209
  and speech difficulties 170, 190, 207, 208
  and urinary difficulties 203, 208
  and writing difficulties 170, 179, 187, 202,
    204–6
  on–off symptoms 172–6
personal identity, memory for 25, 321
personality changes 11; *see also* emotional changes
phenobarbitone 222, 384
phonological agraphia 70
Pitres' rule 57
pituitary lesion 224–5
place disorientation 36
pons 291
positron emission tomography (PET) 15, 32, 57,
  128, 137
post-mortem examination 364–6
post-traumatic amnesia 307
posterior cerebral artery 139–40
procedural memory 17
prosopagnosia 36

Quaerens 360

radiotherapy 226, 229–30, 238–9
reading difficulties 9, 259
recovery of function 408–12
  mechanisms 262–3, 268
recovery of visual function 149–53
recovery of language function 57
recovery of memory function 18, 47
rehabilitation 405–6
  in head injury 338–9
  of language deficits 114–15
  of memory disorders 11–15, 18–19
retrograde amnesia, *see* retrograde memory deficits
retrograde memory deficits 8, 12, 16, 45, 87, 113
  assessment of 25–6, 315
  in epilepsy 384–5
  in head injury 318–20, 335–6
  in hypoxia 8, 16–17

in transient global amnesia 28, 32
  See also amnesia
Riese, Walther 71–4
right hemisphere stroke 251, 272, 277, 283
rivotril 387
Rose, Robert H. 59–70
Ruff, Ronald M. 313–15

salivation, excessive in Parkinson's disease 170,
  187, 201, 203, 208–9
scopolamine 170
scotoma 121–8
seizure 104–5, 137, 220–2, 246, 380, 384
  triggers 372–8
  see also epilepsy
selegiline 201, 203, 204, 207, 209
semantic memory deficits 39, 45, 114
sexual functioning
  in brain tumour 224
  in head injury 329
  in Parkinson's disease 208
sinemet 172, 177, 182–3, 201, 204–5, 207
singing, impairment in Parkinson's disease 206
skills, memory for 17
skills, performance 254
sleeping difficulty in Parkinson's disease 190,
  209
smell
  as an epileptic aura 389
  impaired sense of 221, 304, 321–2
Smithells, P.A. 279–80
social adjustment 114
social interaction 10
sodium valproate 387
speech difficulties
  in Parkinson's disease 170, 190, 207, 208
  in right hemisphere stroke 283
speech therapy 78–9
spreading depression (neuronal) 128, 154
stramonium 170
stroke **243–93**, 403, 410
  and anal sphincter control 291
  and clumsiness 279
  and contractures 275
  and depression 271
  memory disorders in right hemisphere stroke 259
  and neglect, of limbs after 274
  and oedema (peripheral), after 274
  speech difficulties in right hemisphere stroke 283
  and urinary difficulties in 290
  writing difficulties in right hemisphere stroke
    255–8, 269, 279
  see also cerebrovascular disease
suicidal thoughts 95
swallowing difficulties 170, 259, 291

taste, impaired sense of 221, 321–2
tearfulness 285–6
tegretol 387
temperament, *see* emotional changes
temporal lobe 326
temporo-occipital lesions 137